Molecular and Cellular Mechanisms of Preeclampsia

Molecular and Cellular Mechanisms of Preeclampsia

Editor

Berthold Huppertz

MDPI • Basel • Beijing • Wuhan • Barcelona • Belgrade • Manchester • Tokyo • Cluj • Tianjin

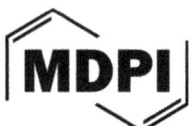

Editor
Berthold Huppertz
Medical University of Graz
Austria

Editorial Office
MDPI
St. Alban-Anlage 66
4052 Basel, Switzerland

This is a reprint of articles from the Special Issue published online in the open access journal *International Journal of Molecular Sciences* (ISSN 1422-0067) (available at: https://www.mdpi.com/journal/ijms/special_issues/Preeclampsia).

For citation purposes, cite each article independently as indicated on the article page online and as indicated below:

LastName, A.A.; LastName, B.B.; LastName, C.C. Article Title. *Journal Name* **Year**, *Volume Number*, Page Range.

ISBN 978-3-0365-2528-0 (Hbk)
ISBN 978-3-0365-2529-7 (PDF)

Cover image courtesy of Berthold Huppertz

© 2021 by the authors. Articles in this book are Open Access and distributed under the Creative Commons Attribution (CC BY) license, which allows users to download, copy and build upon published articles, as long as the author and publisher are properly credited, which ensures maximum dissemination and a wider impact of our publications.
The book as a whole is distributed by MDPI under the terms and conditions of the Creative Commons license CC BY-NC-ND.

Contents

About the Editor ix

Berthold Huppertz
Special Issue "Molecular and Cellular Mechanisms of Preeclampsia"
Reprinted from: *Int. J. Mol. Sci.* **2020**, *21*, 4801, doi:10.3390/ijms21134801 1

Berthold Huppertz
Traditional and New Routes of Trophoblast Invasion and Their Implications for
Pregnancy Diseases
Reprinted from: *Int. J. Mol. Sci.* **2020**, *21*, 289, doi:10.3390/ijms21010289 5

Padma Murthi, Anita A. Pinar, Evdokia Dimitriadis and Chrishan S. Samuel
Inflammasomes—A Molecular Link for Altered Immunoregulation and Inflammation
Mediated Vascular Dysfunction in Preeclampsia
Reprinted from: *Int. J. Mol. Sci.* **2020**, *21*, 1406, doi:10.3390/ijms21041406 17

**Akitoshi Nakashima, Sayaka Tsuda, Tae Kusabiraki, Aiko Aoki, Akemi Ushijima,
Tomoko Shima, Shi-Bin Cheng, Surendra Sharma and Shigeru Saito**
Current Understanding of Autophagy in Pregnancy
Reprinted from: *Int. J. Mol. Sci.* **2019**, *20*, 2342, doi:10.3390/ijms20092342 35

Polina Vishnyakova, Andrey Elchaninov, Timur Fatkhudinov and Gennady Sukhikh
Role of the Monocyte–Macrophage System in Normal Pregnancy and Preeclampsia
Reprinted from: *Int. J. Mol. Sci.* **2019**, *20*, 3695, doi:10.3390/ijms20153695 49

Anna Ridder, Veronica Giorgione, Asma Khalil and Basky Thilaganathan
Preeclampsia: The Relationship between Uterine Artery Blood Flow and Trophoblast Function
Reprinted from: *Int. J. Mol. Sci.* **2019**, *20*, 3263, doi:10.3390/ijms20133263 67

**Marei Sammar, Tijana Drobnjak, Maurizio Mandala, Sveinbjörn Gizurarson,
Berthold Huppertz and Hamutal Meiri**
Galectin 13 (PP13) Facilitates Remodeling and Structural Stabilization of Maternal Vessels
during Pregnancy
Reprinted from: *Int. J. Mol. Sci.* **2019**, *20*, 3192, doi:10.3390/ijms20133192 81

Clara Apicella, Camino S.M. Ruano, Céline Méhats, Francisco Miralles and Daniel Vaiman
The Role of Epigenetics in Placental Development and the Etiology of Preeclampsia
Reprinted from: *Int. J. Mol. Sci.* **2019**, *20*, 2837, doi:10.3390/ijms20112837 99

Weronika Dymara-Konopka and Marzena Laskowska
The Role of Nitric Oxide, ADMA, and Homocysteine in The Etiopathogenesis of
Preeclampsia—Review
Reprinted from: *Int. J. Mol. Sci.* **2019**, *20*, 2757, doi:10.3390/ijms20112757 145

Suchismita Dutta, Sathish Kumar, Jon Hyett and Carlos Salomon
Molecular Targets of Aspirin and Prevention of Preeclampsia and Their Potential Association
with Circulating Extracellular Vesicles during Pregnancy
Reprinted from: *Int. J. Mol. Sci.* **2019**, *20*, 4370, doi:10.3390/ijms20184370 165

Thajasvarie Naicker, Wendy N. Phoswa, Onankoy A. Onyangunga, Premjith Gathiram and Jagidesa Moodley
Angiogenesis, Lymphangiogenesis, and the Immune Response in South African Preeclamptic Women Receiving HAART
Reprinted from: *Int. J. Mol. Sci.* **2019**, *20*, 3728, doi:10.3390/ijms20153728 191

Rahana Abd Rahman, Padma Murthi, Harmeet Singh, Seshini Gurungsinghe, Bryan Leaw, Joanne C. Mockler, Rebecca Lim and Euan M. Wallace
Hydroxychloroquine Mitigates the Production of 8-Isoprostane and Improves Vascular Dysfunction: Implications for Treating Preeclampsia
Reprinted from: *Int. J. Mol. Sci.* **2020**, *21*, 2504, doi:10.3390/ijms21072504 207

Kristin Kräker, Till Schütte, Jamie O'Driscoll, Anna Birukov, Olga Patey, Florian Herse, Dominik N. Müller, Basky Thilaganathan, Nadine Haase and Ralf Dechend
Speckle Tracking Echocardiography: New Ways of Translational Approaches in Preeclampsia to Detect Cardiovascular Dysfunction
Reprinted from: *Int. J. Mol. Sci.* **2020**, *21*, 1162, doi:10.3390/ijms21031162 221

Stacey J. Ellery, Padma Murthi, Paul A. Della Gatta, Anthony K. May, Miranda L. Davies-Tuck, Greg M. Kowalski, Damien L. Callahan, Clinton R. Bruce, Euan M. Wallace, David W. Walker, Hayley Dickinson and Rod J. Snow
The Effects of Early-Onset Pre-Eclampsia on Placental Creatine Metabolism in the Third Trimester
Reprinted from: *Int. J. Mol. Sci.* **2020**, *21*, 806, doi:10.3390/ijms21030806 235

Alexander Mocker, Marius Schmidt, Hanna Huebner, Rainer Wachtveitl, Nada Cordasic, Carlos Menendez-Castro, Andrea Hartner and Fabian B. Fahlbusch
Expression of Retinoid Acid Receptor-Responsive Genes in Rodent Models of Placental Pathology
Reprinted from: *Int. J. Mol. Sci.* **2020**, *21*, 242, doi:10.3390/ijms21010242 249

Juria Akasaka, Katsuhiko Naruse, Toshiyuki Sado, Tomoko Uchiyama, Mai Makino, Akiyo Yamauchi, Hiroyo Ota, Sumiyo Sakuramoto-Tsuchida, Asako Itaya-Hironaka, Shin Takasawa and Hiroshi Kobayashi
Involvement of Receptor for Advanced Glycation Endproducts in Hypertensive Disorders of Pregnancy
Reprinted from: *Int. J. Mol. Sci.* **2019**, *20*, 5462, doi:10.3390/ijms20215462 265

Ashtin B. Giambrone, Omar C. Logue, Qingmei Shao, Gene L. Bidwell III and Junie P. Warrington
Perinatal Micro-Bleeds and Neuroinflammation in E19 Rat Fetuses Exposed to Utero-Placental Ischemia
Reprinted from: *Int. J. Mol. Sci.* **2019**, *20*, 4051, doi:10.3390/ijms20164051 283

Helmut K. Lackner, Ilona Papousek, Karin Schmid-Zalaudek, Mila Cervar-Zivkovic, Vassiliki Kolovetsiou-Kreiner, Olivia Nonn, Miha Lucovnik, Isabella Pfniß and Manfred G. Moertl
Disturbed Cardiorespiratory Adaptation in Preeclampsia: Return to Normal Stress Regulation Shortly after Delivery?
Reprinted from: *Int. J. Mol. Sci.* **2019**, *20*, 3149, doi:10.3390/ijms20133149 297

Zahra Masoumi, Gregory E. Maes, Koen Herten, Álvaro Cortés-Calabuig, Abdul Ghani Alattar, Eva Hanson, Lena Erlandsson, Eva Mezey, Mattias Magnusson, Joris R Vermeesch, Mary Familari and Stefan R Hansson
Preeclampsia Is Associated with Sex-Specific Transcriptional and Proteomic Changes in Fetal Erythroid Cells
Reprinted from: *Int. J. Mol. Sci.* **2019**, *20*, 2038, doi:10.3390/ijms20082038 . . . . **315**

Ilona Hromadnikova, Katerina Kotlabova, Lenka Dvorakova, Ladislav Krofta and Jan Sirc
Postnatal Expression Profile of microRNAs Associated with Cardiovascular and Cerebrovascular Diseases in Children at the Age of 3 to 11 Years in Relation to Previous Occurrence of Pregnancy-Related Complications
Reprinted from: *Int. J. Mol. Sci.* **2019**, *20*, 654, doi:10.3390/ijms20030654 . . . . **335**

About the Editor

Berthold Huppertz is PhD and professor of cell biology at the Medical University of Graz, Austria. Since more than 25 years, Berthold is working in reproductive biology and medicine and specifically on the human placenta. He is working on the developmental pathways and biomarkers of pregnancy pathologies, especially preeclampsia and fetal growth restriction (FGR). Berthold pioneered the research on trophoblast turnover and introduced the apoptosis cascade to the human placenta. He focuses particularly on the regulation of trophoblast biology in preeclampsia and FGR, where he developed a new concept on the etiology of preeclampsia. Berthold has published more than 230 papers and has received the IFPA Award in Placentology (2009), recognizing outstanding achievements in the field of placental research. Berthold belongs to the most cited German-speaking scientists in the field of reproductive biology and is among the top 20 world's top experts on preeclampsia (www.expertscape.com).

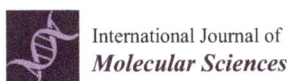

Editorial

Special Issue "Molecular and Cellular Mechanisms of Preeclampsia"

Berthold Huppertz

Professor of Cell Biology, Chair, Division of Cell Biology, Histology and Embryology, Gottfried Schatz Research Center, Medical University of Graz, Neue Stiftingtalstr. 6/II, 8010 Graz, Austria; berthold.huppertz@medunigraz.at; Tel.: +43-316-385-71897

Received: 3 July 2020; Accepted: 6 July 2020; Published: 7 July 2020

Over the last few decades, massive research efforts have been put into deciphering the etiology of the pregnancy pathology preeclampsia. However, this syndrome has remained what it was fifty years ago: the syndrome of hypotheses. Even today, the pathways and etiologies, as well as the real origin of the syndrome, all of which result in the clinical symptoms of preeclampsia, remain obscure. With the new definition of preeclampsia, where only hypertension remains as a constant value, it becomes more and more difficult to compare samples and studies with each other, as each and every one may choose different ways to define the syndrome.

During the last two decades, a number of very promising hypotheses and theories have been developed, ranging from a pure placental origin to a pure maternal origin. Most of them are comprehensible, while others are outdated and have already been falsified [1]. In these times where data are collected and theories are created on a daily basis, we need to keep up with this development. Hence, we need to understand and agree that a hypothesis we have been working on for some time, is now no longer valid, and thus we need to adapt to a new thinking [1–3].

This Special Issue is a compilation of 19 research papers and reviews, all on a joint topic: "Molecular and Cellular Mechanisms of Preeclampsia". It is a fascinating journey through the complex world of science, all meant to add another piece to the picture. The original papers range from new technologies for identifying changes in the maternal system to putative new therapies, the effect of the syndrome on the placenta, rodent models of preeclampsia, effects of the syndrome on the cardiovascular system, sex-specific differences and the effect on the children born from a preeclamptic pregnancy [4–12]. The reviews of this Special Issue range from immunoregulation and macrophages during preeclampsia and molecular targets of therapeutics to trophoblast invasion, uterine blood flow and angiogenesis, they touch on specific protein families and oxidative stress related to preeclampsia, and finally deal with autophagy in preeclampsia and the role of epigenetics in the etiology of the syndrome [13–22].

With these diverse topics, it becomes obvious why it is so difficult to identify the real origin of the disease—we simply do not know where to look. Additionally, we do not have the chance to look at the tissues of interest at the time of onset, which is supposed to be very early in pregnancy. Additionally, no good animal model exists that mimics all facets of the human syndrome. The combination of all the above leaves us with the hope that in the near future, the combination of all the data collected so far will be sufficient to identify how and why some women develop preeclampsia—and, of course, how we can prevent it.

Funding: This research received no external funding.

Conflicts of Interest: The author declares no conflict of interest.

References

1. Huppertz, B. Placental origins of preeclampsia: Challenging the current hypothesis. *Hypertension* **2008**, *51*, 970–975. [CrossRef] [PubMed]

2. Huppertz, B. An updated view on the origin and use of angiogenic biomarkers for preeclampsia. *Expert Rev. Mol. Diagn.* **2018**, *18*, 1053–1061. [CrossRef] [PubMed]
3. Huppertz, B. Biology of preeclampsia: Combined actions of angiogenic factors, their receptors and placental proteins. *Biochim. Biophys. Acta Mol. Basis Dis.* **2020**, *1866*, 165349. [CrossRef] [PubMed]
4. Rahman, R.; Murthi, P.; Singh, H.; Gurungsinghe, S.; Leaw, B.; Mockler, J.; Lim, R.; Wallace, E. Hydroxychloroquine Mitigates the Production of 8-Isoprostane and Improves Vascular Dysfunction: Implications for Treating Preeclampsia. *Int. J. Mol. Sci.* **2020**, *21*, 2504. [CrossRef]
5. Kräker, K.; Schütte, T.; O'Driscoll, J.; Birukov, A.; Patey, O.; Herse, F.; Müller, D.; Thilaganathan, B.; Haase, N.; Dechend, R. Speckle Tracking Echocardiography: New Ways of Translational Approaches in Preeclampsia to Detect Cardiovascular Dysfunction. *Int. J. Mol. Sci.* **2020**, *21*, 1162. [CrossRef] [PubMed]
6. Ellery, S.; Murthi, P.; Della Gatta, P.; May, A.; Davies-Tuck, M.; Kowalski, G.; Callahan, D.; Bruce, C.; Wallace, E.; Walker, D.; et al. The Effects of Early-Onset Pre-Eclampsia on Placental Creatine Metabolism in the Third Trimester. *Int. J. Mol. Sci.* **2020**, *21*, 806. [CrossRef]
7. Mocker, A.; Schmidt, M.; Huebner, H.; Wachtveitl, R.; Cordasic, N.; Menendez-Castro, C.; Hartner, A.; Fahlbusch, F. Expression of Retinoid Acid Receptor—Responsive Genes in Rodent Models of Placental Pathology. *Int. J. Mol. Sci.* **2020**, *21*, 242. [CrossRef]
8. Akasaka, J.; Naruse, K.; Sado, T.; Uchiyama, T.; Makino, M.; Yamauchi, A.; Ota, H.; Sakuramoto-Tsuchida, S.; Itaya-Hironaka, A.; Takasawa, S.; et al. Involvement of Receptor for Advanced Glycation Endproducts in Hypertensive Disorders of Pregnancy. *Int. J. Mol. Sci.* **2019**, *20*, 5462. [CrossRef]
9. Giambrone, A.; Logue, O.; Shao, Q.; Bidwell, G.; Warrington, J. Perinatal Micro-Bleeds and Neuroinflammation in E19 Rat Fetuses Exposed to Utero-Placental Ischemia. *Int. J. Mol. Sci.* **2019**, *20*, 4051. [CrossRef]
10. Lackner, H.; Papousek, I.; Schmid-Zalaudek, K.; Cervar-Zivkovic, M.; Kolovetsiou-Kreiner, V.; Nonn, O.; Lucovnik, M.; Pfniß, I.; Moertl, M. Disturbed Cardiorespiratory Adaptation in Preeclampsia: Return to Normal Stress Regulation Shortly after Delivery? *Int. J. Mol. Sci.* **2019**, *20*, 3149. [CrossRef]
11. Masoumi, Z.; Maes, G.; Herten, K.; Cortés-Calabuig, Á.; Alattar, A.; Hanson, E.; Erlandsson, L.; Mezey, E.; Magnusson, M.; Vermeesch, J.; et al. Preeclampsia is Associated with Sex-Specific Transcriptional and Proteomic Changes in Fetal Erythroid Cells. *Int. J. Mol. Sci.* **2019**, *20*, 2038. [CrossRef] [PubMed]
12. Hromadnikova, I.; Kotlabova, K.; Dvorakova, L.; Krofta, L.; Sirc, J. Postnatal Expression Profile of microRNAs Associated with Cardiovascular and Cerebrovascular Diseases in Children at the Age of 3 to 11 Years in Relation to Previous Occurrence of Pregnancy-Related Complications. *Int. J. Mol. Sci.* **2019**, *20*, 654. [CrossRef] [PubMed]
13. Murthi, P.; Pinar, A.; Dimitriadis, E.; Samuel, C. Inflammasomes—A Molecular Link for Altered Immunoregulation and Inflammation Mediated Vascular Dysfunction in Preeclampsia. *Int. J. Mol. Sci.* **2020**, *21*, 1406. [CrossRef] [PubMed]
14. Huppertz, B. Traditional and New Routes of Trophoblast Invasion and Their Implications for Pregnancy Diseases. *Int. J. Mol. Sci.* **2020**, *21*, 289. [CrossRef] [PubMed]
15. Dutta, S.; Kumar, S.; Hyett, J.; Salomon, C. Molecular Targets of Aspirin and Prevention of Preeclampsia and Their Potential Association with Circulating Extracellular Vesicles during Pregnancy. *Int. J. Mol. Sci.* **2019**, *20*, 4370. [CrossRef] [PubMed]
16. Naicker, T.; Phoswa, W.; Onyangunga, O.; Gathiram, P.; Moodley, J. Angiogenesis, Lymphangiogenesis, and the Immune Response in South African Preeclamptic Women Receiving HAART. *Int. J. Mol. Sci.* **2019**, *20*, 3728. [CrossRef]
17. Vishnyakova, P.; Elchaninov, A.; Fatkhudinov, T.; Sukhikh, G. Role of the Monocyte—Macrophage System in Normal Pregnancy and Preeclampsia. *Int. J. Mol. Sci.* **2019**, *20*, 3695. [CrossRef]
18. Ridder, A.; Giorgione, V.; Khalil, A.; Thilaganathan, B. Preeclampsia: The Relationship between Uterine Artery Blood Flow and Trophoblast Function. *Int. J. Mol. Sci.* **2019**, *20*, 3263. [CrossRef]
19. Sammar, M.; Drobnjak, T.; Mandala, M.; Gizurarson, S.; Huppertz, B.; Meiri, H. Galectin 13 (PP13) Facilitates Remodeling and Structural Stabilization of Maternal Vessels during Pregnancy. *Int. J. Mol. Sci.* **2019**, *20*, 3192. [CrossRef]
20. Apicella, C.; Ruano, C.; Méhats, C.; Miralles, F.; Vaiman, D. The Role of Epigenetics in Placental Development and the Etiology of Preeclampsia. *Int. J. Mol. Sci.* **2019**, *20*, 2837. [CrossRef]
21. Dymara-Konopka, W.; Laskowska, M. The Role of Nitric Oxide, ADMA, and Homocysteine in The Etiopathogenesis of Preeclampsia—Review. *Int. J. Mol. Sci.* **2019**, *20*, 2757. [CrossRef] [PubMed]

22. Nakashima, A.; Tsuda, S.; Kusabiraki, T.; Aoki, A.; Ushijima, A.; Shima, T.; Cheng, S.; Sharma, S.; Saito, S. Current Understanding of Autophagy in Pregnancy. *Int. J. Mol. Sci.* **2019**, *20*, 2342. [CrossRef] [PubMed]

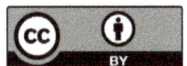

© 2020 by the author. Licensee MDPI, Basel, Switzerland. This article is an open access article distributed under the terms and conditions of the Creative Commons Attribution (CC BY) license (http://creativecommons.org/licenses/by/4.0/).

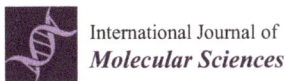

Review

Traditional and New Routes of Trophoblast Invasion and Their Implications for Pregnancy Diseases

Berthold Huppertz

Division of Cell Biology, Histology and Embryology, Gottfried Schatz Research Center, Medical University of Graz, 8010 Graz, Austria; berthold.huppertz@medunigraz.at; Tel.: +43-316-385-71897

Received: 6 December 2019; Accepted: 30 December 2019; Published: 31 December 2019

Abstract: Historically, invasion of placental trophoblasts was thought to be extremely specific, only invading into the connective tissues of the maternal uterus and finally reaching and transforming the uterine spiral arteries. Only recently, identification of new routes of trophoblast invasion into different structures of the maternal uterus has been achieved. Thorough morphological analysis has resulted in the identification of trophoblasts invading into glands, veins, and lymph vessels of the uterine wall. These new routes pave the way for a re-evaluation of trophoblast invasion during normal placental development. Of course, such new routes of trophoblast invasion may well be altered, especially in pregnancy pathologies such as intra-uterine growth restriction, preeclampsia, early and recurrent pregnancy loss, stillbirth, and spontaneous abortion. Maybe one or more of these pregnancy pathologies show alterations in different pathways of trophoblast invasion, and, thus, etiologies may need to be redefined, and new therapies may be developed.

Keywords: trophoblast; invasion; placenta; uterine glands; uterine milk; intra-uterine growth restriction; pregnancy outcome

1. Introduction

Proper and strictly controlled invasion of extravillous trophoblasts is mandatory for placental development, enabling the normal growth of a fetus in the maternal uterus. The trophoblast cell line develops at the time of blastocyst formation and divides into two main cell populations, (1) the villous trophoblast with villous cytotrophoblasts and the multinucleated syncytiotrophoblast, forming the outer cover of all placental villi; and (2) the extravillous trophoblast that invades into the maternal uterine tissues, reaching down to the inner third of the myometrium.

Extravillous trophoblasts start their journey at trophoblast cell columns that develop at the tips of anchoring villi that attach to the uterine wall. Within these cell columns the trophoblast cells in direct contact to the villous basement membrane proliferate and build the source for all extravillous trophoblasts. Their daughter cells leave the cell cycle and are pushed toward maternal tissues by the proliferative pressure of the cells at the basement membrane. After a transitional phase, the daughter cells start their active migration and invade into the uterine connective tissues. This is why these cells have been termed "interstitial trophoblasts" [1].

Traditionally, the visualization of extravillous trophoblasts has been achieved by using antibodies against cytokeratin isoforms, such as cytokeratins 8 and 18 [2], and mostly cytokeratin 7 [3–5]. Although trophoblast staining for cytokeratin was always referred to as highly specific, especially in the placenta of a first-trimester placenta, other fetal and maternal cells display immunostaining for these cytoskeletal proteins, including epithelial cells of the embryonic amnion or epithelial cells of maternal uterine glands [6]. With the identification of the highly specific expression of the major histocompatibility complex protein HLA-G on extravillous trophoblasts [7–9] followed by the development of suitable antibodies that specifically bind to only this type of HLA proteins, a new era of identification of extravillous trophoblasts began [6,10].

As will be described below, alterations of trophoblast invasion have been associated with pregnancy pathologies, including preeclampsia, intra-uterine growth restriction (IUGR), spontaneous abortion, and placenta accrete/increta/percreta [11]. So far, scientists tried to link all the above pathologies with trophoblast invasion in total or invasion into uterine arteries only. In specific cases, hypotheses finding associations between pathology and trophoblast invasion were developed but failed testing due to conceptual challenges [12]. Similarly, the placental expression and release of growth factors such as sFlt-1 and/or PlGF were associated with specific pregnancy pathologies, but also, here, the direct link between placental growth factor expression and pathology development could not be established [12,13].

So far, the new routes of trophoblast invasion have not been investigated regarding their impact on placental and thus fetal development. Hence, there is a great knowledge gap that needs to be filled.

2. Historical Thinking of Trophoblast Invasion

Early descriptions of uterine spiral arteries during pregnancy date back to 1774, when William Hunter described "convoluted arteries that passed between the womb and the placenta" [14]. At that time, no one thought of placental cells invading into the maternal uterus. About a century later, Friedländer (1870) was the first to describe "endovascular cells" in these spiral arteries, without mentioning any information on the source of these cells. This observation of Friedländer was described in a book that was published another 50 years later, by Grosser (1927) [15]. This author was the one who first imagined that the endovascular cells in spiral arteries during pregnancy are not necessarily derived from the maternal decidua but rather could well be of trophoblastic/placental/fetal origin.

It was not until the 1950s and 1960s that the aspect of arterial transformation was revisited, and major observations on spiral artery transformation were published by Harris and Ramsey [16,17], as well as Boyd and Hamilton [18,19]. Both groups described perivascular trophoblast in the decidual stroma surrounding arteries, mural trophoblasts in the walls of these arteries, and intraluminal trophoblasts residing in the vessel lumen. Already at this time, it was speculated that the trophoblast cells within the lumen of spiral arteries may well be washed out into the intervillous space of the placenta.

Interestingly, both groups missed any other route of trophoblast invasion into other luminal structures of the decidua. One of the reasons for this may be the fact that, at that time, an identification of cells by using specific probes, e.g., antibodies, was not possible. Moreover, only few specimens were available at the time; and hence, knowledge on changes of spiral arteries until delivery, even during normal pregnancy, was very sparse.

This became obvious when the first studies dealt with alterations of trophoblast invasion into arteries in pregnancy pathologies. In one of these early studies the authors stated the following: "The examination of the spiral arteries in pregnancy associated with hypertension has not been easy because of two factors. The first was the difficulty of obtaining suitable material and the second the occurrence in the same spiral arteries of extensive morphological changes due to pregnancy itself" [20]. Thus, at the time when scientists and clinicians became aware of structural alterations of invaded spiral arteries in pathological cases, they realized that there was not enough knowledge on how a normal placental bed with invaded structures looks like.

The combination of the following facts may be the reason why, even today, the knowledge on trophoblast invasion is very restricted:

(1) In the very beginning, only very few groups looked into changes of uterine vessels, in particular focusing on spiral arteries.

(2) These groups visualized arteries and the entrance of blood into the intervillous space of the placenta by dye injection and thus missed the veins.

(3) These groups visualized arteries and the infiltrating trophoblasts mostly in monkeys and only a few human cases, and thus may have missed the differences between monkeys and humans.

(4) These groups had no tools in hands to specifically identify invading trophoblasts.

(5) Maybe due to the combination of the above facts, trophoblast invasion into other luminal structures never came into focus.

(6) Scientists following these initial studies simply used this knowledge as a basis and did not scrutinize the real variety of structures invaded by extravillous trophoblast.

3. Looking into Invaded Uterine Structures from the Embryo's Nutritional Point of View

Looking from the side of the embryo in terms of nutritional support from the mother, shortly after implantation, there is the need to increase nutritional support due to the massively increasing volumes of embryo and placenta in the absence of any supporting blood vessel. Within the endometrium of the human uterus, this is best performed by eroding uterine glands in direct vicinity to the placenta, allowing direct contact of the syncytiotrophoblast to the glandular secretion products. Hence, it looks as if histiotrophic nutrition of the embryo already starts a few days after implantation [21].

In the collection of images of Allen Enders at the Centre for Trophoblast Research in Cambridge, there are images from case 8020, which is considered the earliest specimen in the Carnegie collection, probably of day one after initiation of implantation. In one of the images from case 8020, the margin of the trophoblastic plate is displayed (Figure 1A). Here, the initially invading syncytiotrophoblast has already invaded uterine glands underlying the embryo. This is the earliest description of glandular invasion by trophoblast. In a later-stage case of the early lacunar stage (Figure 1B), invasion into a uterine gland can be seen again [22].

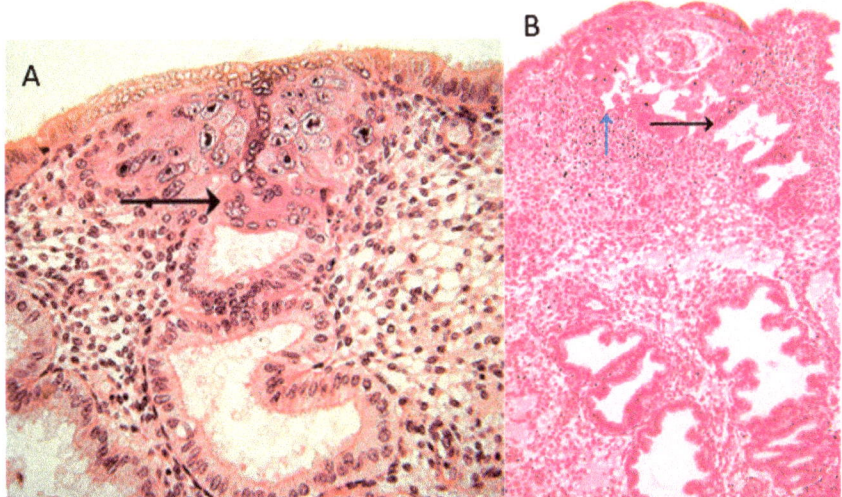

Figure 1. (**A**) Image #7 of case 8020: Margin of the trophoblastic plate. Allen Enders explained: "Syncytial trophoblast with small nuclei has invaded the underlying endometrial gland. It is not known whether the small nuclear syncytium is synctiotrophoblast or is partially a heterokaryon involving fusion of trophoblast and uterine cells." The black arrow points to invasion into a uterine gland. (**B**) Image #13 of case 8171: Early lacunar stage (stage 5B). Allen Enders' explained: "Note that the appearance of endometrial glands is similar to that seen in one of the stage 5A sites." He further explained (under image #14 of case 8171): "Note continuity of a capillary with a lacuna that anastomoses with other lacunae. Trophoblast appears to be invading a gland in the upper right." The black arrow points to invasion into a uterine gland, while the blue arrow points to invasion into a uterine blood vessel. Image are provided by courtesy of Allen C. Enders and the Carnegie Collection.

Following this early invasion by the initially invasive syncytiotrophoblast, the extravillous trophoblast population takes over and further invades into uterine glands, resulting in opening these luminal structures toward the developing intervillous space of the placenta [21]. As soon as the intervillous space of the placenta is established, the glandular secretion products flow into this space and are transferred from the placenta to the embryo [23]. At the same time, the remaining secretion products and the respective fluids need to be drained back into the maternal system. Hence, erosion and connection of uterine veins to the intervillous space of the placenta needs to take place next (Figure 2A) [24–26]. Other images of the Enders collection show the junctional zone of trophoblast invasion at the secondary villus stage. Here, invasion into veins and glands can be found, while arteries next to these two luminal structures do not show any signs of invasion [22].

Finally, around mid-first trimester spiral arteries are the next target of the invading extravillous trophoblasts. While glands and veins have thin walls and only need to be eroded and connected to the placenta (Figure 2A), the arterial walls need to be prepared prior to invasion into them. Finally, the spiral arteries are invaded as well, and their lumen is plugged until the beginning of the second trimester (Figure 2B) [27,28].

Hence, during the first trimester, a plasma flow from the plugged arteries, plus a flow of glandular secretion products, enters the intervillous space of the placenta, which is drained back into the maternal system by the utero-placental veins (Figure 2B). This allows the nutritional support of the embryo during the first trimester of pregnancy with substances in maternal plasma, plus the secretion products of the uterine glands. This has been termed histiotrophic nutrition by glands rather than vessels [23].

While the histiotrophic nutrition seems to be sufficient in the first trimester of pregnancy, with the massive growth of the fetus later in pregnancy, a different nutritional support is needed. With the dissolution of the plugs from the arteries and the establishment of the flow of maternal blood into the placenta at the beginning of the second trimester, the nutritional supply of the fetus changes from a histiotrophic to a hemotrophic nutrition (Figure 2C) [23,29]. At the same time, the number and the input of uterine glands diminish, while, of course, the veins remain, to drain back maternal blood into the maternal circulation. Due to the lack of normal placental-bed specimens of the time around mid-gestation, it is not clear when the glandular connection to the placenta disappears. It seems as if this occurs around week 20 of pregnancy, but this still needs further elucidation.

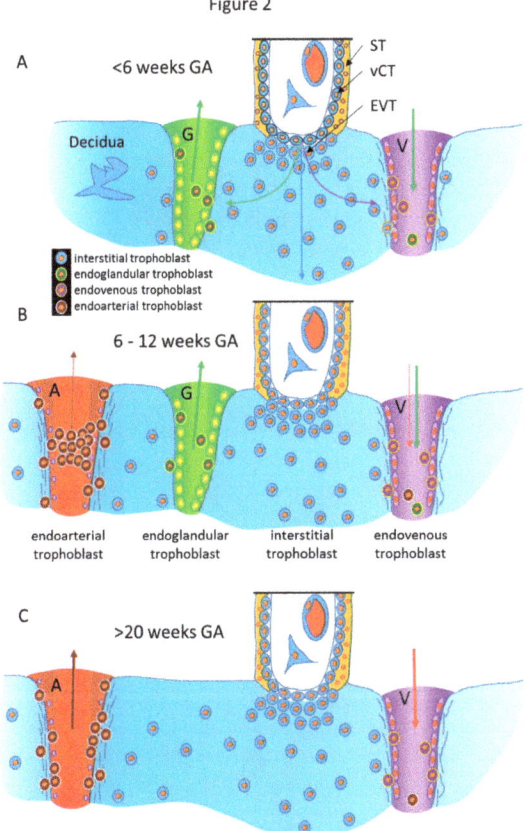

Figure 2. Schematic representation of the routes of trophoblast invasion during normal pregnancy. (**A**) Very early in pregnancy, prior to six weeks of gestation, invasion of the early invading syncytiotrophoblast during implantation, as well as invasion of early extravillous trophoblasts, results in opening uterine glands and veins toward the intervillous space of the placenta. Endoglandular trophoblasts open uterine glands, to enable the flow of "uterine milk" toward the placenta. This is followed by invasion of endovenous trophoblasts into uterine veins, to enable backflow of fluids into the maternal system, including villous material and endoglandular trophoblasts (shown in vein). The arrows in gland and vein represent the material transported in these structures (green arrow: glandular secretion products). (**B**) Later, during the first trimester, endoarterial trophoblasts invade into uterine spiral arteries, transform their walls, and plug their lumen, to hinder flow of maternal blood into the placenta. At that stage, only blood plasma is seeping through the plugs (indicated by the dashed red arrow). During this stage of pregnancy, the backflow via utero–placental veins comprises glandular secretion products, plus plasma from the spiral arteries (green arrow plus dashed red arrow), including villous material plus endoglandular and endoarterial trophoblasts (shown in vein). (**C**) At the beginning of the second trimester, the arterial plugs disintegrate, and the flow of maternal blood into the placenta is finally established. So far, it is not clear at which time point the glandular input diminishes and disappears, but in the second half of pregnancy, respective glands can hardly be found. Hence, this schematic drawing only shows arteries and veins (red arrows: maternal blood). Now, the venous backflow contains villous material, as well as endoarterial trophoblasts (shown in vein). A, artery; G, gland; V, vein; GA, gestational age; ST, syncytiotrophoblast; vCT, villous cytotrophoblast; EVT, extravillous trophoblast.

4. New Routes of Trophoblast Invasion

All the above considerations are only conceivable due to the recent progress in the identification of new routes of invasion of extravillous trophoblasts (Figure 2) [30]. Interestingly, the identification of these new types of cellular pathways can only be performed by using the original tissue organization. Any dissolution of the tissue would have destroyed the possibility to identify these routes.

Of course, this is a purely descriptive approach, which needs to be followed by the elucidation of the functional differences of the cells in the different routes and pathways. It needs to be clarified whether the cells already "know" from the beginning where to go and which luminal structure they will go for or whether they just invade uterine tissues and reach a luminal structure simply by chance.

4.1. Endoglandular Trophoblast

The aspect of histiotrophic nutrition raised the question of how glands should release their secretion products into the placenta when there is no connection between glands and placenta [23]. Also, histiotrophic nutrition of the embryo/fetus by secretion products of uterine glands was referred to as "uterine milk" in those eutherians with an epitheliochorial placentation, including animals such as the sheep, cow, and pig [31]. So far, histiotrophic nutrition has not been described in eutherians with a hemochorial placentation, such as in humans, rats, and mice.

The identification of a subpopulation of extravillous trophoblasts invading into uterine glands allowed the aspect of histiotrophic nutrition to come into focus also in the human [5,32]. The new subpopulation of endoglandular trophoblasts does not only invade into uterine glands but also connects them to the placenta (Figure 2A) [33], thus allowing early nutritive support of the embryo by using the secretion products of the uterine glands. This is the first description of the "uterine milk" in a eutherian with hemochorial placentation, the human.

As outlined above, invasion into uterine glands already starts prior to the establishment of the extravillous trophoblast cell population. Images from very early time points of human implantation depict invasion of the early invasive syncytiotrophoblast into uterine glands as early as one day after implantation [21,22,32]. Hence, it seems important for the embryo to have this histiotrophic supply right from the beginning of pregnancy, before other means to nutritive support take over at the end of the first trimester.

Another aspect of endoglandular invasion is the interesting observation of the escape of these trophoblast cells from the placental bed. As outlined above, during the first half of pregnancy, endoglandular trophoblasts invade into uterine glands. This also takes place at the outer margin of the growing placenta. At this site, some of the uterine glands may already have been invaded and connected to the intervillous space of the placenta, while other glands are still open to their normal target, the uterine cavity. If endoglandular invasion takes place into glands that are already connected to the intervillous space of the placenta, then trophoblast cells that are washed out from the glands enter into the intervillous space and are then drained into the vascular system of the mother. However, if glands are invaded that are still connected to the uterine cavity, endoglandular trophoblasts that invade into such glands and are washed out may end up being flushed into the uterine cavity. From here, they can easily reach the cervix, from where they can be isolated and used for noninvasive prenatal testing [34]. Interestingly, the cervix during the first half of pregnancy seems to be the site with the highest density of extravillous trophoblasts, and hence it is tempting to use these cells for noninvasive prenatal testing [33].

4.2. Endovenous Trophoblast

Following invasion into uterine glands, it seems as if the next route of invasion guides extravillous trophoblasts toward uterine veins (Figure 2A) [24–26]. The secretion products of the uterine glands need to be removed from the growing intervillous space. With the invasion of uterine veins by endovenous trophoblasts and the connection of the veins to the placenta, this removal is assured

(Figure 2A). The connection of the veins prior to the connection of the arteries is physiologically allegeable as removal of the blood plasma flowing into the placenta needs to be secured prior to floating of the intervillous space (Figure 2B). As outlined above, respective findings have been obtained already during very early stages of placentation [22].

4.3. Endoarterial Trophoblast

The next route of invasion is the one that has been identified centuries ago, invasion into spiral arteries by endoarterial trophoblasts (Figure 2B) [21]. Here, invasion is much more complex than that into glands and veins. In the latter two, invasion simply needs to connect these thin-walled luminal structures to the placenta. In case of the arteries, the walls of these arteries need to be restructured and invasion goes much deeper than in veins and glands—as far as we know today (Figure 2C). There is no need for the invading trophoblasts to restructure the walls of glands and veins; there is only the need to open and connect these luminal structures to the intervillous space of the placenta. However, this is different for uterine arteries, where the muscle layer of their walls needs to be restructured and the arteries need to become large tubes that have lost their contractile abilities.

4.4. Endolymphatic Trophoblast

Finally, invasion into uterine lymph vessels is described (endolymphatic trophoblast) [24,26]. The function of this route of invasion is unclear so far. It may simply show that trophoblast invasion is not specific at all, and, thus, extravillous trophoblasts simply invade all luminal structures within the placental bed. However, it may well serve a function such as connecting lymph vessels to the placenta, as well to serve as additional regulatory structure to adapt intra-placental fluid pressure. In both cases, it will be interesting to see whether endolymphatic trophoblasts can be retrieved from local lymph nodes. The first data showing a respective localization have already been published [26].

5. Alterations of Trophoblast Invasion and the Putative Effects on Pregnancy Outcome

First insight into alterations of the migratory routes of extravillous trophoblast in pathological pregnancies is slowly evolving. Since trophoblast invasion and its alterations have only been recognized in arteries so far [34], there is only very little data available on how altered invasion into other luminal structures of the placental bed may affect pregnancy outcomes. Of course, it is easily comprehensible that failure in connecting uterine veins to the placenta leads to spontaneous abortion of the embryo early in gestation. However, the complex interplay between the different luminal structures and their invasion opens a much broader field to finally understand the effects of altered trophoblast invasion.

5.1. One Example of Non-Arterial Changes of Trophoblast Invasion in a Pregnancy Pathology

So far, there is only one example available, which is based on new data in the field of recurrent spontaneous abortion. In this pregnancy pathology, alterations of trophoblast invasion have been shown to be related to vascular changes. In cases with idiopathic recurrent spontaneous abortion, a role for alterations of trophoblast invasion into spiral arteries has been described; however, this role is still debated today, with no final conclusion whether or not there is a direct relation between altered arterial invasion and the etiology of recurrent spontaneous abortion [35–37].

Windsperger et al. (2017) [26] recently analyzed decidual placental bed tissues from cases with recurrent spontaneous abortion. These authors quantified the spatial distribution of extravillous trophoblasts in placental bed spiral arteries, veins, and lymph vessels. They identified alterations in vascular invasion only in veins and lymph vessels, hence, in non-arterial vessels [26], while invasion into spiral arteries was not affected. In cases with recurrent spontaneous abortion, there were fewer invaded lymph vessels and veins compared to the total number of such vessels in healthy controls [26].

As for all such cases with alterations of trophoblast invasion, it still needs to be clarified whether the defect is directly related to a respectively dysregulated trophoblast phenotype or whether the dysregulation is found in the uterine (micro-) environment. The study above also revealed that the decidual tissues of cases with recurrent spontaneous abortion comprise a significantly higher number of all types of vessels compared to gestational-age-matched controls [26]. This is in line with data from Quenby et al. (2009) [38], who showed an enhanced density of blood vessels in the nonpregnant secretory endometrium of women diagnosed with recurrent spontaneous abortion. Thus, more thorough and specific analyses of vessel types and subtypes of extravillous trophoblast need to be performed to decipher the still blurry picture of trophoblast invasion in pregnancy pathologies, such as recurrent spontaneous abortion.

5.2. General Considerations of Changes of Trophoblast Invasion and Their Effects on Pregnancy Outcome

Other examples of non-arterial changes of trophoblast invasion in pregnancy pathologies have not yet been published, as the identification of the new routes of trophoblast invasion with all its aspects has only recently been published. At the same time, the new routes of invasion open new avenues to decipher if pregnancy pathologies, such as intra-uterine growth restriction (IUGR), preeclampsia, early or recurrent pregnancy loss, stillbirth, and spontaneous abortion, may at least be partly related to abnormal trophoblast invasion into one or more uterine luminal structures. Table 1 gives an overview of which invasion failure may be related to what type of pregnancy pathology. Of course, biology always goes the most complex way; hence, it may be the balance between, e.g., invaded arteries versus invaded veins, that makes the pathology rather than the simple total number of invaded vessels per vessel type. To make the story even more complex, there is much more to look at that needs to be taken into account, including the depth of invasion in arteries, the number of connected (not only invaded) luminal structures, and the development of invasion during the whole duration of pregnancy.

Table 1. Simplified representation of the putative effects of dysregulated trophoblast invasion for the different subtypes of extravillous trophoblast.

Extravillous Trophoblast Subtype	Invaded Structure	Putative Alteration	Putative Effect	Possibly Involved Pathologies
Interstitial trophoblast	Uterine tissues (decidua & myometrium)	Reduced	Less cells invading the uterus in general	IUGR w and w/o preeclampsia
		Enhanced	Deeper invasion than normal	Placenta accreta/increta/percreta OR Maternal anemia, pregnancy at high altitude
Endoarterial trophoblast	Uterine spiral arteries	Reduced	Faster blood flow into the placenta	IUGR w and w/o preeclampsia
		Enhanced	Further widening of the arteries	Maternal anemia, pregnancy at high altitude
Endovenous trophoblast	Uterine veins	Reduced	Decreased backflow of maternal blood into the maternal system	Early pregnancy loss, IUGR, spontaneous abortion, stillbirth
		Enhanced	Increased backflow of blood into the maternal system	Mild IUGR
Endoglandular trophoblast	Uterine glands	Reduced	Decreased nutrition of the embryo	Early pregnancy loss, spontaneous abortion
		Enhanced	Increased nutrition of the embryo	LGA
Endolymphatic trophoblast	Uterine lymph vessels	Reduced	Decreased regulation of placental fluid pressure	Spontaneous abortion
		Enhanced	?	?

?, not known so far.

6. New Omics Technologies and Morphological Assessment of Tissues

The recent development of new omics technologies has revolutionized our understanding of different cell types within a tissue. This is especially true for the RNA level, including technologies such as single-nucleus RNA sequencing per droplet (DroNc-Seq) [39] or single-cell combinatorial indexing RNA sequencing (sci-RNA-seq) [40]. Over the last few years, the respective technologies have been introduced to and have been used in the placenta field as well. Surveys on the cellular composition of the first-trimester placenta and decidua have now added new information on the different cell types within these tissues [41–43].

At the same time, the preparation of the single-cell suspensions needed for RNA sequencing technologies includes the dissociation of tissues to allow single-cell RNA sequencing. It needs to be stressed at this point that this dissociation step hinders the visualization of the single-cell microenvironment and thus the identification of the direct cell–cell interactome. In the survey publications, e.g., [41–43], cells are grouped based on the similarities in their RNA expression profiles. Hence, in vivo tissue neighborhoods, the original microenvironment and the direct cell–cell interactome can no longer be identified and taken into consideration. Especially in such a complex organ as the placenta, cells with a similar RNA expression profile may localize at different sites within the organ.

To identify the direct cell–cell interactome, the classical morphological analysis with immunohistochemistry for proteins or techniques such as the in situ padlock method for RNA [44,45] need to be performed. A first publication based on the use of in situ padlock probes to visualize the distribution of single mRNA species in cells still residing within their original tissues was recently published [46]. Only the combination of the RNA profile of single cells, plus their morphological mapping, will allow the correct interpretation of the cellular interactomes.

Moreover, even today, the routine morphological analysis of a tissue is performed on a section of the tissue, i.e., in only two dimensions. However, the information on the third dimension is of course crucial to fully understand the structural and thus functional interactions of cells and their surrounding matrices within a tissue. The field of 3D analysis of placental tissues is just starting to emerge, and it will take some time until the techniques used in this field can be applied to reach quantitative results. An example was recently published by Perazollo et al. (2017) [47].

Hence, even in the times of all the new omics technologies, a direct correlation of single-cell RNA profiles and the exact morphological localization of a cell is yet to be established.

7. Conclusions

New morphological data identified new routes of trophoblast invasion, and, thus, there is room to speculate over new and different subtypes of extravillous trophoblast. So far, it is not clear whether the extravillous trophoblast simply invades all luminal structures of the placental bed using a single phenotype, or whether there are specific trophoblast phenotypes invading arteries, veins, glands, and lymph vessels.

As the new routes of trophoblast invasion have only discovered very recently, information on effect of these routes on normal placentation and, thus, fetal development is scarce. The next years need to show how altered invasion into the different types of uterine structures may affect pregnancy outcome. There may be a large variety of pregnancy pathologies that is directly related to alterations of trophoblast invasion in arteries, veins, glands, or lymph vessels. This may not only increase our knowledge on basic processes of human development; it may also result in new therapeutic interventions based on this knowledge.

Funding: This research received no external funding.

Conflicts of Interest: The author declares no conflicts of interest.

References

1. Benirschke, K.; Burton, G.J.; Baergen, R.N. Nonvillous Parts and Trophoblast Invasion. In *Pathology of the Human Placenta*, 6th ed.; Springer: New York, NY, USA, 2012; pp. 157–240.
2. Kadyrov, M.; Schmitz, C.; Black, S.; Kaufmann, P.; Huppertz, B. Pre-eclampsia and maternal anaemia display reduced apoptosis and opposite invasive phenotypes of extravillous trophoblast. *Placenta* **2003**, *24*, 540–548. [CrossRef] [PubMed]
3. Goffin, F.; Munaut, C.; Malassiné, A.; Evain-Brion, D.; Frankenne, F.; Fridman, V.; Dubois, M.; Uzan, S.; Merviel, P.; Foidart, J.M. Evidence of a limited contribution of feto-maternal interactions to trophoblast differentiation along the invasive pathway. *Tissue Antigens* **2003**, *62*, 104–116. [CrossRef] [PubMed]
4. Lian, I.A.; Toft, J.H.; Olsen, G.D.; Langaas, M.; Bjørge, L.; Eide, I.P.; Børdahl, P.E.; Austgulen, R. Matrix metalloproteinase 1 in pre-eclampsia and fetal growth restriction: Reduced gene expression in decidual tissue and protein expression in extravillous trophoblasts. *Placenta* **2010**, *31*, 615–620. [CrossRef] [PubMed]
5. Moser, G.; Gauster, M.; Orendi, K.; Glasner, A.; Theuerkauf, R.; Huppertz, B. Endoglandular trophoblast, an alternative route of trophoblast invasion? Analysis with novel confrontation co-culture models. *Hum. Reprod.* **2010**, *25*, 1127–1136. [CrossRef] [PubMed]
6. Moser, G.; Orendi, K.; Gauster, M.; Siwetz, M.; Helige, C.; Huppertz, B. The art of identification of extravillous trophoblast. *Placenta* **2011**, *32*, 197–199. [CrossRef] [PubMed]
7. Apps, R.; Gardner, L.; Moffett, A. A critical look at HLA-G. *Trends Immunol.* **2008**, *29*, 313–321. [CrossRef]
8. McMaster, M.T.; Librach, C.L.; Zhou, Y.; Lim, K.H.; Janatpour, M.J.; DeMars, R.; Kovats, S.; Damsky, C.; Fisher, S.J. Human placental HLA-G expression is restricted to differentiated cytotrophoblasts. *J. Immunol.* **1995**, *154*, 3771–3778.
9. Weetman, A.P. The immunology of pregnancy. *Thyroid* **1999**, *9*, 643–646. [CrossRef]
10. James, J.L.; Chamley, L.W. A caution on the use of HLA-G isoforms as markers of extravillous trophoblasts. *Placenta* **2008**, *29*, 305–306. [CrossRef]
11. Huppertz, B. The critical role of abnormal trophoblast development in the etiology of preeclampsia. *Curr. Pharm. Biotechnol.* **2018**, *19*, 771–780. [CrossRef]
12. Huppertz, B. Placental origins of preeclampsia: Challenging the current hypothesis. *Hypertension* **2008**, *51*, 970–975. [CrossRef] [PubMed]
13. Huppertz, B. An updated view on the origin and use of angiogenic biomarkers for preeclampsia. *Expert Rev. Mol. Diagn.* **2018**, *18*, 1053–1061. [CrossRef] [PubMed]
14. Hunter, W. *Anatomia uteri humani gravidi tabulis illustrata [The Anatomy of the Human Gravid Uterus Exhibited in Figures]*; John Baskerville: Birmingham, UK, 1774.
15. Grosser, O. *Frühentwicklung, Eihautbildung und Placentation des Menschen und der Säugetiere*; J.F. Bergmann: München, Germany, 1927; p. 454.
16. Ramsey, E.M.; Harris, J.W.S. Comparison of uteroplacental vasculature and circulation in the rhesus monkey and man. *Contrib. Embryol. Carnegie Inst. Wash.* **1966**, *38*, 59e70.
17. Harris, J.W.S.; Ramsey, E.M. The morphology of human uteroplacental vasculature. *Contrib. Embryol. Carnegie Inst. Wash.* **1966**, *38*, 43e58.
18. Boyd, J.D.; Hamilton, W.J. Cells in the spiral arteries of the pregnant uterus. *J. Anat.* **1956**, *90*, 595.
19. Hamilton, W.J.; Boyd, J.D. Trophoblast in human utero-placental arteries. *Nature* **1966**, *212*, 906–908. [CrossRef]
20. Robertson, W.B.; Brosens, I.; Dixon, H.G. The pathological response of the vessels of the placental bed to hypertensive pregnancy. *J. Pathol.* **1967**, *93*, 581–592. [CrossRef]
21. Moser, G.; Huppertz, B. Implantation and extravillous trophoblast invasion: From rare archival specimens to modern biobanking. *Placenta* **2017**, *56*, 19–26. [CrossRef]
22. Enders, A. Available online: https://www.trophoblast.cam.ac.uk/Resources/enders (accessed on 25 October 2019).
23. Burton, G.J.; Watson, A.L.; Hempstock, J.; Skepper, J.N.; Jauniaux, E. Uterine glands provide histiotrophic nutrition for the human fetus during the first trimester of pregnancy. *J. Clin. Endocrinol. Metab.* **2002**, *87*, 2954–2959. [CrossRef]

24. He, N.; van Iperen, L.; de Jong, D.; Szuhai, K.; Helmerhorst, F.M.; van der Westerlaken, L.A.J.; Chuva de Sousa Lopes, S.M. Human extravillous trophoblasts penetrate decidual veins and lymphatics before remodeling spiral arteries during early pregnancy. *PLoS ONE* **2017**, *12*, e0169849. [CrossRef]
25. Moser, G.; Weiss, G.; Sundl, M.; Gauster, M.; Siwetz, M.; Lang-Olip, I.; Huppertz, B. Extravillous trophoblasts invade more than uterine arteries: Evidence for the invasion of uterine veins. *Histochem. Cell Biol.* **2017**, *147*, 353–366. [CrossRef] [PubMed]
26. Windsperger, K.; Dekan, S.; Pils, S.; Golletz, C.; Kunihs, V.; Fiala, C.; Kristiansen, G.; Knöfler, M.; Pollheimer, J. Extravillous trophoblast invasion of venous as well as lymphatic vessels is altered in idiopathic, recurrent, spontaneous abortions. *Hum. Reprod.* **2017**, *32*, 1208–1217. [CrossRef] [PubMed]
27. Kaufmann, P.; Black, S.; Huppertz, B. Endovascular trophoblast invasion: Implications for the pathogenesis of intrauterine growth retardation and preeclampsia. *Biol. Reprod.* **2003**, *69*, 1–7. [CrossRef] [PubMed]
28. Weiss, G.; Sundl, M.; Glasner, A.; Huppertz, B.; Moser, G. The trophoblast plug during early pregnancy: A deeper insight. *Histochem. Cell Biol.* **2016**, *146*, 749–756. [CrossRef] [PubMed]
29. Jauniaux, E.; Watson, A.L.; Hempstock, J.; Bao, Y.P.; Skepper, J.N.; Burton, G.J. Onset of maternal arterial blood flow and placental oxidative stress. *Am. J. Pathol.* **2000**, *157*, 2111–2122. [CrossRef]
30. Moser, G.; Windsperger, K.; Pollheimer, J.; de Sousa Lopes, S.C.; Huppertz, B. Human trophoblast invasion: New and unexpected routes and functions. *Histochem. Cell Biol.* **2018**, *150*, 361–370. [CrossRef]
31. Vogel, P. The current molecular phylogeny of Eutherian mammals challenges previous interpretations of placental evolution. *Placenta* **2005**, *26*, 591–596. [CrossRef]
32. Moser, G.; Weiss, G.; Gauster, M.; Sundl, M.; Huppertz, B. Evidence from the very beginning: Endoglandular trophoblasts penetrate and replace uterine glands in situ and in vitro. *Hum. Reprod.* **2015**, *30*, 2747–2757. [CrossRef]
33. Moser, G.; Drewlo, S.; Huppertz, B.; Armant, D.R. Trophoblast retrieval and isolation from the cervix: Origins of cervical trophoblasts and their potential value for risk assessment of ongoing pregnancies. *Hum. Reprod. Update* **2018**, *24*, 484–496. [CrossRef]
34. Burton, G.J.; Woods, A.W.; Jauniaux, E.; Kingdom, J.C.P. Rheological and physiological consequences of conversion of the maternal spiral arteries for uteroplacental blood flow during human pregnancy. *Placenta* **2009**, *30*, 473–482. [CrossRef]
35. Ball, E.; Robson, S.C.; Ayis, S.; Lyall, F.; Bulmer, J.N. Early embryonic demise: No evidence of abnormal spiral artery transformation or trophoblast invasion. *J. Pathol.* **2006**, *208*, 528–534. [CrossRef] [PubMed]
36. Michel, M.Z.; Khong, T.Y.; Clark, D.A.; Beard, R.W. A morphological and immunological study of human placental bed biopsies in miscarriage. *BJOG Int. J. Obstet. Gynaecol.* **1990**, *97*, 984–988. [CrossRef] [PubMed]
37. Sebire, N.J.; Fox, H.; Backos, M.; Rai, R.; Paterson, C.; Regan, L. Defective endovascular trophoblast invasion in primary antiphospholipid antibody syndrome-associated early pregnancy failure. *Hum. Reprod.* **2002**, *17*, 1067–1071. [CrossRef] [PubMed]
38. Quenby, S.; Nik, H.; Innes, B.; Lash, G.; Turner, M.; Drury, J.; Bulmer, J. Uterine natural killer cells and angiogenesis in recurrent reproductive failure. *Hum. Reprod.* **2009**, *24*, 45–54. [CrossRef]
39. Habib, N.; Avraham-Davidi, I.; Basu, A.; Burks, T.; Shekhar, K.; Hofree, M.; Choudhury, S.R.; Aguet, F.; Gelfand, E.; Ardlie, K.; et al. Massively parallel single-nucleus RNA-seq with DroNc-seq. *Nat. Methods* **2017**, *14*, 955–958. [CrossRef]
40. Cao, J.; Packer, J.S.; Ramani, V.; Cusanovich, D.A.; Huynh, C.; Daza, R.; Qiu, X.; Lee, C.; Furlan, S.N.; Steemers, F.J.; et al. Comprehensive single-cell transcriptional profiling of a multicellular organism. *Science* **2017**, *357*, 661–667. [CrossRef]
41. Liu, Y.; Fan, X.; Wang, R.; Lu, X.; Dang, Y.L.; Wang, H.; Lin, H.Y.; Zhu, C.; Ge, H.; Cross, J.C.; et al. Single-cell RNA-seq reveals the diversity of trophoblast subtypes and patterns of differentiation in the human placenta. *Cell Res.* **2018**, *28*, 819–832. [CrossRef]
42. Suryawanshi, H.; Morozov, P.; Straus, A.; Sahasrabudhe, N.; Max, K.E.A.; Garzia, A.; Kustagi, M.; Tuschl, T.; Williams, Z. A single-cell survey of the human first-trimester placenta and decidua. *Sci. Adv.* **2018**, *4*, eaau4788. [CrossRef]
43. Vento-Tormo, R.; Efremova, M.; Botting, R.A.; Turco, M.Y.; Vento-Tormo, M.; Meyer, K.B.; Park, J.E.; Stephenson, E.; Polański, K.; Goncalves, A.; et al. Single-cell reconstruction of the early maternal-fetal interface in humans. *Nature* **2018**, *563*, 347–353. [CrossRef]

44. Mezger, A.; Öhrmalm, C.; Herthnek, D.; Blomberg, J.; Nilsson, M. Detection of rotavirus using padlock probes and rolling circle amplification. *PLoS ONE* **2014**, *9*, e111874. [CrossRef]
45. El-Heliebi, A.; Kashofer, K.; Fuchs, J.; Jahn, S.W.; Viertler, C.; Matak, A.; Sedlmayr, P.; Hoefler, G. Visualization of tumor heterogeneity by in situ padlock probe technology in colorectal cancer. *Histochem. Cell Biol.* **2017**, *148*, 105–115. [CrossRef] [PubMed]
46. Siwetz, M.; Blaschitz, A.; El-Heliebi, A.; Hiden, U.; Desoye, G.; Huppertz, B.; Gauster, M. TNF-α alters the inflammatory secretion profile of human first trimester placenta. *Lab. Investig.* **2016**, *96*, 428–438. [CrossRef] [PubMed]
47. Perazzolo, S.; Lewis, R.M.; Sengers, B.G. Modelling the effect of intervillous flow on solute transfer based on 3D imaging of the human placental microstructure. *Placenta* **2017**, *60*, 21–27. [CrossRef] [PubMed]

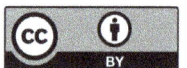

© 2019 by the author. Licensee MDPI, Basel, Switzerland. This article is an open access article distributed under the terms and conditions of the Creative Commons Attribution (CC BY) license (http://creativecommons.org/licenses/by/4.0/).

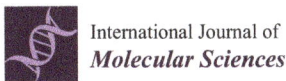

Review

Inflammasomes—A Molecular Link for Altered Immunoregulation and Inflammation Mediated Vascular Dysfunction in Preeclampsia

Padma Murthi [1,2,3,*,†], Anita A. Pinar [1,†], Evdokia Dimitriadis [3] and Chrishan S. Samuel [1]

[1] Cardiovascular Disease Program, Monash Biomedicine Discovery Institute and Department of Pharmacology, Monash University, Victoria 3168, Australia; anita.pinar@monash.edu (A.A.P.); chrishan.samuel@monash.edu (C.S.S.)
[2] Hudson Institute of Medical Research, Clayton, Victoria 3168, Australia
[3] Department of Obstetrics and Gynaecology, University of Melbourne, Parkville, Victoria 3168, Australia; evdokia.dimitriadis@unimelb.edu.au
* Correspondence: padma.murthi@monash.edu; Tel.: +61-03-99059917
† These authors were contributed equally to this work.

Received: 31 December 2019; Accepted: 17 February 2020; Published: 19 February 2020

Abstract: Preeclampsia (PE) is a pregnancy-specific multisystem disorder and is associated with maladaptation of the maternal cardiovascular system and abnormal placentation. One of the important characteristics in the pathophysiology of PE is a dysfunction of the placenta. Placental insufficiency is associated with poor trophoblast uterine invasion and impaired transformation of the uterine spiral arterioles to high capacity and low impedance vessels and/or abnormalities in the development of chorionic villi. Significant progress in identifying potential molecular targets in the pathophysiology of PE is underway. The human placenta is immunologically functional with the trophoblast able to generate specific and diverse innate immune-like responses through their expression of multimeric self-assembling protein complexes, termed inflammasomes. However, the type of response is highly dependent upon the stimuli, the receptor(s) expressed and activated, the downstream signaling pathways involved, and the timing of gestation. Recent findings highlight that inflammasomes can act as a molecular link for several components at the syncytiotrophoblast surface and also in maternal blood thereby directly influencing each other. Thus, the inflammasome molecular platform can promote adverse inflammatory effects when chronically activated. This review highlights current knowledge in placental inflammasome expression and activity in PE-affected pregnancies, and consequently, vascular dysfunction in PE that must be addressed as an interdependent interactive process.

Keywords: preeclampsia; placental insufficiency; inflammasomes

1. Introduction

Placental development is complex and is spatio-temporally regulated by an array of factors including placentally- and maternally-derived growth factors, hormones, and cytokines [1]. Uterine spiral arteries are remodeled into highly dilated vessels by the invasion of the extravillous trophoblasts (EVT). Invaded EVTs disrupt the vascular smooth cell layer and replace the endothelium, converting muscular wall arteries into wide bore low-resistance vessels ensuring a local increase in blood supply, which allows for sufficient maternal blood flow into the intervillous space for the nutritional requirements of the fetus [2]. These cellular and physiological homeostatic processes are critical steps in the establishment of a successful pregnancy and occurs in association with an increase in blood volume over the course of pregnancy [3]. Concomitant to the normal physiological adaptation, vascular resistance is also reduced via decreased vascular tone that takes place as the placenta is being formed [4]. An abnormality in the physiological adaptation to normal pregnancy occurs in the common pregnancy-related disorder that endangers the proper development of the embryo/fetus, as well as the health of the mother is preeclampsia (PE). PE is a complex pathophysiological condition where vascular resistance is abnormally increased and contributes to maternal hypertension (Figure 1). Concurrent maladaptation of the maternal cardiovascular system along with abnormal placentation predisposes an individual to PE [5]. There are no cures for PE and removal of the placenta leads to resolution of symptoms of PE, and thus its management mainly relies on delivery, often preterm. Despite the importance of the placenta and the maternal cardiovascular maladaptation in the development of PE, exploring the key molecular pathways is critical for the maintenance of homeostasis in pregnancy and also for identifying novel targets for the prevention and management of PE. This review thereby highlights the importance of inflammasomes as potential molecular links of the key inflammatory pathways underlying the development of PE.

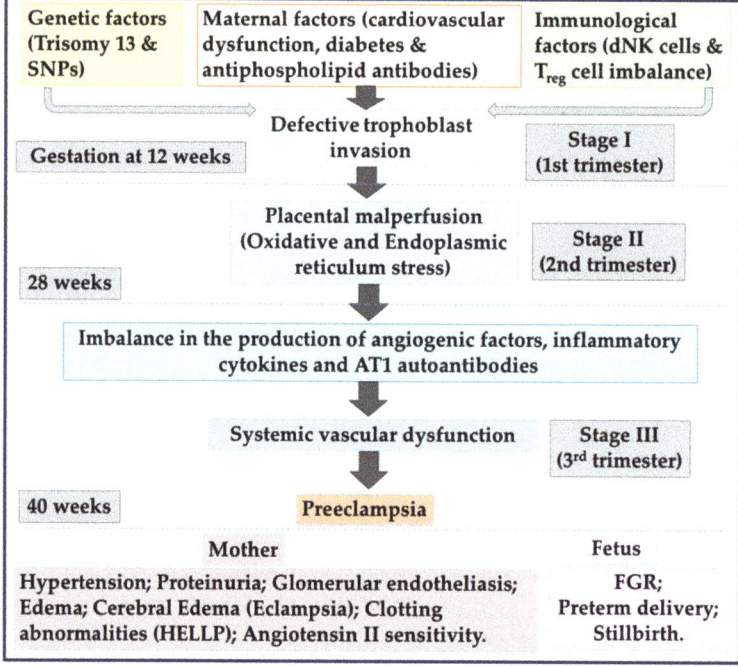

Figure 1. Depicts the complex gestation and stage specific pathophysiological processes associated with preeclampsia. Genetic factors, maternal factors, and immunological factors may cause placental dysfunction (stage I), which in turn leads to the release of anti-angiogenic and other inflammatory mediators that induce preeclampsia (PE) (stage II). AT1: Angiotensin II type I receptor; dNK: Decidual natural killer; HELLP: Haemolysis, elevated liver enzymes and low platelet count; SNP: Single-nucleotide polymorphism; Treg: Regulatory T-cell.

1.1. Human Trophoblast Differentiation Establishes the Maternal–Fetal Interface

In a normal pregnancy, the complex architecture at the boundary of the maternal uterus and the fetally-derived placental tissue is governed largely by the differentiation of immunocompetent cytotrophoblasts. Cytotrophoblasts readily undergo differentiation by emigrating from the anchoring villi and joining the cell columns as extravillous cytotrophoblasts (EVTs), serving as conduits to the uterine wall [2,6]. Briefly, the process of invasion of the EVTs in the maternal decidua and inner third of the myometrium occurs via two spatial routes. Firstly, migration and invasion through the decidual layer gives rise to interstitial EVTs that interact with specialized populations of maternal immune cells present within the decidua. Secondly, the EVTs that move up and target the lumen of the spiral arteries become endovascular EVT, adopt an endothelial-like phenotype, and intercalate within the smooth muscle cells of the tunica media. The remodeling of the spiral arterial wall involves loss of normal musculoelastic structure and replacement of the vascular media with fibrinoid material. This results in converting the originally low capacitance/high resistance uterine arteries into high capacitance low resistance channels that perfuse the surface of the placenta, which is enveloped by multinucleated transport epithelium, namely syncytiotrophoblast (STB) [1]. The invading EVTs exhibit a major transformation at both the cellular and molecular levels. Cytotrophoblasts attached to the chorionic villi initially express adhesion molecules characteristic of epithelial cells such as integrins $\alpha 6/\beta 1$, $\alpha v/\beta 5$. As cytotrophoblasts enter the cell columns and adopt the invasive pathway, the expression of epithelial cell-like adhesion molecules decrease, whilst the expression of endothelial cell adhesion markers such as integrins $\alpha 1/\beta 1$, $\alpha v/\beta 3$, and VE-cadherin is upregulated to promote vascular mimicry [2,7].

1.2. Preeclampsia

Preeclampsia (PE) is a serious human pregnancy-specific disorder, although clinically defined as a new onset of hypertension and proteinuria, in the absence of proteinuria, PE may be diagnosed with any of the following features: Thrombocytopenia (platelet count less than $100,000 \times 10^9$/L); impaired liver function as indicated by abnormally elevated blood concentrations of liver enzymes (to twice the upper limit of normal concentration); severe persistent right upper quadrant or epigastric pain and not accounted for by alternative diagnoses; renal insufficiency (serum creatinine concentration greater than 1.1 mg/dL or a doubling of the serum creatinine concentration in the absence of other renal disease); pulmonary edema; or new-onset headache unresponsive to acetaminophen and not accounted for by alternative diagnoses or visual disturbances. It should also be noted that these criteria must be met after the 20th week of gestation, otherwise this would be classed as chronic hypertension.

PE affects 2%–8% of pregnancies, is associated with 12% of infants with fetal growth restriction (FGR) and approximately 20% of preterm deliveries [8]. PE remains lacking reliable means of diagnosis and prediction, with no effective therapy or pharmacological agents available to treat the disease. The only solution is the removal of the placenta by early delivery and often preterm delivery. As depicted in Figure 1, if left untreated, PE can lead to life threatening systemic vascular dysfunction and may progress to eclampsia with complications of the HELLP syndrome (elevated liver enzymes, haemolysis, and low platelets), placental abruption, acute renal failure, and pulmonary edema [9]. Although maternal symptoms appear to be largely resolved with the delivery of the placenta and the fetus, accumulating evidence suggests that PE is associated with long-term maternal cardiovascular and other complications such as renal diseases [10–14].

1.2.1. Placental Ischemia

Poor placentation resulting from the insufficient EVT invasion and reduced uterine blood flow leading to placental ischemia have been proposed to be one of the leading causes of PE. Specifically, placental ischemia is associated with an imbalance of immune function and chronic inflammation similar to autoimmune diseases [15–17]. This immune imbalance creates a state of chronically uncontrolled inflammation due to an increase in the production of pro-inflammatory factors and the abnormal activation of immune cells and production of cytokines, whilst decreasing the abundance of regulatory immune cells and cytokines [18,19]. These alterations lead to progressive pathophysiological changes including an enhanced production of reactive oxygen species [20], increased oxidative and endoplasmic reticulum stress, endothelin-1 expression, production of potent pro-inflammatory mediators [21], anti-angiogenic factors at the implantation site, and the production of autoantibodies such as angiotensin-II type I receptor (AT1-AA) [22], thus culminating in the development of hypertension during pregnancy. Therefore, insight into how different components of the innate immune system and inflammatory cytokines are regulated and contribute to the progression of development of PE will be useful in developing targeted therapies that are necessary to improve pregnancy outcomes.

1.2.2. The Immunology of Pregnancy

Human pregnancy is an immunological paradox [23]. Maintenance of pregnancy relies on finely tuned immune adaptations at the maternal-fetal interface where the two distinct genomes of the mother and the fetus commingle to maintain tolerance to the fetal allograft while preserving innate and adaptive immune mechanisms for protection against microbial challenges. Studies by Co et al. [23] have reported that trophoblast interaction with the decidual natural killer cells (dNK) is crucial for the maternal-fetal immune tolerance early in pregnancy. Combinations of signals and responses originating from the maternal and fetal-placental immune systems are critical for a successful placentation, as well as for pregnancy outcome [24]. The signals that originate from the placenta has the ability to sense the infectious and non-infectious triggers and generate innate, immune-like responses [25]. The placenta not only uses several mechanisms to regulate immune tolerance and adaptation, but it may also modulate the way the maternal immune system adapts in the presence of potential dangerous signals [25,26]. Immunologic miscommunications that have origins at the placenta or in the mother may contribute to disruption to the regulatory and protective mechanisms leading to pregnancy complications including PE.

1.2.3. Inflammation in the Development of PE

A generalized systemic inflammatory response is common to all pregnancies, as highlighted by Redman et al. [27] which proposed that PE is intrinsically similar to normal pregnancy and is characterized by the extreme end of a continuous spectrum of inflammatory responses. In PE, a deviation in the physiological immunoregulatory adaption to pregnancy has been described for promoting inhibitory reactivity to the fetus. Furthermore, in PE-affected pregnancies, an increase in immune cells has been demonstrated in response to activation of the innate immune system and inflammation in the maternal circulation and uteroplacental unit [28]. These events in turn contribute to the shallow invasion of EVT in the uterine wall and insufficient spiral arteriole remodeling leading to placental ischemia (Figure 1).

As a consequence of placental ischemia, oxidative stress is augmented with an excessive release of placental factors, such as STB knots/debris, soluble fms-like tyrosine kinase-1 (sFlt-1), the soluble receptor for vascular endothelial growth factor (VEGF) into the maternal circulation, which collectively contribute to the development of hypertension [29,30]. These angiogenic factors are also critical inflammatory mediators which contribute to maternal inflammation associated with PE [31]. Villous cytotrophoblasts mediate inflammation via the secretion of inflammatory cytokines including interleukins (ILs)-1β, -2, -4, -6, -8, -10, -12, and -18, transforming growth factor (TGF)-β1, IFN-γ-inducible protein 10/IP-10, tumor necrosis factor (TNF)-α, interferon (IFN)-γ, monocyte chemotactic protein (MCP)1, intercellular adhesion molecule (ICAM)-1, and vascular cell adhesion molecule (VCAM)-1 [6,28,32–34], which contribute to the development of PE. This role is particularly important for cytotrophoblasts, which fuses to form STB, and is the site for maternal–fetal interactions. Several cytokines including IL-1β and IL-18 have also been correlated with maternal endothelial dysfunction [34]. These inflammatory cytokines can activate several downstream pathways both directly or indirectly to contribute to the clinical manifestations and progression of PE. Several triggers including elevated maternal serum concentrations of cholesterol and uric acid in PE have been shown to contribute to a heightened inflammatory response through STB [35]. Depending on the stimulant or physiological change(s) that occur during pregnancy, placental cells may mount either a regulated protective response that maintains and promotes a healthy pregnancy, or alternatively, promotes a damaging response that adversely impacts the outcome of pregnancy, as observed in PE. One such molecular mechanism by which inflammatory responses are regulated in the human placenta is via the molecular inflammasome platform [36], which are known producers of IL-1β and IL-18. A greater understanding of the precise molecular pathways governed by inflammasomes in the placental sensing mechanisms is therefore critical for drug discovery and therapeutic targeting.

As a consequence of placental ischemia, oxidative stress is augmented with an excessive release of placental factors, such as STB knots/debris, soluble fms-like tyrosine kinase-1 (sFlt-1), the soluble receptor for vascular endothelial growth factor (VEGF) into the maternal circulation, which collectively contribute to the development of hypertension [29,30]. These angiogenic factors are also critical inflammatory mediators which contribute to maternal inflammation associated with PE [31]. Villous cytotrophoblasts mediate inflammation via the secretion of inflammatory cytokines including interleukins (ILs)-1β, -2, -4, -6, -8, -10, -12, and -18, transforming growth factor (TGF)-β1, IFN-γ-inducible protein 10/IP-10, tumor necrosis factor (TNF)-α, interferon (IFN)-γ, monocyte chemotactic protein (MCP)1, intercellular adhesion molecule (ICAM)-1, and vascular cell adhesion molecule (VCAM)-1 [6,28,32–34], which contribute to the development of PE. This role is particularly important for cytotrophoblasts, which fuses to form STB, and is the site for maternal–fetal interactions. Several cytokines including IL-1β and IL-18 have also been correlated with maternal endothelial dysfunction [34]. These inflammatory cytokines can activate several downstream pathways both directly or indirectly to contribute to the clinical manifestations and progression of PE. Several triggers including elevated maternal serum concentrations of cholesterol and uric acid in PE have been shown to contribute to a heightened inflammatory response through STB [35]. Depending on the stimulant or physiological change(s) that occur during pregnancy, placental cells may mount either a regulated protective response that maintains and promotes a healthy pregnancy, or alternatively, promotes a damaging response that adversely impacts the outcome of pregnancy, as observed in PE. One such molecular mechanism by which inflammatory responses are regulated in the human placenta is via the molecular inflammasome platform [36], which are known producers of IL-1β and IL-18. A greater understanding of the precise molecular pathways governed by inflammasomes in the placental sensing mechanisms is therefore critical for drug discovery and therapeutic targeting.

2. Inflammasomes

The ability to activate immune cells depends on the presence of molecular multiprotein inflammasome complexes [37,38]. Inflammasomes are high molecular-weight multimeric self-assembling protein complexes of the innate immune system, which are not only important for initiating the inflammatory response and release of IL-1β and IL-18 (Figure 2), but also in regulating cellular apoptosis [38]. As shown in the schematic diagram, signaling for inflammasome activation occurs in two stages. Priming in stage 1 is followed by activation of inflammasome complex by interaction with several components. The inflammasome complex contains a sensor molecule, an adaptor protein and the pro-inflammatory caspase-1 [37,39]. Inflammasomes act as a finely tuned alarm, triggering and amplifying systems in response to cellular stresses and/or infections. Placental trophoblasts, endothelial cells and macrophages can sense and respond to a variety of infectious agents by the presence of the pattern recognition receptors (PRRs). The PRRs have the ability to sense pathogen-associated molecular patterns (PAMPs) that are expressed by microbes, as well as noninfectious (sterile inflammation) host-derived damage associated molecular patterns (DAMPs) including reactive oxygen species, uric acid, cholesterol, microparticles, and exosomes (namely alarmins) [40,41] (Figure 2). When activated, the inflammasome machinery has the potential to promote maturation and release of pro-inflammatory cytokines including the release of danger signals, as well as pyroptosis, a rapid, pro-inflammatory form of cell death [42].

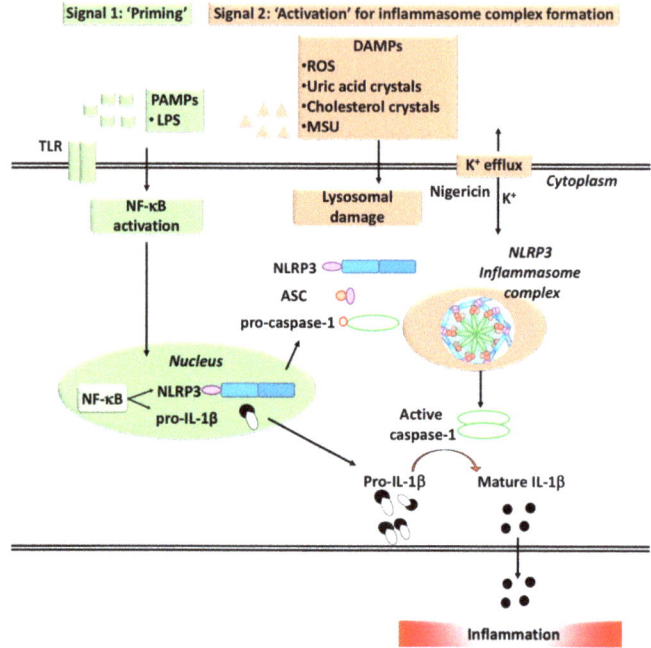

Figure 2. Activation and formation of inflammasome complex. Two-step signaling mechanisms are involved in the formation inflammasome complexes: The first "priming" signal initiated by infectious agents such as LPS, enhances the expression of inflammasome components and target proteins via activation of transcription factor NF-κB. The second "activation" signal promotes the assembly of inflammasome components. The second signal also involves three major mechanisms, including lysosomal damage, and the potassium efflux. Nigericin is a microbial toxin that alters potassium efflux. Abbreviations: LPS: Lipopolysaccharide; TLR: Toll-like receptor; PAMPs: Pathogen-associated molecular patterns; DAMPs: Danger-associated molecular patterns; ROS: Reactive oxygen species.

2.1. Pattern Recognition Receptors (PRRs)

The potential for a cell to promote inflammation is evident by its expression of a repertoire of PRRs. Two major families of PRRs are the Toll-like receptors (TLRs) and the nucleotide-binding domain leucine-rich repeat containing receptors [37], also known as Nod-like receptors (NLRs) (Figure 3). TLRs are transmembrane receptors, which allow for the sensing of PAMPs or DAMPs either at the cell surface or within endosomal compartments. There are 10 human TLRs that have been identified, each with distinct specificities to activate downstream cascade of events in response to Gram-positive/Gram-negative bacterial infection or viral RNA [43,44]. NLRs are cytoplasmic-based PRRs, which provides an intracellular recognition system for sensing PAMPs or DAMPs. Endogenous danger signals initiate and maintain inflammatory responses through activation of NLRs (Figure 3).

Multiple NLRs and NLR-dependent inflammasomes have been identified including pyrin-domain containing the initiator proteins including NLRP-1, NLRP3, NLR family caspase activation, and recruitment domain (CARD) domain-containing protein-4 (NLRC4) and the adaptor protein called ASC (apoptosis-associated speck-like protein containing a CARD) [45]. Additionally, NLR-independent inflammasomes that are driven by sensor molecules such as absent in melanoma-2 (AIMS2) and pyrin have also been described [46]. In the absence of TLRs or reduced signaling of TLRs, NLRs synergize with TLRs for a greater response or provide a compensatory system [46]. Several of the sensor molecules of the inflammasomes such as NLRP1, NLRP3, NLRP7, NLRC4, AIM2, and pyrin have been well characterized for their specific ligands, mechanisms of action, and roles in disease pathogenesis (reviewed in Strowig et al. [47]). However, inflammasomes such as NLRP6, NLRP12, retinoic-acid inducible gene-1 (RIG-I), and interferon-γ inducible protein-16 (INFI16) are yet to be fully characterized in health and disease.

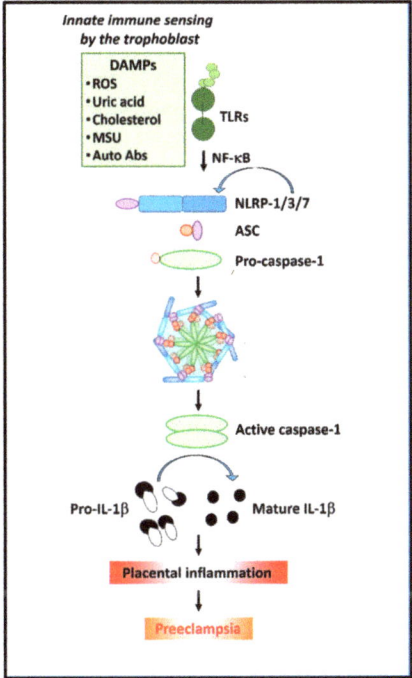

Figure 3. Depicts the role of inflammasomes in placental inflammation in preeclampsia. Cholesterol or uric acid crystals (alarmins) and extracellular vesicles/microparticles can trigger NLRP (1/3/7) inflammasomes in the placenta, which releases active caspase-1 and mature IL-1β and increases inflammation.

2.2. Inflammasome Components in the Gestational Tissues during Normal Pregnancy

An inflammatory environment is mandatory in order to ensure an adequate reconstruction of the uterine epithelium, elimination of cellular debris, and tissue remodeling during implantation, placentation, maintenance of pregnancy throughout gestation and in parturition [48–50]. Inflammasome components have been identified in both maternal and fetal compartments throughout gestation. The mRNA transcripts, as well as the protein expression of NLRP1-4; the adaptor protein ASC (or PYCARD) and the caspases (1 and 4) have all been detected in the human placental trophoblasts, myometrium, and in the amniotic membranes throughout gestation [51–57]. Hyperactivity of inflammasomes has also been reported in the choriodecidua, myometrium, and cervix during term parturition (reviewed in [36]). Specifically, several studies indicate that the activation of NLRP3 inflammasome leads to the pyroptosis as part of the sterile inflammatory milieu during physiological labour in term pregnancies [58]. Emerging studies describing inflammasome expression and activation in physiological inflammation associated with uncomplicated human pregnancies provide important knowledge on their role in the pathophysiology of pregnancy complications such as PE [35] and FGR [59].

2.3. Activation of Inflammasomes in Preeclampsia-Affected Pregnancies

Activation of inflammasomes are an essential element of the innate immune system and disturbances in these processes have been implicated in various inflammatory diseases including placental inflammation associated with PE [35], FGR [59], and gestational diabetes mellitus [60]. Inflammasome hyperactivity has been reported in placental tissues from pregnant women with PE [35,41,61]. Mulla et al. [62] reported that inflammasome activation in STB could be a possible mechanism of induction of inflammation at the maternal–fetal interface that causes adverse pregnancy outcomes, including PE. To further support this, elevated levels of TLR2, TLR4, NLRP3, and IL-1β have been reported in the neutrophils of women with PE, when compared to normal pregnant women [44]. Furthermore, Pontillo et al. [52] reported enhanced gene transcripts for NLRP1, NLRP3, NLRC4, ASC, caspase-1, and IL-1β following stimulation with lipopolysaccharide (LPS) in human first-trimester cytotrophoblasts, decidual stromal cells, and endothelial cells in vitro. Anti-angiogenic factor (sFlt-1) in the syncytial knots and TNFα release from the STB were also implicated in inducing higher inflammasome activation in the placental tissues from PE pregnancies [35,41]. Further to this, an association between higher levels of TNFα and NLRP3 activation in peripheral blood monocytes from PE pregnancies demonstrated a direct involvement of TNFα in inflammasome activation [63].

Recent studies by Nunes et al. reported that alterations in STB functions as a consequence of the imbalance between pro- and antioxidant properties may also cause cellular stress and injury to activate inflammasomes [64]. Although the molecular mechanism involved in placental inflammasome activation in PE is largely unknown, it is possible that the inappropriate inflammatory response observed in PE may have its origin in the placenta. Potential mechanisms may include shedding of STB-derived micro or nanovesicles (that can act as DAMPs) into the maternal circulation, which are known to exert pro-inflammatory, procoagulant, and anti-endothelial activity in vitro [40,65]. Recent studies [41,65] also demonstrated that oxidative stress induced increase in the release of high-mobility group box 1 protein (HMGB1) from STB that may contribute to the pathogenesis of PE. Furthermore, Ivernsen (2013) [66] reported that the inflammatory molecules such as heat shock protein 70 (Hsp70), HMGB1, Galectin 3, and Synctin 1 carried by microvesicles in PE pregnancies may also act as DAMPS in the placenta and in the peripheral blood mononuclear cells (PBMC) in patients with PE. Thus, as illustrated in Figure 3, placental milieu resultant from the STB activation by inflammatory cytokines/or release of microparticles from injured or necrotic cells or complement primed and endogenous uric acid accumulation can activate the inflammasome machinery [35,61–63,67].

Although PE has been considered the disease of the primigravid for many years, a robust evidence for this important observation has never been reported. Several studies have also reported that there is a role for the immune system during pregnancy reacting against and/or tolerating the paternal antigens of the conceptus [68–74]. It was suggested that that increased exposure to the father's semen assists this immunological tolerance [68]. In addition to these benefits, although semen is not sterile, microbial tolerance mechanisms may exist [75]. Recent reports [68,75] have shown evidence that semen may be responsible for inoculating the developing conceptus, including the placenta with microbes, not all of which are infectious. It was suggested that when they are infectious, it may cause PE [68]. Furthermore, a variety of epidemiological and other evidence is entirely consistent with this, not least correlations between semen infection and PE [71,76]. Overall, these studies strongly suggest a significant paternal role in the development of PE through microbial infection of the mother via insemination.

Taken together, the above studies suggest that inflammasome activation may play a central role in the placental inflammatory processes that are associated with the pathophysiology of pregnancy complications including PE. However, further studies are required to investigate whether the inhibition of inflammasomes can be considered as a potential therapeutic strategy to prevent placental inflammation-induced development of PE.

3. Inflammasome-Mediated Downstream Molecular Pathways in Long-Term Vascular Functions

There is evidence that women who have PE and pregnancy-induced hypertension or who deliver a preterm baby have an increased risk of developing cardiovascular disease later in life [10,77]. Several systematic reviews and meta-analyses have determined that after a diagnosis of PE the relative risks for developing hypertension, cardiometabolic disorders are significantly increased in both mother and in child [78–80]. Follow-up studies of children who were born prematurely show evidence of an increased risk of high blood pressure and insulin resistance in their adulthood [81]. Thus, these reports suggest that the pregnancies associated with PE, pregnancy hypertension; as well as pregnancies associated with preterm delivery show evidence of significant changes in vascular function (detailed below) at the time of the pregnancy. These changes greatly impact the cardiovascular health of both the mother and child later in life. The cascade of events downstream of inflammasomes may play a critical role in changes associated with vascular functions in hypertensive disorders [82] including PE; however, the molecular mechanisms by which inflammasomes promote pathogenesis of PE is yet to be investigated. In the following section, we provide possible mechanisms of inflammasome-mediated alterations observed in hypertensive disorders, which may provide a foundation for developing improved management and treatment strategies to reduce pregnancy specific burden of vascular dysfunction associated with PE.

3.1. Activation of Inflammasomes in Hypertensive Disorders

Hypertension, defined as individuals presenting with blood pressure greater than 140/90 mmHg [83], represents a worldwide-spread cardiovascular abnormality and is a major cause of subsequent end-organ damage observed in affected patients. Numerous studies have detailed the pathogenesis of hypertensive disorders and reported that the molecular inflammasome platform represents a central pathogenic mechanism in initiating and promoting organ damage attributed to hypertension. Eight-week-old male Dahl salt-sensitive rats fed with a high-salt diet (8% NaCl) for six weeks were found to have higher levels of NLRP3 and IL-1β in the hypothalamic paraventricular nucleus when compared to rats fed a normal diet (0.3% NaCl) [84]. Similarly, bilateral hypothalamic paraventricular nucleus injection of an IL-1β inhibitor, gevokizumab (1 µL of 10 µg), reduced the mean arterial pressure, heart rate, and levels of plasma norepinephrine, as well as, attenuated the levels of oxidative stress (NOX-2 and NOX-4) and restored the levels of NLRP3, IL-1β, and IL-10 [84]. Additionally, via inhibiting NLRP3-induced inflammation and idiopathic pulmonary fibrosis, the clinically used TGF- β blocker, pirfenidone protected against thoracic aortic constriction (TAC)-induced hypertension and left ventricular hypertrophy, collectively contributing to myocardial fibrosis, via blocking NLRP3-mediated inflammation and fibrosis [85].

Furthermore, the ASC adaptor protein of the NLRP3 inflammasome, was shown to be critical in hypoxia-induced pulmonary hypertension and right ventricular remodeling which was associated with increased protein levels of caspase-1, IL-18, and IL-1β [86]. Moreover, Asc$^{-/-}$ mice demonstrated reduced collagen deposition and muscularization around arteries [86]. Collectively, the findings from this study indicate that hypoxia promotion of right ventricular pressure and remodeling were attenuated in mice lacking Asc, but not in mice lacking Nlrp3, indicating that the inflammasome molecular platform plays a critical role in the pathogenesis of pulmonary hypertension [86]. Another study reported that 1K/DOCA/salt-induced hypertensive mice demonstrated increased expression of renal Nlrp3, Asc, and pro-caspase-1, as well as IL-1β and IL-18 mRNA [87]. Additionally, Asc$^{-/-}$ mice in the same model were protected from an increase in the renal inflammatory profile (IL-6, IL-17A, CCL2, ICAM-1, and VCAM-1) and accumulation of macrophages and collagen [87]. These studies suggested that the cascade of events downstream of inflammasomes play a critical role in disease progression; their mechanism of actions include both a central nervous and a peripheral modulation of the inflammatory pathways.

3.2. Inflammasomes: A Potential Molecular Link for Long-Term Vascular Dysfunction and End-Organ Failure in Preeclampsia

The villous stroma of the placenta provides the microenvironment for placental vascular development where immune cells reside and serve as a barrier to induce inflammatory (inflammasome)- mediated responses [88]. PE involves the excessive activation of inflammatory immune cells [63], including monocytes, fibroblasts, and granulocytes and their exacerbated production of pro-inflammatory cytokines, IL-1β, IL-6, and IL-8 [89,90], and reduced production of regulatory cytokines such as IL-10 and TGF-α [91]. In this setting, TGF-β-promoted extracellular matrix (ECM) proteins, such as collagens, laminins, and fibronectin, play a key modulatory role in tissue remodeling [88,92,93]. Placental fibroblasts modulate the expression of ECM proteins (collagens I and IV, fibronectin, and fibrillin I) more prominently in the first trimester and term tissue [88]. Placental ischemia primes aberrant vascular and uteroplacental remodeling via the release of pro-inflammatory factors cytokines such as TNF-α in the maternal circulation [94–97]. Li et al. quantified the levels and distribution of MMPs measured in the aorta, uterus, and placenta of normal versus pregnant rats with reduced uterine perfusion pressure (RUPP) [94]. Gelatin zymography showed marked levels of uterine MMP-2 and MMP-9, whereas casein zymography demonstrated upregulated MMP-1 and MMP-7 in the aorta, uterus, and placenta of pregnant rats with reduced uterine perfusion pressure, compared with that from normal pregnant rats. Supplementary organ culture work in the same study demonstrated that TNF-α stimulation upregulated the levels of MMP-1 and MMP-7 in the aorta, uterus, and placenta of normal pregnant rats, whereas a TNF-α inhibitor antagonized the increased tissue MMP levels in rats with RUPP [94].

Collectively, these findings suggest that placenta ischemia, via TNF-α mediated signal transduction and potentially through priming of the inflammasome platform, could lead to inadequate uteroplacental and aberrant vascular remodeling in pregnancies associated with hypertension and PE. Targeting MMP-1 and MMP-7, and/or the TNF receptor upstream of that, may also present a novel avenue in the therapeutic modulation of inflammasome priming that promotes hypertension and PE [94]. As previously discussed, women with PE also demonstrate an elevated hyperuricemia profile associated with proteinuria, suggesting that increased levels of uric acid promote the disease severity and pathogenesis associated with PE, via inducers of the NLRP3 inflammasome [90]. Uric acid is known to promote inflammation and endothelial dysfunction [98] and its crystals, monosodium urate (MSU) promote the release of IL-1β via activation of the NLRP3 inflammasome (Figure 2) [35,38,63,87]. Monocytes from PE women were activated and hence released higher levels of TNF-α, superoxide anion (O_2^-), and H_2O_2 compared to monocytes derived from normotensive pregnant women [99]. These findings indicated that monocytes from the maternal peripheral blood are a key source of reactive oxygen species, free radicals, and pro-inflammatory cytokines. Collectively, these studies suggest that the production of IL-1β, via activation of the inflammasome cascade, is key to driving the pathogenesis of PE. To date, research is trying to design inflammasome antagonists or equivalent inhibition strategies.

4. Therapeutic Targeting for the Components of Inflammasomes

Due to the wide range of hypertension-driven inflammatory diseases, a number of targeted therapies have been investigated for antagonizing the effects of the inflammatory (inflammasome)-pathway. Pharmacological blockade of human cord blood leukocytes demonstrated that ATP released as a result of tissue injury can further promote the secretion of IL-1β from laboring and nonlaboring women [100], indicating that inhibition of the P2X7 receptor may protect from inflammation induced vascular injury during pregnancy. A separate study evaluated pharmacological blockade using a P2X7 receptor inhibitor and pannexin-1 blocker carbenoxolone, was shown to attenuate the LPS-induced increase in the levels of secreted IL-1β [101]. Silibinin (SB) is a flavonoid complex medicinal herb with anti-inflammatory, hepatoprotective, antioxidant, and antifibrotic properties. The antioxidant and anti-inflammatory properties of SB were assessed via dose-dependent inhibition of H_2O_2 release, production of TNF-α, IL-10, TGF-β, and prostaglandin E2 (PGE2) following LPS stimulation of peripheral blood monocytes from healthy individuals. Monocytes were treated with SB to determine whether SB can modulate the NLRP1 and NLRP3 inflammasomes, as well as influence upstream TLR-4/NF-κB activation [99]. Administration of SB to MSU-stimulated monocytes reduced the degree of NLRP1 and NLRP3 inflammasome activation, as well as TLR-4/NF-kB activation [99]. Furthermore, administration of SB to pregnant rats in an experimental model of PE, induced by nitric oxide synthase inhibition (with N-omega-nitro-l-arginine methyl (l-NAME)) protected reproductive outcomes, normalized blood pressure, reduced proteinuria, and also serum levels of pro-inflammatory cytokines [102]. Additional studies have examined targeting of the NLRP3 sensor itself, via administration of the small and highly selective NLRP3 inflammasome inhibitor, MCC950, a diarylsulfonylurea-containing compound [103]. The mechanism of action of MCC950 is via its ability to inhibit NLRP3-induced ASC oligomerization to subsequently block the secretion of IL-1β [103], where MCC950 was recently shown to attenuate the high deoxycorticosterone (DOCA)-induced hypertensive effects [87,104]. Krishnan et al. [87] demonstrated an increased DOCA/salt-induced renal inflammatory profile (IL-6, IL-17A, CCL2, ICAM-1, and VCAM-1), fibrosis (assessed via extent of renal collagen accumulation), via an inflammasome/IL-1β-dependent mechanism.

As a follow-up study, Krishnan et al. [104], showed that pharmacological inhibition of the NLRP3 inflammasome, with MCC950, significantly lowered the 1K/DOCA/salt-induced increase in blood pressure, renal expression of inflammasome markers (NLRP3, ASC, pro-caspase-1, pro-IL-1β and pro-IL-18), and markers associated with renal inflammation and injury (IL-17A, TNF-α, osteopontin, ICAM-1, VCAM-1, CCL2, and vimentin). A MCC950-induced reduction in these 1K/DOCA/salt-induced measures was accompanied by an additional marked attenuation in the levels of renal interstitial collagen and renal albuminuria (by up to 25%) in C57Bl/6 mice [104]. Similarly, by blocking the ability of the NLRP3 inflammasome components to assemble and oligomerize, as well as inhibiting K$^+$ efflux, β-hydroxybutyrate (BHB) was shown to reduce the production of both IL-1β and IL-18 [105]. A separate study also demonstrated that treatment with EMD638683, a specific glucocorticoid-inducible kinase (SGK1) inhibitor, significantly reduced hypertension induced cardiac damage [106]. Taken together, these studies provide proof-of-concept that pharmacological inhibition of upstream, as well as downstream targets of the NLRP3 inflammasome signaling cascade; and the inflammasome platform, present a viable anti-hypertensive strategy in attenuating the pathogenesis of PE with an underpinning inflammatory component.

5. Conclusions

There is consistent evidence for activation of inflammasomes in physiological inflammatory processes during pregnancy. Inflammasomes are implicated in both normal physiological and in the pathophysiological processes that occur in response to inflammatory milieu throughout gestation. This suggests that the placenta is immunologically functional and able to generate specific and diverse innate immune-like responses through the expression of specific components of inflammasomes. However, the type of response is highly dependent upon the timing of gestation, as well as the type of stimuli, the expression and activation of status of the specific type of receptors, and the downstream signaling pathways that are altered in response to the stimuli. Furthermore, it is in the pathological inflammatory processes as seen in PE, that premature activation of inflammasomes as a consequence of placental ischemia (Figure 4) could contribute to increased fibrosis resulting in end organ damage in the heart, liver, and kidneys. Therefore, research findings in these areas will be critical for developing targeted therapies for the prevention of poor pregnancy outcomes of PE affected pregnancies.

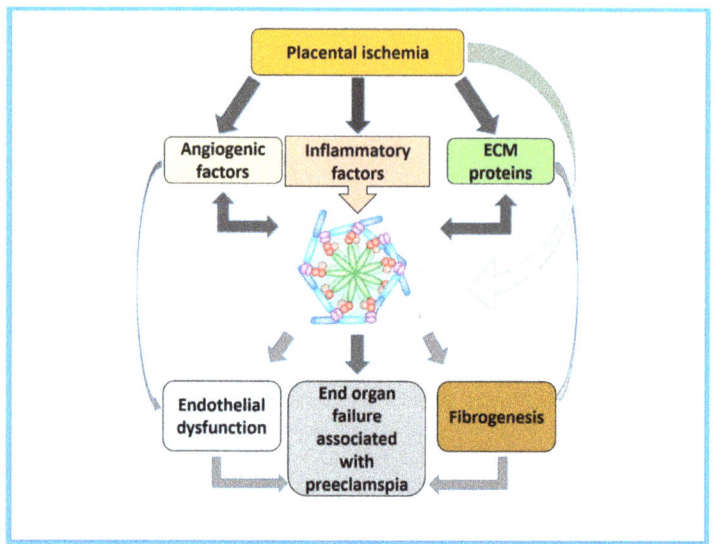

Figure 4. Summarizes the central role of inflammasomes in the pathogenesis of preeclampsia. Premature activation of inflammasomes following placental ischemia in preeclampsia affected pregnancies may lead to changes in vascular structure and function and enhanced fibrosis contributing to end stage organ failure.

Author Contributions: This review was conceptualized by P.M. in collaboration with A.A.P. and C.S.S.; P.M. and A.A.P. wrote the original draft and was extensively reviewed by C.S.S.; E.D. reviewed and edited the manuscript. All authors have read and agreed to the published version of the manuscript.

Funding: This research received no external funding.

Conflicts of Interest: The authors declare no conflict of interest.

Abbreviations

PE	preeclampsia
AIM2	absent melanoma-2
DAMP	danger-associated molecular pattern
NLR	nucleotide-binding oligomerization domain leucine-rich repeat containing protein
PRR	pattern recognition receptors
PAMP	pathogen-associated molecular pattern
CARD	caspase-activation and recruitment domain
ASC	apoptosis-associated speck-like protein containing a caspase recruitment domain
IL	interleukin
NLRP	nucleotide binding oligomerization domain leucine-rich repeat containing protein and pyrin domain containing protein
IFI16	interferon-gamma inducible protein-16
TLR	Toll-like receptor
STB	syncytiotrophoblast
EVT	extravillous cytotrophoblast

References

1. Evain-Brion, D.; Malassine, A. Human placenta as an endocrine organ. *Growth Horm. IGF Res.* **2003**, *13*, S34–S37. [CrossRef]
2. Zhou, Y.; Fisher, S.J.; Janatpour, M.; Genbacev, O.; Dejana, E.; Wheelock, M.; Damsky, C.H. Human cytotrophoblasts adopt a vascular phenotype as they differentiate. A strategy for successful endovascular invasion? *J. Clin. Investig.* **1997**, *99*, 2139–2151. [CrossRef]
3. Pijnenborg, R.; Vercruysse, L.; Hanssens, M. The uterine spiral arteries in human pregnancy: Facts and controversies. *Placenta* **2006**, *27*, 939–958. [CrossRef] [PubMed]
4. Boeldt, D.S.; Bird, I.M. Vascular adaptation in pregnancy and endothelial dysfunction in preeclampsia. *J. Endocrinol.* **2017**, *232*, R27–R44. [CrossRef] [PubMed]
5. Vinayagam, D.; Leslie, K.; Khalil, A.; Thilaganathan, B. Preeclampsia-What is to blame? The placenta, maternal cardiovascular system or both? *World J. Obstet. Gynecol.* **2015**, *4*, 77–85. [CrossRef]
6. Roth, I.; Corry, D.B.; Locksley, R.M.; Abrams, J.S.; Litton, M.J.; Fisher, S.J. Human placental cytotrophoblasts produce the immunosuppressive cytokine interleukin 10. *J. Exp. Med.* **1996**, *184*, 539–548. [CrossRef]
7. Pijnenborg, R. Establishment of uteroplacental circulation. *Reprod. Nutr. Dev.* **1988**, *28*, 1581–1586. [CrossRef]
8. Duley, L. The global impact of pre-eclampsia and eclampsia. *Semin. Perinatol.* **2009**, *33*, 130–137. [CrossRef]
9. Arulkumaran, N.; Lightstone, L. Severe pre-eclampsia and hypertensive crises. *Best Pract. Res. Clin. Obstet. Gynaecol.* **2013**, *27*, 877–884. [CrossRef]
10. Smith, G.C.; Pell, J.P.; Walsh, D. Pregnancy complications and maternal risk of ischaemic heart disease: A retrospective cohort study of 129,290 births. *Lancet* **2001**, *357*, 2002–2006. [CrossRef]
11. Saxena, A.R.; Karumanchi, S.A.; Brown, N.J.; Royle, C.M.; McElrath, T.F.; Seely, E.W. Increased sensitivity to angiotensin II is present postpartum in women with a history of hypertensive pregnancy. *Hypertension* **2010**, *55*, 1239–1245. [CrossRef] [PubMed]
12. Craici, I.M.; Wagner, S.J.; Hayman, S.R.; Garovic, V.D. Pre-eclamptic pregnancies: An opportunity to identify women at risk for future cardiovascular disease. *Womens Health* **2008**, *4*, 133–135. [CrossRef] [PubMed]
13. Garovic, V.D.; Hayman, S.R. Hypertension in pregnancy: An emerging risk factor for cardiovascular disease. *Nat. Clin. Pract. Nephrol.* **2007**, *3*, 613–622. [CrossRef] [PubMed]
14. Veerbeek, J.H.; Brouwers, L.; Koster, M.P.; Koenen, S.V.; van Vliet, E.O.; Nikkels, P.G.; Franx, A.; van Rijn, B.B. Spiral artery remodeling and maternal cardiovascular risk: The spiral artery remodeling (SPAR) study. *J. Hypertens.* **2016**, *34*, 1570–1577. [CrossRef]
15. Cornelius, D.C.; Hogg, J.P.; Scott, J.; Wallace, K.; Herse, F.; Moseley, J.; Wallukat, G.; Dechend, R.; LaMarca, B. Administration of interleukin-17 soluble receptor C suppresses TH17 cells, oxidative stress, and hypertension in response to placental ischemia during pregnancy. *Hypertension* **2013**, *62*, 1068–1073. [CrossRef]
16. Irani, R.A.; Zhang, Y.; Zhou, C.C.; Blackwell, S.C.; Hicks, M.J.; Ramin, S.M.; Kellems, R.E.; Xia, Y. Autoantibody-mediated angiotensin receptor activation contributes to preeclampsia through tumor necrosis factor-alpha signaling. *Hypertension* **2010**, *55*, 1246–1253. [CrossRef]
17. Redman, C.W.; Sargent, I.L. The pathogenesis of pre-eclampsia. *Gynecol. Obstet. Fertil.* **2001**, *29*, 518–522. [CrossRef]
18. LaMarca, B.; Cornelius, D.; Wallace, K. Elucidating immune mechanisms causing hypertension during pregnancy. *Physiology* **2013**, *28*, 225–233. [CrossRef]
19. Wallace, K.; Richards, S.; Dhillon, P.; Weimer, A.; Edholm, E.S.; Bengten, E.; Wilson, M.; Martin, J.N., Jr.; LaMarca, B. CD4+ T-helper cells stimulated in response to placental ischemia mediate hypertension during pregnancy. *Hypertension* **2011**, *57*, 949–955. [CrossRef]
20. Conrad, K.P.; Benyo, D.F. Placental cytokines and the pathogenesis of preeclampsia. *Am. J. Reprod. Immunol.* **1997**, *37*, 240–249. [CrossRef]
21. LaMarca, B.B.; Cockrell, K.; Sullivan, E.; Bennett, W.; Granger, J.P. Role of endothelin in mediating tumor necrosis factor-induced hypertension in pregnant rats. *Hypertension* **2005**, *46*, 82–86. [CrossRef] [PubMed]
22. LaMarca, B.; Wallukat, G.; Llinas, M.; Herse, F.; Dechend, R.; Granger, J.P. Autoantibodies to the angiotensin type I receptor in response to placental ischemia and tumor necrosis factor alpha in pregnant rats. *Hypertension* **2008**, *52*, 1168–1172. [CrossRef] [PubMed]

23. Co, E.C.; Gormley, M.; Kapidzic, M.; Rosen, D.B.; Scott, M.A.; Stolp, H.A.; McMaster, M.; Lanier, L.L.; Barcena, A.; Fisher, S.J. Maternal decidual macrophages inhibit NK cell killing of invasive cytotrophoblasts during human pregnancy. *Biol. Reprod.* **2013**, *88*, 155. [CrossRef] [PubMed]
24. Mor, G.; Cardenas, I.; Abrahams, V.; Guller, S. Inflammation and pregnancy: The role of the immune system at the implantation site. *Ann. N Y Acad. Sci.* **2011**, *1221*, 80–87. [CrossRef] [PubMed]
25. Tong, M.; Abrahams, V.M. Immunology of the Placenta. *Obstet. Gynecol. Clin. N. Am.* **2020**, *47*, 49–63. [CrossRef]
26. Mor, G.; Cardenas, I. The immune system in pregnancy: A unique complexity. *Am. J. Reprod. Immunol.* **2010**, *63*, 425–433. [CrossRef]
27. Redman, C.W.; Sargent, I.L. Immunology of pre-eclampsia. *Am. J. Reprod. Immunol.* **2010**, *63*, 534–543. [CrossRef]
28. Cornelius, D.C. Preeclampsia: From Inflammation to Immunoregulation. *Clin. Med. Insights Blood Disord.* **2018**, *11*. [CrossRef]
29. Borzychowski, A.M.; Sargent, I.L.; Redman, C.W. Inflammation and pre-eclampsia. *Semin. Fetal Neonatal Med.* **2006**, *11*, 309–316. [CrossRef]
30. Sargent, I.L.; Borzychowski, A.M.; Redman, C.W. NK cells and human pregnancy-an inflammatory view. *Trends Immunol.* **2006**, *27*, 399–404. [CrossRef]
31. Tangeras, L.H.; Stodle, G.S.; Olsen, G.D.; Leknes, A.H.; Gundersen, A.S.; Skei, B.; Vikdal, A.J.; Ryan, L.; Steinkjer, B.; Myklebost, M.F.; et al. Functional Toll-like receptors in primary first-trimester trophoblasts. *J. Reprod. Immunol.* **2014**, *106*, 89–99. [CrossRef] [PubMed]
32. LaMarca, B.D.; Ryan, M.J.; Gilbert, J.S.; Murphy, S.R.; Granger, J.P. Inflammatory cytokines in the pathophysiology of hypertension during preeclampsia. *Curr. Hypertens Rep.* **2007**, *9*, 480–485. [CrossRef] [PubMed]
33. Szarka, A.; Rigo, J., Jr.; Lazar, L.; Beko, G.; Molvarec, A. Circulating cytokines, chemokines and adhesion molecules in normal pregnancy and preeclampsia determined by multiplex suspension array. *BMC Immunol.* **2010**, *11*, 59. [CrossRef]
34. Rusterholz, C.; Hahn, S.; Holzgreve, W. Role of placentally produced inflammatory and regulatory cytokines in pregnancy and the etiology of preeclampsia. *Semin. Immunopathol.* **2007**, *29*, 151–162. [CrossRef]
35. Stodle, G.S.; Silva, G.B.; Tangeras, L.H.; Gierman, L.M.; Nervik, I.; Dahlberg, U.E.; Sun, C.; Aune, M.H.; Thomsen, L.C.V.; Bjorge, L.; et al. Placental inflammation in pre-eclampsia by Nod-like receptor protein (NLRP)3 inflammasome activation in trophoblasts. *Clin. Exp. Immunol.* **2018**, *193*, 84–94. [CrossRef]
36. Gomez-Lopez, N.; Motomura, K.; Miller, D.; Garcia-Flores, V.; Galaz, J.; Romero, R. Inflammasomes: Their Role in Normal and Complicated Pregnancies. *J. Immunol.* **2019**, *203*, 2757–2769. [CrossRef]
37. Broz, P.; Dixit, V.M. Inflammasomes: Mechanism of assembly, regulation and signalling. *Nat. Rev. Immunol.* **2016**, *16*, 407–420. [CrossRef]
38. Martinon, F.; Burns, K.; Tschopp, J. The inflammasome: A molecular platform triggering activation of inflammatory caspases and processing of proIL-beta. *Mol. Cell.* **2002**, *10*, 417–426. [CrossRef]
39. Tschopp, J.; Martinon, F.; Burns, K. NALPs: A novel protein family involved in inflammation. *Nat. Rev. Mol. Cell. Biol.* **2003**, *4*, 95–104. [CrossRef]
40. Khan, R.N.; Hay, D.P. A clear and present danger: Inflammasomes DAMPing down disorders of pregnancy. *Hum. Reprod. Update* **2015**, *21*, 388–405. [CrossRef]
41. C Weel, I.; Romao-Veiga, M.; Matias, M.L.; Fioratti, E.G.; Peracoli, J.C.; Borges, V.T.; Araujo, J.P., Jr.; Peracoli, M.T. Increased expression of NLRP3 inflammasome in placentas from pregnant women with severe preeclampsia. *J. Reprod. Immunol.* **2017**, *123*, 40–47. [CrossRef]
42. Liu, X.; Zhang, Z.; Ruan, J.; Pan, Y.; Magupalli, V.G.; Wu, H.; Lieberman, J. Inflammasome-activated gasdermin D causes pyroptosis by forming membrane pores. *Nature* **2016**, *535*, 153–158. [CrossRef] [PubMed]
43. Ilekis, J.V.; Tsilou, E.; Fisher, S.; Abrahams, V.M.; Soares, M.J.; Cross, J.C.; Zamudio, S.; Illsley, N.P.; Myatt, L.; Colvis, C.; et al. Placental origins of adverse pregnancy outcomes: Potential molecular targets: An Executive Workshop Summary of the Eunice Kennedy Shriver National Institute of Child Health and Human Development. *Am. J. Obstet. Gynecol.* **2016**, *215*, S1–S46. [CrossRef]
44. Xie, F.; Hu, Y.; Turvey, S.E.; Magee, L.A.; Brunham, R.M.; Choi, K.C.; Krajden, M.; Leung, P.C.; Money, D.M.; Patrick, D.M.; et al. Toll-like receptors 2 and 4 and the cryopyrin inflammasome in normal pregnancy and pre-eclampsia. *BJOG* **2010**, *117*, 99–108. [CrossRef]

45. Lu, A.; Magupalli, V.G.; Ruan, J.; Yin, Q.; Atianand, M.K.; Vos, M.R.; Schroder, G.F.; Fitzgerald, K.A.; Wu, H.; Egelman, E.H. Unified polymerization mechanism for the assembly of ASC-dependent inflammasomes. *Cell* **2014**, *156*, 1193–1206. [CrossRef]
46. Abrahams, V.M. The role of the Nod-like receptor family in trophoblast innate immune responses. *J. Reprod. Immunol.* **2011**, *88*, 112–117. [CrossRef] [PubMed]
47. Strowig, T.; Henao-Mejia, J.; Elinav, E.; Flavell, R. Inflammasomes in health and disease. *Nature* **2012**, *481*, 278–286. [CrossRef] [PubMed]
48. Orsi, N.M.; Tribe, R.M. Cytokine networks and the regulation of uterine function in pregnancy and parturition. *J. Neuroendocrinol.* **2008**, *20*, 462–469. [CrossRef] [PubMed]
49. Evans, J.; Salamonsen, L.A.; Winship, A.; Menkhorst, E.; Nie, G.; Gargett, C.E.; Dimitriadis, E. Fertile ground: Human endometrial programming and lessons in health and disease. *Nat. Rev. Endocrinol.* **2016**, *12*, 654–667. [CrossRef]
50. Romero, R.; Espinoza, J.; Goncalves, L.F.; Kusanovic, J.P.; Friel, L.A.; Nien, J.K. Inflammation in preterm and term labour and delivery. *Semin. Fetal Neonatal Med.* **2006**, *11*, 317–326. [CrossRef]
51. Yin, Y.; Yan, Y.; Jiang, X.; Mai, J.; Chen, N.C.; Wang, H.; Yang, X.F. Inflammasomes are differentially expressed in cardiovascular and other tissues. *Int. J. Immunopathol. Pharmacol.* **2009**, *22*, 311–322. [CrossRef]
52. Pontillo, A.; Girardelli, M.; Agostinis, C.; Masat, E.; Bulla, R.; Crovella, S. Bacterial LPS differently modulates inflammasome gene expression and IL-1beta secretion in trophoblast cells, decidual stromal cells, and decidual endothelial cells. *Reprod. Sci.* **2013**, *20*, 563–566. [CrossRef]
53. Tilburgs, T.; Meissner, T.B.; Ferreira, L.M.R.; Mulder, A.; Musunuru, K.; Ye, J.; Strominger, J.L. NLRP2 is a suppressor of NF-kB signaling and HLA-C expression in human trophoblastsdagger, double dagger. *Biol. Reprod.* **2017**, *96*, 831–842. [CrossRef]
54. Bryant, A.H.; Bevan, R.J.; Spencer-Harty, S.; Scott, L.M.; Jones, R.H.; Thornton, C.A. Expression and function of NOD-like receptors by human term gestation-associated tissues. *Placenta* **2017**, *58*, 25–32. [CrossRef]
55. Gomez-Lopez, N.; Romero, R.; Panaitescu, B.; Leng, Y.; Xu, Y.; Tarca, A.L.; Faro, J.; Pacora, P.; Hassan, S.S.; Hsu, C.D. Inflammasome activation during spontaneous preterm labor with intra-amniotic infection or sterile intra-amniotic inflammation. *Am. J. Reprod. Immunol.* **2018**, *80*, e13049. [CrossRef]
56. Panaitescu, B.; Romero, R.; Gomez-Lopez, N.; Xu, Y.; Leng, Y.; Maymon, E.; Pacora, P.; Erez, O.; Yeo, L.; Hassan, S.S.; et al. In vivo evidence of inflammasome activation during spontaneous labor at term. *J Matern. Fetal Neonatal Med.* **2019**, *32*, 1978–1991. [CrossRef]
57. Romero, R.; Xu, Y.; Plazyo, O.; Chaemsaithong, P.; Chaiworapongsa, T.; Unkel, R.; Than, N.G.; Chiang, P.J.; Dong, Z.; Xu, Z.; et al. A Role for the Inflammasome in Spontaneous Labor at Term. *Am. J. Reprod. Immunol.* **2018**, *79*, e12440. [CrossRef]
58. Gomez-Lopez, N.; Romero, R.; Xu, Y.; Garcia-Flores, V.; Leng, Y.; Panaitescu, B.; Miller, D.; Abrahams, V.M.; Hassan, S.S. Inflammasome assembly in the chorioamniotic membranes during spontaneous labor at term. *Am. J. Reprod. Immunol.* **2017**, *77*. [CrossRef]
59. Abi Nahed, R.; Reynaud, D.; Borg, A.J.; Traboulsi, W.; Wetzel, A.; Sapin, V.; Brouillet, S.; Dieudonne, M.N.; Dakouane-Giudicelli, M.; Benharouga, M.; et al. NLRP7 is increased in human idiopathic fetal growth restriction and plays a critical role in trophoblast differentiation. *J. Mol. Med.* **2019**, *97*, 355–367. [CrossRef]
60. Han, C.S.; Herrin, M.A.; Pitruzzello, M.C.; Mulla, M.J.; Werner, E.F.; Pettker, C.M.; Flannery, C.A.; Abrahams, V.M. Glucose and metformin modulate human first trimester trophoblast function: A model and potential therapy for diabetes-associated uteroplacental insufficiency. *Am. J. Reprod. Immunol.* **2015**, *73*, 362–371. [CrossRef]
61. Kohli, S.; Ranjan, S.; Hoffmann, J.; Kashif, M.; Daniel, E.A.; Al-Dabet, M.M.; Bock, F.; Nazir, S.; Huebner, H.; Mertens, P.R.; et al. Maternal extracellular vesicles and platelets promote preeclampsia via inflammasome activation in trophoblasts. *Blood* **2016**, *128*, 2153–2164. [CrossRef]
62. Mulla, M.J.; Weel, I.C.; Potter, J.A.; Gysler, S.M.; Salmon, J.E.; Peracoli, M.T.S.; Rothlin, C.V.; Chamley, L.W.; Abrahams, V.M. Antiphospholipid Antibodies Inhibit Trophoblast Toll-Like Receptor and Inflammasome Negative Regulators. *Arthritis Rheumatol.* **2018**, *70*, 891–902. [CrossRef]
63. Matias, M.L.; Romao, M.; Weel, I.C.; Ribeiro, V.R.; Nunes, P.R.; Borges, V.T.; Araujo, J.P.J.; Peracoli, J.C.; de Oliveira, L.; Peracoli, M.T. Endogenous and Uric Acid-Induced Activation of NLRP3 Inflammasome in Pregnant Women with Preeclampsia. *PLoS ONE* **2015**, *10*, e0129095. [CrossRef] [PubMed]

64. Nunes, P.R.; Peracoli, M.T.S.; Romao-Veiga, M.; Matias, M.L.; Ribeiro, V.R.; Da Costa Fernandes, C.J.; Peracoli, J.C.; Rodrigues, J.R.; De Oliveira, L. Hydrogen peroxide-mediated oxidative stress induces inflammasome activation in term human placental explants. *Pregnancy Hypertens* **2018**, *14*, 29–36. [CrossRef] [PubMed]
65. Chen, Q.; Yin, Y.X.; Wei, J.; Tong, M.; Shen, F.; Zhao, M.; Chamley, L. Increased expression of high mobility group box 1 (HMGB1) in the cytoplasm of placental syncytiotrophoblast from preeclamptic placentae. *Cytokine* **2016**, *85*, 30–36. [CrossRef] [PubMed]
66. Ivernsen, A. Inflammatory mechanisms in preeclampsia. *Pregnancy Hypertens.* **2013**, *3*, 58.
67. Shirasuna, K.; Usui, F.; Karasawa, T.; Kimura, H.; Kawashima, A.; Mizukami, H.; Ohkuchi, A.; Nishimura, S.; Sagara, J.; Noda, T.; et al. Nanosilica-induced placental inflammation and pregnancy complications: Different roles of the inflammasome components NLRP3 and ASC. *Nanotoxicology* **2015**, *9*, 554–567. [CrossRef]
68. Kenny, L.C.; Kell, D.B. Immunological Tolerance, Pregnancy, and Preeclampsia: The Roles of Semen Microbes and the Father. *Front. Med.* **2017**, *4*, 239. [CrossRef]
69. Dekker, G. The partner's role in the etiology of preeclampsia. *J. Reprod. Immunol.* **2002**, *57*, 203–215. [CrossRef]
70. Dekker, G.; Robillard, P.Y.; Roberts, C. The etiology of preeclampsia: The role of the father. *J. Reprod. Immunol.* **2011**, *89*, 126–132. [CrossRef]
71. Dekker, G.A.; Robillard, P.Y.; Hulsey, T.C. Immune maladaptation in the etiology of preeclampsia: A review of corroborative epidemiologic studies. *Obstet. Gynecol. Surv.* **1998**, *53*, 377–382. [CrossRef] [PubMed]
72. Johansson, M.; Bromfield, J.J.; Jasper, M.J.; Robertson, S.A. Semen activates the female immune response during early pregnancy in mice. *Immunology* **2004**, *112*, 290–300. [CrossRef] [PubMed]
73. Moldenhauer, L.M.; Diener, K.R.; Thring, D.M.; Brown, M.P.; Hayball, J.D.; Robertson, S.A. Cross-presentation of male seminal fluid antigens elicits T cell activation to initiate the female immune response to pregnancy. *J. Immunol.* **2009**, *182*, 8080–8093. [CrossRef] [PubMed]
74. Robertson, S.A.; Sharkey, D.J. The role of semen in induction of maternal immune tolerance to pregnancy. *Semin. Immunol.* **2001**, *13*, 243–254. [CrossRef] [PubMed]
75. Kell, D.B.; Kenny, L.C. A Dormant Microbial Component in the Development of Preeclampsia. *Front. Med.* **2016**, *3*, 60. [CrossRef]
76. Robillard, P.Y.; Dekker, G.; Chaouat, G.; Hulsey, T.C.; Saftlas, A. Epidemiological studies on primipaternity and immunology in preeclampsia–a statement after twelve years of workshops. *J. Reprod. Immunol.* **2011**, *89*, 104–117. [CrossRef]
77. Catov, J.M.; Newman, A.B.; Roberts, J.M.; Kelsey, S.F.; Sutton-Tyrrell, K.; Harris, T.B.; Colbert, L.; Rubin, S.M.; Satterfield, S.; Ness, R.B.; et al. Preterm delivery and later maternal cardiovascular disease risk. *Epidemiology* **2007**, *18*, 733–739. [CrossRef]
78. Kirollos, S.; Skilton, M.; Patel, S.; Arnott, C. A Systematic Review of Vascular Structure and Function in Pre-eclampsia: Non-invasive Assessment and Mechanistic Links. *Front. Cardiovasc. Med.* **2019**, *6*, 166. [CrossRef]
79. Ray, J.G.; Vermeulen, M.J.; Schull, M.J.; Redelmeier, D.A. Cardiovascular health after maternal placental syndromes (CHAMPS): Population-based retrospective cohort study. *Lancet* **2005**, *366*, 1797–1803. [CrossRef]
80. Rana, S.; Lemoine, E.; Granger, J.P.; Karumanchi, S.A. Preeclampsia: Pathophysiology, Challenges, and Perspectives. *Circ. Res.* **2019**, *124*, 1094–1112. [CrossRef]
81. Dalziel, S.R.; Parag, V.; Rodgers, A.; Harding, J.E. Cardiovascular risk factors at age 30 following pre-term birth. *Int. J. Epidemiol.* **2007**, *36*, 907–915. [CrossRef] [PubMed]
82. Pasqua, T.; Pagliaro, P.; Rocca, C.; Angelone, T.; Penna, C. Role of NLRP-3 Inflammasome in Hypertension: A Potential Therapeutic Target. *Curr. Pharm. Biotechnol.* **2018**, *19*, 708–714. [CrossRef] [PubMed]
83. Drummond, G.R.; Vinh, A.; Guzik, T.J.; Sobey, C.G. Immune mechanisms of hypertension. *Nat. Rev. Immunol.* **2019**, *19*, 517–532. [CrossRef] [PubMed]
84. Qi, J.; Zhao, X.F.; Yu, X.J.; Yi, Q.Y.; Shi, X.L.; Tan, H.; Fan, X.Y.; Gao, H.L.; Yue, L.Y.; Feng, Z.P.; et al. Targeting Interleukin-1 beta to Suppress Sympathoexcitation in Hypothalamic Paraventricular Nucleus in Dahl Salt-Sensitive Hypertensive Rats. *Cardiovasc. Toxicol.* **2016**, *16*, 298–306. [CrossRef]
85. Wang, Y.; Wu, Y.; Chen, J.; Zhao, S.; Li, H. Pirfenidone attenuates cardiac fibrosis in a mouse model of TAC-induced left ventricular remodeling by suppressing NLRP3 inflammasome formation. *Cardiology* **2013**, *126*, 1–11. [CrossRef]

86. Cero, F.T.; Hillestad, V.; Sjaastad, I.; Yndestad, A.; Aukrust, P.; Ranheim, T.; Lunde, I.G.; Olsen, M.B.; Lien, E.; Zhang, L.; et al. Absence of the inflammasome adaptor ASC reduces hypoxia-induced pulmonary hypertension in mice. *Am. J. Physiol. Lung Cell. Mol. Physiol.* **2015**, *309*, L378–L387. [CrossRef]
87. Krishnan, S.M.; Dowling, J.K.; Ling, Y.H.; Diep, H.; Chan, C.T.; Ferens, D.; Kett, M.M.; Pinar, A.; Samuel, C.S.; Vinh, A.; et al. Inflammasome activity is essential for one kidney/deoxycorticosterone acetate/salt-induced hypertension in mice. *Br. J. Pharmacol.* **2016**, *173*, 752–765. [CrossRef]
88. Chen, C.P.; Aplin, J.D. Placental extracellular matrix: Gene expression, deposition by placental fibroblasts and the effect of oxygen. *Placenta* **2003**, *24*, 316–325. [CrossRef]
89. Luppi, P.; Deloia, J.A. Monocytes of preeclamptic women spontaneously synthesize pro-inflammatory cytokines. *Clin. Immunol.* **2006**, *118*, 268–275. [CrossRef]
90. Peracoli, J.C.; Rudge, M.V.; Peracoli, M.T. Tumor necrosis factor-alpha in gestation and puerperium of women with gestational hypertension and pre-eclampsia. *Am. J. Reprod. Immunol.* **2007**, *57*, 177–185. [CrossRef]
91. Cristofalo, R.; Bannwart-Castro, C.F.; Magalhaes, C.G.; Borges, V.T.; Peracoli, J.C.; Witkin, S.S.; Peracoli, M.T. Silibinin attenuates oxidative metabolism and cytokine production by monocytes from preeclamptic women. *Free Radic. Res.* **2013**, *47*, 268–275. [CrossRef]
92. Brubaker, D.B.; Ross, M.G.; Marinoff, D. The function of elevated plasma fibronectin in preeclampsia. *Am. J. Obstet. Gynecol.* **1992**, *166*, 526–531. [CrossRef]
93. Caceres, F.T.; Gaspari, T.A.; Samuel, C.S.; Pinar, A.A. Serelaxin inhibits the profibrotic TGF-beta1/IL-1beta axis by targeting TLR-4 and the NLRP3 inflammasome in cardiac myofibroblasts. *FASEB J.* **2019**, *33*, 14717–14733. [CrossRef] [PubMed]
94. Li, W.; Cui, N.; Mazzuca, M.Q.; Mata, K.M.; Khalil, R.A. Increased vascular and uteroplacental matrix metalloproteinase-1 and -7 levels and collagen type I deposition in hypertension in pregnancy: Role of TNF-alpha. *Am. J. Physiol. Heart Circ. Physiol.* **2017**, *313*, H491–H507. [CrossRef] [PubMed]
95. LaMarca, B.; Speed, J.; Fournier, L.; Babcock, S.A.; Berry, H.; Cockrell, K.; Granger, J.P. Hypertension in response to chronic reductions in uterine perfusion in pregnant rats: Effect of tumor necrosis factor-alpha blockade. *Hypertension* **2008**, *52*, 1161–1167. [CrossRef]
96. LaMarca, B.B.; Bennett, W.A.; Alexander, B.T.; Cockrell, K.; Granger, J.P. Hypertension produced by reductions in uterine perfusion in the pregnant rat: Role of tumor necrosis factor-alpha. *Hypertension* **2005**, *46*, 1022–1025. [CrossRef] [PubMed]
97. Chen, J.; Khalil, R.A. Matrix Metalloproteinases in Normal Pregnancy and Preeclampsia. *Prog. Mol. Biol. Transl. Sci.* **2017**, *148*, 87–165. [CrossRef]
98. Zhao, J.; Zheng, D.Y.; Yang, J.M.; Wang, M.; Zhang, X.T.; Sun, L.; Yun, X.G. Maternal serum uric acid concentration is associated with the expression of tumour necrosis factor-alpha and intercellular adhesion molecule-1 in patients with preeclampsia. *J. Hum. Hypertens* **2016**, *30*, 456–462. [CrossRef]
99. Matias, M.L.; Gomes, V.J.; Romao-Veiga, M.; Ribeiro, V.R.; Nunes, P.R.; Romagnoli, G.G.; Peracoli, J.C.; Peracoli, M.T.S. Silibinin Downregulates the NF-kappaB Pathway and NLRP1/NLRP3 Inflammasomes in Monocytes from Pregnant Women with Preeclampsia. *Molecules* **2019**, *24*, 1548. [CrossRef]
100. Warren, A.Y.; Harvey, L.; Shaw, R.W.; Khan, R.N. Interleukin-1 beta secretion from cord blood mononuclear cells in vitro involves P2X 7 receptor activation. *Reprod. Sci.* **2008**, *15*, 189–194. [CrossRef]
101. Lappas, M. Caspase-1 activation is increased with human labour in foetal membranes and myometrium and mediates infection-induced interleukin-1beta secretion. *Am. J. Reprod. Immunol.* **2014**, *71*, 189–201. [CrossRef] [PubMed]
102. Souza, C.O.; Peracoli, M.T.; Weel, I.C.; Bannwart, C.F.; Romao, M.; Nakaira-Takahagi, E.; Medeiros, L.T.; Silva, M.G.; Peracoli, J.C. Hepatoprotective and anti-inflammatory effects of silibinin on experimental preeclampsia induced by L-NAME in rats. *Life Sci.* **2012**, *91*, 159–165. [CrossRef] [PubMed]
103. Coll, R.C.; Robertson, A.A.; Chae, J.J.; Higgins, S.C.; Munoz-Planillo, R.; Inserra, M.C.; Vetter, I.; Dungan, L.S.; Monks, B.G.; Stutz, A.; et al. A small-molecule inhibitor of the NLRP3 inflammasome for the treatment of inflammatory diseases. *Nat. Med.* **2015**, *21*, 248–255. [CrossRef]
104. Krishnan, S.M.; Ling, Y.H.; Huuskes, B.M.; Ferens, D.M.; Saini, N.; Chan, C.T.; Diep, H.; Kett, M.M.; Samuel, C.S.; Kemp-Harper, B.K.; et al. Pharmacological inhibition of the NLRP3 inflammasome reduces blood pressure, renal damage, and dysfunction in salt-sensitive hypertension. *Cardiovasc. Res.* **2019**, *115*, 776–787. [CrossRef] [PubMed]

105. Youm, Y.H.; Nguyen, K.Y.; Grant, R.W.; Goldberg, E.L.; Bodogai, M.; Kim, D.; D'Agostino, D.; Planavsky, N.; Lupfer, C.; Kanneganti, T.D.; et al. The ketone metabolite beta-hydroxybutyrate blocks NLRP3 inflammasome-mediated inflammatory disease. *Nat. Med.* **2015**, *21*, 263–269. [CrossRef]
106. Gan, W.; Ren, J.; Li, T.; Lv, S.; Li, C.; Liu, Z.; Yang, M. The SGK1 inhibitor EMD638683, prevents Angiotensin II-induced cardiac inflammation and fibrosis by blocking NLRP3 inflammasome activation. *Biochim. Biophys. Acta Mol. Basis Dis.* **2018**, *1864*, 1–10. [CrossRef]

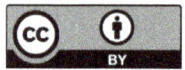

© 2020 by the authors. Licensee MDPI, Basel, Switzerland. This article is an open access article distributed under the terms and conditions of the Creative Commons Attribution (CC BY) license (http://creativecommons.org/licenses/by/4.0/).

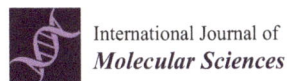

Review

Current Understanding of Autophagy in Pregnancy

Akitoshi Nakashima [1], Sayaka Tsuda [1], Tae Kusabiraki [1], Aiko Aoki [1], Akemi Ushijima [1], Tomoko Shima [1], Shi-Bin Cheng [2], Surendra Sharma [2] and Shigeru Saito [1,*]

[1] Department of Obstetrics and Gynecology, University of Toyama, Toyama 930-0194, Japan; akinaka@med.u-toyama.ac.jp (A.N.); syk3326jp@yahoo.co.jp (S.T.); tae.kusabiraki@gmail.com (T.K.); aikoyuzu8829@yahoo.co.jp (A.A.); au@med.u-toyama.ac.jp (A.U.); shitoko@med.u-toyama.ac.jp (T.S.)

[2] Departments of Pediatrics, Women and Infants Hospital of Rhode Island, Warren Alpert Medical School of Brown University, Providence, RI 02905, USA; shibin_cheng@brown.edu (S.-B.C.); ssharma@wihri.org (S.S.)

* Correspondence: s30saito@med.u-toyama.ac.jp; Tel.: +81-76-434-7357

Received: 12 April 2019; Accepted: 10 May 2019; Published: 11 May 2019

Abstract: Autophagy is an evolutionarily conserved process in eukaryotes to maintain cellular homeostasis under environmental stress. Intracellular control is exerted to produce energy or maintain intracellular protein quality controls. Autophagy plays an important role in embryogenesis, implantation, and maintenance of pregnancy. This role includes supporting extravillous trophoblasts (EVTs) that invade the decidua (endometrium) until the first third of uterine myometrium and migrate along the lumina of spiral arterioles under hypoxic and low-nutrient conditions in early pregnancy. In addition, autophagy inhibition has been linked to poor placentation—a feature of preeclamptic placentas—in a placenta-specific autophagy knockout mouse model. Studies of autophagy in human placentas have revealed controversial results, especially with regard to preeclampsia and gestational diabetes mellitus (GDM). Without precise estimation of autophagy flux, wrong interpretation would lead to fixed tissues. This paper presents a review of the role of autophagy in pregnancy and elaborates on the interpretation of autophagy in human placental tissues.

Keywords: Atg7; autophagy; lysosomes; placenta; preeclampsia; protein aggregation; p62/SQSTM1

1. Introduction

Cellular homeostasis is maintained through protein quality controls that balance synthesis and degradation. Although turnover rate varies in each cellular component, eukaryotic cells degrade proteins using two intracellular degradation systems—the autophagy-lysosomal system and the ubiquitin-proteasome system. Proteasomal degradation selectively recognizes ubiquitinated proteins, which mainly consist of short-lived proteins. Lysosomal-mediated degradation targets long-lived proteins in a complex process [1–3]: cytosolic components, including damaged organelles, are delivered to lysosomes through autophagosomes, while extracellular materials are delivered via endocytosis. Macroautophagy, a non-selective physiological process producing cellular energy, is involved in the delivery of cargo to lysosomes.

There are several types of selective autophagy that behave like a vacuum cleaner in cells [2]. Impaired mitophagy, selective mitochondrial autophagy, has been linked to familial Parkinson's disease [4]. If damaged mitochondria are not eliminated through mitophagy, they accumulate causing oxidative stress, which results in neuron loss. Recently, other targets for selective autophagy have been uncovered: peroxisomes, endoplasmic reticulum (ER), endosomes, lysosomes, lipid droplets, secretory granules, cytoplasmic aggregates, ribosomes, invading pathogens, and viruses [5]. Autophagosomes function in numerous biological processes independent of lysosomal degradation, including phagocytosis, exocytosis, secretion, antigen presentation, and regulation of inflammation [6]. Chaperone-mediated autophagy (CMA), another type of autophagy, directly translocates cytosolic proteins into lysosomes via chaperones. Chaperone-mediated autophagy and macroautophagic activities decline with age [7]. When RUN (RPIP8, UNC-14, NESCA) and a cysteine-rich domain containing beclin1 interacting protein (Rubicon), a negative regulator of autophagy, were suppressed, lifespan was extended and age-related pathologies were reduced [8]. Thus, autophagy is thought to be deeply related to aging. The terms "autophagy" and "macroautophagy" are used interchangeably for the purposes of this paper.

2. The Molecular Mechanism of Autophagy

There are three types of autophagy: macroautophagy, microautophagy, and CMA [2]. Macroautophagy is triggered by a stimulus, such as starvation, hypoxia, mammalian target of rapamycin (mTOR) inhibition, or infection. An isolation membrane derived from the ER-mitochondria contact site, appears in the cytoplasm, elongates, engulfs the target, and closes, forming a vesicle with a double membrane called an autophagosome [9]. Autolysosomes, the autophagosome–lysosome complex, degrade the contents in the inner membrane through lysosomal hydrolases (Figure 1).

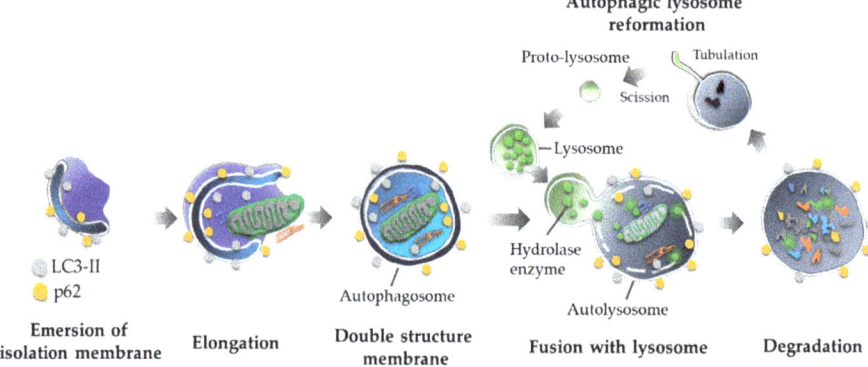

Figure 1. Autophagy cascade. An isolation membrane is merging in cytoplasm via PI3K complex. After elongation of the membrane, the isolation membrane closes and completes the autophagosome, which is formed with double membranes. Finally, the autophagosome forms the autolysosome by fusing with the lysosome and digests the contents the inner membrane. Following with the degradation, autophagy provides matured lysosomes by a recycling of proto-lysosomal membrane components.

Multiple autophagy-related (Atg) proteins intertwine to form autophagosomes after induction. The ULK1 complex, which includes Atg13, Atg101, and FAK family kinase-interacting protein of 200 kDa (FIP200), translocates to the ER regulating class III phosphatidylinositol 3-kinase complex (PI3K), which is involved in the early stage of autophagosome formation. Next, pro-MAP1LC3 (Microtubule associated protein 1 light chain 3) is converted to MAP1LC3-I by Atg4B proteins, a cysteine protease [10], the complex of Atg5-Atg12-Atg16L1, as well as MAP1LC3 (Atg8-homolog)-phosphatidylethanolamine (PE)-conjugate, which play an important role in the elongation and completion, are maturated through Atg7 proteins [2]. Autolysosome formation involves numerous proteins, some of which are common to the endocytic pathway. This process is mediated by Rab GTPases, soluble N-ethylmaleimide-sensitive factor attachment protein receptors (SNAREs), and vacuole protein sorting (HOPS) complexes, which function as a tethering factor for autophagosomal fusion [11]. Conversely, Rubicon blocks the fusion of autophagosomes to lysosomes upon interacting with phosphatidylinositol 3-kinase catalytic subunit type 3 (PIK3C3) [12]. Autophagy substrates are degraded by lysosomal hydrolases dependently of V-type ATPase [13]. Finally, the autophagic lysosome reforms through the reactivation of mTOR, which inhibits autophagy, and produces mature lysosomes by recycling proto-lysosomal membrane components [14].

3. Autophagy in Reproduction

Functions of oocytes, including ovulation, fertilization, and implantation, were not affected by autophagy inhibition in the ovary-specific Beclin1 knockout mouse model [15]. Atg7 was found to protect against ovarian follicle loss in germ cell-specific Atg7 knockout mice [16]. This suggests that Atg proteins are more involved in downstream—rather than upstream—regulation of the ovarian reserve of primordial follicles. Autophagy is not essential for oogenesis or fertilization. Oocytes lacking Atg5, which like Atg7, are involved in autophagosome formation, were fertilized normally in vivo [17]. Although autophagy activation was observed in fertilized oocytes at the two-cell stage, it was not observed in unfertilized oocytes [17]. Autophagy-deficient embryos, derived from Atg5-null oocytes, do not develop beyond the four- and eight-cell stages when fertilized with Atg5-null sperm, but develop normally if fertilized with an Atg5-plus sperm. Transient autophagy activation, which negatively regulates endoplasmic reticulum (ER) stress, increased the blastocyst development rate, trophectoderm cell number, and blastomere survival in bovine embryos [18]. Thus, autophagy seems to aid the development of zygotes (fertilized embryos), by refining excessive maternal factors during early embryonal development in mammals. In most eukaryotic species, the autophagy receptors p62 and gamma-aminobutyric acid receptor-associated protein (GABARAP) eliminate the mitochondria of sperm through mitophagy after fertilization [19]. The sperm mitochondrial proteins are degraded by the ubiquitin-proteasome system, but selective autophagy is partially used in this process. Autophagy activation in blastocysts, which is mediated by 17β-estradiol (E2), may contribute to delayed implantation, because E2-mediated autophagy activation allows dormant blastocysts to survive longer than those not treated with E2 [20]. In addition, progesterone, like E2, activates autophagy via suppression of mTOR in bovine mammary epithelial cells [21].

4. Autophagy in Placentation

The MAP1LC3 protein families: MAP1LC3A, MAP1LC3B, and MAP1LC3C, are expressed in both the labyrinth zone and decidua basalis in mouse models. Expression of MAP1LC3A and MAP1LC3B were higher in the decidua basalis than in the labyrinth layer [22]. Autophagy activation was observed in human EVTs, which invade the maternal decidua basalis at the implantation site, at week 7 of gestation [23]. Autophagy plays an important role in trophoblast functions, including invasion and vascular remodeling in EVTs, for normal placental development [23]. This was confirmed using a mouse model, in which the Atg7 gene, essential for autophagy, was deleted in trophoblast cells, but not fetuses, by a lentiviral vector [24]. The Atg7 knockout placentas were smaller than the wild, suggesting autophagy deficiency mediates poor placentation, a feature of preeclamptic placentas (Figure 2) [24]. The Atg7 knockout placentas were characterized by shallow trophoblast invasion and failure of vascular remodeling. This functional impairment was confirmed by autophagy-deficient human EVT cell lines, which are constructed by stably transfecting Atg4B^{C74A}, an inactive mutant of Atg4B that inhibits autophagic degradation and lipidation of MAP1LC3B paralogs in hypoxia [23,25]. Physiological hypoxia during early pregnancy, with approximately 2% oxygen tension, induces autophagy in primary trophoblasts [23,26]. Although hypoxia inducible factor1α (HIF1α) is required for EVT invasion regardless of oxygen tension; failure of EVT invasion was provoked by hyper-expression of HIF1α by cobalt chloride, and excessive autophagy activation by glucose oxidase in HTR8/SVneo cells, an EVT cell line [27–29]. Thus, physiological hypoxia regulates autophagy by adjusting trophoblasts to cope with harsh conditions during early placentation.

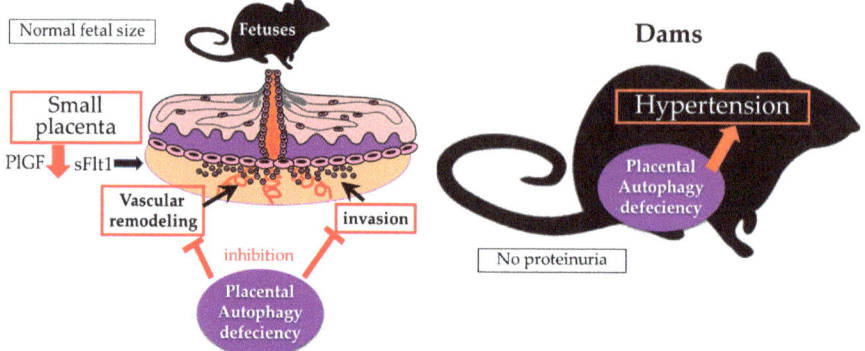

Figure 2. Placental autophagy inhibition inducing gestational hypertension and poor placentation. (Left figure) Trophoblast-invasion and vascular remodeling are fundamental for normal placentation (the black arrows indicate the place of invasion and vascular remodeling). Autophagy deficiency impairs the functions of trophoblasts in the trophoblast-specific Atg7 knockout mouse model, resulting in poor placentation (the red "T" bars indicate the inhibition). PlGF mRNA levels, but not sFlt1 mRNA levels, are decreased in the knockout placentas (the red arrow indicates the decrease, and the black arrow indicates the stable). (Right figure) Also, the dams bearing the knockout placentas showed hypertension, but not proteinuria (the red arrow indicates the induction of hypertension by the placenta).

Trophoblastic stem cells differentiate to syncytiotrophoblasts as well as EVTs. Autophagy regulates the differentiation of invasive trophoblasts via reduction of galectin-4, which is required for normal placental development, as seen in a rat model [30,31]. Autophagy activation is expected during syncytialisation of BeWo cells, a choriocarcinoma cell line [32,33]. During this process, p53 negatively regulates autophagy activation based on high levels of p53 in the nuclei of cytotrophoblasts, but not in syncytiotrophoblasts [33]. However, as these experiments used choriocarcinoma cell lines, this experiment should be replicated using the primary human trophoblast differentiation model [34].

HIF1α is a key factor for EVT invasion. HIF1α expression, induced by hypoxia, was not affected by autophagy suppression in trophoblast cells [23]. Interestingly, CMA partially controls HIF1α expression in lysosomes [35]. Hypoxia stabilizes HIF1α by blocking proteasome-mediated degradation, but HIF1α is degraded via CMA in response to nutrient deprivation, but not hypoxia in the liver of rats [35]. CMA may be important for EVT invasion via modulating HIF1α expression levels, because the placenta, especially in intervillous space, develops under in conditions of hypoxia and low glucose during the first trimester [36,37].

5. Autophagy in Pregnancy-Related Complications

5.1. Preeclampsia or Fetal Growth Restriction (FGR)

It has been reported that the expression of BECN1, involved in autophagosome formation in mammalian placentas, is higher in the presence of FGR without preeclampsia, but not when preeclampsia is present [38,39]. However, BECN1 increase has been reported recently in preeclamptic placentas compared to those in age-matched controls [40]. A substrate of autophagy, p62, is highly expressed in EVT cells in human placental bed biopsies obtained from preeclampsia, suggesting that autophagy inhibition is present in EVTs of preeclamptic placentas. Sera from preeclamptic patients induce hypertension and proteinuria in pregnant interleukin 10 (IL-10) knockout mice, suggesting that factors in blood, including soluble endoglin (sENG) and soluble fms-like tyrosine kinase (sFlt1), induce preeclampsia-like features in mice [41]. The sera from normotensive women, but not from women with preeclampsia, induced autophagy in peripheral blood mononuclear cells [42]. In the sera of preeclamptic women, sENG, which blocks transforming growth factor-β1 (TGF-β1) signals, suppressed invasion and vascular remodeling via autophagy inhibition in EVT cell lines. This effect was reversed by administration of TGF-β [23]. Pregnant women with donor oocytes would be at a greater risk of preeclampsia and gestational hypertension than pregnant women with their own oocytes [43–45]. Accumulation of p62, an indicator of autophagy inhibition, in EVTs was significantly higher in women with donor oocytes, suggesting autophagy inhibition correlates with preeclampsia [46]. Conversely, some reports suggest activation of autophagy in preeclamptic placentas. An electron microscopic study showed autophagic vacuoles in both syncytial layers and endothelium in preeclamptic placentas [40]. An increase in MAP1LC3-II and decrease in p62 were reported in the placentas of women with hypertensive disorder, compared to those in normotensive pregnancies, which indicates autophagy activation [47]. Ceramide overload-induced autophagy impaired placental function in preeclampsia in cooperated with oxidative stress-reduced hydrolase activity [48]. Autophagy is clearly involved in the pathophysiology of preeclampsia, but the effect on preeclamptic placentas remains unclear. As mentioned earlier, it is still impossible to accurately estimate autophagy flux in fixed tissues because autophagy is a dynamic mechanism to maintain homeostasis in cells. A placental autophagy-deficient model is required to solve this problem. Dams bearing Atg7-knockout placentas, which were smaller than wild dams, showed hypertension without proteinuria, suggesting that autophagy deficiency in placentas, but not in maternal bodies, induced gestational hypertension [24]. Autophagy deficient placentas, in which mRNA levels of placental growth factor (PlGF), but not sFlt1, decreased, appear to affect maternal circulation, but not endothelial dysfunction [24]. Atg9a mediates autophagosome formation and is ubiquitous in multiple human organs. Atg9b, a homolog of Atg9a, is found only in the placenta and pituitary gland [49]. The role of autophagy under preeclamptic dams was reported using Atg9a knockout mice mated with heterozygous p57^{Kip2} mice, which develop hypertension and proteinuria in dams [50]. The incidence of fetal death increased in pups with hetero- or homozygous deletion of Atg9a compared to that in the wild type [51]. In addition, the body weights in Atg9a homozygous knockout pups were significantly lower than those in Atg9a heterozygous knockout or wild type pups. Taken together, autophagy protects placental and fetal growth from stress under preeclampsia.

Autophagic vacuoles are more likely to be present in the syncytiotrophoblast layer of human FGR placentas, which indicates autophagy activation [52,53]. Higher expression of BCLN1 in FGR placentas might support this notion [38]. On the other hand, a recent paper reported that the birth weight of fetuses delivered from dams with labyrinth layer-specific Atg7-deleted placentas were significantly lower than the birth weight of dams with normal placentas, indicating that inhibition of autophagy was also related to FGR [54]. In addition, Hirota et al. reported that an autophagy inducer, rapamycin, which is used for preventing preterm birth, did not affect the body weight of pups [55]. There is still some controversy for autophagy status in placentas with FGR between human and mouse.

Protein aggregation caused by autophagy suppression has been reported in several neurodegenerative diseases, including Alzheimer's disease, Parkinson's disease, and Huntington's disease [56,57]. Recently, protein aggregation has been reported in preeclampsia [58]. Transthyretin, a transporter of thyroxine and retinol, and amyloid precursor proteins; which are proteins that accumulate in neurodegenerative diseases are also seen in preeclamptic placentas [59,60]. Furthermore, aggregated amyloid proteins were detected in higher levels in the urine of women with preeclampsia than in healthy pregnant women [59,61]. Thus, autophagy would prevent protein aggregation in trophoblasts. Aggregated proteins might disturb placental development through induction of apoptosis, and cellular senescence. Cellular senescence is known to be triggered by aging or autophagy suppression, in trophoblasts, and results in telomere shortening or dysfunction. This process is seen in early onset preeclampsia and FGR and is related to placental aging that accompanies the pro-inflammatory phenotype [62]. Senescent cells also alter their microenvironment by the secretion of proinflammatory cytokines, chemokines, growth factors, and proteases, collectively known as the senescence-associated secretory phenotype (SASP) [63]. Three pathways have been proposed for cellular senescence with

DNA damage: the p16^{INK4a} pathway, the p53 pathway, and the autophagy-mediated GATA Binding Protein 4 (GATA4) pathway. Increased expression of p53, p21, and p16^{INK4a} proteins has been reported in preeclampsia [64,65]. GATA Binding Protein 4, which is essential for embryonic development, is selectively degraded by p62 [66,67]. Therefore, GATA4 stabilization mediated by autophagy inhibition may contribute to cellular senescence with inflammation in preeclampsia.

5.2. Gestational Diabetes Mellitus (GDM) and Obesity

Gestational diabetes mellitus (GDM) is a type of diabetes that develops during pregnancy and affects 3–30% of pregnant women [68–70]. Gestational diabetes mellitus increases the risk of fetal morbidity and mortality, as well as incidence of preeclampsia in mothers [69]. The role of autophagy in GDM remains controversial. Ji et al. reported that autophagy activation, manifested by increases in MAP1LC3-II and Atg5, and a decrease in p62, was observed in GDM placentas [71]. In addition, high glucose increased autophagy in HTR8/SVneo cells. Although the opposite result has also been reported, which included a decrease in BCLN1, and increases in MAP1LC3-II and p62 [72]. Placentas from obese women with GDM showed downregulation of protein kinase AMP-activated catalytic subunit alpha 2 (PRKAA2, also known as AMPK) and upregulation of mTOR which caused an increase in ribosomal protein S6 kinase B1 (RPS6KB1), suggesting autophagy inhibition in GDM placentas [73]. Muralimanoharan et al. constructed a labyrinth layer-specific Atg7 knockout mouse model on the basis of findings that autophagic activity decreased in the placentas of obese women [54]. Interestingly, weight gain in the offspring of animals with these knockout placentas was significantly greater than that in the wild type counterparts and was accompanied by hyperglycemia. This was thought to be due to greater sensitivity to a high-fat diet. Placental autophagy deficiency in this context supports the developmental origins of health and disease (DOHaD) hypothesis correlating poor fetal nutrition in utero with chronic diseases in adulthood such as obesity and certain cancers [74].

5.3. Preterm Labor

Atg16L1 is essential for forming autophagosomes with the Atg5-Atg12 complex, which is associated with Crohn's disease [75]. Atg16L1-knockout macrophages produced high levels of inflammatory cytokines such as IL-1β and IL-18 via the TIR-domain containing adaptor-inducing interferon-β (TRIF)-dependent signaling pathway, indicating that autophagy suppresses intestinal inflammation [76]. Atg16L1 knockout mice gave birth prematurely in response to lipopolysaccharide (LPS) [32]. Thus, autophagy is involved in resistance to infection by removing inflammasomes to regulate inflammation. Turnover of organelles mediated by selective autophagy would be an important mechanism by which autophagy prevents inflammation [77]. If it does not work properly, accumulation of damaged organelles induces activation of NLRP3 inflammasomes. Uric acid, which increases in preeclampsia, activates inflammasomes via activation of NLRP3 inflammasomes in monocytes [78]. Paradoxically, a treatment of either LPS, a Toll-like receptor (TLR) 4 ligand, or peptidoglycan with poly(I:C), TLR2 and TLR3 ligands, inhibited autophagy via decrease of Atg4c and Atg7 proteins in placentas using inflammation-induced preterm labor models [79]. This might be a consequence of excessive autophagy activation; in other words, autophagic capacity might be exhausted with continuous infection. As for the other type of premature delivery model, in which p53 knockout induced senescence in uterine decidual cells with activation of mTOR signaling, rapamycin treatment, which activates autophagy, reduced preterm birth as well as the incidence of neonatal death [55,80]. Thus, autophagy restoration has a positive effect on premature delivery; mTOR-mediated autophagy inhibition is related with premature delivery. As for spontaneous deliveries at term, little evidence is provided for the role of autophagy in humans. One important caution is given for the study; we have to consider at least the mode of delivery, in which labor pain might affect autophagy status in the placentas, when comparing autophagy status in human placentas [81].

6. Caution When Interpreting Autophagy-Related Experiments

The importance of estimating autophagy is to precisely calculate the velocity of autophagy flow. Estimating autophagy using a single method is impossible, and is more difficult in vivo—and in humans—than in vitro, or in animal models [82,83]. In western blot analyses of cell cultures, the increase in the MAP1LC3-II/actin ratio, sometimes replaced with the MAP1LC3-II/MAP1LC3-I ratio, indicated autophagy activation in response to lysosomal inhibitors, such as bafilomycin A1 or chloroquine, compared with cell cultures without inhibitors. Thus, the dynamics of autophagy flux are comparable to autophagy inhibitors in living cells. Autophagy cannot be precisely estimated from "human" fixed tissues. Some studies, however, reported increases of MAP1LC3 mRNA and protein as an indicator of autophagic activity in placental tissues, but the increase does not imply activation of autophagy in other tissues [82,83]. Though numbers of MAP1LC3 puncta in immunofluorescence analysis are equal to the number of autophagosomes, the increase of MAP1LC3 puncta could be the result of the fusion of an autophagosome and lysosome being blocked, as well as autophagy activation. To precisely estimate autophagy in an organ or tissue, Kaizuka et al. developed a new method using MAP1LC3 fluorescent probes, in which one is degradative and the other is not [84]. However, autophagy activation still remains difficult to measure in human tissues. In fixed tissues, the number of autophagosomes and autolysosomes should be evaluated. A step in the formation of an autolysosome, co-localization of MAP1LC3 dots, and lysosomal-associated membrane protein 1 (LAMP1), which are composed of autophagosomes and lysosomes, can be useful in confirming the formation of the autolysosome. The ratio of autolysosomes to autophagosomes could be used to estimate autophagy in fixed tissues. A marked accumulation of p62, which was seen in liver-specific autophagy-deficient mice, would be useful as well [85]. This is because the accumulation of p62 in cytoplasmic inclusion bodies impair cellular viability [86]. Accumulation of p62 was seen in some trophoblast cell lines, in which autophagy was suppressed by an Atg4B^{C74A} mutation, and EVTs in biopsies taken from the placental bed of women with preeclampsia [23]. This would be a marker of autophagy inhibition in placental tissues. Rubicon inhibited autophagic flux, which led to the accumulation of p62 in a mouse model. Increased expression of Rubicon in nonalcoholic fatty liver disease would increase autophagy inhibition and lead to complications [87]. Taken together; the ratio of autolysosomes to autophagosomes, p62 accumulation, and Rubicon may allow an estimation of autophagy in placental tissues.

7. Conclusions

Autophagy mediates a variety of life process, including cancer development, immune response, and aging pathophysiology [88]. Autophagy decreases with age, which coincides with the increases in neurodegenerative diseases we observe in the elderly. Because aging is an independent risk factor for preeclampsia, these concepts may be linked. The decrease of autophagic activity with aging, which results in susceptibility to endotoxin-induced inflammation, and the inflammation related to preeclampsia, might gradually increase risk for systemic inflammation in older pregnant women [89]. This suggests pharmacological manipulation of autophagy may treat preeclampsia. In addition, autophagy activation might prevent premature labor not caused by bacterial infection. However, these theories are untested, so it remains unclear whether autophagy activation is favorable or unfavorable for preeclampsia, FGR, and other pregnancy-related diseases. To solve this question, the placental characteristics that regulate autophagy may need to be segmentalized: age, body mass index, severity, time of onset, genetic background, microvesicles, immune status, and origin of eggs. Finally, technical advances are needed to enable precise measurement of autophagy before it can be manipulated in clinical research.

Funding: The series of this study was supported by AMED-CREST from the Japan Agency for Medical Research and Development, AMED 16gk0110018h0001, grants from the Kanzawa Medical Research Foundation, Tamura Science and Technology Foundation, Yamaguchi Endocrine Research Foundation, First Bank of Toyama, Toyama University Hospital Grant, 040200-59200003502, and JSPS KAKENHI Grant Numbers JP17K11221 and JP19K09750.

Conflicts of Interest: The authors declare no conflict of interests. The funders had no role in the design of the study; in the collection, analyses, or interpretation of data; in the writing of the manuscript, or in the decision to publish the results.

Abbreviations

Atg	Autophagy-related
BECN1	Beclin 1
CMA	Chaperone-mediated autophagy
DOHaD	Developmental origins of health and disease
ER	Endoplasmic reticulum
E2	17β-estradiol
EVTs	Extravillous trophoblasts
FIP200	FAK family kinase-interacting protein of 200 kDa
FGR	Fetal growth restriction
GABARAP	Gamma-aminobutyric acid receptor-associated protein
GATA4	GATA binding protein 4Gestational diabetes mellitus
GDM	Gestational diabetes mellitus
HIF1α	Hypoxia inducible factor-1α
HOPS	Homotypic fusion and vacuole protein sorting
LAMP1	Lysosomal-associated membrane protein 1
LPS	Lipopolysaccharide
MAP1LC3	Microtubule associated protein 1 light chain 3
mTOR	Mammalian target of rapamycin
NLRP3	NLR family pyrin domain containing 3
PIK3C3	Phosphatidylinositol 3-kinase catalytic subunit type 3
PI3K	Class III phosphatidylinositol 3-kinase complex
PlGF	Placental growth factor
PRKAA2	Protein kinase AMP-activated catalytic subunit alpha 2
RPS6KB1	Ribosomal protein S6 kinase B1
Rubicon	RUN and cysteine-rich domain containing beclin1 interacting protein
SASP	Senescence-associated secretory phenotype
TGF-β	Transforming growth factor-β
TRIF	TIR-domain-containing adapter-inducing interferon-β
sENG	Soluble endoglin
sFlt1	Soluble Fms-like tyrosine kinase
SNAREs	Soluble N-ethylmaleimidesensitive factor attachment protein receptors
TLR	Toll-like receptor

References

1. Klionsky, D.J.; Emr, S.D. Autophagy as a regulated pathway of cellular degradation. *Science* **2000**, *290*, 1717–1721. [CrossRef] [PubMed]
2. Mizushima, N.; Komatsu, M. Autophagy: Renovation of cells and tissues. *Cell* **2011**, *147*, 728–741. [CrossRef] [PubMed]
3. Mizushima, N.; Ohsumi, Y.; Yoshimori, T. Autophagosome formation in mammalian cells. *Cell Struct. Funct.* **2002**, *27*, 421–429. [CrossRef]
4. Youle, R.J.; Narendra, D.P. Mechanisms of mitophagy. *Nat. Rev. Mol. Cell Biol.* **2011**, *12*, 9–14. [CrossRef] [PubMed]
5. Reggiori, F.; Komatsu, M.; Finley, K.; Simonsen, A. Autophagy: More than a nonselective pathway. *Int. J. Cell Biol.* **2012**, *2012*, 219625. [CrossRef]
6. Boya, P.; Reggiori, F.; Codogno, P. Emerging regulation and functions of autophagy. *Nat. Cell Biol.* **2013**, *15*, 713–720. [CrossRef]
7. Cuervo, A.M.; Dice, J.F. Age-related decline in chaperone-mediated autophagy. *J. Biol. Chem.* **2000**, *275*, 31505–31513. [CrossRef]

8. Nakamura, S.; Oba, M.; Suzuki, M.; Takahashi, A.; Yamamuro, T.; Fujiwara, M.; Ikenaka, K.; Minami, S.; Tabata, N.; Yamamoto, K.; et al. Suppression of autophagic activity by Rubicon is a signature of aging. *Nat. Commun.* **2019**, *10*, 847. [CrossRef]
9. Hamasaki, M.; Furuta, N.; Matsuda, A.; Nezu, A.; Yamamoto, A.; Fujita, N.; Oomori, H.; Noda, T.; Haraguchi, T.; Hiraoka, Y.; et al. Autophagosomes form at ER-mitochondria contact sites. *Nature* **2013**, *495*, 389–393. [CrossRef]
10. Marino, G.; Uria, J.A.; Puente, X.S.; Quesada, V.; Bordallo, J.; Lopez-Otin, C. Human autophagins, a family of cysteine proteinases potentially implicated in cell degradation by autophagy. *J. Biol. Chem.* **2003**, *278*, 3671–3678. [CrossRef]
11. Nakamura, S.; Yoshimori, T. New insights into autophagosome-lysosome fusion. *J. Cell Sci.* **2017**, *130*, 1209–1216. [CrossRef]
12. Matsunaga, K.; Saitoh, T.; Tabata, K.; Omori, H.; Satoh, T.; Kurotori, N.; Maejima, I.; Shirahama-Noda, K.; Ichimura, T.; Isobe, T.; et al. Two Beclin 1-binding proteins, Atg14L and Rubicon, reciprocally regulate autophagy at different stages. *Nat. Cell Biol.* **2009**, *11*, 385–396. [CrossRef]
13. Mindell, J.A. Lysosomal acidification mechanisms. *Annu. Rev. Physiol.* **2012**, *74*, 69–86. [CrossRef]
14. Yu, L.; McPhee, C.K.; Zheng, L.; Mardones, G.A.; Rong, Y.; Peng, J.; Mi, N.; Zhao, Y.; Liu, Z.; Wan, F.; et al. Termination of autophagy and reformation of lysosomes regulated by mTOR. *Nature* **2010**, *465*, 942–946. [CrossRef] [PubMed]
15. Gawriluk, T.R.; Ko, C.; Hong, X.; Christenson, L.K.; Rucker, E.B., 3rd. Beclin-1 deficiency in the murine ovary results in the reduction of progesterone production to promote preterm labor. *Proc. Natl. Acad. Sci. USA* **2014**, *111*, E4194–E4203. [CrossRef] [PubMed]
16. Song, Z.H.; Yu, H.Y.; Wang, P.; Mao, G.K.; Liu, W.X.; Li, M.N.; Wang, H.N.; Shang, Y.L.; Liu, C.; Xu, Z.L.; et al. Germ cell-specific Atg7 knockout results in primary ovarian insufficiency in female mice. *Cell Death. Dis.* **2015**, *6*, e1589. [CrossRef] [PubMed]
17. Tsukamoto, S.; Kuma, A.; Murakami, M.; Kishi, C.; Yamamoto, A.; Mizushima, N. Autophagy is essential for preimplantation development of mouse embryos. *Science* **2008**, *321*, 117–120. [CrossRef]
18. Song, B.S.; Yoon, S.B.; Kim, J.S.; Sim, B.W.; Kim, Y.H.; Cha, J.J.; Choi, S.A.; Min, H.K.; Lee, Y.; Huh, J.W.; et al. Induction of autophagy promotes preattachment development of bovine embryos by reducing endoplasmic reticulum stress. *Biol. Reprod.* **2012**, *87*, 8, 1–11. [CrossRef] [PubMed]
19. Song, W.H.; Yi, Y.J.; Sutovsky, M.; Meyers, S.; Sutovsky, P. Autophagy and ubiquitin-proteasome system contribute to sperm mitophagy after mammalian fertilization. *Proc. Natl. Acad. Sci. USA* **2016**, *113*, E5261–E5270. [CrossRef]
20. Lee, J.E.; Oh, H.A.; Song, H.; Jun, J.H.; Roh, C.R.; Xie, H.; Dey, S.K.; Lim, H.J. Autophagy regulates embryonic survival during delayed implantation. *Endocrinology* **2011**, *152*, 2067–2075. [CrossRef]
21. Sobolewska, A.; Gajewska, M.; Zarzynska, J.; Gajkowska, B.; Motyl, T. IGF-I, EGF, and sex steroids regulate autophagy in bovine mammary epithelial cells via the mTOR pathway. *Eur. J. Cell Biol.* **2009**, *88*, 117–130. [CrossRef] [PubMed]
22. Hiyama, M.; Kusakabe, K.T.; Takeshita, A.; Sugi, S.; Kuniyoshi, N.; Imai, H.; Kano, K.; Kiso, Y. Nutrient starvation affects expression of LC3 family at the feto-maternal interface during murine placentation. *J. Vet. Med. Sci.* **2015**, *77*, 305–311. [CrossRef] [PubMed]
23. Nakashima, A.; Yamanaka-Tatematsu, M.; Fujita, N.; Koizumi, K.; Shima, T.; Yoshida, T.; Nikaido, T.; Okamoto, A.; Yoshimori, T.; Saito, S. Impaired autophagy by soluble endoglin, under physiological hypoxia in early pregnant period, is involved in poor placentation in preeclampsia. *Autophagy* **2013**, *9*, 303–316. [CrossRef] [PubMed]
24. Aoki, A.; Nakashima, A.; Kusabiraki, T.; Ono, Y.; Yoshino, O.; Muto, M.; Kumasawa, K.; Yoshimori, T.; Ikawa, M.; Saito, S. Trophoblast-Specific Conditional Atg7 Knockout Mice Develop Gestational Hypertension. *Am. J. Pathol.* **2018**, *188*, 2474–2486. [CrossRef]
25. Fujita, N.; Noda, T.; Yoshimori, T. Atg4B(C74A) hampers autophagosome closure: A useful protein for inhibiting autophagy. *Autophagy* **2009**, *5*, 88–89. [CrossRef] [PubMed]
26. Chen, B.; Longtine, M.S.; Nelson, D.M. Hypoxia induces autophagy in primary human trophoblasts. *Endocrinology* **2012**, *153*, 4946–4954. [CrossRef] [PubMed]
27. Choi, J.H.; Lee, H.J.; Yang, T.H.; Kim, G.J. Effects of hypoxia inducible factors-1alpha on autophagy and invasion of trophoblasts. *Clin. Exp. Reprod. Med.* **2012**, *39*, 73–80. [CrossRef] [PubMed]

28. Gao, L.; Qi, H.B.; Kamana, K.C.; Zhang, X.M.; Zhang, H.; Baker, P.N. Excessive autophagy induces the failure of trophoblast invasion and vasculature: Possible relevance to the pathogenesis of preeclampsia. *J. Hypertens* **2015**, *33*, 106–117. [CrossRef] [PubMed]
29. Yamanaka-Tatematsu, M.; Nakashima, A.; Fujita, N.; Shima, T.; Yoshimori, T.; Saito, S. Autophagy induced by HIF1alpha overexpression supports trophoblast invasion by supplying cellular energy. *PLoS ONE* **2013**, *8*, e76605. [CrossRef]
30. Arikawa, T.; Liao, S.; Shimada, H.; Inoue, T.; Sakata-Haga, H.; Nakamura, T.; Hatta, T.; Shoji, H. Galectin-4 expression is down-regulated in response to autophagy during differentiation of rat trophoblast cells. *Sci. Rep.* **2016**, *6*, 32248. [CrossRef]
31. Arikawa, T.; Simamura, E.; Shimada, H.; Nishi, N.; Tatsuno, T.; Ishigaki, Y.; Tomosugi, N.; Yamashiro, C.; Hata, T.; Takegami, T.; et al. Expression pattern of Galectin 4 in rat placentation. *Placenta* **2012**, *33*, 885–887. [CrossRef]
32. Cao, B.; Macones, C.; Mysorekar, I.U. ATG16L1 governs placental infection risk and preterm birth in mice and women. *JCI Insight* **2016**, *1*, e86654. [CrossRef]
33. Gauster, M.; Maninger, S.; Siwetz, M.; Deutsch, A.; El-Heliebi, A.; Kolb-Lenz, D.; Hiden, U.; Desoye, G.; Herse, F.; Prokesch, A. Downregulation of p53 drives autophagy during human trophoblast differentiation. *Cell Mol. Life Sci.* **2018**, *75*, 1839–1855. [CrossRef] [PubMed]
34. Motomura, K.; Okada, N.; Morita, H.; Hara, M.; Tamari, M.; Orimo, K.; Matsuda, G.; Imadome, K.I.; Matsuda, A.; Nagamatsu, T.; et al. A Rho-associated coiled-coil containing kinases (ROCK) inhibitor, Y-27632, enhances adhesion, viability and differentiation of human term placenta-derived trophoblasts in vitro. *PLoS ONE* **2017**, *12*, e0177994. [CrossRef]
35. Ferreira, J.V.; Fofo, H.; Bejarano, E.; Bento, C.F.; Ramalho, J.S.; Girao, H.; Pereira, P. STUB1/CHIP is required for HIF1A degradation by chaperone-mediated autophagy. *Autophagy* **2013**, *9*, 1349–1366. [CrossRef] [PubMed]
36. Jauniaux, E.; Hempstock, J.; Teng, C.; Battaglia, F.C.; Burton, G.J. Polyol concentrations in the fluid compartments of the human conceptus during the first trimester of pregnancy: Maintenance of redox potential in a low oxygen environment. *J. Clin. Endocrinol. Metab.* **2005**, *90*, 1171–1175. [CrossRef] [PubMed]
37. Jauniaux, E.; Watson, A.; Burton, G. Evaluation of respiratory gases and acid-base gradients in human fetal fluids and uteroplacental tissue between 7 and 16 weeks' gestation. *Am. J. Obstet. Gynecol.* **2001**, *184*, 998–1003. [CrossRef]
38. Hung, T.H.; Chen, S.F.; Lo, L.M.; Li, M.J.; Yeh, Y.L.; Hsieh, T.T. Increased autophagy in placentas of intrauterine growth-restricted pregnancies. *PLoS ONE* **2012**, *7*, e40957. [CrossRef] [PubMed]
39. Oh, S.Y.; Choi, S.J.; Kim, K.H.; Cho, E.Y.; Kim, J.H.; Roh, C.R. Autophagy-related proteins, LC3 and Beclin-1, in placentas from pregnancies complicated by preeclampsia. *Reprod. Sci.* **2008**, *15*, 912–920. [CrossRef] [PubMed]
40. Kalkat, M.; Garcia, J.; Ebrahimi, J.; Melland-Smith, M.; Todros, T.; Post, M.; Caniggia, I. Placental autophagy regulation by the BOK-MCL1 rheostat. *Autophagy* **2013**, *9*, 2140–2153. [CrossRef]
41. Kalkunte, S.; Boij, R.; Norris, W.; Friedman, J.; Lai, Z.; Kurtis, J.; Lim, K.H.; Padbury, J.F.; Matthiesen, L.; Sharma, S. Sera from preeclampsia patients elicit symptoms of human disease in mice and provide a basis for an in vitro predictive assay. *Am. J. Pathol.* **2010**, *177*, 2387–2398. [CrossRef]
42. Kanninen, T.T.; Jayaram, A.; Jaffe Lifshitz, S.; Witkin, S.S. Altered autophagy induction by sera from pregnant women with pre-eclampsia: A case-control study. *BJOG* **2014**, *121*, 958–964. [CrossRef]
43. Keegan, D.A.; Krey, L.C.; Chang, H.C.; Noyes, N. Increased risk of pregnancy-induced hypertension in young recipients of donated oocytes. *Fertil. Steril.* **2007**, *87*, 776–781. [CrossRef] [PubMed]
44. Salha, O.; Sharma, V.; Dada, T.; Nugent, D.; Rutherford, A.J.; Tomlinson, A.J.; Philips, S.; Allgar, V.; Walker, J.J. The influence of donated gametes on the incidence of hypertensive disorders of pregnancy. *Hum. Reprod.* **1999**, *14*, 2268–2273. [CrossRef]
45. Wiggins, D.A.; Main, E. Outcomes of pregnancies achieved by donor egg in vitro fertilization–a comparison with standard in vitro fertilization pregnancies. *Am. J. Obstet. Gynecol.* **2005**, *192*, 2002–2006. [CrossRef] [PubMed]
46. Nakabayashi, Y.; Nakashima, A.; Yoshino, O.; Shima, T.; Shiozaki, A.; Adachi, T.; Nakabayashi, M.; Okai, T.; Kushima, M.; Saito, S. Impairment of the accumulation of decidual T cells, NK cells, and monocytes, and the poor vascular remodeling of spiral arteries, were observed in oocyte donation cases, regardless of the presence or absence of preeclampsia. *J. Reprod. Immunol.* **2016**, *114*, 65–74. [CrossRef]

47. Akaishi, R.; Yamada, T.; Nakabayashi, K.; Nishihara, H.; Furuta, I.; Kojima, T.; Morikawa, M.; Fujita, N.; Minakami, H. Autophagy in the placenta of women with hypertensive disorders in pregnancy. *Placenta* **2014**, *35*, 974–980. [CrossRef] [PubMed]
48. Melland-Smith, M.; Ermini, L.; Chauvin, S.; Craig-Barnes, H.; Tagliaferro, A.; Todros, T.; Post, M.; Caniggia, I. Disruption of sphingolipid metabolism augments ceramide-induced autophagy in preeclampsia. *Autophagy* **2015**, *11*, 653–669. [CrossRef]
49. Yamada, T.; Carson, A.R.; Caniggia, I.; Umebayashi, K.; Yoshimori, T.; Nakabayashi, K.; Scherer, S.W. Endothelial nitric-oxide synthase antisense (NOS3AS) gene encodes an autophagy-related protein (APG9-like2) highly expressed in trophoblast. *J. Biol. Chem.* **2005**, *280*, 18283–18290. [CrossRef]
50. Kanayama, N.; Takahashi, K.; Matsuura, T.; Sugimura, M.; Kobayashi, T.; Moniwa, N.; Tomita, M.; Nakayama, K. Deficiency in p57Kip2 expression induces preeclampsia-like symptoms in mice. *Mol. Hum. Reprod.* **2002**, *8*, 1129–1135. [CrossRef]
51. Kojima, T.; Yamada, T.; Akaishi, R.; Furuta, I.; Saitoh, T.; Nakabayashi, K.; Nakayama, K.I.; Nakayama, K.; Akira, S.; Minakami, H. Role of the Atg9a gene in intrauterine growth and survival of fetal mice. *Reprod. Biol.* **2015**, *15*, 131–138. [CrossRef] [PubMed]
52. Curtis, S.; Jones, C.J.; Garrod, A.; Hulme, C.H.; Heazell, A.E. Identification of autophagic vacuoles and regulators of autophagy in villous trophoblast from normal term pregnancies and in fetal growth restriction. *J. Matern. Fetal. Neonatal. Med.* **2013**, *26*, 339–346. [CrossRef]
53. Hung, T.H.; Hsieh, T.T.; Chen, S.F.; Li, M.J.; Yeh, Y.L. Autophagy in the human placenta throughout gestation. *PLoS ONE* **2013**, *8*, e83475. [CrossRef] [PubMed]
54. Muralimanoharan, S.; Gao, X.; Weintraub, S.; Myatt, L.; Maloyan, A. Sexual dimorphism in activation of placental autophagy in obese women with evidence for fetal programming from a placenta-specific mouse model. *Autophagy* **2016**, *12*, 752–769. [CrossRef] [PubMed]
55. Hirota, Y.; Cha, J.; Yoshie, M.; Daikoku, T.; Dey, S.K. Heightened uterine mammalian target of rapamycin complex 1 (mTORC1) signaling provokes preterm birth in mice. *Proc. Natl. Acad. Sci. USA* **2011**, *108*, 18073–18078. [CrossRef] [PubMed]
56. Nixon, R.A. The role of autophagy in neurodegenerative disease. *Nat. Med.* **2013**, *19*, 983–997. [CrossRef]
57. Soto, C. Unfolding the role of protein misfolding in neurodegenerative diseases. *Nat. Rev. Neurosci.* **2003**, *4*, 49–60. [CrossRef]
58. Cheng, S.B.; Nakashima, A.; Sharma, S. Understanding Pre-Eclampsia Using Alzheimer's Etiology: An Intriguing Viewpoint. *Am. J. Reprod. Immunol.* **2016**, *75*, 372–381. [CrossRef]
59. Buhimschi, I.A.; Nayeri, U.A.; Zhao, G.; Shook, L.L.; Pensalfini, A.; Funai, E.F.; Bernstein, I.M.; Glabe, C.G.; Buhimschi, C.S. Protein misfolding, congophilia, oligomerization, and defective amyloid processing in preeclampsia. *Sci. Transl. Med.* **2014**, *6*, 245ra92. [CrossRef]
60. Kalkunte, S.S.; Neubeck, S.; Norris, W.E.; Cheng, S.B.; Kostadinov, S.; Vu Hoang, D.; Ahmed, A.; von Eggeling, F.; Shaikh, Z.; Padbury, J.; et al. Transthyretin is dysregulated in preeclampsia, and its native form prevents the onset of disease in a preclinical mouse model. *Am. J. Pathol.* **2013**, *183*, 1425–1436. [CrossRef]
61. McCarthy, F.P.; Adetoba, A.; Gill, C.; Bramham, K.; Bertolaccini, M.; Burton, G.J.; Girardi, G.; Seed, P.T.; Poston, L.; Chappell, L.C. Urinary congophilia in women with hypertensive disorders of pregnancy and preexisting proteinuria or hypertension. *Am. J. Obstet. Gynecol.* **2016**, *215*, 464.e1–464.e7. [CrossRef]
62. Cox, L.S.; Redman, C. The role of cellular senescence in ageing of the placenta. *Placenta* **2017**, *52*, 139–145. [CrossRef]
63. Coppe, J.P.; Patil, C.K.; Rodier, F.; Sun, Y.; Munoz, D.P.; Goldstein, J.; Nelson, P.S.; Desprez, P.Y.; Campisi, J. Senescence-associated secretory phenotypes reveal cell-nonautonomous functions of oncogenic RAS and the p53 tumor suppressor. *PLoS Biol.* **2008**, *6*, 2853–2868. [CrossRef]
64. Nuzzo, A.M.; Giuffrida, D.; Masturzo, B.; Mele, P.; Piccoli, E.; Eva, C.; Todros, T.; Rolfo, A. Altered expression of G1/S phase cell cycle regulators in placental mesenchymal stromal cells derived from preeclamptic pregnancies with fetal-placental compromise. *Cell Cycle* **2017**, *16*, 200–212. [CrossRef]
65. Sharp, A.N.; Heazell, A.E.; Baczyk, D.; Dunk, C.E.; Lacey, H.A.; Jones, C.J.; Perkins, J.E.; Kingdom, J.C.; Baker, P.N.; Crocker, I.P. Preeclampsia is associated with alterations in the p53-pathway in villous trophoblast. *PLoS ONE* **2014**, *9*, e87621. [CrossRef]

66. Kang, C.; Xu, Q.; Martin, T.D.; Li, M.Z.; Demaria, M.; Aron, L.; Lu, T.; Yankner, B.A.; Campisi, J.; Elledge, S.J. The DNA damage response induces inflammation and senescence by inhibiting autophagy of GATA4. *Science* **2015**, *349*, aaa5612. [CrossRef] [PubMed]
67. Lentjes, M.H.; Niessen, H.E.; Akiyama, Y.; de Bruine, A.P.; Melotte, V.; van Engeland, M. The emerging role of GATA transcription factors in development and disease. *Expert Rev. Mol. Med.* **2016**, *18*, e3. [CrossRef]
68. American Diabetes, A. Gestational diabetes mellitus. *Diabetes Care* **2000**, *23*, S77–S79.
69. American Diabetes, A. 15. Diabetes Advocacy: Standards of Medical Care in Diabetes-2018. *Diabetes Care* **2018**, *41*, S152–S153. [CrossRef]
70. American Diabetes, A. Standards of Medical Care in Diabetes-2018 Abridged for Primary Care Providers. *Clin. Diabetes* **2018**, *36*, 14–37.
71. Ji, L.; Chen, Z.; Xu, Y.; Xiong, G.; Liu, R.; Wu, C.; Hu, H.; Wang, L. Systematic Characterization of Autophagy in Gestational Diabetes Mellitus. *Endocrinology* **2017**, *158*, 2522–2532. [CrossRef] [PubMed]
72. Avagliano, L.; Massa, V.; Terraneo, L.; Samaja, M.; Doi, P.; Bulfamante, G.P.; Marconi, A.M. Gestational diabetes affects fetal autophagy. *Placenta* **2017**, *55*, 90–93. [CrossRef]
73. Martino, J.; Sebert, S.; Segura, M.T.; Garcia-Valdes, L.; Florido, J.; Padilla, M.C.; Marcos, A.; Rueda, R.; McArdle, H.J.; Budge, H.; et al. Maternal Body Weight and Gestational Diabetes Differentially Influence Placental and Pregnancy Outcomes. *J. Clin. Endocrinol. Metab.* **2016**, *101*, 59–68. [CrossRef] [PubMed]
74. Haugen, A.C.; Schug, T.T.; Collman, G.; Heindel, J.J. Evolution of DOHaD: The impact of environmental health sciences. *J. Dev. Orig. Health Dis.* **2015**, *6*, 55–64. [CrossRef]
75. Roberts, R.L.; Gearry, R.B.; Hollis-Moffatt, J.E.; Miller, A.L.; Reid, J.; Abkevich, V.; Timms, K.M.; Gutin, A.; Lanchbury, J.S.; Merriman, T.R.; et al. IL23R R381Q and ATG16L1 T300A are strongly associated with Crohn's disease in a study of New Zealand Caucasians with inflammatory bowel disease. *Am. J. Gastroenterol.* **2007**, *102*, 2754–2761. [CrossRef]
76. Saitoh, T.; Akira, S. Regulation of inflammasomes by autophagy. *J. Allergy Clin. Immunol.* **2016**, *138*, 28–36. [CrossRef] [PubMed]
77. Shi, C.S.; Shenderov, K.; Huang, N.N.; Kabat, J.; Abu-Asab, M.; Fitzgerald, K.A.; Sher, A.; Kehrl, J.H. Activation of autophagy by inflammatory signals limits IL-1beta production by targeting ubiquitinated inflammasomes for destruction. *Nat. Immunol.* **2012**, *13*, 255–263. [CrossRef] [PubMed]
78. Matias, M.L.; Romao, M.; Weel, I.C.; Ribeiro, V.R.; Nunes, P.R.; Borges, V.T.; Araujo, J.P., Jr.; Peracoli, J.C.; de Oliveira, L.; Peracoli, M.T. Endogenous and Uric Acid-Induced Activation of NLRP3 Inflammasome in Pregnant Women with Preeclampsia. *PLoS ONE* **2015**, *10*, e0129095. [CrossRef] [PubMed]
79. Agrawal, V.; Jaiswal, M.K.; Mallers, T.; Katara, G.K.; Gilman-Sachs, A.; Beaman, K.D.; Hirsch, E. Altered autophagic flux enhances inflammatory responses during inflammation-induced preterm labor. *Sci. Rep.* **2015**, *5*, 9410. [CrossRef]
80. Hirota, Y.; Daikoku, T.; Tranguch, S.; Xie, H.; Bradshaw, H.B.; Dey, S.K. Uterine-specific p53 deficiency confers premature uterine senescence and promotes preterm birth in mice. *J. Clin. Investig.* **2010**, *120*, 803–815. [CrossRef] [PubMed]
81. Oh, S.Y.; Roh, C.R. Autophagy in the placenta. *Obstet. Gynecol. Sci.* **2017**, *60*, 241–259. [CrossRef] [PubMed]
82. Klionsky, D.J.; Cuervo, A.M.; Seglen, P.O. Methods for monitoring autophagy from yeast to human. *Autophagy* **2007**, *3*, 181–206. [CrossRef]
83. Mizushima, N.; Yoshimori, T.; Levine, B. Methods in mammalian autophagy research. *Cell* **2010**, *140*, 313–326. [CrossRef] [PubMed]
84. Kaizuka, T.; Morishita, H.; Hama, Y.; Tsukamoto, S.; Matsui, T.; Toyota, Y.; Kodama, A.; Ishihara, T.; Mizushima, T.; Mizushima, N. An Autophagic Flux Probe that Releases an Internal Control. *Mol. Cell* **2016**, *64*, 835–849. [CrossRef] [PubMed]
85. Inami, Y.; Waguri, S.; Sakamoto, A.; Kouno, T.; Nakada, K.; Hino, O.; Watanabe, S.; Ando, J.; Iwadate, M.; Yamamoto, M.; et al. Persistent activation of Nrf2 through p62 in hepatocellular carcinoma cells. *J. Cell Biol.* **2011**, *193*, 275–284. [CrossRef] [PubMed]
86. Komatsu, M.; Waguri, S.; Koike, M.; Sou, Y.S.; Ueno, T.; Hara, T.; Mizushima, N.; Iwata, J.; Ezaki, J.; Murata, S.; et al. Homeostatic levels of p62 control cytoplasmic inclusion body formation in autophagy-deficient mice. *Cell* **2007**, *131*, 1149–1163. [CrossRef] [PubMed]

87. Tanaka, S.; Hikita, H.; Tatsumi, T.; Sakamori, R.; Nozaki, Y.; Sakane, S.; Shiode, Y.; Nakabori, T.; Saito, Y.; Hiramatsu, N.; et al. Rubicon inhibits autophagy and accelerates hepatocyte apoptosis and lipid accumulation in nonalcoholic fatty liver disease in mice. *Hepatology* **2016**, *64*, 1994–2014. [CrossRef]
88. Kroemer, G. Autophagy: A druggable process that is deregulated in aging and human disease. *J. Clin. Investig.* **2015**, *125*, 1–4. [CrossRef]
89. Saitoh, T.; Fujita, N.; Jang, M.H.; Uematsu, S.; Yang, B.G.; Satoh, T.; Omori, H.; Noda, T.; Yamamoto, N.; Komatsu, M.; et al. Loss of the autophagy protein Atg16L1 enhances endotoxin-induced IL-1beta production. *Nature* **2008**, *456*, 264–268. [CrossRef] [PubMed]

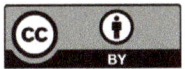

© 2019 by the authors. Licensee MDPI, Basel, Switzerland. This article is an open access article distributed under the terms and conditions of the Creative Commons Attribution (CC BY) license (http://creativecommons.org/licenses/by/4.0/).

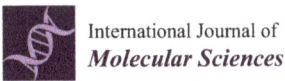

Review

Role of the Monocyte–Macrophage System in Normal Pregnancy and Preeclampsia

Polina Vishnyakova [1,*,†], **Andrey Elchaninov** [1,2,†], **Timur Fatkhudinov** [2,3] and **Gennady Sukhikh** [1]

1. National Medical Research Center for Obstetrics, Gynecology and Perinatology Named after Academician V.I. Kulakov of Ministry of Healthcare of Russian Federation, 4 Oparina Street, 117997 Moscow, Russia
2. Peoples' Friendship University of Russia, 6 Miklukho-Maklaya Street, 117198 Moscow, Russia
3. Scientific Research Institute of Human Morphology, 3 Tsurupa Street, 117418 Moscow, Russia
* Correspondence: vpa2002@mail.ru
† These authors contributed equally to this work.

Received: 12 June 2019; Accepted: 26 July 2019; Published: 28 July 2019

Abstract: The proper functioning of the monocyte–macrophage system, an important unit of innate immunity, ensures the normal course of pregnancy. In this review, we present the current data on the origin of the monocyte–macrophage system and its functioning in the female reproductive system during the ovarian cycle, and over the course of both normal and complicated pregnancy. Preeclampsia is a crucial gestation disorder characterized by pronounced inflammation in the maternal body that affects the work of the monocyte–macrophage system. The effects of inflammation at preeclampsia manifest in changes in monocyte counts and their subset composition, and changes in placental macrophage counts and their polarization. Here we summarize the recent data on this issue for both the maternal organism and the fetus. The influence of estrogen on macrophages and their altered levels in preeclampsia are also discussed.

Keywords: preeclampsia; monocyte; macrophage; placenta; decidua; inflammation

1. Introduction

The prevalence, main symptoms, and classification of preeclampsia (PE) are well established and can be found in every article devoted to this multisystem pregnancy complication. Hundreds of studies devoted to the cell and animal models of PE, as well as biological samples from patients with PE are published every year. However, the scientific community is still wondering what are the main causes of PE and is it possible to predict and prevent the development of this widespread pregnancy disorder?

It is now clear that PE is a multifactorial syndrome, but not an isolated disease. PE occurs in the second half of pregnancy (after the 20th week) and is characterized by arterial hypertension (depending on the severity of PE) in combination with proteinuria (≥ 0.3 g/L in daily urine) and/or manifestations of multi-organ or multisystem dysfunction/failure [1]. The frequency of PE depends on the country; it is estimated at 8% on average [2]. PE is associated with insufficiently deep placentation, which may be associated with the impairment of spiral arteries remodeling and the presence of obstructive injuries in myometrium. PE is characterized by systemic immune activation associated with elevated levels of inflammatory cytokines produced by various cell types in blood and tissues [3].

Today, a large amount of accumulated data suggests that the dysfunctional maternal immune response in the mother's organism at PE is manifested by altered functional activity of monocyte–macrophage system, which is the most important unit of innate immunity. According to the modern classification, there are three groups of monocytes—classical, intermediate, and non-classical. Each subpopulation has its own function and characteristic markers, as detailed below. Tissue macrophages are usually divided into proinflammatory (M1) and anti-inflammatory (M2), although the distinction between these types is currently being revised. In this regard, several questions remain open, notably which subpopulations of monocytes are predominantly destined to become M1- or M2-polarized macrophages and whether identical monocytes from the same subpopulation can undergo differential polarization in tissues. It is now known that polarization is triggered by local concentrations of certain cytokines. However, it is not clear whether selective depletion of a particular monocyte population will affect the composition of tissue macrophage populations. The answers will provide a relevant support to identification of early predictors for PE.

This article attempts to link the knowledge on developmental origins of the monocyte–macrophage system to the ways of its functioning during normal pregnancy and in PE. Having addressed the key differential characteristics of monocytes we ultimately discuss their possible relevance as predictors in the prevention and diagnosis of PE. The review is focused on studies published over the last few years in order to provide the most up-to-date information on the topic.

2. Monocyte–Macrophage System during Pregnancy

2.1. Monocyte–Macrophage System: Developmental Origins and Cell Lineage

Macrophages play a key role in the maintenance of tissue homeostasis, regulation of inflammatory processes and tissue repair. In accordance with modern concepts, tissue macrophages in mammalian ontogenesis develop from three sources that correspond to three generations of hematopoietic progenitor cells [4,5].

The first generation of hematopoietic cells is specified within the wall of the yolk sac. It is important to note that these hematopoietic cells have a different origin than progenitor cells developing from hematopoietic islets in the endothelium of yolk sac capillaries [5]. It is supposed that microglial cells of the central nervous system descend from these very first hematopoietic progenitors [6]. Life cycle of a macrophage usually involves a migratory stage represented by monocytes circulating in the blood; this stage is absent in microglia development. Microglial precursors migrate directly to the central nervous system and mature within [6].

The second generation, erythro-myeloid progenitor cells, is formed from the hematogenic endothelium of the yolk sac capillaries. These cells subsequently colonize the embryo's liver. By the profile of molecular markers, macrophages derived from these progenitors are very similar to macrophages derived from the first generation of progenitors; however, their maturation involves the stage of monocytes [5,6].

The third generation of hematopoietic progenitors develops from the hematogenic endothelium of the aorta–gonad–mesonephros zone; these cells subsequently migrate to the liver and red bone marrow. Macrophages derived from this generation colonize almost all organs of the embryo except the central nervous system [5].

Thus, macrophage populations of most organs in the prenatal period consist of hematopoietic cells descending from the second and third generations. In most of them, the proportion of macrophages descending from erythro-myeloid progenitor cells of the yolk sac is being gradually decreased, and accordingly the proportion of macrophages descending from hematopoietic cells of the third generation is increased [4,5]. However, there are three exceptions. First of them is the central nervous system (which is apparently inaccessible to monocytes and macrophages except for the macrophages of the first generation). The other two are the liver and the epidermis, where only macrophages descending from the second generation of hematopoietic cells are normally found, named Kupffer cells and Langerhans cells, respectively [5]. Eventually, macrophages of embryonic origin (descendants of the second generation of hematopoietic progenitors) completely disappear from connective tissues of skin dermis and intestinal tract mucosae, being replaced by macrophages of bone marrow origin [4,5,7]. The reasons for such particular macrophage distribution within the mammal organism are unknown.

Macrophages of the second and third generation undergo the stage of monocytes in their development. In the postnatal period, based on CD14 (lipopolysaccharide coreceptor (LPS) and CD16 expression patterns (Fc receptor-FcγRIII), there are three subpopulations of blood monocytes: classical (CD14++, about 90%), non-classical (CD16++, about 10%), and a small intermediate population of monocytes expressing high levels of CD14 and CD16 [8]. These subpopulations have different properties. CD14++ monocytes are considered mature; they show pronounced phagocytic activity and are capable of producing reactive oxygen species and cytokines through activation of TLR signaling pathway [9]. CD16++ cells do not produce reactive oxygen species but are better at production of pro-inflammatory cytokines. CD16++ cells are the patrolling monocytes which perpetually assess the state of the endothelium and infiltrate tissues under normal conditions and during inflammatory processes [8,9]. The role of the intermediate population of monocytes is poorly understood, but given the high expression level of MHC-II they probably participate in antigen presentation and activation of T lymphocytes [10].

The data on the ontogenesis of mammalian macrophages were obtained mainly on various lines of laboratory mice. The number of works concerning studies dealing with the development of macrophage populations in humans are few. It is reasonably supposed that the program of tissue macrophage development in humans is generally consistent with that in mice [11,12].

Macrophages are a heterogeneous population of cells, not only in terms of the source of their development but also in their functional characteristics. Macrophages are capable of rapid adaptation by changing their phenotype and functions under the influence of various signaling molecules. Activation of macrophages in situ can be directed towards either pro-inflammatory M1 or anti-inflammatory M2 polarized macrophages, which differ not only by expression of specific markers but also by their roles in immune response [13]. A local shift of the M1/M2 balance towards M2 in the area of damage significantly improves the dynamics and efficiency of reparative processes; it has been convincingly demonstrated for skin wounds [14], spinal cord injuries [15], myocardial infarction, and cardiomyopathy [16] among other models. Macrophages could be polarized using specific inductors (what is often called the direct polarization), or using an indirect method: blockage the undesired phenotype and get the reverse, desired, phenotype. At the same time, a part of macrophages may remain in a non-activated state [17]. Thus, the in vivo M2 phenotype could be achieved by blocking IL-6-signaling [15] or by adding IL-4 [18] and IL-10 what induced M2a and M2c polarization, respectively [13]. However, it is often emphasized that phenotypes of activated macrophages should be seen as a continuum, with M1 and M2 being its extremum variants [19]. The common markers of M1 macrophages are CD80/86, CD11c, and iNOS, whereas M2 phenotype is usually characterized by expression of CD163, CD206, and Arginase 1 (Arg1) [20,21]. At the same time, CD68- and CD14-specific staining is a common approach for identification of total macrophage population in tissue and the number of positive cells often serves as a normalization value for M1 and M2 cell counts.

2.2. The Role of Monocytes in Pregnancy

During normal pregnancy, an increase in the number of blood monocytes and their activation are observed. These events are accompanied by a change in the ratio of blood monocyte subpopulations: an increase in the number of intermediate monocytes with high levels of CD14 and CD16, and a decrease in the number of the classical monocyte population (CD14++) [22]. Another study revealed an increase in the number of classical monocytes and a decrease in the number of non-classical monocytes [23].

The high heterogeneity of monocyte populations is well known; however, most of the studies have been performed on CD14++ monocytes. An increase in CD11b, CD14, and CD64 monocyte markers in the blood of pregnant women is observed along with high levels of the oxygen free radical production and a decrease in phagocytic activity [24]. The data on cytokine production by unstimulated monocytes are controversial, which may reflect the influence of methods used for monocyte isolation. However, LPS stimulation promotes a decrease in cytokine production in the blood of pregnant women as compared to non-pregnant [25,26]. Another shortcoming of the studies on monocytes in pregnancy is related to the term of gestation: most of the studies have been carried out on blood monocytes collected at the third trimester of pregnancy, the corresponding data for other terms are largely missing [25,26].

The exact mechanisms of monocyte activation during pregnancy are unknown. It is assumed that the placenta plays a leading role in this process. Monocytes, circulating with the blood through placental lacunae, come into contact with syncytiotrophoblast which can activate them towards pro-inflammatory phenotype [27,28]. In addition to the direct contacts, monocytes can be activated indirectly by cytokines [29,30], by microvesicles and exosomes released from syncytiotrophoblast into the maternal blood [31–34] and by pregnancy hormones, e.g., estrogens. A number of studies indicate that estrogens exert anti-inflammatory effect on monocytes [35–38]. Estrogens downregulate the expression of chemokine receptors CCR2 and CXCR3 and suppress the monocyte migration capacity evoked by MIP-1α and MCP-1/JE stimulation [35,36,39]. Estrogens also downregulate production of IL-1 by LPS-stimulated monocytes [40]. In blood, high levels of 17-estradiol are associated with increased numbers of monocytes expressing the markers of M2 macrophages [41]. The anti-inflammatory effect of estrogens on monocytes is believed to be mediated by a specific splice variant of the ERα36 receptor [42]. In vitro, estrogens induce monocyte apoptosis by increasing FasL expression [43]. There is still no data on the possible influence of preeclamptic hypoestrogenemia on the counts and population structure of monocytes. However, it has been established that reduced concentrations of 17-estradiol facilitate the expression of CD16 and boost the production of pro-inflammatory cytokines TNFalpha (Tumor necrosis factor), IL-1, and IL-6 [37].

2.3. The Role of Macrophages in Female Reproductive System Prior to and during Pregnancy

Macrophages are found in all organs of the female reproductive system, their populations being represented by both the monocyte-derived macrophages and the resident macrophages that colonize organs in the prenatal period [44]. Macrophages are unevenly distributed in the endometrium; their numbers and density vary depending on the stage of the menstrual cycle. Within the endometrium, several macrophage populations are distinguished. One of them is located closer to the uterine lumen and is supposed to be involved in the processes of desquamation and regeneration; another population is found mainly around the uterine glands [45]. During the proliferative phase, endometrial macrophages express surface proteins (Transferrin receptor protein 1 (TFRC), CD69 and intracellular adhesion molecule 1), matrix remodeling factors, cytokines, and growth factors that prepare endometrium for possible implantation or the induction of desquamation [45].

During the proliferative phase, macrophages are located within the stroma of superficial layer of endometrium, surrounding and penetrating the lumens of uterine glands. During the secretory phase, the number of macrophages in the endometrium increases dramatically [46]. It is shown that the number of CD14+ macrophages increases by about 45% [47]. During the proliferative phase and in the beginning of the secretory phase, the number of macrophages increases due to proliferation of the resident macrophages; at the end of the secretory phase, migration of monocyte–macrophages to endometrium is observed. It is assumed that during desquamation endometrial macrophages partially migrate from endometrium to lymph nodes or die by apoptosis [48]. In the case of fertilization, the trophoblast invasion occurs at the site of placentation accompanied by accumulation of macrophages in decidua, the pregnancy-modified endometrium. The main functions of decidual macrophages are secretion of cytokines and growth factors for successful placentation, providing immune tolerance to the semi-allogeneic fetus and protection of the fetus against infections. Decidual macrophages mostly originate from monocytes circulating in the blood. Macrophages that reside in the placenta amount to no less than 20%–30% of the total macrophages in the body; they play a key role in the establishment of the immunological aspects of mother–fetus interaction [49,50]. Remodeling of the spiral arteries in maternal uterus is also supported by local decidual macrophages. The involvement of macrophages in the remodeling of spiral arteries is determined by the fact that macrophages secrete many factors universally involved in angiogenesis and tissue remodeling [51,52]. Angiogenic factors secreted by decidual macrophages include angiogenin, keratinocyte growth factor, fibroblast growth factor B, vascular endothelial growth factor A, and angiopoietins 1 and 2. Remodeling factors synthesized by decidual macrophages include matrix metalloproteinases 1, 2, 7, 9, and 10 [52,53]. At the same time, the high phagocytic activity of decidual macrophages is indispensable for the uptake of dead cells that undergo apoptosis during the remodeling of spiral arteries and decidual membrane. The timely disposal of apoptotic cells has been shown to prevent the risks of endothelium activation and excessive attraction of monocytes [54]. Modulation of immune reactions occurs in the placenta throughout pregnancy with macrophages playing a central role in this process [55]. Placentation in the first and second trimesters of pregnancy is characterized by pro-inflammatory environment (favoring M1 polarization), which ensures the correct restoration of the uterine epithelium and protection against infections. The second and third trimesters are the periods of rapid growth of the fetus at the advanced stages of its development, and the prevailing immunological profile is anti-inflammatory (favoring the alternative M2 polarization). A similar immunological shift is observed for other immune cell types including T helper 2 cells (Th2) and a subset of suppressor CD4+ T cells (regulatory T cells, Treg). Th2 and Treg cells are responsible for maintaining peripheral immune tolerance during pregnancy [56]. Successful course of pregnancy is accompanied by activation of anti-inflammatory Th2 and a decrease in Th1/Th2 cytokine ratio [57–59]. Treg cells play a principal role in the protection against recognition of semiallogeneic fetus by the immune system of maternal organism. Deviations in Treg cell counts are associated with different pregnancy complications [60]. During delivery, the immune profile returns to pro-inflammatory state which is necessary for the uterine contraction and fetal movement [61].

The above-mentioned polarization lability of macrophages is mediated by the ability to respond to changing levels of estrogen and estrogen-related factors. It ensures participation of macrophages in maintaining the homeostasis of female reproductive system during the ovarian-uterine cycle and pregnancy. The estrogen group includes several hormones: estradiol, estriol, and estrone [62,63]. A gradual increase in the estrogen blood levels during healthy pregnancy is mainly defined by increasing concentrations of estradiol [62]. At the beginning of pregnancy, estrogens are synthesized by the corpus luteum. From about the 9th week of gestation, the placenta becomes the main source of estradiol; it is produced predominantly by syncytiotrophoblast [63] and to a much lesser extent by Hofbauer cells [64,65]. The synthesis of estrogen in placenta depends on the adrenal glands of the mother and the fetus, since the placenta itself lacks some of the key enzymes of steroidogenesis [62]. Estrogens act on cells through two intracellular estrogen receptors ESR1 (ERα) and ESR2 (ERβ), as well as through G protein-coupled estrogen receptor 1 (GPER1). In human placental macrophages, expression of *Esr1* and *Gper1* is detectable, but ESR2 and the progesterone receptor are absent [66].

Although the estrogen receptors have been found in macrophages, it is believed that estrogens do not directly cause macrophage chemotaxis to the endometrium. It is rather that estrogen stimulates other cells (mostly fibroblasts) to produce cytokines which attract macrophages [44]. However, estrogens have multiple effects on macrophages. It is assumed that estradiol can stimulate macrophage proliferation directly or through other cells that produce mitogens EGF and IGF-1) [44]. Even in the absence of inflammatory mediators, estrogens cause the expression of early and late response genes in macrophages. In inflammation, estrogens promote polarization of macrophages to M2 phenotype and stimulate the synthesis of molecules involved in the extracellular matrix remodeling (proteases and their inhibitors) [67]. Estrogens can enhance or suppress the phagocytic ability of macrophages depending on the prevailing activation factors. Macrophages are capable of absorbing iron through the transferrin receptor 1 (TFRC) and CD163; estrogens enhance the absorption of iron ions through activation of TFRC, as well as by suppressing synthesis of hepcidin in the liver [44].

Some authors suggest that estrogens play a key role in the pathogenesis of PE, since they regulate angiogenesis and cause vasodilation [62]. A decrease in the level of estrogen in the blood of preeclamptic women is evident [68–72]. In PE, estradiol levels are decreased in the blood [69,71,73] and in the placenta [74]. Plasma concentrations of estrone and estriol in severe PE are also reduced, although in some of the studies such changes have not been detected [69,71]; there is also an evidence of reduced estriol levels in the placenta [70]. Androgens are another important group of hormones whose level is important for the normal course of pregnancy. It is supposed that they are responsible for cervical remodeling at term via regulation of cervical collagen fibril organization [75]. As for PE, it has been shown that testosterone level in women with PE is greatly increased [76]. It does not, however, answer the question of how it affects macrophages of placenta. Testosterone receptors have been found on the surface of macrophages and it was shown that the signal cascade triggered by testosterone includes the fluctuation of cytosolic calcium [77,78]. In another work, it was shown that androgens induce polarization of the lung macrophages towards the M2 phenotype [79].

Despite the large body of data concerning this topic, it is difficult to find a study addressing the role of estrogen- and androgen-dependent polarization of macrophages in PE. This area needs further research.

2.4. Monocytes in Preeclampsia

In considering the pathogenesis of PE, great emphasis is being made on oxidative stress and endothelial dysfunction occurring in the maternal body. Insufficient placentation causes abnormally regulated blood pressure in the maternal cardiovascular system, followed by blood supply shortages and, as a consequence, ischemia/reperfusion of the placenta. It is believed that under these conditions the hypoxic placenta synthesizes and secretes increased quantities of vasoactive substances promoting the release of a the number of signal factors such as placental debris, exosomes, microvesicles, cell-free nucleic acids, and pro-inflammatory cytokines into maternal blood flow. The presence of these markers is well described and highly symptomatic [80–82]. The situation eventually leads to a pronounced inflammatory response, oxidative stress and enhances apoptosis of placental cells [83]. Elevated levels of pro-inflammatory cytokines produced by various cell types lead to dramatic changes in the patterns of surface molecules of the endothelium and result in systemic endothelial dysfunction and subsequent hypertension [84–86]. Detailed reviews concerning the delicate immune balance in normal pregnancy and in PE are available from scientific databases [3,87].

Inflammation is a pronounced feature of PE; it involves cells of both adaptive and innate immunity. Due to the fact that monocytes circulate in the blood only for a few days, their quantity and composition reflect the severity of the patient's clinical condition. Since generalized inflammation is a well-known feature of PE, changes in monocyte quantity and subset profile should be expected. Indeed, Wang and colleagues analyzed clinical records of more than three hundred patients with PE and found that in PE group the absolute monocyte count and the monocyte-lymphocyte ratio were significantly higher as compared with the control group (Table 1) [88]. As revealed by ROC-analysis, the monocyte-lymphocyte ratio has good diagnostic accuracy to distinguish between the normal condition and PE. In the work of Brien and colleagues, an increase in monocyte counts was also found typical for PE; the authors used CD14 marker to identify monocytes [89].

Table 1. Summary observations concerning monocyte–macrophage system in preeclampsia (PE).

Subject	Observation in PE	Quantity: Control vs. PE	Reference
Monocyte	↑ Monocyte count ↑ Monocyte-lymphocyte ratio	161/302	[88]
	↑ Monocyte count	20/20	[89]
	↓ CD14++CD16−, ↑ CD14+CD16++	11/17	[23]
		40/35	[90]
		8/4 (umbilical cord blood)	[91]
	↓ CD14++CD16−; ↑ (CD14+CD16++ and CD14++CD16+)	24/9	[92]
	↑ CD14+CD11c+CD163-	23/26	[22]
		30/22	[93]
Macrophages in placenta Hofbauer cells	↓ CD14+	30/10	[94]

Table 1. Cont.

Subject	Observation in PE	Quantity: Control vs. PE	Reference
Decidual macrophages	↓ CD68+	11/10	[95]
	↑ CD68+	20/20	[96]
		6/6	[97]
	↑ Hofbauer cells number	50/50	[98]
	↓ CD163+	30/10	[94]
	↓ CD163+	11/10	[95]
	↓ CD74+	28/24	[99]
	↓ CD11b+Arg1+ ↑ CD11b+ iNOS+	22/30	[93]
	↑ CD14+	5/6	[50]
	↑ CD68+	20/30	[100]
		6/6	[97]
	↓ CD14+	12/12	[101]
		6/6	[102]
	↓ CD163/CD14	5/6	[50]

Characterization of monocyte subpopulations in PE became a subject of interest after 2010 [22,23]. Recent investigations confirm the previous findings on its relevance. In recent work of Alahakoon and colleagues, the authors estimated quantities of classical, intermediate and non-classical monocytes in blood samples from preeclamptic patients (with or without intrauterine growth restriction, IUGR) and uncomplicated pregnancies [92]. The authors observed a significantly lower content of classical monocytes for both PE groups (with or without IUGR), while the number of inflammatory monocytes which combined intermediate and non-classical subsets for these groups was significantly increased as compared with the control. Similar results were obtained by Jabalie et al. who observed a decline in the percentage of classical monocytes paralleled by an increase in the percentage of intermediate and non-classical monocytes in blood samples from preeclamptic women with or without metabolic syndrome [90].

Ma and colleagues analyzed cytokine profiles of serum from women with PE and also estimated the percentage of blood monocytes positive for M1 and M2 macrophage markers [93]. The counts of CD14+CD11c+CD163-(M1) monocytes in PE group were significantly increased, which correlated with the increased level of pro-inflammatory factors (IL-1, IL-6, and MCP-1). However, the works concerning M1 and M2 macrophage markers in the blood of women with PE are few, which indicates the necessity of further studies in this field.

Several studies focused on the composition of umbilical cord blood in PE have obvious scientific novelty since fetal participation is rarely considered in the context of PE. Interestingly, the authors come to the same observation: a significant reduction in the classical monocyte subset and a significant increase in non-classical monocyte subset were observed for the cord blood in PE group [91].

Summarizing these data leads to a general conclusion that the observed PE-associated changes in counts and composition of blood monocytes towards the prevalence of non-classical subset indicate progression of the inflammation symptoms in the maternal organism. The upheaval of inflammatory reaction during PE is possibly caused by extracellular agents, which appear in blood, and cytokines, which activate monocytes [103]. Since monocyte counts are included in routine clinical blood tests, and given that phenotyping of monocytes by flow cytometry is a straightforward procedure, appearance of monocyte-based tests for PE prediction as a routine practice may be expected. Surely it would require a prospective study to assess the prognostic value of monocyte profile indicators in the blood of a pregnant woman who would have PE and absolute standardization of all manipulations. To date, none of the existing tests reliably evaluates the risks of PE. At present, only a few markers associated with PE, such as endoglin, placental growth factor (PlGF) and sFlt-1 (soluble fms-like tyrosine kinase 1), have been sufficiently studied.

2.5. Macrophages in Preeclampsia

The increase in non-classical monocyte subset may affect the composition of tissue macrophages in the endometrium and be responsible for the poor placentation in PE [104]. Appropriate balance between pro- and anti-inflammatory macrophages in the placenta is essential for healthy pregnancy and its optimal outcome. It has been suggested that transition to the M2 profile, which normally occurs in the second trimester, is blocked in PE; more specifically, it is canceled at the early stages of the disease [105]. As a consequence, M1 responses remain unsuppressed, and cytokines exhibit a pro-inflammatory profile with elevated levels of IFN-γ, TNFalpha, IL6 and reduced levels of IL-4 and IL-10 [105,106].

Behavior of resident placental macrophages in PE has not received the proper attention of the researchers as yet. This can be possibly explained by the complexity of the biomaterial collection and the time-consuming procedure of isolation and phenotyping of the cells from this material in contrast to the easily obtained blood samples. However, this subject requires a comprehensive study. In the context of any pregnancy complication, placental macrophages should be considered as two populations: Hofbauer cells of the fetal placenta and decidual macrophages of the maternal placental part.

Recently published works comprise somewhat controversial numerical estimates for both Hofbauer cells and decidual macrophages in preeclamptic placentas. Yang and colleagues observed significantly lower numbers of CD14+ Hofbauer cells in PE placenta as compared with the healthy control but no corresponding significant difference in CD68+ cell numbers was found [94]. Tang et al. observed significantly declined numbers of CD68+ Hofbauer cells in PE group in comparison with the gestation age-matched preterm birth control group [95]. By contrast, Evsen and colleagues, on the contrary, observed increased Hofbauer cell numbers in PE complicated by HELLP syndrome group compared to the control group; the authors also used CD68 as a macrophage marker [96]. Saeed et al. report a two-fold increase in the Hofbauer cell number in preeclamptic placentas in comparison to normotensive pregnancy [98]. As for decidual macrophages, their comparative abundance in the preeclamptic placenta is also a controversial subject. Schonkeren and colleagues reported an increase in number of CD14+ cells in the decidua basalis for preterm preeclamptic pregnancies compared with preterm control pregnancies [50]. Milosevic-Stevanovic et al. observed higher numbers of CD68+ decidual cells in PE compared to healthy control placentas [100]. In one study, a significant increase in number of CD68+ cells, in both fetal and decidual parts of placenta, was observed in preeclamptic group as compared to controls [97]. At the same time, several research groups report that decidual macrophage numbers in PE placentas are reduced [94,101,102]. Apparent inconsistencies between the studies may be explained by the use of different technical approaches (cell markers, antibodies, signal detection protocols, etc.) and the difference in the formation of studied groups.

The issue of macrophage polarization in preeclamptic placenta looks less ambiguous. Yang and colleagues showed that the level of CD163+ Hofbauer cells is significantly downregulated in PE compared with healthy pregnancies [94]. In work of Tang's and colleagues they also observed a decrease in CD163+ cell numbers compared with the preterm control [95]. Przybyl et al. reported reduced CD74+ cell numbers in preeclamptic placentas; according to the proposed model, this may lead to a pro-inflammatory signature [99]. Ma et al. observed an increase in the percentage of CD11b-iNOS co-labeled cells and a concomitant decrease in the percentage of CD11b-Arg1 co-labeled cells in preeclamptic placentas as compared with normal ones [93]; the combinations of markers reflect M1 and M2 phenotypes, respectively. The ratio of CD163/CD14 decidual cells was also found to be declined in placental samples collected from women with PE [50].

The shift in the balance of M2/M1 macrophages towards M1 is explained by high levels of pro-inflammatory cytokines and low levels of anti-inflammatory cytokines within the preeclamptic placenta [107,108]. In addition to the altered cytokine production, there is also a cellular axis in the process of polarization. A number of studies suggest an essential role of placental mesenchymal stem cells in macrophage polarization and their ability to affect their activation [109,110]. Wang and colleagues revealed the role of hyaluronan in maintaining normal pregnancy. Their findings indicate that high levels of hyaluronan induce M2 polarization and regulate production of cytokines (e.g., IL-10) by decidual macrophages [111].

The summarizing scheme is presented in Figure 1. Despite the large body of available data, several questions are still remaining unanswered. When do the observed changes in macrophage polarization really emerge—at the early stages of pregnancy or after the PE manifestation? At what gestational age could they be valid as markers? Can we use macrophages and monocytes for therapeutic purposes?

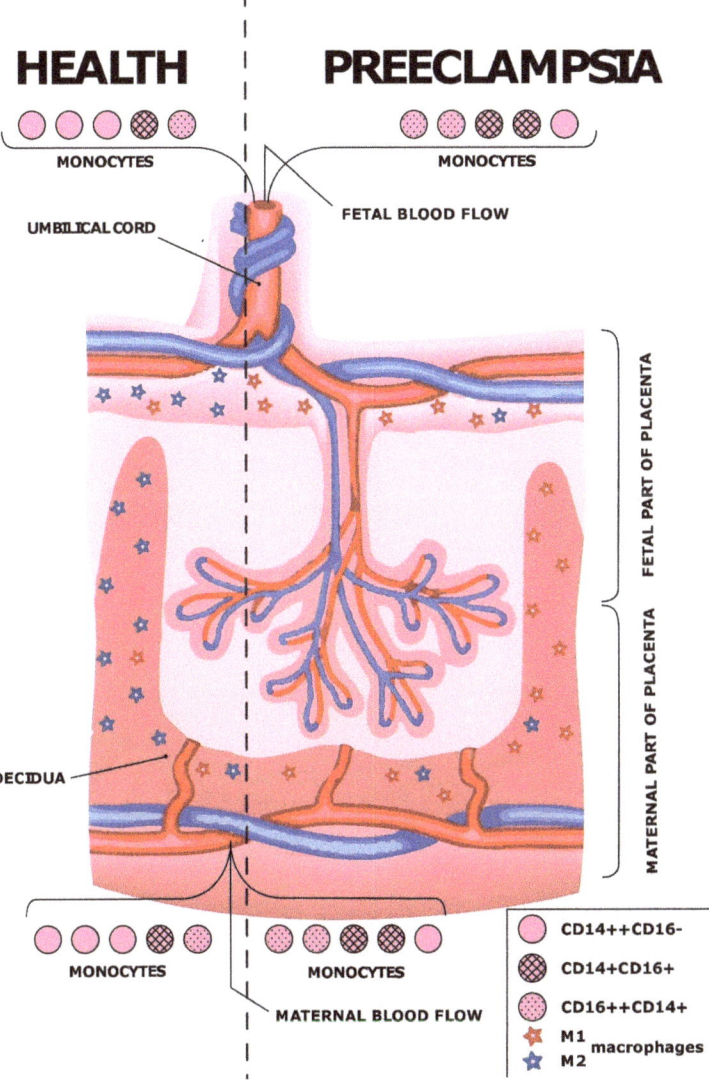

Figure 1. Summarizing scheme. Monocyte–macrophage system in decidua, fetal and maternal placental parts and blood flow of mother and fetus. Classical (CD14++CD16−), non-classical (CD16++CD14+) and intermediate (CD14+CD16+) monocyte populations as well as proinflammatory (M1) and anti-inflammatory (M2) macrophages are shown. Modified from [26] (distributed under CC-BY).

2.6. Potential Therapeutic Approaches

Reprogramming of macrophages seems to be an attractive therapeutic strategy. A number of FDA approved approaches involving cellular and gene therapy are now used in clinical practice [112]. Macrophages derived from monocytes can be activated in different ways by varying combinations of external stimuli. The ex vivo reprogramming of macrophages conventionally aims to polarize them towards the anti-inflammatory phenotype in order to make the M2 polarized macrophages confront inflammation in maternal body. The idea of ex vivo reprogramming of autologous macrophages has been developed since the 1980s [113]. By now, the reprogrammed macrophages have been successfully used in a number of therapeutic cases including treatment of cancer, transplantation, and stimulation of regeneration [114–116]. Common approaches for the ex vivo macrophage polarization are stimulation of the cells with cytokine cocktails, genetic manipulation, or using specific low-molecular inhibitors of transcription factors [117,118]. iPS-ML, the macrophage-like myelomonocytic cells generated from the human induced pluripotent stem cells, are also amenable to ex vivo polarization [119]. Injection of the autologous monocyte-derived M2-polarized macrophages at a certain time of gestation (or at the stage of its planning by taking into account the risks of PE) may evolve into a new strategy for PE treatment. Such therapy seems to be promising due to reports about the absence of adverse reactions and long-term side effects after macrophages transplantation in other diseases [120,121]. A possible side effect of the proposed therapy may be the phenomenon of maternal–fetal cellular trafficking—the ability of mother and fetus cells pass the placental barrier [122]. The presence of fetal cells in the maternal circulation is known as fetal microchimerism, while the presence maternal cells in the fetal organism is known as maternal microchimerism. Indeed, in a number of works it was shown that fetuses with severe congenital diaphragmatic hernia have increased levels of maternal microchimerism [122,123]. However, this does not mean that the activated *ex vivo* auto-monocytes will necessarily penetrate the placenta. This question has not been sufficiently investigated.

3. Summary and Conclusions

Compared to other pregnancy complications, PE is the main cause of maternal morbidity and mortality. For several decades, researchers have been trying to understand the causes of PE, considering the disorder from different points of view. An important aspect of PE development is the response of maternal innate immunity to various proinflammatory stimuli from the placenta. Normally, the maternal organism adapts to the presence of the fetus; however, at PE, a pronounced inflammatory process occurs. The consequences of this process are manifested in the increased monocyte numbers and altered subset composition, including changes in counts and polarization of placental macrophages. The recent examples of observations listed in this review suggest that monitoring of blood composition and phenotyping of monocytes over the course of pregnancy might be considered as screening tests for PE. However, such tests must be used in combination with other PE prognostic markers because the symptoms of some other complications and conditions (e.g., stress, infections or cancer) occasionally could mimic the PE-associated monocyte changes [8]. Monocytes and tissue macrophages are the extremely important cell types involved in PE pathogenesis. Their possible application as PE predictors and/or therapeutics agents holds great promise.

Author Contributions: Writing—original draft preparation, P.V., A.E., T.F.; writing—review and editing, T.F., G.S.; supervision, T.F., G.S.; project administration, G.S.

Funding: This research was funded by President Grant for Government Support of Young Russian Scientists No. 075-15-2019-1120, P.V. was supported by the President's Scholarship (SP-4132.2018.4).

Acknowledgments: We are very grateful to Priluchnyi Vlad for the help in illustration of the article.

Conflicts of Interest: The authors declare no conflict of interest.

Abbreviations

PE	Preeclampsia
IUGR	Intrauterine growth restriction
Arg1	Arginase 1
Treg	Regulatory T cells
Th2	T helper 2

References

1. World Health Organization WHO Recommendations for Prevention and Treatment of Pre-Eclampsia and Eclampsia. Available online: http://www.ncbi.nlm.nih.gov/books/NBK140561/ (accessed on 23 May 2016).
2. Saito, S. *Preeclampsia Basic, Genomic, and Clinical*; Springer Nature Singapore Pte Ltd.: Singapore, 2018.
3. Cornelius, D.C. Preeclampsia: From inflammation to immunoregulation. *Clin. Med. Insights Blood Disord.* **2018**, *11*. [CrossRef] [PubMed]
4. Chazaud, B. Macrophages: Supportive cells for tissue repair and regeneration. *Immunobiology* **2014**, *219*, 172–178. [CrossRef] [PubMed]
5. Perdiguero, E.G.; Geissmann, F. The development and maintenance of resident macrophages. *Nat. Immunol.* **2016**, *17*, 2–8. [CrossRef] [PubMed]
6. Hoeffel, G.; Chen, J.; Lavin, Y.; Low, D.; Almeida, F.F.; See, P.; Beaudin, A.E.; Lum, J.; Low, I.; Forsberg, E.C.; et al. C-Myb(+) erythro-myeloid progenitor-derived fetal monocytes give rise to adult tissue-resident macrophages. *Immunity* **2015**, *42*, 665–678. [CrossRef] [PubMed]
7. Epelman, S.; Lavine, K.J.; Randolph, G.J. Origin and Functions of Tissue Macrophages. *Immunity* **2014**, *41*, 21–35. [CrossRef] [PubMed]
8. Ziegler-Heitbrock, L. Monocyte subsets in man and other species. *Cell. Immunol.* **2014**, *289*, 135–139. [CrossRef]
9. Mildner, A.; Marinkovic, G.; Jung, S. Murine Monocytes: Origins, Subsets, Fates, and Functions. *Microbiol. Spectr.* **2016**, *4*.
10. Wong, K.L.; Tai, J.J.; Wong, W.C.; Han, H.; Sem, X.; Yeap, W.H.; Kourilsky, P.; Wong, S.C. Gene expression profiling reveals the defining features of the classical, intermediate, and nonclassical human monocyte subsets. *Blood* **2011**, *118*, e16–e31. [CrossRef]
11. Godin, I.; Cumano, A. The hare and the tortoise: An embryonic haematopoietic race. *Nat. Rev. Immunol.* **2002**, *2*, 593–604. [CrossRef]
12. Röszer, T. Understanding the Biology of Self-Renewing Macrophages. *Cells* **2018**, *7*, 103. [CrossRef]
13. Martinez, F.O.; Gordon, S. The M1 and M2 paradigm of macrophage activation: Time for reassessment. *F1000Prime Rep.* **2014**, *6*, 13. [CrossRef] [PubMed]
14. Okizaki, S.; Ito, Y.; Hosono, K.; Oba, K.; Ohkubo, H.; Amano, H.; Shichiri, M.; Majima, M. Suppressed recruitment of alternatively activated macrophages reduces TGF-β1 and impairs wound healing in streptozotocin-induced diabetic mice. *Biomed. Pharmacother.* **2015**, *70*, 317–325. [CrossRef] [PubMed]
15. Nakajima, H.; Uchida, K.; Guerrero, A.R.; Watanabe, S.; Sugita, D.; Takeura, N.; Yoshida, A.; Long, G.; Wright, K.T.; Johnson, W.E.B.; et al. Transplantation of Mesenchymal Stem Cells Promotes an Alternative Pathway of Macrophage Activation and Functional Recovery after Spinal Cord Injury. *J. Neurotrauma* **2012**, *29*, 1614–1625. [CrossRef] [PubMed]
16. Singla, D.K.; Singla, R.D.; Abdelli, L.S.; Glass, C. Fibroblast Growth Factor-9 Enhances M2 Macrophage Differentiation and Attenuates Adverse Cardiac Remodeling in the Infarcted Diabetic Heart. *PLoS ONE* **2015**, *10*, e0120739. [CrossRef] [PubMed]
17. Murray, P.J.; Wynn, T.A. Obstacles and opportunities for understanding macrophage polarization. *J. Leukoc. Biol.* **2011**, *89*, 557–563. [CrossRef] [PubMed]
18. Kiguchi, N.; Kobayashi, Y.; Saika, F.; Sakaguchi, H.; Maeda, T.; Kishioka, S. Peripheral interleukin-4 ameliorates inflammatory macrophage-dependent neuropathic pain. *Pain* **2015**, *156*, 684–693. [CrossRef]
19. Malyshev, I.; Malyshev, Y. Current Concept and Update of the Macrophage Plasticity Concept: Intracellular Mechanisms of Reprogramming and M3 Macrophage "Switch" Phenotype. *Biomed. Res. Int.* **2015**, *2015*, 1–22. [CrossRef] [PubMed]
20. Mills, C.D. Anatomy of a Discovery: M1 and M2 Macrophages. *Front. Immunol.* **2015**, *6*, 212. [CrossRef]

21. Yao, Y.; Xu, X.H.; Jin, L. Macrophage Polarization in Physiological and Pathological Pregnancy. *Front. Immunol.* **2019**, *10*, 792. [CrossRef]
22. Melgert, B.N.; Spaans, F.; Borghuis, T.; Klok, P.A.; Groen, B.; Bolt, A.; de Vos, P.; van Pampus, M.G.; Wong, T.Y.; van Goor, H.; et al. Pregnancy and Preeclampsia Affect Monocyte Subsets in Humans and Rats. *PLoS ONE* **2012**, *7*, e45229. [CrossRef]
23. Al-ofi, E.; Coffelt, S.B.; Anumba, D.O. Monocyte subpopulations from pre-eclamptic patients are abnormally skewed and exhibit exaggerated responses to toll-like receptor ligands. *PLoS ONE* **2012**, *7*, e42217. [CrossRef] [PubMed]
24. Lampé, R.; Kövér, Á.; Szűcs, S.; Pál, L.; Árnyas, E.; Ádány, R.; Póka, R. Phagocytic index of neutrophil granulocytes and monocytes in healthy and preeclamptic pregnancy. *J. Reprod. Immunol.* **2015**, *107*, 26–30. [CrossRef] [PubMed]
25. Faas, M.M.; de Vos, P. Maternal monocytes in pregnancy and preeclampsia in humans and in rats. *J. Reprod. Immunol.* **2017**, *119*, 91–97. [CrossRef] [PubMed]
26. Faas, M.M.; Spaans, F.; De Vos, P. Monocytes and macrophages in pregnancy and pre-eclampsia. *Front. Immunol.* **2014**, *5*, 298. [CrossRef] [PubMed]
27. Nonn, O.; Güttler, J.; Forstner, D.; Maninger, S.; Zadora, J.; Balogh, A.; Frolova, A.; Glasner, A.; Herse, F.; Gauster, M. Placental CX3CL1 is Deregulated by Angiotensin II and Contributes to a Pro-Inflammatory Trophoblast-Monocyte Interaction. *Int. J. Mol. Sci.* **2019**, *20*, 641. [CrossRef] [PubMed]
28. Siwetz, M.; Sundl, M.; Kolb, D.; Hiden, U.; Herse, F.; Huppertz, B.; Gauster, M. Placental fractalkine mediates adhesion of THP-1 monocytes to villous trophoblast. *Histochem. Cell Biol.* **2015**, *143*, 565–574. [CrossRef]
29. Hung, T.-H.; Charnock-Jones, D.S.; Skepper, J.N.; Burton, G.J. Secretion of tumor necrosis factor-alpha from human placental tissues induced by hypoxia-reoxygenation causes endothelial cell activation in vitro: A potential mediator of the inflammatory response in preeclampsia. *Am. J. Pathol.* **2004**, *164*, 1049–1061. [CrossRef]
30. Sacks, G.P.; Clover, L.M.; Bainbridge, D.R.J.; Redman, C.W.G.; Sargent, I.L. Flow Cytometric Measurement of Intracellular Th1 and Th2 Cytokine Production by Human Villous and Extravillous Cytotrophoblast. *Placenta* **2001**, *22*, 550–559. [CrossRef]
31. Dragovic, R.A.; Collett, G.P.; Hole, P.; Ferguson, D.J.P.; Redman, C.W.; Sargent, I.L.; Tannetta, D.S. Isolation of syncytiotrophoblast microvesicles and exosomes and their characterisation by multicolour flow cytometry and fluorescence Nanoparticle Tracking Analysis. *Methods* **2015**, *87*, 64–74. [CrossRef]
32. Göhner, C.; Fledderus, J.; Fitzgerald, J.S.; Schleußner, E.; Markert, U.R.; Scherjon, S.A.; Plösch, T.; Faas, M.M. Syncytiotrophoblast exosomes guide monocyte maturation and activation of monocytes and granulocytes. *Placenta* **2015**, *36*, A47–A48. [CrossRef]
33. Sokolov, D.I.; Ovchinnikova, O.M.; Korenkov, D.A.; Viknyanschuk, A.N.; Benken, K.A.; Onokhin, K.V.; Selkov, S.A. Influence of peripheral blood microparticles of pregnant women with preeclampsia on the phenotype of monocytes. *Transl. Res.* **2016**, *170*, 112–123. [CrossRef] [PubMed]
34. Tannetta, D.; Collett, G.; Vatish, M.; Redman, C.; Sargent, I. Syncytiotrophoblast extracellular vesicles–Circulating biopsies reflecting placental health. *Placenta* **2017**, *52*, 134–138. [CrossRef] [PubMed]
35. Lang, T.J. Estrogen as an immunomodulator. *Clin. Immunol.* **2004**, *113*, 224–230. [CrossRef] [PubMed]
36. Janis, K.; Hoeltke, J.; Nazareth, M.; Fanti, P.; Poppenberg, K.; Aronica, S.M. Estrogen decreases expression of chemokine receptors, and suppresses chemokine bioactivity in murine monocytes. *Am. J. Reprod. Immunol.* **2004**, *51*, 22–31. [CrossRef] [PubMed]
37. Kramer, P.R.; Kramer, S.F.; Guan, G. 17?-estradiol regulates cytokine release through modulation of CD16 expression in monocytes and monocyte-derived macrophages. *Arthritis Rheum.* **2004**, *50*, 1967–1975. [CrossRef] [PubMed]
38. Margaryan, S.; Hyusyan, A.; Martirosyan, A.; Sargsian, S.; Manukyan, G. Differential modulation of innate immune response by epinephrine and estradiol. *Horm. Mol. Biol. Clin. Investig.* **2017**, *30*. [CrossRef] [PubMed]
39. Lee, D.-H.; Kim, S.-C.; Joo, J.-K.; Kim, H.-G.; Na, Y.-J.; Kwak, J.-Y.; Lee, K.-S. Effects of 17β-estradiol on the release of monocyte chemotactic protein-1 and MAPK activity in monocytes stimulated with peritoneal fluid from endometriosis patients. *J. Obstet. Gynaecol. Res.* **2012**, *38*, 516–525. [CrossRef] [PubMed]
40. Morishita, M.; Miyagi, M.; Iwamoto, Y. Effects of Sex Hormones on Production of Interleukin-1 by Human Peripheral Monocytes. *J. Periodontol.* **1999**, *70*, 757–760. [CrossRef]

41. Habib, P.; Dreymueller, D.; Rösing, B.; Botung, H.; Slowik, A.; Zendedel, A.; Habib, S.; Hoffmann, S.; Beyer, C. Estrogen serum concentration affects blood immune cell composition and polarization in human females under controlled ovarian stimulation. *J. Steroid Biochem. Mol. Biol.* **2018**, *178*, 340–347. [CrossRef]
42. Pelekanou, V.; Kampa, M.; Kiagiadaki, F.; Deli, A.; Theodoropoulos, P.; Agrogiannis, G.; Patsouris, E.; Tsapis, A.; Castanas, E.; Notas, G. Estrogen anti-inflammatory activity on human monocytes is mediated through cross-talk between estrogen receptor ERα36 and GPR30/GPER1. *J. Leukoc. Biol.* **2016**, *99*, 333–347. [CrossRef]
43. Mor, G.; Sapi, E.; Abrahams, V.M.; Rutherford, T.; Song, J.; Hao, X.-Y.; Muzaffar, S.; Kohen, F. Interaction of the estrogen receptors with the Fas ligand promoter in human monocytes. *J. Immunol.* **2003**, *170*, 114–122. [CrossRef] [PubMed]
44. Pepe, G.; Locati, M.; Della Torre, S.; Mornata, F.; Cignarella, A.; Maggi, A.; Vegeto, E. The estrogen–macrophage interplay in the homeostasis of the female reproductive tract. *Hum. Reprod. Update* **2018**, *24*, 652–672. [CrossRef] [PubMed]
45. Thiruchelvam, U.; Dransfield, I.; Saunders, P.T.K.; Critchley, H.O.D. The importance of the macrophage within the human endometrium. *J. Leukoc. Biol.* **2013**, *93*, 217–225. [CrossRef] [PubMed]
46. Cousins, F.L.; Kirkwood, P.M.; Saunders, P.T.K.; Gibson, D.A. Evidence for a dynamic role for mononuclear phagocytes during endometrial repair and remodelling. *Sci. Rep.* **2016**, *6*, 36748. [CrossRef]
47. Hunt, J.S.; Robertson, S.A. Uterine macrophages and environmental programming for pregnancy success. *J. Reprod. Immunol.* **1996**, *32*, 1–25. [CrossRef]
48. Wira, C.R.; Fahey, J.V.; Rodriguez-Garcia, M.; Shen, Z.; Patel, M.V. Regulation of Mucosal Immunity in the Female Reproductive Tract: The Role of Sex Hormones in Immune Protection Against Sexually Transmitted Pathogens. *Am. J. Reprod. Immunol.* **2014**, *72*, 236–258. [CrossRef]
49. PrabhuDas, M.; Bonney, E.; Caron, K.; Dey, S.; Erlebacher, A.; Fazleabas, A.; Fisher, S.; Golos, T.; Matzuk, M.; McCune, J.M.; et al. Immune mechanisms at the maternal-fetal interface: Perspectives and challenges. *Nat. Immunol.* **2015**, *16*, 328–334. [CrossRef]
50. Schonkeren, D.; Van Der Hoorn, M.L.; Khedoe, P.; Swings, G.; Van Beelen, E.; Claas, F.; Van Kooten, C.; De Heer, E.; Scherjon, S. Differential distribution and phenotype of decidual macrophages in preeclamptic versus control pregnancies. *Am. J. Pathol.* **2011**, *178*, 709–717. [CrossRef]
51. Smith, S.D.; Dunk, C.E.; Aplin, J.D.; Harris, L.K.; Jones, R.L. Evidence for Immune Cell Involvement in Decidual Spiral Arteriole Remodeling in Early Human Pregnancy. *Am. J. Pathol.* **2009**, *174*, 1959–1971. [CrossRef]
52. Lash, G.E.; Pitman, H.; Morgan, H.L.; Innes, B.A.; Agwu, C.N.; Bulmer, J.N. Decidual macrophages: Key regulators of vascular remodeling in human pregnancy. *J. Leukoc. Biol.* **2016**, *100*, 315–325. [CrossRef]
53. Hazan, A.D.; Smith, S.D.; Jones, R.L.; Whittle, W.; Lye, S.J.; Dunk, C.E. Vascular-Leukocyte Interactions. *Am. J. Pathol.* **2010**, *177*, 1017–1030. [CrossRef]
54. Chen, Q.; Guo, F.; Jin, H.Y.; Lau, S.; Stone, P.; Chamley, L. Phagocytosis of apoptotic trophoblastic debris protects endothelial cells against activation. *Placenta* **2012**, *33*, 548–553. [CrossRef]
55. Mor, G.; Cardenas, I.; Abrahams, V.; Guller, S. Inflammation and pregnancy: The role of the immune system at the implantation site. *Ann. N. Y. Acad. Sci.* **2011**, *1221*, 80–87. [CrossRef]
56. Vargas-Rojas, M.I.; Solleiro-Villavicencio, H.; Soto-Vega, E. Th1, Th2, Th17 and Treg levels in umbilical cord blood in preeclampsia. *J. Matern. Neonatal Med.* **2016**, *29*, 1642–1645. [CrossRef]
57. Reinhard, G.; Noll, A.; Schlebusch, H.; Mallmann, P.; Ruecker, A.V. Shifts in the TH1/TH2 Balance during Human Pregnancy Correlate with Apoptotic Changes. *Biochem. Biophys. Res. Commun.* **1998**, *245*, 933–938. [CrossRef]
58. Piccinni, M.P.; Lombardelli, L.; Logiodice, F.; Kullolli, O.; Romagnani, S.; Bouteiller, P. Le T helper cell mediated-tolerance towards fetal allograft in successful pregnancy. *Clin. Mol. Allergy* **2015**, *13*, 9. [CrossRef]
59. Bogdanova, I.M.; Boltovskaya, M.N. Immune control of reproduction, the role of regulatory t-cells in the induction of immunological tolerance during pregnancy. *Clin. Exp. Morphol.* **2015**, *3*, 59–67.
60. La Rocca, C.; Carbone, F.; Longobardi, S.; Matarese, G. The immunology of pregnancy: Regulatory T cells control maternal immune tolerance toward the fetus. *Immunol. Lett.* **2014**, *162*, 41–48. [CrossRef]
61. Sykes, L.; MacIntyre, D.A.; Yap, X.J.; Teoh, T.G.; Bennett, P.R. The Th1:Th2 Dichotomy of Pregnancy and Preterm Labour. *Mediat. Inflamm.* **2012**, *2012*, 1–12. [CrossRef]

62. Berkane, N.; Liere, P.; Oudinet, J.-P.; Hertig, A.; Lefèvre, G.; Pluchino, N.; Schumacher, M.; Chabbert-Buffet, N. From Pregnancy to Preeclampsia: A Key Role for Estrogens. *Endocr. Rev.* **2017**, *38*, 123–144. [CrossRef]
63. Napso, T.; Yong, H.E.J.; Lopez-Tello, J.; Sferruzzi-Perri, A.N. The Role of Placental Hormones in Mediating Maternal Adaptations to Support Pregnancy and Lactation. *Front. Physiol.* **2018**, *9*, 1091. [CrossRef]
64. Schmidt, M.; Kreutz, M.; Löffler, G.; Schölmerich, J.; Straub, R.H. Conversion of dehydroepiandrosterone to downstream steroid hormones in macrophages. *J. Endocrinol.* **2000**, *164*, 161–169. [CrossRef]
65. Tang, Z.; Tadesse, S.; Norwitz, E.; Mor, G.; Abrahams, V.M.; Guller, S. Isolation of hofbauer cells from human term placentas with high yield and purity. *Am. J. Reprod. Immunol.* **2011**, *66*, 336–348. [CrossRef]
66. Trenti, A.; Tedesco, S.; Boscaro, C.; Trevisi, L.; Bolego, C.; Cignarella, A. Estrogen, Angiogenesis, Immunity and Cell Metabolism: Solving the Puzzle. *Int. J. Mol. Sci.* **2018**, *19*, 859. [CrossRef]
67. Villa, A.; Rizzi, N.; Vegeto, E.; Ciana, P.; Maggi, A. Estrogen accelerates the resolution of inflammation in macrophagic cells. *Sci. Rep.* **2015**, *5*, 15224. [CrossRef]
68. Salas, S.P.; Marshall, G.; Gutiérrez, B.L.; Rosso, P. Time Course of Maternal Plasma Volume and Hormonal Changes in Women With Preeclampsia or Fetal Growth Restriction. *Hypertension* **2006**, *47*, 203–208. [CrossRef]
69. Hertig, A.; Liere, P.; Chabbert-Buffet, N.; Fort, J.; Pianos, A.; Eychenne, B.; Cambourg, A.; Schumacher, M.; Berkane, N.; Lefevre, G.; et al. Steroid profiling in preeclamptic women: Evidence for aromatase deficiency. *Am. J. Obstet. Gynecol.* **2010**, *203*, e1–e477. [CrossRef]
70. Bussen, S.; Bussen, D. Influence of the vascular endothelial growth factor on the development of severe pre-eclampsia or HELLP syndrome. *Arch. Gynecol. Obstet.* **2011**, *284*, 551–557. [CrossRef]
71. Jobe, S.O.; Tyler, C.T.; Magness, R.R. Aberrant synthesis, metabolism, and plasma accumulation of circulating estrogens and estrogen metabolites in preeclampsia implications for vascular dysfunction. *Hypertens. (Dallas, Tex. 1979)* **2013**, *61*, 480–487. [CrossRef]
72. Yin, G.; Zhu, X.; Guo, C.; Yang, Y.; Han, T.; Chen, L.; Yin, W.; Gao, P.; Zhang, H.; Geng, J.; et al. Differential expression of estradiol and estrogen receptor α in severe preeclamptic pregnancies compared with normal pregnancies. *Mol. Med. Rep.* **2013**, *7*, 981–985. [CrossRef]
73. Zhang, Y.; Wang, T.; Shen, Y.; Wang, X.; Baker, P.N.; Zhao, A. 2-Methoxyestradiol deficiency is strongly related to hypertension in early onset severe pre-eclampsia. *Pregnancy Hypertens.* **2014**, *4*, 215–219. [CrossRef]
74. Açıkgöz, Ş.; Özmen Bayar, Ü.; Can, M.; Güven, B.; Mungan, G.; Doğan, S.; Sümbüloğlu, V. Levels of Oxidized LDL, Estrogens, and Progesterone in Placenta Tissues and Serum Paraoxonase Activity in Preeclampsia. *Mediat. Inflamm.* **2013**, *2013*, 1–6. [CrossRef]
75. Makieva, S.; Saunders, P.T.K.; Norman, J.E. Androgens in pregnancy: Roles in parturition. *Hum. Reprod. Update* **2014**, *20*, 542–559. [CrossRef]
76. Kallak, T.K.; Hellgren, C.; Skalkidou, A.; Sandelin-Francke, L.; Ubhayasekhera, K.; Bergquist, J.; Axelsson, O.; Comasco, E.; Campbell, R.E.; Poromaa, I.S. Maternal and female fetal testosterone levels are associated with maternal age and gestational weight gain. *Eur. J. Endocrinol.* **2017**, *177*, 379–388. [CrossRef]
77. Benten, W.P.M.; Guo, Z.; Krücken, J.; Wunderlich, F. Rapid effects of androgens in macrophages. *Steroids* **2004**, *69*, 585–590. [CrossRef]
78. Wunderlich, F.; Benten, W.P.M.; Lieberherr, M.; Guo, Z.; Stamm, O.; Wrehlke, C.; Sekeris, C.E.; Mossmann, H. Testosterone signaling in T cells and macrophages. *Steroids* **2002**, *67*, 535–538. [CrossRef]
79. Becerra-Díaz, M.; Strickland, A.B.; Keselman, A.; Heller, N.M. Androgen and Androgen Receptor as Enhancers of M2 Macrophage Polarization in Allergic Lung Inflammation. *J. Immunol.* **2018**, *201*, 2923–2933. [CrossRef]
80. Biró, O.; Fóthi, Á.; Alasztics, B.; Nagy, B.; Orbán, T.I.; Rigó, J. Circulating exosomal and Argonaute-bound microRNAs in preeclampsia. *Gene* **2019**, *692*, 138–144. [CrossRef]
81. Shen, L.; Li, Y.; Li, R.; Diao, Z.; Yany, M.; Wu, M.; Sun, H.; Yan, G.; Hu, Y. Placenta-associated serum exosomal miR-155 derived from patients with preeclampsia inhibits eNOS expression in human umbilical vein endothelial cells. *Int. J. Mol. Med.* **2018**, *41*, 1731–1739. [CrossRef]
82. Sammar, M.; Dragovic, R.; Meiri, H.; Vatish, M.; Sharabi-Nov, A.; Sargent, I.; Redman, C.; Tannetta, D. Reduced placental protein 13 (PP13) in placental derived syncytiotrophoblast extracellular vesicles in preeclampsia–A novel tool to study the impaired cargo transmission of the placenta to the maternal organs. *Placenta* **2018**, *66*, 17–25. [CrossRef]
83. Aouache, R.; Biquard, L.; Vaiman, D.; Miralles, F.; Aouache, R.; Biquard, L.; Vaiman, D.; Miralles, F. Oxidative Stress in Preeclampsia and Placental Diseases. *Int. J. Mol. Sci.* **2018**, *19*, 1496. [CrossRef]

84. Brownfoot, F.C.; Hannan, N.J.; Cannon, P.; Nguyen, V.; Hastie, R.; Parry, L.J.; Senadheera, S.; Tuohey, L.; Tong, S.; Kaitu'u-Lino, T.J. Sulfasalazine reduces placental secretion of antiangiogenic factors, up-regulates the secretion of placental growth factor and rescues endothelial dysfunction. *EBioMedicine* **2019**, *41*, 636–648. [CrossRef]
85. Valencia-Ortega, J.; Zárate, A.; Saucedo, R.; Hernández-Valencia, M.; Cruz, J.G.; Puello, E. Placental Proinflammatory State and Maternal Endothelial Dysfunction in Preeclampsia. *Gynecol. Obstet. Invest.* **2019**, *84*, 12–19. [CrossRef]
86. Harmon, A.C.; Ibrahim, T.; Cornelius, D.C.; Amaral, L.M.; Cunningham, M.W.; Wallace, K.; LaMarca, B. Placental CD4 + T cells isolated from preeclamptic women cause preeclampsia-like symptoms in pregnant nude-athymic rats. *Pregnancy Hypertens.* **2019**, *15*, 7–11. [CrossRef]
87. Geldenhuys, J.; Rossouw, T.M.; Lombaard, H.A.; Ehlers, M.M.; Kock, M.M. Disruption in the Regulation of Immune Responses in the Placental Subtype of Preeclampsia. *Front. Immunol.* **2018**, *9*, 1659. [CrossRef]
88. Wang, J.; Zhu, Q.W.; Cheng, X.Y.; Liu, J.Y.; Zhang, L.L.; Tao, Y.M.; Cui, Y.B.; Wei, Y. Assessment efficacy of neutrophil-lymphocyte ratio and monocyte-lymphocyte ratio in preeclampsia. *J. Reprod. Immunol.* **2019**, *132*, 29–34. [CrossRef]
89. Brien, M.E.; Boufaied, I.; Soglio, D.D.; Rey, E.; Leduc, L.; Girard, S. Distinct inflammatory profile in preeclampsia and postpartum preeclampsia reveal unique mechanisms. *Biol. Reprod.* **2019**, *100*, 187–194. [CrossRef]
90. Jabalie, G.; Ahmadi, M.; Koushaeian, L.; Eghbal-Fard, S.; Mehdizadeh, A.; Kamrani, A.; Abdollahi-Fard, S.; Farzadi, L.; Hojjat-Farsangi, M.; Nouri, M.; et al. Metabolic syndrome mediates proinflammatory responses of inflammatory cells in preeclampsia. *Am. J. Reprod. Immunol.* **2019**, *81*, e13086. [CrossRef]
91. Alahakoon, T.I.; Medbury, H.; Williams, H.; Fewings, N.; Wang, X.M.; Lee, V.W. Characterization of fetal monocytes in preeclampsia and fetal growth restriction. *J. Perinat. Med.* **2019**. [CrossRef]
92. Alahakoon, T.I.; Medbury, H.; Williams, H.; Fewings, N.; Wang, X.M.; Lee, V.W. Distribution of monocyte subsets and polarization in preeclampsia and intrauterine fetal growth restriction. *J. Obstet. Gynaecol. Res.* **2018**, *44*, 2135–2148. [CrossRef]
93. Ma, Y.; Ye, Y.; Zhang, J.; Ruan, C.-C.; Gao, P.-J. Immune imbalance is associated with the development of preeclampsia. *Medicine (Baltimore)* **2019**, *98*, e15080. [CrossRef]
94. Yang, S.W.; Cho, E.H.; Choi, S.Y.; Lee, Y.K.; Park, J.H.; Kim, M.K.; Park, J.Y.; Choi, H.J.; Lee, J.I.; Ko, H.M.; et al. DC-SIGN expression in Hofbauer cells may play an important role in immune tolerance in fetal chorionic villi during the development of preeclampsia. *J. Reprod. Immunol.* **2017**, *124*, 30–37. [CrossRef]
95. Tang, Z.; Buhimschi, I.A.; Buhimschi, C.S.; Tadesse, S.; Norwitz, E.; Niven-Fairchild, T.; Huang, S.-T.J.; Guller, S. Decreased Levels of Folate Receptor-β and Reduced Numbers of Fetal Macrophages (Hofbauer Cells) in Placentas from Pregnancies with Severe Pre-Eclampsia. *Am. J. Reprod. Immunol.* **2013**, *70*, 104–115. [CrossRef]
96. Evsen, M.S.; Kalkanli, S.; Deveci, E.; Sak, M.E.; Ozler, A.; Baran, O.; Erdem, E.; Seker, U. Human placental macrophages (Hofbauer cells) in severe preeclampsia complicated by HELLP syndrome: Immunohistochemistry of chorionic villi. *Anal. Quant. Cytopathol. Histopathol.* **2013**, *35*, 283–288.
97. Al-Khafaji, L.A.; Al-Yawer, M.A. Localization and counting of CD68-labelled macrophages in placentas of normal and preeclamptic women. In *AIP Conference Proceedings*; AIP Publishing: Melville, NY, USA, 2017; Volume 1888, p. 20011.
98. Saeed, I.; Yousaf, A.; Ali, S. Number of Hofbauer Cells in Placentae from Normal and Pre Eclamptic Gestation. *J. Rawalpindi Med. Coll.* **2018**, *22*, 76–78.
99. Przybyl, L.; Haase, N.; Golic, M.; Rugor, J.; Solano, M.E.; Arck, P.C.; Gauster, M.; Huppertz, B.; Emontzpohl, C.; Stoppe, C.; et al. CD74-downregulation of placental macrophage-trophoblastic interactions in preeclampsia. *Circ. Res.* **2016**, *119*, 55–68. [CrossRef]
100. Milosevic-Stevanovic, J.; Krstic, M.; Radovic-Janosevic, D.; Popovic, J.; Tasic, M.; Stojnev, S. Number of decidual natural killer cells & macrophages in pre-eclampsia. *Indian J. Med. Res.* **2016**, *144*, 823–830.
101. Williams, P.J.; Bulmer, J.N.; Searle, R.F.; Innes, B.A.; Robson, S.C. Altered decidual leucocyte populations in the placental bed in pre-eclampsia and foetal growth restriction: A comparison with late normal pregnancy. *Reproduction* **2009**, *138*, 177–184. [CrossRef]
102. Bürk, M.R.; Troeger, C.; Brinkhaus, R.; Holzgreve, W.; Hahn, S. Severely reduced presence of tissue macrophages in the basal plate of pre-eclamptic placentae. *Placenta* **2001**, *22*, 309–316. [CrossRef]

103. Brien, M.-E.; Baker, B.; Duval, C.; Gaudreault, V.; Jones, R.L.; Girard, S. Alarmins at the maternal–fetal interface: Involvement of inflammation in placental dysfunction and pregnancy complications. *Can. J. Physiol. Pharmacol.* **2018**, *97*, 206–212. [CrossRef]
104. Conrad, K.P.; Rabaglino, M.B.; Post Uiterweer, E.D. Emerging role for dysregulated decidualization in the genesis of preeclampsia. *Placenta* **2017**, *60*, 119–129. [CrossRef]
105. Sargent, I.L.; Borzychowski, A.M.; Redman, C.W.G. Immunoregulation in normal pregnancy and pre-eclampsia: An overview. *Reprod. Biomed. Online* **2006**, *13*, 680–686. [CrossRef]
106. Pinheiro, M.B.; Gomes, K.B.; Dusse, L.M.S. Fibrinolytic system in preeclampsia. *Clin. Chim. Acta* **2013**, *416*, 67–71. [CrossRef]
107. Xu, J.; Gu, Y.; Sun, J.; Zhu, H.; Lewis, D.F.; Wang, Y. Reduced CD200 expression is associated with altered Th1/Th2 cytokine production in placental trophoblasts from preeclampsia. *Am. J. Reprod. Immunol.* **2018**, *79*, 1–8. [CrossRef]
108. Aggarwal, R.; Jain, A.K.; Mittal, P.; Kohli, M.; Jawanjal, P.; Rath, G. Association of pro- and anti-inflammatory cytokines in preeclampsia. *J. Clin. Lab. Anal.* **2019**, 1–10. [CrossRef]
109. Abumaree, M.H.; Al Harthy, S.; Al Subayyil, A.M.; Alshabibi, M.A.; Abomaray, F.M.; Khatlani, T.; Kalionis, B.; El-Muzaini, M.F.; Al Jumah, M.A.; Jawdat, D.; et al. Decidua Basalis Mesenchymal Stem Cells Favor Inflammatory M1 Macrophage Differentiation In Vitro. *Cells* **2019**, *8*, 173. [CrossRef]
110. Abumaree, M.H.; Al Jumah, M.A.; Kalionis, B.; Jawdat, D.; Al Khaldi, A.; Abomaray, F.M.; Fatani, A.S.; Chamley, L.W.; Knawy, B.A. Human Placental Mesenchymal Stem Cells (pMSCs) Play a Role as Immune Suppressive Cells by Shifting Macrophage Differentiation from Inflammatory M1 to Anti-inflammatory M2 Macrophages. *Stem Cell Rev. Rep.* **2013**, *9*, 620–641. [CrossRef]
111. Wang, S.; Sun, F.; Han, M.; Liu, Y.; Zou, Q.; Wang, F.; Tao, Y.; Li, D.; Du, M.; Li, H.; et al. Trophoblast-derived hyaluronan promotes the regulatory phenotype of decidual macrophages. *Reproduction* **2019**, *157*, 189–198. [CrossRef]
112. FDA Approved Cellular and Gene Therapy Products. Available online: https://www.fda.gov/vaccines-blood-biologics/cellular-gene-therapy-products/approved-cellular-and-gene-therapy-products (accessed on 5 June 2019).
113. Fidler, I.J. Inhibition of pulmonary metastasis by intravenous injection of specifically activated macrophages. *Cancer Res.* **1974**, *34*, 1074–1078.
114. Liu, M.; Connor, R.S.O.; Trefely, S.; Graham, K.; Snyder, N.W.; Beatty, G.L. Metabolic rewiring of macrophages by CpG potentiates clearance of cancer cells and overcomes tumor-expressed CD47-mediated 'don't-eat-me' signal. *Nat. Immunol.* **2019**, *20*, 265–275. [CrossRef]
115. Van den Bosch, T.P.P.; Kannegieter, N.M.; Hesselink, D.A.; Baan, C.C.; Rowshani, A.T. Targeting the Monocyte–macrophage Lineage in Solid Organ Transplantation. *Front. Immunol.* **2017**, *8*, 153. [CrossRef]
116. Wynn, T.A.; Vannella, K.M. Macrophages in Tissue Repair, Regeneration, and Fibrosis. *Immunity* **2016**, *44*, 450–462. [CrossRef]
117. Weagel, E.; Smith, C.; Liu, P.G.; Robison, R.; O'Neill, K. Macrophage Polarization and Its Role in Cancer. *J. Clin. Cell. Immunol.* **2015**, *6*, 4–11.
118. Herold, J.; Pipp, F.; Fernandez, B.; Xing, Z.; Heil, M.; Tillmanns, H.; Braun-dullaeus, R.C. Transplantation of Monocytes: A Novel Strategy for In Vivo Augmentation of Collateral Vessel Growth. *Hum. Gene Ther.* **2004**, *12*, 1–12. [CrossRef]
119. Tsuboki, J.; Komohara, Y.; Nishimura, Y.; Imamura, Y.; Senju, S.; Haruta, M.; Tashiro, H.; Ohba, T.; Takaishi, K.; Dashdemberel, N.; et al. Novel therapeutic strategies for advanced ovarian cancer by using induced pluripotent stem cell-derived myelomonocytic cells producing interferon beta. *Cancer Sci.* **2018**, *109*, 3403–3410.
120. Chernykh, E.; Shevela, E.; Kafanova, M.; Sakhno, L.; Polovnikov, E.; Ostanin, A. Monocyte-derived macrophages for treatment of cerebral palsy: A study of 57 cases. *J. Neurorestoratology* **2018**, *6*, 41–47. [CrossRef]
121. Li, J.; Li, C.; Zhuang, Q.; Peng, B.; Zhu, Y.; Ye, Q.; Ming, Y. The Evolving Roles of Macrophages in Organ Transplantation. *J. Immunol. Res.* **2019**, *2019*, 5763430. [CrossRef]

122. Jeanty, C.; Derderian, S.C.; Mackenzie, T.C. Maternal-fetal cellular trafficking: Clinical implications and consequences. *Curr. Opin. Pediatr.* **2014**, *26*, 377–382. [CrossRef]
123. Fleck, S.; Bautista, G.; Keating, S.M.; Lee, T.H.; Keller, R.L.; Moon-Grady, A.J.; Gonzales, K.; Norris, P.J.; Busch, M.P.; Kim, C.J.; et al. Fetal production of growth factors and inflammatory mediators predicts pulmonary hypertension in congenital diaphragmatic hernia. *Pediatr. Res.* **2013**, *74*, 290–298. [CrossRef]

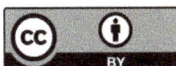

© 2019 by the authors. Licensee MDPI, Basel, Switzerland. This article is an open access article distributed under the terms and conditions of the Creative Commons Attribution (CC BY) license (http://creativecommons.org/licenses/by/4.0/).

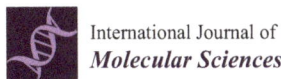

Review

Preeclampsia: The Relationship between Uterine Artery Blood Flow and Trophoblast Function

Anna Ridder [1,†], Veronica Giorgione [1,†], Asma Khalil [1,2] and Basky Thilaganathan [1,2,*]

1. Vascular Biology Research Centre, Molecular and Clinical Sciences Research Institute, St. George's University of London, London SW17 0RE, UK
2. Fetal Medicine Unit, St. George's University Hospitals NHS Foundation Trust, Blackshaw Road, London SW17 0RE, UK
* Correspondence: basky@pobox.com; Tel.: +44-20-8725-0071
† Joint first authors.

Received: 15 May 2019; Accepted: 28 June 2019; Published: 2 July 2019

Abstract: Maternal uterine artery blood flow is critical to maintaining the intrauterine environment, permitting normal placental function, and supporting fetal growth. It has long been believed that inadequate transformation of the maternal uterine vasculature is a consequence of primary defective trophoblast invasion and leads to the development of preeclampsia. That early pregnancy maternal uterine artery perfusion is strongly associated with placental cellular function and behaviour has always been interpreted in this context. Consistently observed changes in pre-conceptual maternal and uterine artery blood flow, abdominal pregnancy implantation, and late pregnancy have been challenging this concept, and suggest that abnormal placental perfusion may result in trophoblast impairment, rather than the other way round. This review focuses on evidence that maternal cardiovascular function plays a significant role in the pathophysiology of preeclampsia.

Keywords: preeclampsia; uterine artery; maternal cardiovascular system

1. Introduction

Maternal uterine artery blood flow is one of the critical factors that contribute to the preservation of the intrauterine environment, which permits normal placental function to support fetal growth and development. This is so, not only because maternal blood carries nutrition and removes waste, but also because oxygen delivered to the developing fetoplacental unit is directly limited by uterine blood flow. Spiral arterioles that perfuse the intervillous space undergo significant morphologic changes during this process, with uterine vascular adaptations resulting in five to 10-fold dilatation to meet the requirements of the fetoplacental unit [1]. It has long been believed that inadequate development of the uterine vasculature may be a consequence of primary defective placentation, which may lead to the development of both preeclampsia and fetal growth restriction. Understanding the relationship between uterine artery blood flow and placental development is fundamental to understanding normal placentation and its disruption in both preeclampsia and fetal growth restriction. This review focuses on the relationship between uterine artery blood flow and the trophoblast function, and discusses the insights provided into the pathophysiology of preeclampsia.

2. Uterine Artery Blood Flow Assessment

Maternal uterine arteries can be readily and reliably identified via ultrasound by the use of a color Doppler and the pulsatility index (resistance to blood flow), assessed concurrently with a pulsed wave Doppler. Resistance to blood flow in the uterine arteries falls with advancing gestation, a finding attributed to progressive trophoblastic invasion and transformation of the uterine spiral arteries into large vessels of low resistance [2]. Failure to transform has been described in preeclampsia and fetal growth restriction, resulting in the use of a uterine artery blood flow Doppler assessment to screen for these pregnancy problems [3]. A recent review of reviews for preeclampsia screening methods demonstrated that uterine artery Doppler assessment as a stand-alone test had the best predictive value for the prediction of early-onset preeclampsia when compared to other tests with a moderate predictive value, such as increased body mass index (BMI), placental growth factor (PLGF), and placental protein 13 (PP13). The analysis also showed that no single biomarker met the standards required for a clinical screening test, but that models, that combined markers, were more promising for the prediction of preeclampsia [4]. In a recent randomized controlled trial, the use of such multimodal screening to determine the risk of preterm preeclampsia, followed by the prescription of low-dose Aspirin prophylaxis before 16 weeks' gestation to the high-risk group, has been shown to halve the risk of preterm preeclampsia [5,6].

3. Uterine Artery Doppler Indices and Trophoblast Biology

The process of implantation, trophoblast development, and spiral artery transformation must involve many cellular and tissue processes to their effect. In view of the strong association between high uterine artery Doppler indices and the subsequent development of preeclampsia and fetal growth restriction, numerous authors have investigated trophoblast biology in samples obtained from pregnancies demonstrating high or low uterine artery Doppler resistance. Persistence of high resistance in the uterine artery Doppler indices in early pregnancy suggests that impaired trophoblast invasion and inadequate spiral artery remodeling has occurred [7].

3.1. Cell Injury and Apoptosis

Several studies have shown that placental tissues obtained from women with high-resistance uterine artery Doppler indices were more sensitive to apoptotic stimuli than placental tissue from women with normal indices [8–10]. Charolidi et al. examined the effect of tumor necrosis factor alpha (TNFα) on placental endothelial cell (PEC) apoptosis in the context of high vs. normal uterine artery Dopplers (Figure 1). They demonstrated that placental endothelial cells (PECs) from the high resistance index (RI) group exposed to TNFα had a 40% reduction in half-life compared to those from the normal RI group which were exposed to TNFα [10].

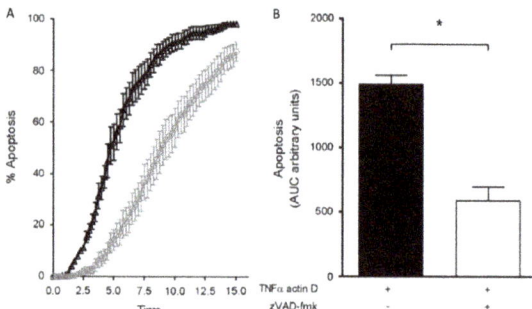

Figure 1. Apoptosis of first-trimester placental endothelial cells (PEC) from normal (normal RI) and high-resistance (high-RI) pregnancies in response to stimulation with TNFα and actinomycin D. First-trimester PEC were cultured with 30 ng/mL TNFα and 800 ng/mL actinomycin D. Images were taken every 15 min over 15 h. (**a**) The kinetics of the induction of apoptosis for PEC, high RI (n = 8 mean ± SEM, black symbols) and normal RI (n = 8 mean ± SEM, grey symbols). (**b**) In a separate cohort, normal-RI PEC were incubated with TNFα and actinomycin D alone (n = 4), as well as in the presence of the broad-spectrum caspase inhibitor, zVAD-fmk (n = 4). The results are expressed as mean ± SEM and * $p < 0.05$. Adapted with permission from Charolidi et al. [9].

3.2. Cell Motility and Penetration

During early placentation, trophoblast cells invade the endometrium and differentiate to form the villous structure of the placenta. Extravillous trophoblast (EVT) migrates from said villi to attach the placenta to the decidual stroma cells (DSC) of the uterus. Interstitial EVT invades through the decidua into the myometrium, while endovascular EVT migrates into the lumen of the spiral arteries, replacing vascular smooth muscle cells, leading to spiral artery transformation [11]. James-Allan et al., assessed DSC function in pregnancies with high or normal uterine artery Doppler resistance indices in the first trimester. Their results showed that the chemoattraction of trophoblast cells by the DSC was dysfunctional when the DSC was gathered from a pregnancy with high uterine artery resistance, thus suggesting that there may be an interplay between the DSC and EVT in early pregnancy which might play a role in impaired trophoblast invasion related to high-resistance uterine artery blood flow [12].

3.3. Cell-Cell Interaction

Decidual natural killer (dNK) cells make up about 70% of the leukocytes found in the decidua in the first trimester [12]. dNK cells secrete a number of factors that disrupt vascular cell interactions and allow for vascular smooth muscle cells to migrate out of the spiral arteries [13–15]. dNK cells have also been shown to increase EVT motility by hepatocyte growth-factor secretion, leading to chemoattraction of the EVT to the sites of remodeling [16]. Wallace et al. demonstrated that dNK cells isolated during the first trimester from pregnancies with high uterine artery Dopplers have decreased ability to chemoattract trophoblast cells and induce the outgrowth of the EVT from the villi when compared to those from pregnancies with normal uterine artery resistance [17].

3.4. Oxidative Stress and Hypoxia

During the first trimester of pregnancy, the placenta develops in an environment with a relatively low oxygen supply of only 20mmHg at 8 weeks, rising to >50 mmHg at 12 weeks, as the maternal uterine artery blood flow increases [18]. Hypoxia-inducible nuclear factors HIF1α and HIF2α are master regulators of the hypoxia response in tissues, and are also expressed in the early-pregnancy placenta [19,20]. Levels of HIF1α are significantly lower in placentas gathered from pregnancies with high uterine artery resistance despite the expectation that placental hypoxia or oxidative stress would be associated with higher levels of HIF1α [8]. The latter tissues expressed an altered balance of antioxidant enzyme activity (lower glutathione peroxidase and higher superoxide dismutase activity) when compared with normal placental tissue. These findings all suggest that hypoxia and oxidative stress appear to be a physiological state in early pregnancy.

3.5. Altered Gene Expression

Two studies of first-trimester placental samples at the time of chorionic villous sampling demonstrated differences in gene expression when the woman subsequently developed preeclampsia or fetal growth restriction compared to those who had a normal pregnancy outcome [21,22]. One study which examined gene expression by microarray in first-trimester placentas demonstrated 26 genes were variably expressed in women with high-resistance uterine artery indices. The genes that were significantly differentially expressed included those mainly responsible for cell death/apoptosis, stress response, inflammatory/immune response, and the metabolic and cyclooxygenase pathways [8].

These findings all suggest a close and likely causative association between early-pregnancy uterine artery Doppler indices, trophoblast invasion, and the subsequent development of preeclampsia (Figure 2). High uterine artery resistance indices are predictive of the development of preeclampsia, and also influence trophoblast cell migration, apoptosis, motility, invasion, cell–cell interaction, response to oxidative stress, and gene expression.

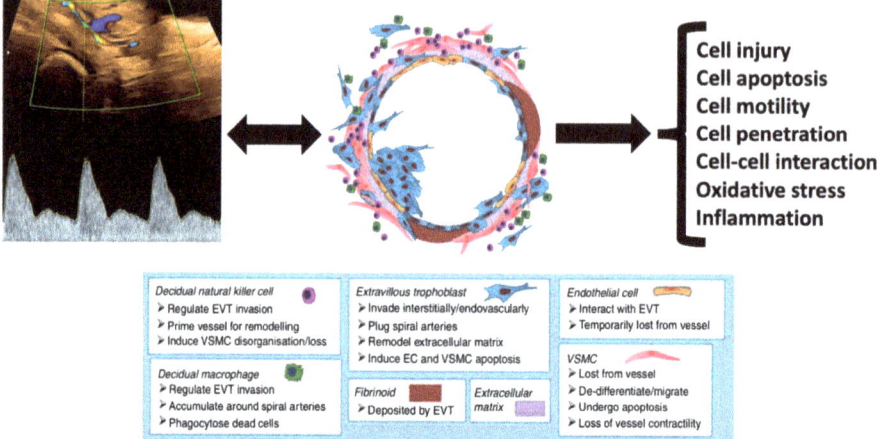

Figure 2. Relationship between uterine artery perfusion and cellular function. There are strong associations between maternal uterine artery perfusion and placental cellular function and behaviour. High-resistance Doppler indices (poor placental perfusion) is related to abnormalities of cell motility, penetration, and cell–cell interaction, as well as increased rates of oxidative stress, inflammation, cellular injury, and apoptosis. Adapted with permission from Cartwright et al. [23].

4. Uterine Artery Blood Flow and Trophoblast Development—A Causality Paradox

The relationships demonstrated in the previous section between uterine artery blood flow and trophoblast cell function/behavior have been conventionally interpreted as reflecting the process of trophoblast invasion, causing decreased resistance to flow in the uterine artery. This hypothesis is propagated by the long-held belief that impaired trophoblast development results in poor spiral artery transformation and creates a predisposition to the development of preeclampsia. However, a number of recent findings have led to the re-evaluation of the cause–effect inference between trophoblast development and spiral artery transformation.

4.1. Abdominal Pregnancy

A recent case report described an advanced abdominal pregnancy where the placenta was implanted outside the uterus in the right-lateral pelvic side wall [24]. The authors took the initiative to describe the uterine artery Doppler findings, which demonstrated a low-resistance waveform consistent with a normal pregnancy placentation. The question this observation raises is how complete spiral artery transformation occurred in order to create the observed low-resistance uterine artery waveform consistent with a normal pregnancy when the placenta was implanted in an extra-uterine site. Case reports are often disregarded by scientists and clinical academics; however, in certain unique situations, the exception observed in a single clinical case may prove (or disprove) the rule. However, the latter finding has previously been consistently reported in extra-uterine pregnancy [25], and suggests that changes observed universally in the maternal uterine and spiral arteries that are reflected by uterine Doppler indices do not occur as a direct consequence of trophoblast invasion.

4.2. Late Pregnancy Uterine Artery Resistance Changes

Binder et al. studied 5887 pregnancies with longitudinal uterine Doppler assessment into the third trimester. They found that one-third of patients demonstrated a de-novo increase in uterine artery resistance in the late third trimester, having previously exhibited normal indices—and that this group had a 30% higher prevalence of preeclampsia [26]. If the conventional paradigm that normal trophoblast invasion causes spiral artery transformation and a decrease in uterine artery resistance is true, then the demonstration of an increase in third-trimester uterine artery resistance would require hypothetical "de-transformation" of the spiral arteries—an implausible biological phenomenon. An alternative explanation for the uterine artery Doppler findings in abdominal or late pregnancy is that observed variations are not caused by localized trophoblast invasion, but may, in fact, reflect maternal systemic vascular resistance changes [27,28].

4.3. Ophthalmic and Radial Artery Doppler Assessment

If, indeed, uterine artery waveform changes reflect maternal systemic hemodynamic perturbations rather than trophoblast invasion, then the Doppler assessment of non-uterine arterial vessels should mirror the findings in the uterine artery. Recent systematic reviews of Doppler assessment of the radial and ophthalmic arteries in pregnancy have demonstrated that these vessels also reduce their resistance with advancing gestation and demonstrate persistent high resistance in the first trimester in pregnancies at increased risk of preeclampsia [29,30]. These vessels seem to have the same ability to predict preeclampsia as the use of the uterine artery Doppler in isolation.

4.4. Pre-Pregnancy Maternal Systemic Vascular Resistance

Above all, the findings suggest that maternal systemic and uterine vascular resistance in pregnancy changes independently of the direct physical consequences of placental invasion and trophoblast cell behavior. If this were the case, it would imply that the biological associations described previously are inversely causal—that is to say, that increased uterine resistance and poor placental perfusion may result in impaired trophoblast invasion and function, rather than the other way around. The hypothesis that maternal systemic and uterine vascular impairment predates placental maldevelopment is supported by a recent prospective study assessing pre-pregnancy cardiovascular function in 530 women [31]. Women who subsequently developed preeclampsia had lower cardiac output and higher systemic vascular resistance in the pre-pregnancy state prior to the development of the trophoblast. The authors concluded that an altered pre-pregnancy hemodynamic phenotype was associated with the subsequent development of preeclampsia and/or fetal growth restriction.

5. Reviewing Evidence Supporting Placental Origins of Preeclampsia

Etiology and pathophysiology are two specific terms referring to distinct processes. The former refers to the origin of the disease, whilst pathophysiology refers to the biological mechanism by which the disease manifests clinical signs and symptoms. Whilst the role of the placenta in the pathophysiology of preeclampsia is indisputable, the observations supporting the hypothesis that abnormal placentation is the etiology of preeclampsia are restricted to spiral artery transformation (discussed above), abnormal placental histology, and fetal size.

5.1. Placental Histology in Preeclampsia

Preeclampsia has been attributed to maternal vascular malperfusion of the placental bed, characterized by myometrial/decidual vascular lesions (incomplete or absent remodeling of maternal spiral arteries) and, more commonly, placental villous lesions, such as accelerated villous maturation, distal villous hypoplasia, increased syncytial knots, and villous infarction [32,33]. Notably, these vascular and villous lesions are not specific to preeclampsia, and are also found in many other pregnancy disorders, such as fetal growth restriction, spontaneous preterm labor, placental abruption, and stillbirth [34,35]. A recent systematic review assessed the prevalence of vascular and villous lesions in preeclamptic and normal pregnancies [36]. The authors demonstrated that placental villous and vascular lesions were not seen in the majority of preeclamptic pregnancies (pooled prevalence of 45.2% and 38.2% in all studies, respectively) and were also seen in 10–20% of normal pregnancies. Interestingly, the authors also reported a three-fold overreporting of placental lesions in preeclampsia when the pathologist was unblinded to the pregnancy diagnosis, compared to blind reporting [37].

These findings show that the placental histological vascular and villous lesions previously presumed to be characteristic of preeclampsia are neither specific nor sensitive markers of the disorder.

5.2. Fetal Size in Preeclampsia

Fetal growth restriction is considered a typical feature of preeclampsia resulting from the primary placental dysfunction that causes the disorder. It is fetal growth restriction and associated hypoxemia that predispose to increased risk of fetal, neonatal, and long-term adverse outcomes [38–40]. Epidemiological studies demonstrate that the majority of preterm preeclampsia cases result in fetal growth restriction. However, over 80% of preeclampsia occurs at a term where the rate of large-for-gestational-age births are as common as small-for-gestational-age births (both 15%), and most neonates are of normal size, even after the exclusion of diabetic pregnancies [41,42]. The finding of normal or excessive fetal growth in the majority of term preeclampsia cases is not consistent with impaired trophoblast invasion with placental dysfunction being the primary etiological process in preeclampsia.

6. Evidence for Cardiovascular Origins of Preeclampsia

Earlier, we outlined the strong associations between uterine artery blood flow and trophoblast cell biology. The data also suggested that trophoblast invasion was not directly responsible for early pregnancy changes in uterine, ophthalmic, and radial artery hemodynamics, leaving us to entertain the alternative possibility that maternal cardiovascular function might be involved. If maternal cardiovascular function plays such an etiological role, this should also be evident from the epidemiology of preeclampsia.

6.1. Predisposing Factors for Preeclampsia

It is not entirely apparent how maternal clinical risk factors for preeclampsia, such as advanced maternal age, ethnicity, obesity, diabetes, hyperlipidemia, renal dysfunction, and chronic hypertension influence trophoblast invasion and spiral artery transformation. However, these are well-recognized risk factors for cardiovascular morbidity, with established and plausible biological mechanisms explaining their pathophysiological roles [43,44]. Apart from these conventional clinical risk factors, systematic reviews of genetic risk factors demonstrated that plasminogen activator inhibitor-1 (PAI-1) and FMS-related tyrosine kinase 1 (FLT1)—known to be linked with risks of coronary heart disease and heart failure—were also strongly associated with preeclampsia [45–47].

6.2. Pre-Pregnancy Cardiovascular Function in Preeclampsia

If maternal risk factors for preeclampsia and adult cardiovascular disease indeed work through the same mechanisms, then there should be evidence for pre-pregnancy cardiovascular impairment in women destined to develop preeclampsia. Although there is a paucity of such pre-conceptual studies, a recent study by Foo et al. longitudinally assessed cardiovascular function in 356 spontaneously conceived pregnancies in apparently healthy women, starting from preconception. The authors noted that the 15 (4.2%) women who developed preeclampsia and fetal growth restriction had lower cardiac output and higher total peripheral resistance before the pre-conceptual period compared to those with uneventful pregnancies [31]. These findings support the concept that suboptimal pre-pregnancy cardiovascular function may predispose the woman to impaired uterine artery blood flow and poor trophoblast development as precursors to the development of preeclampsia. This assertion is supported by pre-conceptual echocardiographic evaluation of formerly preeclamptic women assessing their risk of recurrent preeclampsia. Those with recurrent preeclampsia had lower cardiac left ventricular mass and cardiac stroke volume in the pre-pregnancy period compared to women who had a normal second pregnancy [48].

6.3. Abnormal Cardiovascular Function in Pregnancy and Preeclampsia

First-trimester maternal cardiovascular parameters, such as mean arterial blood pressure and uterine artery resistance, are key biomarkers in the ASPRE (Combined Multimarker Screening and Randomized Patient Treatment with Aspirin for Evidence-Based Preeclampsia Prevention) screening algorithm that have very high accuracy for the prediction of preeclampsia, especially of preterm onset [5]. More sophisticated echocardiographic assessment has shown cardiac remodeling, impaired hemodynamics, and diastolic dysfunction, both in the first trimester and at mid-pregnancy in women destined to develop preeclampsia compared to those with normal outcomes [49–51]. Even in uncomplicated pregnancies, there are well-documented hemodynamic changes which peak in the middle of the third trimester before the cardiac output falls and systemic vascular resistance increases—a paradoxical finding, in view of the fact that maternal respiratory and metabolic demands continue to increase with advancing gestation [52,53]. Echocardiographic studies have demonstrated that in apparently healthy women with normal pregnancies, there are signs of mild cardiac maladaptation to the volume overload, such as an excessive increase in the left ventricular remodeling with associated diastolic dysfunction in a small but significant proportion of cases at term [54,55]. It is apparent that even a normal pregnancy confers a previously unrealized significant workload on the maternal cardiovascular system, and that in some cases, this results in asymptomatic cardiac dysfunction (Figure 3).

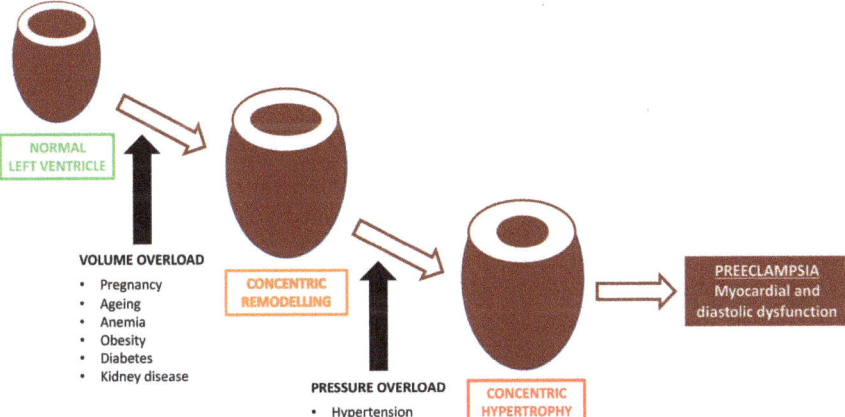

Figure 3. Left ventricle remodelling caused by pregnancy and preeclampsia. Alteration in (volume and pressure) loading conditions and the interaction with mechanical and neurohormonal factors results in ventricular remodeling. At an organ level, remodeling refers to changes in ventricular geometry, volume, and mass. Although remodelling is compensatory in certain pressure and volume overload conditions, progressive ventricular remodeling is ultimately a maladaptive process, contributing to the progression of symptomatic heart failure and an adverse outcome.

6.4. Cardiovascular Function in Preeclampsia

At the clinical onset of preeclampsia, significant hemodynamic impairment, such as lower cardiac output, abnormal ventricular geometry, and diastolic dysfunction have been demonstrated by several maternal echocardiography studies [49,56–58]. Severe preterm disease is associated with a worse cardiovascular profile, which is in turn associated with higher rates of serious peripartum complications, such as pulmonary edema [59–61]. In keeping with these findings, a number of cardiovascular biomarkers, such as ANP-related proteins and Corin, have been shown to be altered in pregnancy in women with preeclampsia [61–63].

6.5. Abnormal Cardiovascular Function Persists after Preeclampsia

Birth is considered to be a "cure" for preeclampsia. While it is not in doubt that the signs, symptoms, and risks of preeclampsia regress in the vast majority of women within days after birth, the paradigm that delivery normalizes maternal health after preeclampsia is not supported by postpartum studies. The risk for developing chronic hypertension postnatally is much higher after preeclampsia than after normotensive pregnancy, with rates of up to 30% for chronic hypertension being reported at one year postpartum [64]. A large register-based study of over a million women confirmed a 20-fold increase in the rate of antihypertensive medication in pregnancies complicated by hypertensive disorders used within the first year after birth [65]. Even in women who are normotensive postpartum, asymptomatic moderate-severe cardiac dysfunction was significantly higher in preterm preeclampsia (56%) compared with term preeclampsia (14%) versus matched controls [66]. The issue of whether the latter findings were caused by preeclampsia or pre-existing was evaluated in a large Norwegian epidemiological study, which suggested that the increased postpartum cardiovascular risk after preeclampsia may most probably be due to pre-existing risk factors, rather than a detrimental effect of preeclampsia on the maternal cardiovascular system [67].

7. Analogy between Preeclampsia and Diabetes in Pregnancy

There are multiple clinical similarities between hypertension and diabetes in pregnancy, despite the fact that one is considered purely of placental origin and the other related to maternal pancreatic dysfunction [68–70]. Both disorders are diagnosed because of new-onset hypertension or hyperglycemia in pregnancy, predisposing risk factors are similar to adult-onset disease, the definitive treatment is birth, and both disorders leave a post-partum legacy of disease (Figure 4). The most convincing alignment between these two disorders is apparent when one considers the phenotypes of the disease. Pre-gestational diabetes and preterm pre-eclampsia both reflect primary organ dysfunction, and as such, are predisposed to pre-pregnancy disease and have a more severe, early-onset phenotype [71,72]. Gestational diabetes and term preeclampsia reflect normal organ function, being overcome by increased vascular/glycemia load late in pregnancy, and as such, are difficult to screen for and present themselves later in pregnancy with a milder phenotype [73].

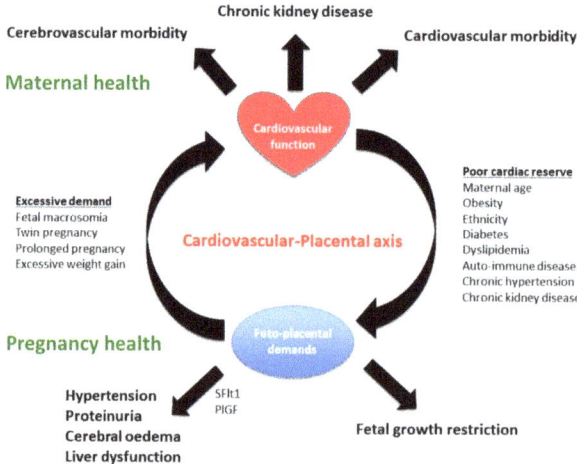

Figure 4. Interaction between maternal cardiovascular function and placental function, maternal health, and fetal well-being. Placental oxidative stress or hypoxia is related to the relative balance of cardiovascular functional reserve and the cardiovascular volume/resistance load of pregnancy. The final common pathway that results in the signs and symptoms of preeclampsia involves the release of placental vasoactive substances. Adapted with permission from Thilaganathan and Kalafat. Hypertension. 2019;73:522–531 [68].

8. Apparent Inconsistencies with Cardiovascular Origin Hypothesis

There are many iconic hypotheses applied to the placental origins of preeclampsia that stem out of clinical or epidemiological associations, such as those involving parity, change in partner, assisted reproductive technology, oocyte donation, and the "protective" effect of smoking. These hypotheses have assumed trophoblast origins of preeclampsia in their development, and a re-examination of their biological plausibility is justified.

8.1. Nulliparity

The risk of preeclampsia is about two times lower in multiparous women, and this has always been attributed to desensitization after exposure to paternal antigens in the placenta during previous pregnancies. Most epidemiological studies that report on parity and prevalence of preeclampsia do not account for the fact that, on average, multiparous women deliver approximately one week earlier than nulliparous women [74]. As shown in a recent randomized trial of induction of labor at 39 weeks' gestation versus expectant management, the effect of this temporal difference is to reduce the prevalence of preeclampsia by about 40%, thereby accounting for a significant proportion of the different rates of preeclampsia with parity [75]. Cardiac assessment of pregnancy has also consistently demonstrated that parous women have a more favorable cardiovascular profile throughout pregnancy compared to nulliparous women [76,77]. Such cardiac programming is a well-accepted phenomenon in non-pregnancy physiology, and provides a biologically plausible rationale for different rates of preeclampsia with parity.

8.2. Change in Partner

Partner change is also considered by many to be a risk factor for preeclampsia, and is attributed to a maternal immune reaction against new paternal antigens expressed in the placenta [78]. Despite original studies indicating the importance of partner change as a risk factor, larger and more recent epidemiological studies in normal and assisted conception pregnancies have demonstrated that partner change is a proxy for lengthening inter-pregnancy intervals and advanced maternal age. Skjaerven and colleagues have demonstrated that a change of partner is not associated with an increased risk of preeclampsia after adjustment for the interval between births and maternal age [79,80].

8.3. Oocyte Donation

The increased risk of preeclampsia with assisted conceptions was shown to be attributable to advanced maternal age and oocyte donation [81,82]. The influence of oocyte donation as a risk factor is in alignment with disrupted immunological tolerance, as previously postulated, until one considers that women who conceive by egg donation tend to be older, affected by premature ovarian failure, or have mosaic Turner syndrome—and all these factors are known to increase cardiovascular risk [83,84].

8.4. Smoking

While it is well-established that smoking increases risk for poor fetal growth, its relation to preeclampsia is more controversial and not consistent with the placental origins hypothesis considering that a meta-analysis showed that smoking is inversely associated with the incidence of preeclampsia [85]. However, smoking is known to increase maternal carbon monoxide levels, which inhibit levels of sFlt-1 and increase those of PlGF—the opposite of what occurs in preeclampsia [86,87]. Furthermore, carbon monoxide also has a protracted hypotensive effect, which would decrease the diagnosis of high blood pressure and, as a consequence, paradoxically reduce the prevalence of preeclampsia whilst increasing the risk of poor fetal growth [88].

9. Conclusions

Placental cellular function and development may be controlled by maternal systemic and local uterine cardiovascular perfusion, rather than vice versa. The key role of the placenta and its discarded products in causing maternal endothelial disfunction during pregnancy is doubtless; nevertheless, the predisposition of women with cardiovascular dysfunction for developing preeclampsia, the development of cardiovascular dysfunction prior to disease onset, the predominance of cardiovascular signs/biology at presentation, and the long-term cardiovascular health risks post-partum all support the assertion that preeclampsia could be a primary cardiovascular disorder. Significant advances in screening, diagnosis, management, and post-partum cardiovascular health after preeclampsia may occur as we acknowledge this paradigm shift in disease causality.

Author Contributions: Conceptualization, B.T.; Writing—Original Draft Preparation, A.R. and V.G.; Writing—Review & Editing, B.T. and A.K.

Funding: Anna Ridder and Veronica Giorgione's are part of the iPLACENTA project, which has received funding from the European Union's Horizon 2020 research and innovation programme under the Marie Skłodowska-Curie grant agreement No 765274.

Conflicts of Interest: The authors declare no conflict of interest. The funder had no role in the design of the study and in the writing of the manuscript.

References

1. Burton, G.J.; Woods, A.W.; Jauniaux, E.; Kingdom, J.C.P. Rheological and Physiological Consequences of Conversion of the Maternal Spiral Arteries for Uteroplacental Blood Flow during Human Pregnancy. *Placenta* **2009**, *30*, 473–482. [CrossRef] [PubMed]
2. Osol, G.; Mandala, M. Maternal uterine vascular remodeling during pregnancy. *Physiology* **2009**, *24*, 58–71. [CrossRef]
3. Cnossen, J.; Morris, R.; ter Riet, G.; Mol, B.W.; van der Post, J.A.; Coomarasamy, A.; Zwinderman, A.H.; Robson, S.C.; Bindels, P.J.; Kleijnen, J.; et al. Use of uterine artery Doppler ultrasonography to predict pre-eclampsia and intrauterine growth restriction: a systematic review and bivariable meta-analysis. *CMAJ* **2008**, *178*, 1–11. [CrossRef] [PubMed]
4. Townsend, R.; Khalil, A.; Premakumar, Y.; Allotey, J.; Snell, K.I.E.; Chan, C.; Chappell, L.C.; Hooper, R.; Green, M.; Mol, B.W.; et al. IPPIC Network. Prediction of pre-eclampsia: review of reviews. *Ultrasound Obstet. Gynecol* **2018**. [CrossRef] [PubMed]
5. Rolnik, D.L.; Wright, D.; Poon, L.C.; O'Gorman, N.; Syngelaki, A.; de Paco Matallana, C.; Akolekar, R.; Cicero, S.; Janga, D.; Singh, M.; et al. Aspirin versus Placebo in Pregnancies at High Risk for Preterm Preeclampsia. *N. Engl. J. Med.* **2017**, *377*, 613–622. [CrossRef] [PubMed]
6. Velauthar, L.; Plana, M.N.; Kalidindi, M.; Zamora, J.; Thilaganathan, B.; Illanes, S.E.; Khan, K.S.; Aquilina, J.; Thangaratinam, S. First-trimester uterine artery Doppler and adverse pregnancy outcome: A meta-analysis involving 55,974 women. *Ultrasound Obstet. Gynecol.* **2014**, *43*, 500–507. [CrossRef] [PubMed]
7. Prefumo, F.; Sebire, N.J.; Thilaganathan, B. Decreased endovascular trophoblast invasion in first trimester pregnancies with high-resistance uterine artery Doppler indices. *Hum. Reprod.* **2004**, *19*, 206–209. [CrossRef]
8. Leslie, K.; Whitley, G.S.J.; Herse, F.; Dechend, R.; Ashton, S.V.; Laing, K.; Thilaganathan, B.; Cartwright, J.E. Increased Apoptosis, Altered Oxygen Signaling, and Antioxidant Defenses in First-Trimester Pregnancies with High-Resistance Uterine Artery Blood Flow. *Am. J. Pathol.* **2015**, *185*, 2731–2741. [CrossRef]
9. Whitley, G.S.J.; Dash, P.R.; Ayling, L.J.; Prefumo, F.; Thilaganathan, B.; Cartwright, J.E. Increased apoptosis in first trimester extravillous trophoblasts from pregnancies at higher risk of developing preeclampsia. *Am. J. Pathol.* **2007**, *170*, 1903–1909. [CrossRef]
10. Charolidi, N.; Host, A.J.; Ashton, S.; Tryfonos, Z.; Leslie, K.; Thilaganathan, B.; Cartwright, J.E.; Whitley, G.S. First trimester placental endothelial cells from pregnancies with abnormal uterine artery Doppler are more sensitive to apoptotic stimuli. *Lab. Investig.* **2018**, *99*, 411–420. [CrossRef]
11. Pijnenborg, R.; Bland, J.M.; Robertson, W.B.; Dixon, G.; Brosens, I. The pattern of interstitial trophoblastic invasion of the myometrium in early human pregnancy. *Placenta* **1981**, *2*, 303–316. [CrossRef]

12. James-Allan, L.B.; Whitley, G.S.; Leslie, K.; Wallace, A.E.; Cartwright, J.E. Decidual cell regulation of trophoblast is altered in pregnancies at risk of pre-eclampsia. *J. Mol. Endocrinol.* **2018**, *60*, 239–246. [CrossRef] [PubMed]
13. James, J.L.; Whitley, G.S.; Cartwright, J.E. Pre-eclampsia: Fitting together the placental, immune and cardiovascular pieces. *J. Pathol.* **2010**, *221*, 363–378. [CrossRef] [PubMed]
14. Smith, S.D.; Dunk, C.E.; Aplin, J.D.; Harris, L.K.; Jones, R.L. Evidence for Immune Cell Involvement in Decidual Spiral Arteriole Remodeling in Early Human Pregnancy. *Am. J. Pathol.* **2009**, *174*, 1959–1971. [CrossRef] [PubMed]
15. Naruse, K.; Lash, G.E.; Innes, B.A.; Otun, H.A.; Searle, R.F.; Robson, S.C.; Bulmer, J.N. Localization of matrix metalloproteinase (MMP)-2, MMP-9 and tissue inhibitors for MMPs (TIMPs) in uterine natural killer cells in early human pregnancy. *Hum. Reprod.* **2008**, *24*, 553–561. [CrossRef]
16. Fraser, R.; Whitley, G.S.; Johnstone, A.P.; Host, A.J.; Sebire, N.J.; Thilaganathan, B.; Cartwright, J.E. Impaired decidual natural killer cell regulation of vascular remodelling in early human pregnancies with high uterine artery resistance. *J. Pathol.* **2012**, *228*, 322–332. [CrossRef]
17. Wallace, A.E.; Host, A.J.; Whitley, G.S.; Cartwright, J.E. Decidual natural killer cell interactions with trophoblasts are impaired in pregnancies at increased risk of preeclampsia. *Am. J. Pathol.* **2013**, *183*, 1853–1861. [CrossRef]
18. Jauniaux, E.; Watson, A.L.; Hempstock, J.; Bao, Y.-P.; Skepper, J.N.; Burton, G.J. Onset of Maternal Arterial Blood Flow and Placental Oxidative Stress. *Am. J. Pathol.* **2000**, *157*, 2111–2122. [CrossRef]
19. Caniggia, I.; Winter, J.; Lye, S.J.; Post, M. Oxygen and placental development during the first trimester: Implications for the pathophysiology of pre-eclampsia. *Placenta* **2000**, *21*, S25–S30. [CrossRef]
20. Semenza, G.L.; Nejfelt, M.K.; Chi, S.M.; Antonarakis, S.E. Hypoxia-inducible nuclear factors bind to an enhancer element located 3′ to the human erythropoietin gene. *Proc. Natl. Acad. Sci USA* **1991**, *88*, 5680. [CrossRef]
21. Founds, S.A.; Conley, Y.P.; Lyons-Weiler, J.F.; Jeyabalan, A.; Allen Hogge, W.; Conrad, K.P. Altered Global Gene Expression in First Trimester Placentas of Women Destined to Develop Preeclampsia. *Placenta* **2009**, *30*, 15–24. [CrossRef] [PubMed]
22. Farina, A.; Sekizawa, A.; De Sanctis, P.; Purwosunu, Y.; Okai, T.; Cha, D.H.; Kang, J.H.; Vicenzi, C.; Tempesta, A.; Wibowo, N.; et al. Gene expression in chorionic villous samples at 11 weeks' gestation from women destined to develop preeclampsia. *Prenat Diagn.* **2008**, *28*, 956–961. [CrossRef]
23. Cartwright, J.E.; Fraser, R.; Leslie, K.; Wallace, A.E.; James, J.L. Remodelling at the maternal–fetal interface: relevance to human pregnancy disorders. *Reproduction.* **2010**, *140*, 803–813. [CrossRef] [PubMed]
24. Collins, S.L.; Grant, D.; Black, R.S.; Vellayan, M.; Impey, L. Abdominal pregnancy: A perfusion confusion? *Placenta* **2011**, *32*, 793–795. [CrossRef] [PubMed]
25. Acácio, G.L. Uterine artery Doppler patterns in abdominal pregnancy. *Ultrasound Obstet. Gynecol.* **2002**, *20*, 194–196. [CrossRef] [PubMed]
26. Binder, J.; Monaghan, C.A.; Carta, S.; Thilaganathan, B.; Khalil, A. OP17.07: Worsening of the uterine artery Doppler is associated with the development of hypertensive disorders of pregnancy. *Ultrasound Obstet. Gynecol.* **2017**, *50*, 104. [CrossRef]
27. Burton, G.J.; Nelson, D.M. Case reports: The exceptions that challenge the rules. *Placenta* **2011**, *32*, 715. [CrossRef]
28. Leslie, K.; Thilaganathan, B. A perfusion confusion? *Placenta* **2012**, *33*, 230. [CrossRef]
29. Kalafat, E.; Laoreti, A.; Khalil, A.; Da Silva Costa, F.; Thilaganathan, B. Ophthalmic artery Doppler for prediction of pre-eclampsia: systematic review and meta-analysis. *Ultrasound Obstet. Gynecol.* **2018**, *51*, 731–737. [CrossRef]
30. Osman, M.W.; Nath, M.; Breslin, E.; Khalil, A.; Webb, D.R.; Robinson, T.G.; Mousa, H.A. Association between arterial stiffness and wave reflection with subsequent development of placental-mediated diseases during pregnancy: Findings of a systematic review and meta-analysis. *J. Hypertens* **2018**, *36*, 1005–1014. [CrossRef]
31. Foo, F.L.; Mahendru, A.A.; Masini, G.; Fraser, A.; Cacciatore, S.; MacIntyre, D.A.; McEniery, C.M.; Wilkinson, I.B.; Bennett, P.R.; Lees, C.C. Association Between Prepregnancy Cardiovascular Function and Subsequent Preeclampsia or Fetal Growth Restriction. *Hypertension.* **2018**, *72*, 442–450. [CrossRef] [PubMed]
32. Khong, T.Y.; Mooney, E.E.; Ariel, I.; Balmus, N.C.; Boyd, T.K.; Brundler, M.A.; Derricott, H.; Evans, M.J.; Faye-Petersen, O.M.; Gillan, J.E.; et al. Sampling and definitions of placental lesions: Amsterdam placental workshop group consensus statement. *Arch. Pathol. Lab. Med.* **2016**, *140*, 698–713. [CrossRef] [PubMed]

33. Parks, W.T. Manifestations of hypoxia in the second and third trimester placenta. *Birth Defects Res.* **2017**, *109*, 1345–1357. [CrossRef]
34. Brosens, I.; Pijnenborg, R.; Vercruysse, L.; Romero, R. The "great obstetrical syndromes" are associated with disorders of deep placentation. *Am. J. Obstet. Gynecol.* **2011**, *204*, 193–201. [CrossRef] [PubMed]
35. Catov, J.M.; Scifres, C.M.; Caritis, S.N.; Bertolet, M.; Larkin, J.; Parks, W.T. Neonatal outcomes following preterm birth classified according to placental features. *Am. J. Obstet. Gynecol* **2017**, *216*, e411–e414. [CrossRef]
36. Falco, M.L.; Sivanathan, J.; Laoreti, A.; Thilaganathan, B.; Khalil, A. Placental histopathology associated with pre-eclampsia: Systematic review and meta-analysis. *Ultrasound Obstet. Gynecol.* **2017**, *50*, 295–301. [CrossRef] [PubMed]
37. Sebire, N.J. Placental histology findings in relation to pre-eclampsia: Implications for interpretation of retrospective studies. *Ultrasound Obstet. Gynecol.* **2017**, *50*, 291–292. [CrossRef]
38. Madden, J.V.; Flatley, C.J.; Kumar, S. Term small-for-gestational-age infants from low-risk women are at significantly greater risk of adverse neonatal outcomes. *Am. J. Obstet. Gynecol* **2018**, *218*, e521–e529. [CrossRef]
39. Lees, C.C.; Marlow, N.; van Wassenaer-Leemhuis, A.; Arabin, B.; Bilardo, C.M.; Brezinka, C.; Calvert, S.; Derks, J.B.; Diemert, A.; Duvekot, J.J.; et al. 2 year neurodevelopmental and intermediate perinatal outcomes in infants with very preterm fetal growth restriction (truffle): A randomised trial. *Lancet* **2015**, *385*, 2162–2172. [CrossRef]
40. Khalil, A.A.; Morales-Rosello, J.; Elsaddig, M.; Khan, N.; Papageorghiou, A.; Bhide, A.; Thilaganathan, B. The association between fetal doppler and admission to neonatal unit at term. *Am. J. Obstet. Gynecol.* **2015**, *213*, e51–e57. [CrossRef]
41. Verlohren, S.; Melchiorre, K.; Khalil, A.; Thilaganathan, B. Uterine artery doppler, birth weight and timing of onset of pre-eclampsia: Providing insights into the dual etiology of late-onset pre-eclampsia. *Ultrasound Obstet Gynecol* **2014**, *44*, 293–298. [CrossRef] [PubMed]
42. Rasmussen, S.; Irgens, L.M.; Espinoza, J. Maternal obesity and excess of fetal growth in pre-eclampsia. *BJOG* **2014**, *121*, 1351–1357. [CrossRef] [PubMed]
43. Tangren, J.S.; Powe, C.E.; Ankers, E.; Ecker, J.; Bramham, K.; Hladunewich, M.A.; Karumanchi, S.A.; Thadhani, R. Pregnancy outcomes after clinical recovery from aki. *J. Am. Soc. Nephrol.* **2017**, *28*, 1566–1574. [CrossRef]
44. Egeland, G.M.; Klungsoyr, K.; Oyen, N.; Tell, G.S.; Naess, O.; Skjaerven, R. Preconception cardiovascular risk factor differences between gestational hypertension and preeclampsia: Cohort norway study. *Hypertension* **2016**, *67*, 1173–1180. [CrossRef] [PubMed]
45. Song, C.; Burgess, S.; Eicher, J.D.; O'Donnell, C.J.; Johnson, A.D. Causal effect of plasminogen activator inhibitor type 1 on coronary heart disease. *J. Am. Heart Assoc.* **2017**, *6*. [CrossRef]
46. Lokki, A.I.; Daly, E.; Triebwasser, M.; Kurki, M.I.; Roberson, E.D.O.; Happola, P.; Auro, K.; Perola, M.; Heinonen, S.; Kajantie, E.; et al. Protective low-frequency variants for preeclampsia in the fms related tyrosine kinase 1 gene in the finnish population. *Hypertension* **2017**, *70*, 365–371. [CrossRef] [PubMed]
47. Giannakou, K.; Evangelou, E.; Papatheodorou, S.I. Genetic and non-genetic risk factors for pre-eclampsia: Umbrella review of systematic reviews and meta-analyses of observational studies. *Ultrasound Obstet. Gynecol.* **2018**, *51*, 720–730. [CrossRef]
48. Ghossein-Doha, C.; Spaanderman, M.E.; Al Doulah, R.; Van Kuijk, S.M.; Peeters, L.L. Maternal cardiac adaptation to subsequent pregnancy in formerly pre-eclamptic women according to recurrence of pre-eclampsia. *Ultrasound Obstet. Gynecol.* **2016**, *47*, 96–103. [CrossRef]
49. Melchiorre, K.; Sutherland, G.; Sharma, R.; Nanni, M.; Thilaganathan, B. Mid-gestational maternal cardiovascular profile in preterm and term pre-eclampsia: A prospective study. *BJOG* **2013**, *120*, 496–504. [CrossRef]
50. Khaw, A.; Kametas, N.A.; Turan, O.M.; Bamfo, J.E.; Nicolaides, K.H. Maternal cardiac function and uterine artery doppler at 11–14 weeks in the prediction of pre-eclampsia in nulliparous women. *BJOG* **2008**, *115*, 369–376. [CrossRef]
51. Ambia, A.M.; Morgan, J.L.; Wells, C.E.; Roberts, S.W.; Sanghavi, M.; Nelson, D.B.; Cunningham, F.G. Perinatal outcomes associated with abnormal cardiac remodeling in women with treated chronic hypertension. *Am. J. Obstet. Gynecol.* **2018**, *218*, e511–e517. [CrossRef]
52. Vinayagam, D.; Thilaganathan, B.; Stirrup, O.; Mantovani, E.; Khalil, A. Maternal hemodynamics in normal pregnancy: Reference ranges and role of maternal characteristics. *Ultrasound Obstet. Gynecol.* **2018**, *51*, 665–671. [CrossRef] [PubMed]

53. Meah, V.L.; Cockcroft, J.R.; Backx, K.; Shave, R.; Stohr, E.J. Cardiac output and related haemodynamics during pregnancy: A series of meta-analyses. *Heart* **2016**, *102*, 518–526. [CrossRef] [PubMed]
54. Savu, O.; Jurcut, R.; Giusca, S.; van Mieghem, T.; Gussi, I.; Popescu, B.A.; Ginghina, C.; Rademakers, F.; Deprest, J.; Voigt, J.U. Morphological and functional adaptation of the maternal heart during pregnancy. *Circ. Cardiovasc Imaging* **2012**, *5*, 289–297. [CrossRef] [PubMed]
55. Melchiorre, K.; Sharma, R.; Khalil, A.; Thilaganathan, B. Maternal cardiovascular function in normal pregnancy: Evidence of maladaptation to chronic volume overload. *Hypertension* **2016**, *67*, 754–762. [CrossRef] [PubMed]
56. Valensise, H.; Vasapollo, B.; Gagliardi, G.; Novelli, G.P. Early and late preeclampsia: Two different maternal hemodynamic states in the latent phase of the disease. *Hypertension* **2008**, *52*, 873–880. [CrossRef] [PubMed]
57. De Haas, S.; Ghossein-Doha, C.; Geerts, L.; van Kuijk, S.M.J.; van Drongelen, J.; Spaanderman, M.E.A. Cardiac remodeling in normotensive pregnancy and in pregnancy complicated by hypertension: Systematic review and meta-analysis. *Ultrasound Obstet. Gynecol.* **2017**, *50*, 683–696. [CrossRef] [PubMed]
58. Castleman, J.S.; Ganapathy, R.; Taki, F.; Lip, G.Y.; Steeds, R.P.; Kotecha, D. Echocardiographic structure and function in hypertensive disorders of pregnancy: A systematic review. *Circ. Cardiovasc Imaging* **2016**, *9*. [CrossRef]
59. Vaught, A.J.; Kovell, L.C.; Szymanski, L.M.; Mayer, S.A.; Seifert, S.M.; Vaidya, D.; Murphy, J.D.; Argani, C.; O'Kelly, A.; York, S.; et al. Acute cardiac effects of severe pre-eclampsia. *J. Am. Coll Cardiol* **2018**, *72*, 1–11. [CrossRef]
60. Melchiorre, K.; Sutherland, G.R.; Watt-Coote, I.; Liberati, M.; Thilaganathan, B. Severe myocardial impairment and chamber dysfunction in preterm preeclampsia. *Hypertens Pregnancy* **2012**, *31*, 454–471. [CrossRef]
61. Borges, V.T.M.; Zanati, S.G.; Peracoli, M.T.S.; Poiati, J.R.; Romao-Veiga, M.; Peracoli, J.C.; Thilaganathan, B. Maternal left ventricular hypertrophy and diastolic dysfunction and brain natriuretic peptide concentration in early- and late-onset pre-eclampsia. *Ultrasound Obstet. Gynecol.* **2018**, *51*, 519–523. [CrossRef] [PubMed]
62. Tihtonen, K.M.; Koobi, T.; Vuolteenaho, O.; Huhtala, H.S.; Uotila, J.T. Natriuretic peptides and hemodynamics in preeclampsia. *Am. J. Obstet. Gynecol.* **2007**, *196*, 328.e1–328.e7. [CrossRef] [PubMed]
63. Khalil, A.; Maiz, N.; Garcia-Mandujano, R.; Elkhouli, M.; Nicolaides, K.H. Longitudinal changes in maternal corin and mid-regional proatrial natriuretic peptide in women at risk of pre-eclampsia. *Ultrasound Obstet. Gynecol.* **2015**, *45*, 190–198. [CrossRef] [PubMed]
64. Benschop, L.; Duvekot, J.J.; Versmissen, J.; van Broekhoven, V.; Steegers, E.A.P.; Roeters van Lennep, J.E. Blood pressure profile 1 year after severe preeclampsia. *Hypertension* **2018**, *71*, 491–498. [CrossRef] [PubMed]
65. Behrens, I.; Basit, S.; Melbye, M.; Lykke, J.A.; Wohlfahrt, J.; Bundgaard, H.; Thilaganathan, B.; Boyd, H.A. Risk of post-pregnancy hypertension in women with a history of hypertensive disorders of pregnancy: Nationwide cohort study. *BMJ* **2017**, *358*, j3078. [CrossRef]
66. Melchiorre, K.; Sutherland, G.R.; Liberati, M.; Thilaganathan, B. Preeclampsia is associated with persistent postpartum cardiovascular impairment. *Hypertension* **2011**, *58*, 709–715. [CrossRef]
67. Romundstad, P.R.; Magnussen, E.B.; Smith, G.D.; Vatten, L.J. Hypertension in pregnancy and later cardiovascular risk: Common antecedents? *Circulation* **2010**, *122*, 579–584. [CrossRef]
68. Thilaganathan, B.; Kalafat, E. Cardiovascular system in preeclampsia and beyond. *Hypertension* **2019**, *73*, 522–531. [CrossRef]
69. Thilaganathan, B. Pre-eclampsia and the cardiovascular-placental axis. *Ultrasound Obstet. Gynecol.* **2018**, *51*, 714–717. [CrossRef]
70. Perry, H.; Khalil, A.; Thilaganathan, B. Preeclampsia and the cardiovascular system: An update. *Trends Cardiovasc Med.* **2018**, *28*, 505–513. [CrossRef]
71. Alexopoulos, A.S.; Blair, R.; Peters, A.L. Management of preexisting diabetes in pregnancy: A review. *JAMA* **2019**, *321*, 1811–1819. [CrossRef] [PubMed]
72. Nzelu, D.; Dumitrascu-Biris, D.; Nicolaides, K.H.; Kametas, N.A. Chronic hypertension: First-trimester blood pressure control and likelihood of severe hypertension, preeclampsia, and small for gestational age. *Am. J. Obstet. Gynecol.* **2018**, *218*, 337.e1–337.e7. [CrossRef] [PubMed]
73. Weissgerber, T.L.; Mudd, L.M. Preeclampsia and diabetes. *Curr. Diab. Rep.* **2015**, *15*, 9. [CrossRef] [PubMed]
74. Smith, G.C. Use of time to event analysis to estimate the normal duration of human pregnancy. *Hum. Reprod* **2001**, *16*, 1497–1500. [CrossRef] [PubMed]

75. Grobman, W.A.; Rice, M.M.; Reddy, U.M.; Tita, A.T.N.; Silver, R.M.; Mallett, G.; Hill, K.; Thom, E.A.; El-Sayed, Y.Y.; Perez-Delboy, A.; et al. Labor induction versus expectant management in low-risk nulliparous women. *N. Engl. J. Med.* **2018**, *379*, 513–523. [CrossRef] [PubMed]
76. Turan, O.M.; De Paco, C.; Kametas, N.; Khaw, A.; Nicolaides, K.H. Effect of parity on maternal cardiac function during the first trimester of pregnancy. *Ultrasound Obstet Gynecol* **2008**, *32*, 849–854. [CrossRef]
77. Ling, H.Z.; Guy, G.; Bisquera, A.; Poon, L.C.; Nicolaides, K.H.; Kametas, N.A. The effect of parity on longitudinal maternal hemodynamics. *Am. J. Obstet. Gynecol.* **2019**. [CrossRef]
78. Li, D.K.; Wi, S. Changing paternity and the risk of preeclampsia/eclampsia in the subsequent pregnancy. *Am. J. Epidemiol.* **2000**, *151*, 57–62. [CrossRef]
79. Tandberg, A.; Klungsoyr, K.; Romundstad, L.B.; Skjaerven, R. Pre-eclampsia and assisted reproductive technologies: Consequences of advanced maternal age, interbirth intervals, new partner and smoking habits. *BJOG* **2015**, *122*, 915–922. [CrossRef]
80. Skjaerven, R.; Wilcox, A.J.; Lie, R.T. The interval between pregnancies and the risk of preeclampsia. *N. Engl. J. Med.* **2002**, *346*, 33–38. [CrossRef]
81. Masoudian, P.; Nasr, A.; de Nanassy, J.; Fung-Kee-Fung, K.; Bainbridge, S.A.; El Demellawy, D. Oocyte donation pregnancies and the risk of preeclampsia or gestational hypertension: A systematic review and metaanalysis. *Am. J. Obstet. Gynecol.* **2016**, *214*, 328–339. [CrossRef] [PubMed]
82. Jeve, Y.B.; Potdar, N.; Opoku, A.; Khare, M. Donor oocyte conception and pregnancy complications: A systematic review and meta-analysis. *BJOG* **2016**, *123*, 1471–1480. [CrossRef] [PubMed]
83. Stochholm, K.; Juul, S.; Juel, K.; Naeraa, R.W.; Gravholt, C.H. Prevalence, incidence, diagnostic delay, and mortality in turner syndrome. *J. Clin. Endocrinol. Metab.* **2006**, *91*, 3897–3902. [CrossRef] [PubMed]
84. Roeters van Lennep, J.E.; Heida, K.Y.; Bots, M.L.; Hoek, A. Collaborators of the Dutch Multidisciplinary Guideline Development Group on Cardiovascular Risk Management after Reproductive, D. Cardiovascular disease risk in women with premature ovarian insufficiency: A systematic review and meta-analysis. *Eur J. Prev. Cardiol.* **2016**, *23*, 178–186. [CrossRef] [PubMed]
85. Wei, J.; Liu, C.X.; Gong, T.T.; Wu, Q.J.; Wu, L. Cigarette smoking during pregnancy and preeclampsia risk: A systematic review and meta-analysis of prospective studies. *Oncotarget* **2015**, *6*, 43667–43678. [CrossRef] [PubMed]
86. Mehendale, R.; Hibbard, J.; Fazleabas, A.; Leach, R. Placental angiogenesis markers sflt-1 and plgf: Response to cigarette smoke. *Am. J. Obstet Gynecol* **2007**, *197*, 363.e1–363.e5. [CrossRef] [PubMed]
87. Cudmore, M.; Ahmad, S.; Al-Ani, B.; Fujisawa, T.; Coxall, H.; Chudasama, K.; Devey, L.R.; Wigmore, S.J.; Abbas, A.; Hewett, P.W.; et al. Negative regulation of soluble flt-1 and soluble endoglin release by heme oxygenase-1. *Circulation* **2007**, *115*, 1789–1797. [CrossRef]
88. Leffler, C.W.; Parfenova, H.; Jaggar, J.H. Carbon monoxide as an endogenous vascular modulator. *Am. J. Physiol Heart Circ. Physiol* **2011**, *301*, H1–H11. [CrossRef]

© 2019 by the authors. Licensee MDPI, Basel, Switzerland. This article is an open access article distributed under the terms and conditions of the Creative Commons Attribution (CC BY) license (http://creativecommons.org/licenses/by/4.0/).

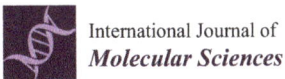

Review

Galectin 13 (PP13) Facilitates Remodeling and Structural Stabilization of Maternal Vessels during Pregnancy

Marei Sammar [1,*], Tijana Drobnjak [2], Maurizio Mandala [3], Sveinbjörn Gizurarson [2], Berthold Huppertz [4,†] and Hamutal Meiri [5,†]

1. Ephraim Katzir Department of Biotechnology Engineering, ORT Braude College, 2161002 Karmiel, Israel
2. Faculty of Pharmaceutical Sciences, School of Health Science, University of Iceland, 107 Reykjavik, Iceland
3. Department of Biology, Ecology and Earth Sciences, University of Calabria, 87030 Rende, Italy
4. Department of Cell Biology, Histology and Embryology, Gottfried Schatz Research Center, Medical University of Graz, 8010 Graz, Austria
5. Hylabs Ltd., Rehovot, 7670606 and TeleMarpe Ltd., 6908742 Tel Aviv, Israel
* Correspondence: sammar@braude.ac.il; Tel.: +972-(4)-9901769
† These authors contributed equally to this work.

Received: 10 June 2019; Accepted: 25 June 2019; Published: 29 June 2019

Abstract: Galectins regulate cell growth, proliferation, differentiation, apoptosis, signal transduction, mRNA splicing, and interactions with the extracellular matrix. Here we focus on the galectins in the reproductive system, particularly on a group of six galectins that first appears in anthropoid primates in conjunction with the evolution of highly invasive placentation and long gestation. Of these six, placental protein 13 (PP13, galectin 13) interacts with glycoproteins and glycolipids to enable successful pregnancy. PP13 is related to the development of a major obstetric syndrome, preeclampsia, a life-threatening complication of pregnancy which affects ten million pregnant women globally. Preeclampsia is characterized by hypertension, proteinuria, and organ failure, and is often accompanied by fetal loss and major newborn disabilities. PP13 facilitates the expansion of uterine arteries and veins during pregnancy in an endothelial cell-dependent manner, via the eNOS and prostaglandin signaling pathways. PP13 acts through its carbohydrate recognition domain that binds to sugar residues of extracellular and connective tissue molecules, thus inducing structural stabilization of vessel expansion. Further, decidual PP13 aggregates may serve as a decoy that induces white blood cell apoptosis, contributing to the mother's immune tolerance to pregnancy. Lower first trimester PP13 level is one of the biomarkers to predict the subsequent risk to develop preeclampsia, while its molecular mutations/polymorphisms that are associated with reduced PP13 expression are accompanied by higher rates of preeclampsia We propose a targeted PP13 replenishing therapy to fight preeclampsia in carriers of these mutations.

Keywords: Placental protein 13; Gal 10; Gal 13; Gal 14; Gal 16; preeclampsia; FGR; polymorphism; risk prediction; biomarkers; eNOS

---

1. Galectins

Galectins are a class of carbohydrate binding proteins with high affinity to β-galactoside sugars that bind to them via their N- or- O-linked glycosylation [1,2]. They share primary structural homology in their carbohydrate-recognition domains (CRDs) included in a canonical sequence of ~130 amino acid backbone. They are synthesized as cytosolic proteins and reside in the cytosol or nucleus for much of their lifetime [3]. They form a β-sandwich [4,5] consisting of five or six anti-parallel β-sheet strands [6], forming a shallow groove for holding a disaccharide or oligosaccharide. Eight amino acids form the CRD motif within this groove to mediate non-covalent binding. Additional amino acids enhance the specific interaction [5–9]. High affinity to the ABO blood groups is responsible for their hemagglutinin activity [10,11]. The galectins are classified into three categories [2]: (1) the prototype homo-dimers (gals 1, 2, 5, 7, 13–17, 19, 20), (2) the "tandem-repeat dimers" (gals 4, 6, 8, 9, 12) with short linkers, and (3) chimera-lectin (gal 3), with a C-terminal CRD and an N-terminal non-lectin for multimerization [12–15]. The multi-valent interaction facilitates crosslinking of signaling pathways, the formation of cell surface lattices, and endocytosis at the cell surface or in intracellular locations [16,17].

Today, we know of 20 members of the galectin family that interact with a plethora of molecules involved in inflammation, immune responses, cell trafficking, apoptosis, autophagy, trans-membrane signaling, and interactions with cytosolic and nuclear targets, nuclear transcription, gene expression, or mRNA splicing [18–21]. Galectins are able to translocate from intra- to extracellular compartments, and back. They affect signal transduction and apoptosis, growth, fibrosis, aggregation, adhesion, and cancer metastasis [22–27]. Hence, galectins are incorporated in the development of new therapeutics [22,27–29], and some are already in clinical development stages (https://galecto.com/ [30]).

2. The Placental Galectins

A variety of galectins are expressed in the reproductive system. They are pleiotropic regulators of key functions in the reproductive tract. Gal-1 and Gal-3 are involved in regulating signaling pathways at the feto-maternal interface [31,32] and are expressed in the endometrium and the decidua. The tandem repeat of Gal-8 acts through spliced variants in various reproductive tissues [1–21]. Gal-9 is abundant via its three encoding genes [33]. In this respect, it is worth mentioning that the Gal 10 protein is also expressed by white blood cells (WBC), while its mRNA is exclusively expressed in bone marrow tissues. However, the WBC reach the reproductive system and influence this system during the process of pregnancy development, especially via generating an immune response against foreign (paternal) genes of the fetus and placenta [34,35]. Other galectins in the reproductive tract such as Gal-13 participate in trophoblast invasion into the decidua, spiral artery remodeling, and immune tolerance of maternal tissues to pregnancy [2].

Here we focus on a placental cluster of six galectins in anthropoid primates in the context of evolution of the highly invasive placentation and long gestation [31]. The expression of these galectins in the placental syncytiotrophoblast is altered in preeclampsia and early fetal growth restriction (FGR) [32]. Three of them, Gal-13, Gal-14, and Gal-16 are uniquely expressed in the placenta, indicating the massive differentiation effort dedicated by nature for assuring the establishment and maintenance of pregnancy in eutherian mammals [36].

3. Galectin 13

3.1. The PP13 Protein and its mRNA

Galectin 13 (Gal-13), also known as LGALS13 and placental protein 13 (PP13), is the most studied galectin of the anthropoid primates. As one of a six cluster primate genes, it is located on chromosome 19q13 [32], and is one of 56 known placental proteins. It was first isolated from human term placenta in 1983 and characterized by Bohn et al. [37]. Normal term placenta has approximately 2.5 mg of PP13, and, according to Bohn, PP13 represents ~7% of the total placental proteins. PP13 shows structural and functional homologies to the ß-galactoside-binding lectins [1], with high homology to the other members of the cluster in their CRD [31,32,38,39]. Although so far no specific individual receptor for PP13 (in the classical sense) has been identified, affinity chromatography and mass spectroscopy determined high affinity binding of PP13 to annexin IIa, a member of Ca2+ and phospholipid binding proteins of the extracellular matrix, and to beta/gamma actin in the cytoplasm [10,40]. PP13 has high affinity to sugar residues, especially to N-acetyl glucose amine, fucose, and N-acetyl galactose amine [10]. It also binds sugar residues of the B and AB antigen of the ABO blood groups [11], a binding that regulates the availability of free PP13 in the blood of pregnant women. This binding has been found to influence the risk assessment and preeclampsia prediction of PP13 [41], as will be further detailed below.

PP13 is expressed from a very early stage of pregnancy, and can be detected in the maternal blood already at week five of gestation [42], or 3 weeks after embryo return in IVF (Meiri, unpublished results). Immunohistochemistry and RNA hybridization studies have pointed to its predominant localization in the placental syncytiotrophoblast layer, placental blood vessels, and specific sites within the placental bed [31,42,43]. Early studies by Than et al. indicated its presence in the syncytiotrophoblast [10]. PP13 is detected in the cytoplasm and mainly along the apical plasma membrane of the syncytiotrophoblast [42,43]. It can also be detected in their nuclei, at least during very early gestation [43]. In cases of oxidative stress, strong staining for PP13 appears in the increasingly appearing syncytiotrophoblast microparticles (STBM, or necrotic bodies) [42,44]. A process of aponecrosis is accompanied by placental shedding of STBM during preeclampsia [42,45].

3.2. Insights on the Gene and Protein Structures

The LGALS13 gene encodes for PP13, and is comprised of a long promoter region at the 5 prime end followed by four exons: E1 (60 bp), E2 (72 bp), E3 (211 bp), and E4 (251 bp) spaced by introns (Figure 1). Intronic regions vary between 499 bp and 1834 bp in length. Exon 4 and part of exon 3 of the LGALS13 gene exclusively code for the entire amino acids included in the CRD domain [6,10,38,46].

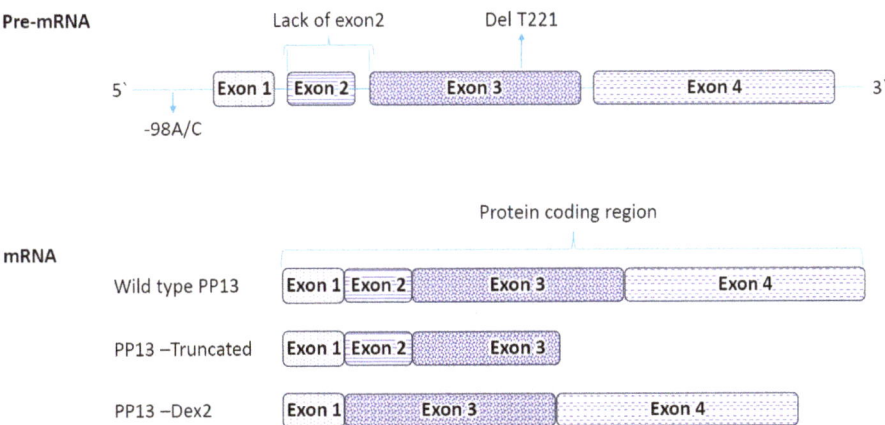

Figure 1. Schematic diagram of the LGALS13 gene and its mRNA variants. Top—The exons and introns are marked by boxes and lines, respectively. Lower panels represent the mRNA and the protein coding region. The wild type Gal-13 (PP13) consists of four full exons. The truncated Gal-13 variant delT$_{221}$ is missing part of exon 3 and the full exon 4, while the Dex-2 variant is missing exon 2. The two variants—the truncated delT$_{221}$ variant and the spliced variant Dex-2 are both naturally occurring variants along with the promoter polymorphic variant of -98 A/C.

The open reading frame of PP13 encodes for 139 amino acids [10,46]. The calculated molecular weight of the monomer is ~ 16.12 kDa. In-vitro studies have shown that its expression is up-regulated by the binding of the TFAP2A transcription factor [32]. Other studies pointed to the link between PP13 expression and human chorionic gonadotropin (hCG) [47] that drives the fusion of villous cytotrophoblasts with the overlying syncytiotrophoblast [48]. Indeed, fusion of differentiating trophoblasts to form the syncytiotrophoblast is accompanied by increased PP13 expression. Fusion also increases PP13 expression in the trophoblast-derived BeWo cell line [47,49].

We engineered several recombinant PP13 variants. Initially, a Histidine-tag (His-PP13) variant was constructed, produced in E. coli, purified, and characterized [10,38]. The resultant His-PP13 fails to dimerize via disulfide bonds since the His-tag prohibits one of its cysteine SH residues from forming a dimer. The molecular conformation of such a monomeric state of PP13 prohibits the formation of the naturally occurring homodimer, and this variant tends to form a long chain of *head-to-tail* linked oligomers, which are characterized by low stability in solutions. Treatment of the His-PP13 variant with the reducing agent dithiothreitol (DTT) keeps the protein in a monomeric form, prohibiting the formation of long chain oligomers. This monomeric form exhibits long stability in solution, and in the presence of DTT lyophilized His-tag PP13 has an estimated shelf-life of 12 years or longer [50]. The second recombinant PP13 variant lacks the histidine tag (rPP13) and is expressed in E. coli [38,51]. The resultant protein was isolated from the inclusion bodies as a monomer that spontaneously homo-dimerizes to form a 32 kDa protein that is very stable in aqueous solutions. Further aggregation to trimers and tetramers is marginal [46]).

3.3. PP13 Secretion from the Placenta

Lacking a signal sequence for transmembrane transport [6], it was estimated that the release of PP13 is accomplished in a manner typical to other galectins, namely via the liberation of extracellular vesicles [12,52,53] (Figure 2). A release of un-packed protein via co-transfer with carrier proteins or endosomes was also suggested to be a calcium dependent mechanism [54,55]. In fact, it has been shown that the PP13 release from immortalized placental cells (BeWo cells) is significantly augmented with the use of a calcium ionophore [44]. Like other galectins, PP13 can re-enter cells by endocytosis via recycling of endocytic vesicles [56].

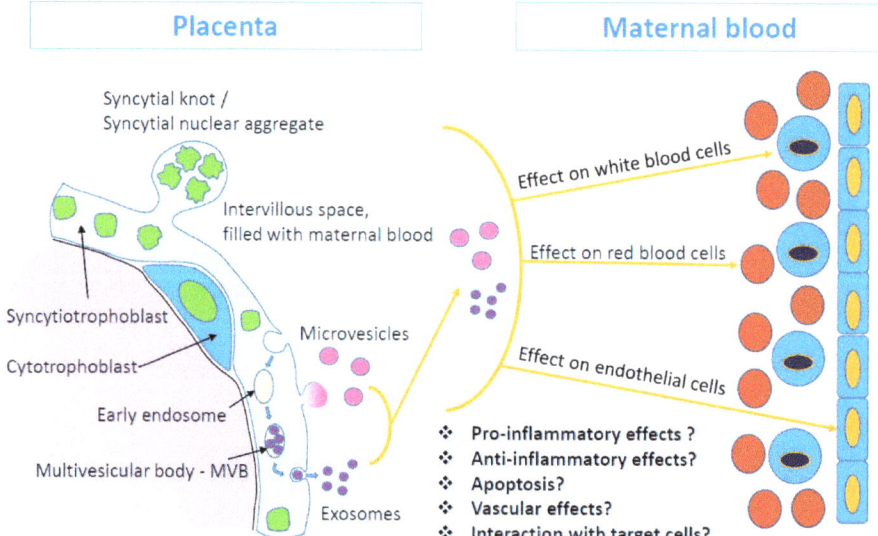

Figure 2. PP13 release from placental syncytiotrophoblast. Extracellular vesicles are cell-derived membrane particles, including exosomes (30–200 nm), microvesicles (100–1000 nm), and apoptotic bodies (>1000 nm). They are released from the placental syncytiotrophoblast layer. During normal turnover, the syncytiotrophoblast releases late-apoptotic syncytial knots (1–5 µm) as large corpuscular structure into the maternal blood. At the same time, microvesicles and exosomes are released and can pass through capillary blood vessels. PP13 cargo of microvesicles and exosomes appears on both types of these extracellular vesicles, on the surface and inside the vesicles. These vesicles may interact with various cell types (red and white blood cells or endothelial cells) and convey different messages to the maternal body.

Sammar et al. [52] discovered a novel pathway for PP13 secretion that may be most relevant to the protein level in maternal blood. PP13 liberation is executed through the release of extracellular vesicles (EVs), mainly microvesicles and exosomes, carrying PP13 on the surface of EVs and/or inside them [52]. The microvesicles and exosomes that carry the PP13 cargo communicate with maternal organs to influence their response, both during normal and complicated pregnancies. Evidence has been obtained for the potential interaction of PP13 in such extracellular vesicles with red and white blood cells, as well as the endothelium (Figure 2).

3.4. PP13 and Preeclampsia

Preeclampsia, a severe life-threatening complication of pregnancy characterized by hypertension, proteinuria and organ failure [57–60] is mainly attributed to impaired placentation [61,62]. It affects ten million pregnant women globally, and is often accompanied by fetal loss and major newborn disabilities ([63]—www.preeclampsia.org). The hunting for serum markers to predict the risk to develop this pregnancy complication was a major challenge in the first decade of the 21st century [64]. We explored the potential use of PP13 as a biomarker for predicting the risk to develop preeclampsia. The availability of the purified native and recombinant PP13 have stimulated the generation of various poly- and monoclonal antibodies, followed by the development of an ELISA immune-diagnostic kit [50]. With these tools in hands, a comparative analysis of PP13 levels in maternal blood was conducted in multiple studies [65–68].

The studies have shown reduced concentrations of maternal blood PP13 in the first trimester in pregnancies that subsequently developed early, preterm and term preeclampsia with and without fetal growth restriction (FGR) [66,69–78]. Longitudinal studies have shown that in preeclampsia there is a sharp increase of PP13 between the first to the third trimester with the slope of change predicting the severity of the subsequent complication [42,75]. Such PP13 increase also predicts severe hemorrhage after delivery [79]. Interestingly, in twin pregnancies that subsequently develop preeclampsia, the level is very high already in the first trimester, indicating accelerated processes of impaired placentation in multiple pregnancy, corresponding with their higher frequency of the disorder [68].

In studies where term placentas were obtained after delivery, the mRNA levels of PP13 were 3.5-fold lower in women who developed PE and the related HELLP syndrome [45,65]. Additional studies have shown that the reduced PP13 mRNA can be determined already in the first trimester in patients who subsequently developed preeclampsia [80–82]. Unlike the protein level that tends to increase near the time of disease, low PP13 mRNA was detected throughout pregnancy. It was subsequently discovered by in-vitro placental explant studies that in a normal pregnancy the release of PP13 from a single placental villus is decreased from the first to the third trimester. During the first trimester of normal pregnancy the level of PP13 in maternal blood increases from 200–300 pg/mL to 400–600 pg/mL [42] due to the increase in the total number of villi during pregnancy [83]. In contrast, villi of preeclamptic placentas showed an elevated PP13 release at the time of disease [83]. It is estimated that aponecrotic release of PP13 from the large number of damaged villi accounts for the sharp slope of the PP13 level in maternal blood during the etiology of preeclampsia [36].

In a meta-analysis of 18 studies that investigated maternal blood levels of PP13 during the first trimester, reduced PP13 levels were found in women who subsequently developed preeclampsia about 20 weeks later. If evaluated in the first trimester as a single biomarker PP13 provided 83% detection rate for 10% false positive rate for early preeclampsia (<34 weeks), 66% for preterm preeclampsia (<37 weeks), and 47% for all cases of preeclampsia [66]. PP13 combined with first trimester Doppler pulsatility index of the blood flow through the maternal uterine arteries and the use of additional markers provides higher detection rates of preeclampsia in the first trimester [66,84].

3.5. PP13 Polymorphism and Preeclampsia

Polymorphic variants of PP13 have been identified [38,66], and three of them are important indicators of a high risk to develop preeclampsia:

(1) The "truncated" variant is a deletion of thymidine in position 221 of the open reading frame of exon 3 [85,86]. It was discovered among black and colored pregnant women in a Cohort of Cape Town,

South African cohort [85]. It is associated with the development of an earlier stop codon coupled to a shorter PP13 variant ("truncated" or "delT221") [38]. The shorter delT221 variant is lacking the entire exon 4 and part of exon 3 [38] (Figure 1). Hence, delT221 is missing 2 of the amino-acids involved in the carbohydrate recognition domain (CRD), and two additional amino acids supporting carbohydrate binding [6,31]. Having this mutation in a heterozygous form is an effective predictor of severe early preeclampsia with 89% positive predictive value. Treatment of human leukocytes derived of the maternal decidua with the wild type of recombinant PP13 but not with the truncated PP13 induced apoptosis [31,43]. From this data it was speculated that one role of PP13 in pregnancy is to render the mother immune-tolerant to pregnancy. The immune tolerance is reached by binding of PP13 via the CRD to glycoproteins and glycolipids. Indeed, pregnancies carrying the homozygous DelT221 mutation are rejected by the mother and are not viable [86].

(2) The promoter variant. The -98 (A/C) promoter genotype displays three genotypes: the "A/A" genotype (homozygous to the adenosine nucleotide), the "C/C" genotype (homozygous to cytosine), or the "A/C" genotype (heterozygous form). In a South African as well as a London cohort of pregnant women, the A/A genotype was found to be associated with decreased expression of PP13 compared to the level of PP13 expression with either A/C or C/C genotypes in the -98 position [51,87]. The reduced expression was contributed in part by the impaired ability of the transcription factor TFAP2A to induce PP13 expression with the A/A genotype [51]. Accordingly, carriers of the A/A variant had an adjusted odds ratio of 3.68 to develop preeclampsia, while the C/C or the A/C genotypes rendered protection from developing preeclampsia. Combining the A/A genotype as a risk factor together with black ethnicity, history of previous preeclampsia, obesity (BMI > 37), and being at advanced maternal age provided an adjusted odds ratio of 14.0 and 7.0, respectively, for developing term or all preeclampsia cases [51].

(3) The Dex-2 variant. Recently, we were able to molecularly engineer a third molecular variant of PP13 that was denoted Dex-2. This mutant completely lacks the second exon (Figure 1). This additional natural PP13 variant was initially isolated in Israel while cloning PP13 DNA from a genomic library. The mutant clones were isolated from a placenta obtained after delivery from a woman with preeclampsia combined with FGR [55]. Burger et al. [55] have shown that PP13 which was isolated from a placenta of preeclampsia with FGR was inferior in inducing the liberation of free fatty acids from trophoblast membranes, and in causing the elevated release of prostaglandins. Further analysis of this mutant is warranted.

In summary, there may well be a link between reduced levels of PP13 during the first trimester of human pregnancy and the elevated risk for a subsequent development of preeclampsia. Preeclampsia patients may be a target population to evaluate if nourishing with the wild-type, full length PP13 can be used as a therapeutic tool to fight preeclampsia.

3.6. PP13 and Immune Tolerance

The syncytiotrophoblast secretes/releases PP13 from the first trimester and the protein reaches the decidua either via diffusion or via the maternal circulation, coinciding with the time of early trophoblast invasion. Kliman et al. [43] have shown the formation of PP13 aggregates closer to areas with increased apoptosis of various maternal immune cells. Killing these cells could enable us to promote extravillous trophoblast invasion of the uterine wall. In this manner, PP13 might serve to establish a decoy inflammatory response, sequestering maternal immune cells away from the site of extravillous trophoblast invading other sites of the uterine wall [31,39,43]. Accordingly, it was proposed that PP13 contributes to the immune tolerance of the mother to the invading trophoblasts. Having low levels of PP13 and/or having a mutated variant may decrease the level of PP13 secretion, thereby contributing to impaired placentation.

3.7. PP13 Replenishing Studies in Animals

The uteroplacental circulation undergoes massive changes during pregnancy, resulting in a vascular system that is directing 20% of the total cardiac output to the uterine vascular bed. This results in more than a ten-fold increase in blood flow over the level present in the non-pregnant state [88]. Since in normal pregnancy there is only a small drop in blood pressure, it is necessary to gain uterine hemodynamic changes by uterine blood vessel expansion and reduced uterine vascular resistance [89]. In pregnancy, extravillous trophoblasts invade all types of luminal structures in the placental bed [90,91]. One of their major targets are spiral arteries and their adjacent stroma. The endoarterial trophoblast subpopulation [92] replaces and reorganizes the vascular smooth muscle and endothelial layers, resulting in the formation of low-resistance vessels that can accommodate a highly increased blood volume flowing towards the placenta [93]. These altered vessels are almost independent of maternal vasoconstriction through a lack of smooth muscle cells [89,94].

Through the invasive processes of the extravillous trophoblast, the vessels towards the intervillous space of the placenta (spiral arteries) and those draining blood back into the maternal system (uteroplacental veins) are connected to the placenta, resulting in a placental blood flow to sufficiently supply the placenta and the growing fetus with nutrients and oxygen [89,91]. This hemochorial type of placentation is present in mammals such as humans, higher order primates, rabbits, guinea pigs, mice, and rats [95–97]. At term there are around 200 spiral arteries opening towards the intervillous space, while the blood flow in the uterine artery is increased in volume with reduced velocity [96]. Impaired trophoblast invasion into spiral arteries results in higher blood flow velocities into the intervillous space of the placenta and thus damage of the fragile villous trees. [98–101].

PP13 appears to have an important role in these hemodynamic changes by facilitating expansion of the uterine vascular system during pregnancy to accommodate the increase of blood flow through the uterus and thus the placenta during pregnancy. The following in vivo data have been obtained using PP13 administration in different animal models:

- Initially, a single PP13 dosage injected intravenously into gravid rats and rabbits resulted in a reversible ~30% reduction in blood pressure [102].
- In a second set of experiments, peristaltic pumps were implanted into gravid rats for a slow release of PP13 for 4 to 7 days from day 15 [102], or from day 8 of pregnancy [103]. rPP13 (compared to saline control) reversibly reduced blood pressure until the pumps released all their content. At delivery, 5 to 7 days after the active release of PP13 was over, treated animals had larger placentas and pups. Both the wild type rPP13 and the truncated variant DelT221 were effective in reducing blood pressure, but the truncated variant failed to sustain uterine artery expansion until the time of delivery [103].
- Isolated uterine mesenteric arteries from both mid-pregnant and non-pregnant rats were placed in arteriographs to measure their diameters and pressure in response to drug perfusion [104]. Uterine arteries of both pregnant and non-pregnant rats were dilated in a dose dependent manner with increasing concentrations of PP13. Half-maximal vasodilation of isolated arteries (EC50) was achieved at a concentration of 1pM PP13 (blood level of pregnant women). The effect was mediated by the endothelial layer, since stripping the vessels off the endothelial layer prohibited blood vessel expansion by PP13. Pharmacological analysis of the signaling pathways revealed that the vasodilation was mediated through signaling of the endothelial nitric oxide synthase (eNOS) and prostaglandin type 2 pathways [104].
- An additional study was performed with non-pregnant rats. Again, surgically implanted pumps released a constant dose of PP13 (rPP13 or His-PP13 variants) or saline over seven days. Some animals were sacrificed immediately after the end of PP13 release (on day 7), while others were sacrificed 6 days later (day 13) to compare the short and long-term impacts of PP13 on vessel growth and size. Both uterine veins and arteries were significantly expanded by rPP13 with a more pronounced effect after 13 days compared to the corresponding vessels after seven days. The long-term effect of treatment by rPP13 was more pronounced in the veins compared to the corresponding arteries. His-PP13 also expanded the blood vessels but the effect remained similar between 7 and 13 days, most

likely since His-tag PP13 has only a monomeric form. This molecular variant does not turn into the natural configuration of a homo-dimer. It is estimated that to exert the structurally stable vascular expansion that is developed with the non His-tag protein, a molecular variant that forms a homo-dimer is required [105].

In conclusion, PP13 appears to play a key role in the remodeling of uterine arteries and veins during pregnancy, facilitating the adjustment of blood flow to and from the placenta. This way, PP13 adapts the uterus to provide increased but slower blood flow towards the placenta and back into the maternal system, necessary for normal pregnancy. PP13 acts via the NO and prostaglandin signaling pathways to provide oxygen and nutrients to the growing fetus (Figure 3).

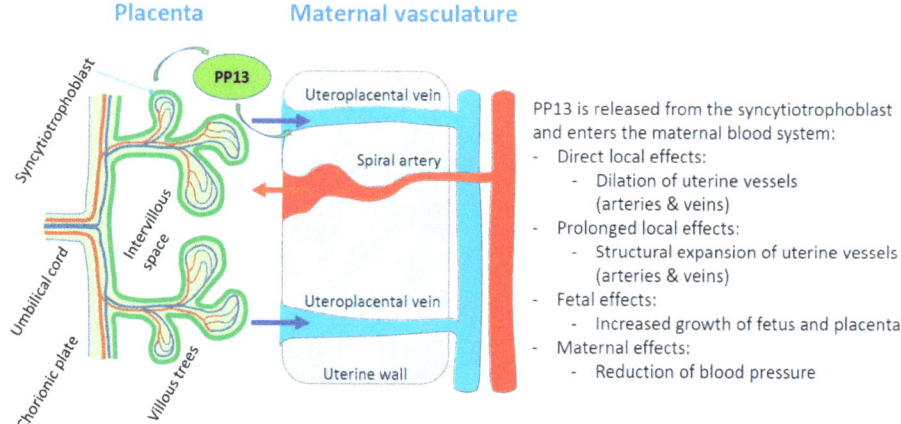

Figure 3. PP13 priming of maternal blood vessels. The scheme displays a comprehensive model of the PP13 effects on the vascular system of the mother. PP13 is released from the syncytiotrophoblast and enters the maternal blood system where it has different effects. The red arrow shows flow of maternal blood into the placenta via invaded spiral arteries, while the blue arrows indicate flow of maternal blood back from the placenta into the maternal vascular system via invaded uterine veins.

3.8. Modeling the Role of PP13 in Pregnancy

The PP13 molecule primes blood vessel expansion to adapt the uterine vascular system to supply oxygen and nutrients to the growing fetus. The effect supports the development of larger placentas and pups, as shown in a rat model [103]. The effect involves a chain of reactions, starting from a physiological effect that involves the endothelial layer through the e-NOS and prostaglandin signaling pathways [103], and continuing through structural stabilization of the surrounding components of the connective tissue around the blood vessels. Connective tissue stabilization requires the CRD component of the PP13 molecules that crosslinks between the endothelial layer and the connective tissue (Figure 4). Finally, PP13 acts as a decoy to attract maternal immune cells and thereby enabling the invasion of extravillous trophoblast into blood vessels [43].

Based on all the above we propose a targeted PP13 therapy to fight preeclampsia in patients with impaired PP13 and high risk to develop preeclampsia [106]. These patients could receive PP13 as a nourishing drug to support uterine vessel expansion and stabilization of blood supply during pregnancy. We are conducting preclinical studies and plan to evaluate the potential clinical impact testing animal models of preeclampsia to explore this hypothesis.

Considering the multifaceted nature of preeclampsia [58–60], the development of PP13 as a novel biological therapy to fight preeclampsia is now evaluated in certain animal models to provide a proof of concept. Among animal models, we plan to test (1) the reduced uterine placenta perfusion (RUPP) model) in rats [107], (2) the transgenic mouse model of STOX-1 [108], and (3) the Baboon uteroplacental ischemia model [109], all identified as important model systems to evaluate novel drugs to fight preeclampsia [110,111].

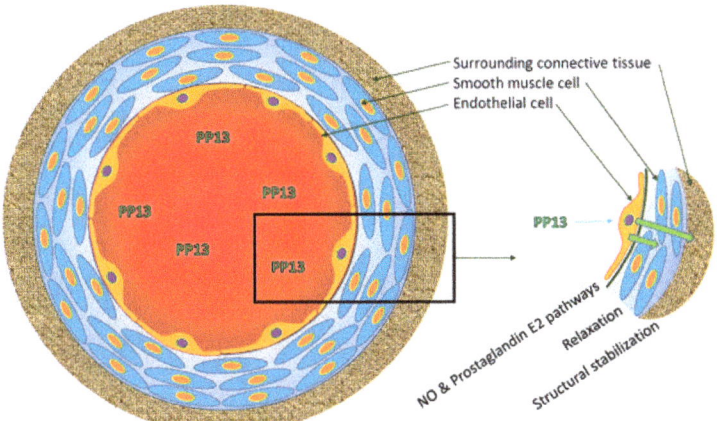

Figure 4. The effect of PP13 on the various layers of blood vessels. PP13 acts on the endothelial layer of the blood vessels and causes vasodilation by muscle relaxation through the signaling pathways of eNOS and prostaglandin 2. Further, PP13 causes stabilization of the surrounding connective tissues. Molecularly, this process requires the carbohydrate recognition domain to cross link between PP13 and molecules on the surface of the connective tissue and extracellular matrix.

4. Multiple Galectins and Deep Placentation

In this article we focus on PP13, a member of the cluster of 6 galectins that emerged during primate evolution, and are only found in anthropoids. These species differ from their strep-sirrhine counterparts by having hemochorial placentas associated with a reduction in the number of offspring, with just one infant being common in monkeys, humans and apes. In all of these species, the newborns have relatively large brains and long gestations [112,113]. As described before, the success of pregnancy is mediated via increased blood flow to and from the placenta, which is achieved via an invasive hemochorial placentation [114–116]. The genetic differences between the mother and the fetal semi-allograft necessitate the development of immune tolerance to reduce the danger of fetal rejection by the mother, considering the alloantigen aspect of eutherian pregnancies [32,114]. We have provided evidence for the crucial role of galectin 13 (PP13) to render the mother immune-tolerant to sustain the hemochorial placentation during the long gestation of anthropoid primates. Interestingly, it has been pointed out that in addition to PP13, the other members of the cluster of galectins of chromosome 19 in anthropoids share high homology in their sequence and placental localization ([117] https://www.ncbi.nlm.nih.gov/kis/ortholog/29124/?scope=9526#genes-tab).

Table 1 indicates that humans have the entire cluster of which 5 are exclusively expressed in the placenta and one (Gal-10) is expressed in the bone marrow, but reaches the placenta via white blood cells, mainly eosinophils [2,31,32,39]. Orangutans, macaque, Sp. monkeys, and marmosets have four of the galectins, chimpanzees have two, and baboons, gorillas, and colobuses have only one galectin [31].

Table 1. Placental galectins in primates.

Species	Gal 10 Eosinophils	Gal 13 Placenta	Gal 14 Placenta	Gal 16 Placenta	Gal 17 Placenta	Gal 20 Placenta	Count	Invasion Level
Chimpanzee							2	3+
Orangutan	10A				17C		4	2+
Baboon							1	1+
Human	10A				17A 17B		5 (with 2 subtypes of Gal 17)	4+
Gorilla							1	3+
Colobus							1	1+
Macaque					17C		4	2+
Marmoset	10A 10B 10C						4 (with 3 subtypes of Gal 10)	2+
Sp. Monkeys	10A 10B 10C						4 (with 3 subtypes of Gal 10)	2+
Total species #	4	8	5	4	3	2		

The presence of placental galectins in primate placenta is provided following the analysis of the evolutionary differentiation tree [31,32,36,39,115] with the exception of Galectin 10 (Gal 10) that is generated in bone-marrow but reaches the placenta via its expression in white blood cells. The letters A, B, and C reflect isoforms of the molecules. In terms of invasion: gorilla, chimpanzee, and human species have the deepest trophoblast invasion (3+ and 4+) reaching the inner myometrium [114–120]. The others have a much shallower implantation (1+ or 2+). The color code indicates in which species the Gal isoforms are expressed. The numbers in "total" refer to the numbers of species in which a specific Gal isoform is expressed. The numbers in "Count" refer to the numbers of Gal isoforms expressed in a given species.

Interestingly, all of the above species with the exception of the baboon, have PP13, most likely reflecting that this protein may be the first to be evolved or is derived from a common ancestor, and potentially it is the most essential one for a successful intrusive pregnancy [31]. The second most frequently found is Gal-14 that appears in four species. Gal-10 and Gal 16 are expressed in three species, while Gal-17 appears in two species and Gal-20 only in one. In terms of sequence homology, all galectins have close to 98% homology in the composition and configuration of their major amino acids of the carbohydrate recognition domain, the CRD. Gal-13 and Gal-16 share 73% amino acid sequence homology, while homology between Gal-13 and Gal-14 and between Gal-13 and Gal-10 is at the level of 68% and 57%, respectively. Interestingly, human Gal-14 and baboon Gal-14 have 98% amino acid sequence homology [34,36].

According to Carter et al. [118] there are different models of placentation among apes. Yet, gorilla, chimpanzee, and human species have the deepest trophoblast invasion and their remodeling of the spiral arteries occurs deep into their inner myometrium [114–120]. All three have Gal-13 (PP13), while baboons with a much shallower trophoblast invasion only express Gal-14. Thus, having multiple co-expression of galectins appears to be essential for successful invasive pregnancy, in which PP13 is pivotal but may not be the only one required. The interplay between the different galectins and their composition is now under study to understand their crucial role in normal pregnancy and pregnancy complications.

Author Contributions: M.S., H.M. and B.H. conceptualized the work; M.S., T.D. and M.M. performed the experiments used as the basis for this work; H.M., M.S. and S.G. provided the resources for this work; M.S. and H.M. did the original draft preparation; all authors reviewed and edited the text; B.H. and M.S. drew the figures; M.S., H.M. and S.G. have lead funding acquisition.

Funding: This research was funded by Daniel Turnberg Fellowship, UK Academy of Medical Sciences and the EU COST action CA16113 – CkiniMark to M.S. This study was also sponsored in part by the European Union (FP7) through the ASPRE project (601852) to H.M., S.G. and T.D. were sponsored by Hananja ehf, and Icelandic Research Fund (Rannís), grant no. 163403-052.

Conflicts of Interest: The funders had no role in the design of the study; in the collection, analyses, or interpretation of data; in the writing of the manuscript, or in the decision to publish the results. Hamutal Meiri and Sveinbjorn Gizurarson have a patent for using PP13 for preeclampsia prevention. The other authors declare no conflict of interest.

Abbreviations

ABO blood groups	Blood group types A, B, AB and O
BP	Base pair
CRD	Carbohydrate-recognition domain
EC_{50}	Effective dose for reaching 50% effect
Enos	Endothelial nitric oxide synthase
Gal 1, Gal 3, etc.	Galectin 1, galectin 3 and other galectins according to their nomenclature
FGR	Fetal growth restriction
kDa	Kilo-Dalton
pMol	Pico molar quantity (10^{-12} M)
PP13	Placental protein 13 also called gal-13 and LGALS13 (gene)
STBM	Syncytiotrophoblast microparticles
WBC	White blood cells

References

1. Barondes, S.H.; Castronovo, V.; Cooper, D.N.W.; Cummings, R.D.; Drickamer, K.; Felzi, T.; Gitt, M.A.; Hirabayashi, J.; Hughes, C.; Kasai, K.; et al. Galectins: A family of animal beta-galactoside-binding lectins. *Cell* **1994**, *76*, 597–598. [CrossRef]
2. Johannes, L.; Jacob, R.; Leffler, H. Galectins at a glance. *J. Cell Sci.* **2018**, *131*, jcs208884. [CrossRef] [PubMed]
3. Lindstedt, R.; Apodaca, G.; Barondes, S.H.; Mostov, K.E.; Leffler, H. Apical secretion of a cytosolic protein by Madin-Darby canine kidney cells. Evidence for polarized release of an endogenous lectin by a nonclassical secretory pathway. *J. Biol. Chem.* **1993**, *268*, 11750–11757. [PubMed]
4. Leffler, H.; Carlsson, S.; Hedlund, M.; Qian, Y.; Poirier, F. Introduction to galectins. *Glycoconj. J.* **2004**, *19*, 433–440. [CrossRef] [PubMed]
5. Visegrády, B.; Than, N.G.; Kilár, F.; Sümegi, B.; Than, G.N.; Bohn, H. Homology modelling and molecular dynamics studies of human placental tissue protein 13 (galectin-13). *Protein Eng.* **2001**, *14*, 875–880. [CrossRef] [PubMed]
6. Di Lella, S.; Sundblad, V.; Cerliani, J.P.; Guardia, C.M.; Estrin, D.A.; Vasta, G.R.; Rabinovich, G.A. When galectins recognize glycans: From biochemistry to physiology and back again. *Biochemistry* **2011**, *50*, 7842–7857. [CrossRef] [PubMed]
7. Hirabayashi, J.; Hashidate, T.; Arata, Y.; Nishi, N.; Nakamura, T.; Hirashima, M.; Urashima, T.; Oka, T.; Futai, M.; Muller, W.E.; et al. Oligosaccharide specificity of galectins: A search by frontal affinity chromatography. *Biochim. Biophys. Acta* **2002**, *1572*, 232–254. [CrossRef]
8. Kamili, N.A.; Arthur, C.M.; Gerner-Smidt, C.; Tafesse, E.; Blenda, A.; Dias-Baruffi, M.; Stowell, S.R. Key regulators of galectin-glycan interactions. *Proteomics* **2016**, *16*, 3111–3125. [CrossRef] [PubMed]
9. Salomonsson, E.; Carlsson, M.C.; Osla, V.; Hendus-Altenburger, R.; Kahl-Knutson, B.; Öberg, C.T.; Sundin, A.; Nilsson, R.; Nordberg-Karlsson, E.; Nilsson, U.J.; et al. Mutational tuning of galectin-3 specificity and biological function. *J. Biol. Chem.* **2010**, *285*, 35079–35091. [CrossRef] [PubMed]
10. Than, N.G.; Pick, E.; Bellyei, S.; Szigeti, A.; Burger, O.; Berente, Z.; Janaky, T.; Boronkai, A.; Kliman, H.; Meiri, H.; et al. Functional analyses of placental protein 13/galectin-13. *Eur. J. Biochem.* **2004**, *71*, 1065–1078. [CrossRef]
11. Than, N.G.; Romero, R.; Meiri, H.; Erez, O.; Xu, Y.; Tarquini, F.; Barna, L.; Szilagyi, A.; Ackerman, R.; Sammar, M.; et al. PP13, maternal ABO blood groups and the risk assessment of pregnancy complications. *PLoS ONE* **2011**, *6*, e21564. [CrossRef] [PubMed]
12. Seelenmeyer, C.; Wegehingel, S.; Tews, I.; Künzler, M.; Aebi, M.; Nickel, W. Cell surface counter receptors are essential components of the unconventional export machinery of galectin-1. *J. Cell Biol.* **2005**, *171*, 373–381. [CrossRef] [PubMed]
13. Hsu, D.K.; Zuberi, R.I.; Liu, F.T. Biochemical and biophysical characterization of human recombinant IgE-binding protein, an S-type animal lectin. *J. Biol. Chem.* **1992**, *267*, 14167–14174. [PubMed]
14. Massa, S.M.; Cooper, D.N.W.; Leffier, H.; Barondes, S.H. L-29, an endogenous lectin, binds to glycoconjugates ligands with positive cooperativity. *Biochemistry* **1993**, *32*, 260–267. [CrossRef] [PubMed]

15. Kuklinski, S.; Probstmeier, R. Homophilic binding properties of galectin-3: Involvement of the carbohydrate recognition domain. *J. Neurochem.* **1998**, *70*, 814–823. [CrossRef] [PubMed]
16. Banani, S.F.; Lee, H.O.; Hyman, A.A.; Rosen, M.K. Biomolecular condensates: Organizers of cellular biochemistry. *Nat. Rev. Mol. Cell Biol.* **2017**, *18*, 285–298. [CrossRef] [PubMed]
17. Dennis, J.W. Many light touches convey the message. *Trends Biochem. Sci.* **2015**, *40*, 673–686. [CrossRef]
18. Dagher, S.F.; Wang, J.L.; Patterson, R.J. Identification of galectin-3 as a factor in pre-mRNA splicing. *Proc. Natl. Acad. Sci. USA* **1995**, *92*, 1213–1217. [CrossRef] [PubMed]
19. Vyakarnam, A.; Dagher, S.F.; Wang, J.L.; Patterson, R.J. Evidence for a role for galectin-1 in pre-mRNA splicing. *Mol. Cell. Biol.* **1997**, *17*, 4730–4737. [CrossRef] [PubMed]
20. Michaud, S.; Reed, R. An ATP-independent complex commits pre-mRNA to the mammalian spliceosome assembly pathway. *Genes Dev.* **1991**, *5*, 2534–2546. [CrossRef] [PubMed]
21. Kang, H.G.; Kim, D.H.; Kim, S.J.; Cho, Y.; Jung, J.; Jang, W.; Chun, K.H. Galectin-3 supports stemness in ovarian cancer stem cells by activation of the Notch1 intracellular domain. *Oncotarget* **2016**, *7*, 68229–68241. [CrossRef] [PubMed]
22. Blidner, A.G.; Méndez-Huergo, S.P.; Cagnoni, A.J.; Rabinovich, G.A. Re-wiring regulatory cell networks in immunity by galectin-glycan interactions. *FEBS Lett.* **2015**, *589*, 3407–3418. [CrossRef] [PubMed]
23. Thiemann, S.; Baum, L.G. Galectins and immune responses-just how do they do those things they do? *Annu. Rev. Immunol.* **2016**, *34*, 243–264. [CrossRef] [PubMed]
24. Glinsky, V.V.; Raz, A. Modified citrus pectin anti-metastatic properties: One bullet, multiple targets. *Carbohydr. Res.* **2009**, *344*, 1788–1791. [CrossRef] [PubMed]
25. Glinsky, V.V.; Glinsky, G.V.; Rittenhouse-Olson, K.; Huflejt, M.E.; Glinskii, O.V.; Deutscher, S.L.; Quinn, T.P. The role of Thomsen-Friedenreich antigen in adhesion of human breast and prostate cancer cells to the endothelium. *Cancer Res.* **2001**, *61*, 4851–4857.
26. Sindrewicz, P.; Lian, L.Y.; Yu, L.G. Interaction of the Oncofetal Thomsen-Friedenreich antigen with galectins in cancer progression and metastasis. *Front. Oncol.* **2016**, *6*, 79. [CrossRef]
27. Li, S.; Wandel, M.P.; Li, F.; Liu, Z.; He, C.; Wu, J.; Shi, Y.; Randow, F. Sterical hindrance promotes selectivity of the autophagy cargo receptor NDP52 for the danger receptor galectin-8 in antibacterial autophagy. *Sci. Signal.* **2013**, *6*, 9. [CrossRef]
28. Chen, W.S.; Cao, Z.; Leffler, H.; Nilsson, U.J.; Panjwani, N. Galectin-3 inhibition by a small-molecule inhibitor reduces both pathological corneal neovascularization and fibrosis. *Investig. Ophthalmol. Vis. Sci.* **2017**, *58*, 9–20. [CrossRef]
29. Delaine, T.; Collins, P.; MacKinnon, A.; Sharma, G.; Stegmayr, J.; Rajput, V.K.; Mandal, S.; Cumpstey, I.; Larumbe, A.; Salameh, B.A.; et al. Galectin-3-binding glycomimetics that strongly reduce bleomycin-induced lung fibrosis and modulate intracellular glycan recognition. *ChemBioChem* **2016**, *17*, 1759–1770. [CrossRef]
30. The Galectin Pharmacology List. Available online: https://galecto.com/ (accessed on 17 August 2018).
31. Than, N.G.; Romero, R.; Goodman, M.; Weckle, A.; Xing, J.; Dong, Z.; Xu, Y.; Tarquini, F.; Szilagyi, A.; Gal, P.; et al. A primate subfamily of galectins expressed at the maternal-fetal interface that promote immune cell death. *Proc. Natl. Acad. Sci. USA* **2009**, *106*, 9731–9736. [CrossRef]
32. Than, N.G.; Romero, R.; Xu, Y.; Erez, O.; Xu, Z.; Bhatti, G.; Leavitt, R.; Chung, T.H.; El-Azzamy, H.; LaJeunesse, C.; et al. Evolutionary origins of the placental expression of chromosome 19 cluster galectins, and their complex dysregulation in preeclampsia. *Placenta* **2014**, *35*, 855–865. [CrossRef]
33. Su, E.U.; Bi, S.; Kane, L.P. Galectin-9 regulates T helper cell function independently of Tim-3. *Glycobiology* **2011**, *21*, 1258–1265. [CrossRef]
34. Ackerman, S.J.; Liu, L.; Kwatia, M.A.; Savage, M.P.; Leonidas, D.D.; Swaminathan, G.J.; Acharya, K.R. Charcot-Leyden crystal protein (galectin-10) is not a dual function galectin with lysophospholipase activity but binds a lysophospholipase inhibitor in a novel structural fashion. *J. Biol. Chem.* **2002**, *277*, 14859–14868. [CrossRef] [PubMed]
35. Su, J. A brief history of Charcot-Leyden Crystal Protein/Galectin-10 research. *Molecules* **2018**, *23*, 2931. [CrossRef] [PubMed]
36. Than, N.G.; Romero, R.; Kim, C.J.; McGowen, M.R.; Papp, Z.; Wildman, D.E. Galectins: Guardians of eutherian pregnancy at the maternal-fetal interface. *Trends Endocrinol. Metab.* **2012**, *23*, 23–31. [CrossRef] [PubMed]

37. Bohn, H.; Kraus, W.; Winckler, W. Purification and characterization of two new soluble placental tissue proteins (PP13 and PP17). *Oncodev. Biol. Med.* **1983**, *4*, 343–350. [PubMed]
38. Sammar, M.; Nisamblatt, S.; Gonen, R.; Huppertz, B.; Gizurarson, S.; Osol, G.; Meiri, H. The role of the carbohydrate recognition domain of placental protein 13 (PP13) in pregnancy evaluated with recombinant PP13 and the DelT221 PP13 variant. *PLoS ONE* **2014**, *9*, e102832. [CrossRef]
39. Than, N.G.; Romero, R.; Balogh, A.; Karpati, E.; Mastrolia, S.A.; Staretz-Chacham, O.; Hahn, S.; Erez, O.; Papp, Z.; Kim, C.J. Galectins: Double-edged swords in the cross-roads of pregnancy complications and female reproductive tract inflammation and neoplasia. *J. Pathol. Transl. Med.* **2015**, *49*, 181–208. [CrossRef]
40. Yang, R.Y.; Rabinovich, G.A.; Liu, F.T. Galectins: Structure, function and therapeutic potential. *Expert Rev. Mol. Med.* **2008**, *10*, e17. [CrossRef] [PubMed]
41. Burgess, A.; Johnson, T.S.; Simanek, A.; Bell, T.; Founds, S. Maternal ABO blood type and factors associated with preeclampsia subtype. *Biol. Res. Nurs.* **2019**, *21*, 264–271. [CrossRef] [PubMed]
42. Huppertz, B.; Sammar, M.; Chefetz, I.; Neumaier-Wagner, P.; Bartz, C.; Meiri, H. Longitudinal determination of serum placental protein 13 during development of preeclampsia. *Fetal Diagn. Ther.* **2008**, *24*, 230–236. [CrossRef] [PubMed]
43. Kliman, H.J.; Sammar, M.; Grimpel, Y.I.; Lynch, S.K.; Milano, K.M.; Pick, E.; Bejar, J.; Arad, A.; Lee, J.J.; Meiri, H.; et al. Placental protein 13 and decidual zones of necrosis: An immunologic diversion that may be linked to preeclampsia. *Reprod. Sci.* **2012**, *19*, 16–30. [CrossRef] [PubMed]
44. Balogh, A.; Pozsgay, J.; Matkó, J.; Dong, Z.; Kim, C.J.; Várkonyi, T.; Sammar, M.; Rigó, J., Jr.; Meiri, H.; Romero, R.; et al. Placental protein 13 (PP13/galectin-13) undergoes lipid raft-associated subcellular redistribution in the syncytiotrophoblast in preterm preeclampsia and HELLP syndrome. *Am. J. Obstet. Gynecol.* **2011**, *205*, 156.e1–156.e14. [CrossRef] [PubMed]
45. Than, N.G.; Abdul Rahman, O.; Magenheim, R.; Nagy, B.; Fule, T.; Hargitai, B.; Sammar, M.; Hupuczi, P.; Tarca, A.L.; Szabo, G.; et al. Placental protein 13 (galectin-13) has decreased placental expression but increased shedding and maternal serum concentrations in patients presenting with preterm pre-eclampsia and HELLP syndrome. *Virchows Arch.* **2008**, *453*, 387–400. [CrossRef] [PubMed]
46. Than, N.G.; Sumegi, B.; Than, G.N.; Berente, Z.; Bohn, H. Isolation and sequence analysis of a cDNA encoding human placental tissue protein 13 (PP13), a new lysophospholipase, homologue of human eosinophil Charcot-Leyden Crystal protein. *Placenta* **1999**, *20*, 703–710. [CrossRef] [PubMed]
47. Orendi, K.; Gauster, M.; Moser, G.; Meiri, H.; Huppertz, B. The choriocarcinoma cell line BeWo: Syncytial fusion and expression of syncytium-specific proteins. *Reproduction* **2010**, *140*, 759–766. [CrossRef] [PubMed]
48. Kliman, H.J.; Nestler, J.E.; Sermasi, E.; Sanger, J.M.; Strauss, J.F., III. Purification, characterization, and in vitro differentiation of cytotrophoblasts from human term placentae. *Endocrinology* **1986**, *118*, 1567–1582. [CrossRef] [PubMed]
49. Orendi, K.; Gauster, M.; Moser, G.; Meiri, H.; Huppertz, B. Effects of vitamins C and E, acetylsalicylic acid and heparin on fusion, beta-hCG and PP13 expression in BeWo cells. *Placenta* **2010**, *31*, 431–438. [CrossRef] [PubMed]
50. Meiri, H.; PP13. PP13. ELISA KIT for IVD of pregnancy complications. IDABC—EUDAMED: European Database on Medical Devices. Available online: http://ec.europa.eu/idabc/en/document/2256/5637.html. (accessed on 31 August 2008).
51. Madar-Shapiro, L.; Karady, I.; Trahtenherts, A.; Syngelaki, A.; Akolekar, R.; Poon, L.; Cohen, R.; Sharabi-Nov, A.; Huppertz, B.; Sammar, M.; et al. Predicting the risk to develop preeclampsia in the first trimester combining promoter variant-98A/C of LGALS13 (Placental Protein 13), black ethnicity, previous preeclampsia, obesity, and maternal age. *Fetal Diagn. Ther.* **2018**, *43*, 250–265. [CrossRef]
52. Sammar, M.; Dragovic, R.; Meiri, H.; Vatish, M.; Sharabi-Nov, A.; Sargent, I.; Redman, C.; Tannetta, D. Reduced placental protein 13 (PP13) in placental derived syncytiotrophoblast extracellular vesicles in preeclampsia—A novel tool to study the impaired cargo transmission of the placenta to the maternal organs. *Placenta* **2018**, *66*, 17–25. [CrossRef]
53. Hughes, R.C. Secretion of the galectin family of mammalian carbohydrate-binding proteins. *Biochim. Biophys. Acta* **1999**, *1473*, 172–185. [CrossRef]
54. Ideo, H.; Hoshi, I.; Yamashita, K.; Sakamoto, M. Phosphorylation and externalization of galectin-4 is controlled by Src family kinases. *Glycobiology* **2013**, *23*, 1452–1462. [CrossRef] [PubMed]

55. Burger, O.; Pick, E.; Zwickel, J.; Kliman, M.; Meiri, H.; Slotky, R.; Mandel, S.; Rabinovitch, L.; Paltieli, Y.; Admon, A.; et al. Placental protein 13 (PP-13): Effects on cultured trophoblasts, and its detection in human body fluids in normal and pathological pregnancies. *Placenta* **2004**, *25*, 608–622. [CrossRef] [PubMed]
56. Furtak, V.; Hatcher, F.; Ochieng, J. Galectin-3 mediates the endocytosis of beta-1 integrins by breast carcinoma cells. *Biochem. Biophys. Res. Commun.* **2001**, *289*, 845–850. [CrossRef] [PubMed]
57. Walker, J.J. Pre-eclampsia. *Lancet* **2000**, *356*, 1260–1265. [CrossRef]
58. Roberts, J.M.; Cooper, H. Pathogenesis and genetics of pre-eclampsia. *Lancet* **2001**, *357*, 53–56. [CrossRef]
59. Redman, C.W.; Sargent, I. Latest advances in understanding preeclampsia. *Science* **2005**, *308*, 1592–1594. [CrossRef] [PubMed]
60. World Health Organization. Maternal Mortality: To Improve Maternal Health, Barriers that Limit Access to Quality Maternal Health Services Must be Identified and Addressed at All Levels of the Health System: Fact Sheet. World Health Organization, 2014. Available online: https://apps.who.int/iris/handle/10665/112318 (accessed on 9 June 2019).
61. Meekins, J.W.; Pijnenborg, R.; Hanssens, M.; McFadyen, I.R.; van Asshe, A. A study of placental bed spiral arteries and trophoblast invasion in normal and severe pre-eclamptic pregnancies. *Br. J. Obstet. Gynaecol.* **1994**, *101*, 669–674. [CrossRef]
62. Huppertz, B. Placental origins of preeclampsia: Challenging the current hypothesis. *Hypertension* **2008**, *51*, 970–975. [CrossRef]
63. The Preeclampsia Foundation. Available online: https://www.preeclampsia.org/ (accessed on 9 June 2019).
64. Cetin, I.; Huppertz, B.; Burton, G.; Cuckle, H.; Gonen, R.; Lapaire, O.; Mandia, L.; Nicolaides, K.; Redman, C.; Soothill, P.; et al. Pregenesys pre-eclampsia markers consensus meeting: What do we require from markers, risk assessment and model systems to tailor preventive strategies? *Placenta* **2011**, *32*, S4–S16. [CrossRef]
65. Sammar, M.; Nisemblat, S.; Fleischfarb, Z.; Golan, A.; Sadan, O.; Meiri, H.; Huppertz, B.; Gonen, R. Placenta-bound and body fluid PP13 and its mRNA in normal pregnancy compared to preeclampsia, HELLP and preterm delivery. *Placenta* **2011**, *32*, S30–S36. [CrossRef] [PubMed]
66. Huppertz, B.; Meiri, H.; Gizurarson, S.; Osol, G.; Sammar, M. Placental protein 13 (PP13): A new biological target shifting individualized risk assessment to personalized drug design combating pre-eclampsia. *Hum. Reprod. Update* **2013**, *19*, 391–405. [CrossRef]
67. Meiri, H.; Sammar, M.; Herzog, A.; Grimpel, Y.I.; Fihaman, G.; Cohen, A.; Kivity, V.; Sharabi-Nov, A.; Gonen, R. Prediction of preeclampsia by placental protein 13 and background risk factors and its prevention by aspirin. *J. Perinat. Med.* **2014**, *42*, 591–601. [CrossRef] [PubMed]
68. Maymon, R.; Trahtenherts, A.; Svirsky, R.; Melcer, Y.; Madar-Shapiro, L.; Klog, E.; Meiri, H.; Cuckle, H. Developing a new algorithm for first and second trimester preeclampsia screening in twin pregnancies. *Hypertens Pregnancy* **2017**, *36*, 108–115. [CrossRef] [PubMed]
69. Nicolaides, K.H.; Bindra, R.; Turan, O.M.; Chefetz, I.; Sammar, M.; Meiri, H.; Tal, J.; Cuckle, H.S. A novel approach to first-trimester screening for early pre-eclampsia combining serum PP-13 and Doppler ultrasound. *Ultrasound Obstet. Gynecol.* **2006**, *27*, 13–17. [CrossRef] [PubMed]
70. Spencer, K.; Cowans, N.J.; Chefetz, I.; Tal, J.; Meiri, H. First-trimester maternal serum PP-13, PAPP-A and second-trimester uterine artery Doppler pulsatility index as markers of pre-eclampsia. *Ultrasound Obstet. Gynecol.* **2007**, *29*, 128–134. [CrossRef] [PubMed]
71. Spencer, K.; Cowans, N.J.; Chefetz, I.; Tal, J.; Kuhnreich, I.; Meiri, H. Second-trimester uterine artery Doppler pulsatility index and maternal serum PP13 as markers of pre-eclampsia. *Prenat. Diagn.* **2007**, *27*, 258–263. [CrossRef]
72. Chafetz, I.; Kuhnreich, I.; Sammar, M.; Tal, Y.; Gibor, Y.; Meiri, H.; Cuckle, H.S.; Wolf, M. First-trimester placental protein 13 screening for preeclampsia and intrauterine growth restriction. *Am. J. Obstet. Gynecol.* **2007**, *197*, e1–e7. [CrossRef] [PubMed]
73. Cowans, N.J.; Spencer, K.; Meiri, H. First-trimester maternal placental protein 13 levels in pregnancies resulting in adverse outcomes. *Prenat. Diagn.* **2008**, *28*, 121–125. [CrossRef]
74. Romero, R.; Kusanovic, J.P.; Than, N.G.; Erez, O.; Gotsch, F.; Espinoza, J.; Edwin, S.; Chefetz, I.; Gomez, R.; Nien, J.K.; et al. First-trimester maternal serum PP13 in the risk assessment for preeclampsia. *Am. J. Obstet. Gynecol.* **2008**, *199*, 122.e1–122.e11. [CrossRef]

75. Gonen, R.; Shahar, R.; Grimpel, Y.I.; Chefetz, I.; Sammar, M.; Meiri, H.; Gibor, Y. Placental protein 13 as an early marker for pre-eclampsia: A prospective longitudinal study. *Br. J. Obstet. Gynaecol.* **2008**, *115*, 1465–1472. [CrossRef] [PubMed]
76. Khalil, A.; Cowans, N.J.; Spencer, K.; Goichman, S.; Meiri, H.; Harrington, K. First trimester maternal serum placental protein 13 for the prediction of pre-eclampsia in women with a priori high risk. *Prenat. Diagn.* **2009**, *29*, 781–789. [CrossRef] [PubMed]
77. Khalil, A.; Cowans, N.J.; Spencer, K.; Goichman, S.; Meiri, H.; Harrington, K. First-trimester markers for the prediction of pre-eclampsia in women with a-priori high risk. *Ultrasound Obstet. Gynecol.* **2010**, *35*, 671–679. [CrossRef] [PubMed]
78. Meiri, H.; Huppertz, B.; Cetin, I. Development of early non-invasive markers and means for the diagnosis and progression monitoring of preeclampsia and tailoring putative therapies (project pregenesys 037244). *Placenta* **2011**, *32*, S1–S3. [CrossRef] [PubMed]
79. Farina, A.; Bernabini, D.; Zucchini, C.; De Sanctis, P.; Quezada, M.S.; Mattioli, M.; Rizzo, N. Elevated maternal placental protein 13 serum levels at term of pregnancy in postpartum major hemorrhage (>1000 mLs). A prospective cohort study. *Am. J. Reprod. Immunol.* **2017**, *78*, e12702. [CrossRef] [PubMed]
80. Shekizawa, A.; Purwosunu, Y.; Yoshimura, S.; Nakamura, M.; Shimizu, H. PP13 mRNA expression in trophoblasts from preeclamptic placentas. *Reprod. Sci.* **2009**, *16*, 408–413. [CrossRef] [PubMed]
81. Shimizu, H.; Sekizawa, A.; Purwosunu, Y.; Nakamura, M.; Farina, A.; Rizzo, N.; Okai, T. PP13 mRNA expression in the cellular component of maternal blood as a marker for preeclampsia. *Prenat. Diagn.* **2009**, *29*, 1231–1236. [CrossRef] [PubMed]
82. Farina, A.; Zucchini, C.; Sekizawa, A.; Purwosunu, Y.; de Sanctis, P.; Santarsiero, G.; Rizzo, N.; Morano, D.; Okai, T. Performance of messenger RNAs circulating in maternal blood in the prediction of preeclampsia at 10–14 weeks. *Am. J. Obstet. Gynecol.* **2010**, *203*, 575.e1-7. [CrossRef]
83. Grimpel, Y.I.; Kivity, V.; Cohen, A.; Meiri, H.; Sammar, M.; Gonen, R.; Huppertz, B. Effects of calcium, magnesium, low-dose aspirin and low-molecular-weight heparin on the release of PP13 from placental explants. *Placenta* **2011**, *32*, S55–S64. [CrossRef]
84. Than, N.G.; Balogh, A.; Romero, R.; Kárpáti, E.; Erez, O.; Szilágyi, A.; Kovalszky, I.; Sammar, M.; Gizurarson, S.; Matkó, J.; et al. Placental Protein 13 (PP13)-A placental immunoregulatory galectin protecting pregnancy. *Front. Immunol.* **2014**, *20*, 348. [CrossRef]
85. Gebhardt, S.; Bruiners, N.; Hillerman, R. A novel exonic variant (221delT) in the LGALS13 gene encoding placental protein 13 (PP13) is associated with preterm labour in a low risk population. *J. Reprod. Immunol.* **2009**, *82*, 166–173. [CrossRef] [PubMed]
86. Than, N.G.; Romero, R.; Hillermann, R.; Cozzi, V.; Nie, G.; Huppertz, B. Prediction of preeclampsia-a workshop report. *Placenta* **2008**, *29*, S83–S85. [CrossRef] [PubMed]
87. Bruiners, N.; Bosman, M.; Postma, A.; Gebhardt, S.; Rebello, G.; Sammar, M.; Meiri, H.; Hillermann, R. Promoter variant-98A-C of the LGALS13 gene and pre-eclampsia. In Proceedings of the 8th World Congress of Prenatal Medicine and Fetal Development, Florence, Italy, 7 September 2007.
88. Palmer, S.K.; Zamudio, S.; Coffin, C.; Parker, S.; Stamm, E.; Moore, L.G. Quantitative estimation of human uterine artery blood flow and pelvic blood flow redistribution in pregnancy. *Obstet. Gynecol.* **1992**, *80*, 1000–1006. [PubMed]
89. Thornburg, K.L.; Jacobson, S.L.; Giraud, G.D.; Morton, M.J. Hemodynamic changes in pregnancy. *Semin. Perinatol.* **2000**, *24*, 11–14. [CrossRef]
90. Moser, G.; Windsperger, K.; Pollheimer, J.; de Sousa Lopes, S.C.; Huppertz, B. Human trophoblast invasion: New and unexpected routes and functions. *Histochem. Cell Biol.* **2018**, *150*, 361–370. [CrossRef]
91. Moser, G.; Drewlo, S.; Huppertz, B.; Armant, D.R. Trophoblast retrieval and isolation from the cervix: Origins of cervical trophoblasts and their potential value for risk assessment of ongoing pregnancies. *Hum. Reprod. Update* **2018**, *24*, 484–496. [CrossRef]
92. Moser, G.; Huppertz, B. Implantation and extravillous trophoblast invasion: From rare archival specimens to modern biobanking. *Placenta* **2017**, *56*, 19–26. [CrossRef]
93. Kaufmann, P.; Black, S.; Huppertz, B. Endovascular trophoblast invasion: Implications for the pathogenesis of intrauterine growth retardation and preeclampsia. *Biol. Reprod.* **2003**, *69*, 1–7. [CrossRef]
94. Gokina, N.I.; Mandala, M.; Osol, G. Induction of localized differences in rat uterine radial artery behavior and structure during gestation. *Am. J. Obstet. Gynecol.* **2003**, *189*, 1489–1493. [CrossRef]

95. Pijnenborg, R.; Vercruysse, L.; Hanssens, M. The uterine spiral arteries in human pregnancy: Facts and controversies. *Placenta* **2006**, *27*, 939–958. [CrossRef]
96. Pijnenborg, R.; Vercruysse, L.; Brosens, I. Deep placentation. *Best Pract. Res. Clin. Obstet. Gynaecol.* **2011**, *25*, 273–285. [CrossRef] [PubMed]
97. Moll, W. Structure adaptation and blood flow control in the uterine arterial system after hemochorial placentation. *Eur. J. Obstet. Gynecol. Reprod. Biol.* **2003**, *110*, S19–S27. [CrossRef]
98. Burton, G.J.; Woods, A.W.; Jauniaux, E.; Kingdom, J.C. Rheological and physiological consequences of conversion of the maternal spiral arteries for uteroplacental blood flow during human pregnancy. *Placenta* **2009**, *30*, 473–482. [CrossRef] [PubMed]
99. Browne, V.A.; Julian, C.G.; Toledo-Jaldin, L.; Cioffi-Ragan, D.; Vargas, E.; Moore, L.G. Uterine artery blood flow, fetal hypoxia and fetal growth. *Philos. Trans. R. Soc. B Biol. Sci.* **2015**, *370*, 20140068. [CrossRef] [PubMed]
100. Konje, J.C.; Kaufmann, P.; Bell, S.C.; Taylor, D.J. A longitudinal study of quantitative uterine blood flow with the use of color power angiography in appropriate for gestational age pregnancies. *Am. J. Obstet. Gynecol.* **2001**, *185*, 608–613. [CrossRef] [PubMed]
101. Mandala, M.; Osol, G. Physiological remodelling of the maternal uterine circulation during pregnancy. *Basic Clin. Pharmacol. Toxicol.* **2012**, *110*, 12–18. [CrossRef] [PubMed]
102. Gizurarson, S.; Huppertz, B.; Osol, G.; Skarphedinsson, J.O.; Mandala, M.; Meiri, H. Effects of placental protein 13 on the cardiovascular system in gravid and non-gravid rodents. *Fetal Diagn. Ther.* **2013**, *33*, 257–264. [CrossRef] [PubMed]
103. Gizurarson, S.; Sigurdardottir, E.R.; Meiri, H.; Huppertz, B.; Sammar, M.; Sharabi-Nov, A.; Mandalá, M.; Osol, G. Placental protein 13 administration to pregnant rats lowers blood pressure and augments fetal growth and venous remodeling. *Fetal Diagn. Ther.* **2016**, *39*, 56–63. [CrossRef] [PubMed]
104. Drobnjak, T.; Gizurarson, S.; Gokina, N.I.; Meiri, H.; Mandalá, M.; Huppertz, B.; Osol, G. Placental protein 13 (PP13)-induced vasodilation of resistance arteries from pregnant and nonpregnant rats occurs via endothelial-signaling pathways. *Hypertens. Pregnancy* **2017**, *36*, 86–95. [CrossRef]
105. Drobnjak, T.; Jónsdóttir, A.M.; Helgadóttir, H.; Runólfsdóttir, M.S.; Meiri, H.; Sammar, M.; Osol, G.; Mandalà, M.; Huppertz, B.; Gizurarson, S. Placental protein 13 (PP13) stimulates rat uterine vessels after slow subcutaneous administration. *Int. J. Womens Health* **2019**, *11*, 213–222. [CrossRef]
106. Meiri, H.; Osol, G.; Cetin, I.; Gizurarson, S.; Huppertz, B. Personalized therapy against preeclampsia by replenishing placental protein 13 (PP13) targeted to patients with impaired PP13 molecule or function. *Comput. Struct. Biotechnol. J.* **2017**, *15*, 433–446. [CrossRef] [PubMed]
107. Li, J.; LaMarca, B.; Reckelhoff, J.F. A model of preeclampsia in rats: The reduced uterine perfusion pressure (RUPP) model. *Am. J. Physiol. Heart Circ. Physiol.* **2012**, *303*, H1–H8. [CrossRef] [PubMed]
108. Collinot, H.; Marchiol, C.; Lagoutte, I.; Lager, F.; Siauve, N.; Autret, G.; Balvay, D.; Renault, G.; Salomon, L.J.; Vaiman, D. Preeclampsia induced by STOX1 overexpression in mice induces intrauterine growth restriction, abnormal ultrasonography and BOLD MRI signatures. *J. Hypertens.* **2018**, *36*, 1399–1406. [CrossRef] [PubMed]
109. Makris, A.; Yeung, K.R.; Shirlene, M.; Lim, S.L.; Sunderland, N.; Heffernan, S.; Thompson, J.F.; Iliopoulos, J.; Killingsworth, M.C.; Yong, J.; et al. Placental growth factor reduces blood pressure in a uteroplacental ischemia model of preeclampsia in non-human primates. *Hypertension* **2016**, *67*, 1263–1272. [CrossRef] [PubMed]
110. Grimes, P.S.; Bombay, K.; Lanes, A.; Walker, M.; Daniel, J.; Corsi, D.J. Potential biological therapies for severe preeclampsia: A systematic review and meta-analysis. *BMC Pregnancy Childbirth* **2019**, *19*, 163. [CrossRef]
111. Gunnarsson, R.; Akerstorm, B.; Hansson, S.R.; Gram, M. Recombinant alpha-1-microglobulin: A potential treatment for preeclampsia. *Drug Dis. Today* **2017**, *22*, 736–743. [CrossRef] [PubMed]
112. Chavatte-Palmer, P.; Tarrade, A. Placentation in different mammalian species. *Ann. Endocrinol.* **2016**, *77*, 67–74. [CrossRef]
113. Enders, A.C.; Carter, A.M. The evolving placenta: Different developmental paths to a hemochorial relationship. *Placenta* **2012**, *3*, S92–S98. [CrossRef]
114. Wildman, D.E.; Chen, C.; Erez, O.; Grossman, L.I.; Goodman, M.; Romero, R. Evolution of the mammalian placenta revealed by phylogenetic analysis. *Proc. Natl. Acad. Sci. USA* **2006**, *103*, 3203–3208. [CrossRef]

115. Wildman, D.E.; Uddin, M.; Romero, R.; Gonzalez, J.M.; Than, N.G.; Murphy, J.; Hou, Z.C.; Fritz, J. Spontaneous abortion and preterm labor and delivery in nonhuman primates: Evidence from a captive colony of chimpanzees (Pan troglodytes). *PLoS ONE* **2011**, *6*, e24509. [CrossRef]
116. Roberts, M.R.; Green, J.A.; Schulz, L.C. The evolution of the placenta. *Reproduction* **2016**, *152*, R179–R189. [CrossRef] [PubMed]
117. Searching for Orthologous Genes at NCBI. Available online: https://www.ncbi.nlm.nih.gov/kis/ortholog/29124/?scope=9526#genes-tab (accessed on 9 June 2019).
118. Carter, A.M. Recent advances in understanding evolution of the placenta: Insights from transcriptomics. *F1000Research* **2018**, *7*. [CrossRef] [PubMed]
119. Hou, Z.C.; Sterner, K.N.; Romero, R.; Than, N.G.; Gonzalez, J.M.; Weckle, A.; Xing, J.; Benirschke, K.; Goodman, M.; Wildman, D.E. Elephant transcriptome provides insights into the evolution of eutherian placentation. *Genome Biol. Evol.* **2012**, *4*, 713–725. [CrossRef] [PubMed]
120. Pijnenborg, R.; Vercruysse, L.; Carter, A.M. Deep trophoblast invasion and spiral artery remodelling in the placental bed of the lowland gorilla. *Placenta* **2011**, *32*, 586–591. [CrossRef] [PubMed]

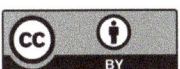

© 2019 by the authors. Licensee MDPI, Basel, Switzerland. This article is an open access article distributed under the terms and conditions of the Creative Commons Attribution (CC BY) license (http://creativecommons.org/licenses/by/4.0/).

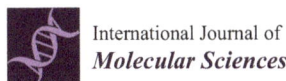

Review

The Role of Epigenetics in Placental Development and the Etiology of Preeclampsia

Clara Apicella †, Camino S. M. Ruano †, Céline Méhats, Francisco Miralles and Daniel Vaiman *

Institut Cochin, U1016 INSERM, UMR8104 CNRS, Université Paris Descartes, 24 rue du faubourg St Jacques, 75014 Paris, France; clara.apicella@inserm.fr (C.A.); camino.ruano@inserm.fr (C.S.M.R.); celine.mehats@inserm.fr (C.M.); francisco.miralles@inserm.fr (F.M.)
* Correspondence: daniel.vaiman@inserm.fr; Tel.: +33-1-4441-2301; Fax: +33-1-4441-2302
† These authors contributed equally to this work.

Received: 3 May 2019; Accepted: 3 June 2019; Published: 11 June 2019

Abstract: In this review, we comprehensively present the function of epigenetic regulations in normal placental development as well as in a prominent disease of placental origin, preeclampsia (PE). We describe current progress concerning the impact of DNA methylation, non-coding RNA (with a special emphasis on long non-coding RNA (lncRNA) and microRNA (miRNA)) and more marginally histone post-translational modifications, in the processes leading to normal and abnormal placental function. We also explore the potential use of epigenetic marks circulating in the maternal blood flow as putative biomarkers able to prognosticate the onset of PE, as well as classifying it according to its severity. The correlation between epigenetic marks and impacts on gene expression is systematically evaluated for the different epigenetic marks analyzed.

Keywords: preeclampsia; epigenetics; DNA methylation; non coding RNAs; miRNAs; histone post translational modifications; HOX genes; H19; miR-210

1. Introduction

PE affects ~2–5% of the pregnancies. This disease, characterized in the classical definition by hypertension and proteinuria, surging from the mid-gestation at the earliest, is often seen as a two-stage disease, where a placental dysfunction occurs, first without observable symptoms and is followed later by a symptomatic phase from the 20th week of gestation at the earliest. The placenta is central to the disease development [1]. During pregnancy, the cytotrophoblasts (CTs) invade and remodel the structure of the spiral arteries of the myometrium [2]. These changes cause a significant increase in blood flow to the placenta. In a classical vision of the disease etiology, it is said that deep invasion is deficient in preeclampsia [3]. It is generally acknowledged that in preeclamptic pregnancies, placentation is disrupted because the CTs fail to properly invade the myometrium and transform the spiral arteries [4]. This decreases the blood flow and alters the oxygenation of the placenta (causing hypoxia and hyperoxia events), triggering oxidative stress, necrosis and inflammation [5]. In a very stimulating paper, B. Huppertz challenges this classical understanding of PE etiology, by dissociating the defect of deep trophoblast invasion from preeclampsia but rather associating this defect with the Fetal Growth Restriction (FGR) phenotype [6]. In this vision, preeclampsia would rather be caused by a combination of *villous* trophoblast defects (which are not involved in invasion, contrary to *extravillous* trophoblast) and maternal susceptibility. He based his reasoning on the fact that invasion defects are actually not histologically visible in many cases of preeclampsia. This may be connected to mouse models of preeclampsia where no obvious fetal growth restriction occurs, consistently with the fact that invasion is not important in rodent [7]. More accepted than this vision, the same paper strengthens the idea that hyperoxia rather than hypoxia is a major actor of the disease [6,8].

The preeclamptic placenta releases vasoactive molecules, pro-inflammatory cytokines, microparticles and syncytial fragments into the maternal circulation which ultimately cause a systemic endothelial dysfunction [9]. Epigenetics plays an important role in the regulation of the development and physiology of the placenta [10]. Besides, substantial epigenetic alterations, in the preeclamptic placenta and other affected tissues have been described and are likely playing a substantial role in the evolution of the disease [11–14].

2. Epigenetics and Normal Placental Development

2.1. Description of the Placenta and Placental Cells

The placenta is a temporary organ connecting the developing fetus to the uterine wall through the umbilical cord, to allow for nutrient absorption, thermal regulation, waste disposal and gas exchange via the mother's blood supply. In addition, the placenta produces hormones that support pregnancy and it acts as a barrier to fight against internal infection [15].

The human placenta at term has a discoid shape, an average diameter of 15–20 cm, a thickness of 2.5 cm in the center and a weight of about 500 g. Its surfaces are the chorionic plate on the fetus side and to which the umbilical cord is attached and the basal plate facing the maternal endometrium. Between the endometrium and the basal plate there is a cavity filled with maternal blood, the intervillous space, into which branched chorionic villi project. The chorionic villi are the structural and functional unit of the placenta. Their core is made of fibroblasts, mesenchymal cells, endothelial cells, immune cells such as Hofbauer cells (supposed to be macrophage-like) and fetal-placental vessels. The villi are covered by two layers of trophoblasts. The inner layer is composed of villous cytotrophoblasts (vCTs), which are highly proliferative and can differentiate into either outer layer villous syncytiotrophoblasts (SCT), which are in direct contact with the maternal blood or extravillous trophoblasts (EVTs), as shown in Figure 1.

2.2. Human Placental Development

The development of the human placenta has been described in detail elsewhere [16–18]. Briefly, the blastocyst implants into the uterine endometrium (decidua) via the trophectoderm cells adjacent to the inner cell mass (ICM). From the trophectoderm, the syncytium (SCT) emerges and spreads. Subsequently, CTs proliferate rapidly to form large finger-like projections (villi) that penetrate the entire depth of the SCT. Ultimately, the villi become filled with mesenchyme originated from the extraembryonic mesoderm. This mesenchyme will form fetal blood vessels which connect to the fetal circulation via the umbilical cord. The intervillous space subsequently becomes filled with maternal blood. The vCTs situated at the tips of the anchoring villi proliferate and stratify, forming highly compact cell columns breached only by channels carrying maternal blood toward and away from the placenta (Figure 1). The trophoblast cells within this structure are referred to as EVTs, according to their external location relative to the chorionic villi. EVTs situated close to the decidua, stop proliferating and develop invasive properties. These invasive EVTs migrate deeply into the decidua, where they transform the uterine vasculature in order to supply the placenta maternal blood, a critical step in establishing uteroplacental circulation. As pregnancy progresses, the number of vCTs decreases and few is observable at term underneath the SCT.

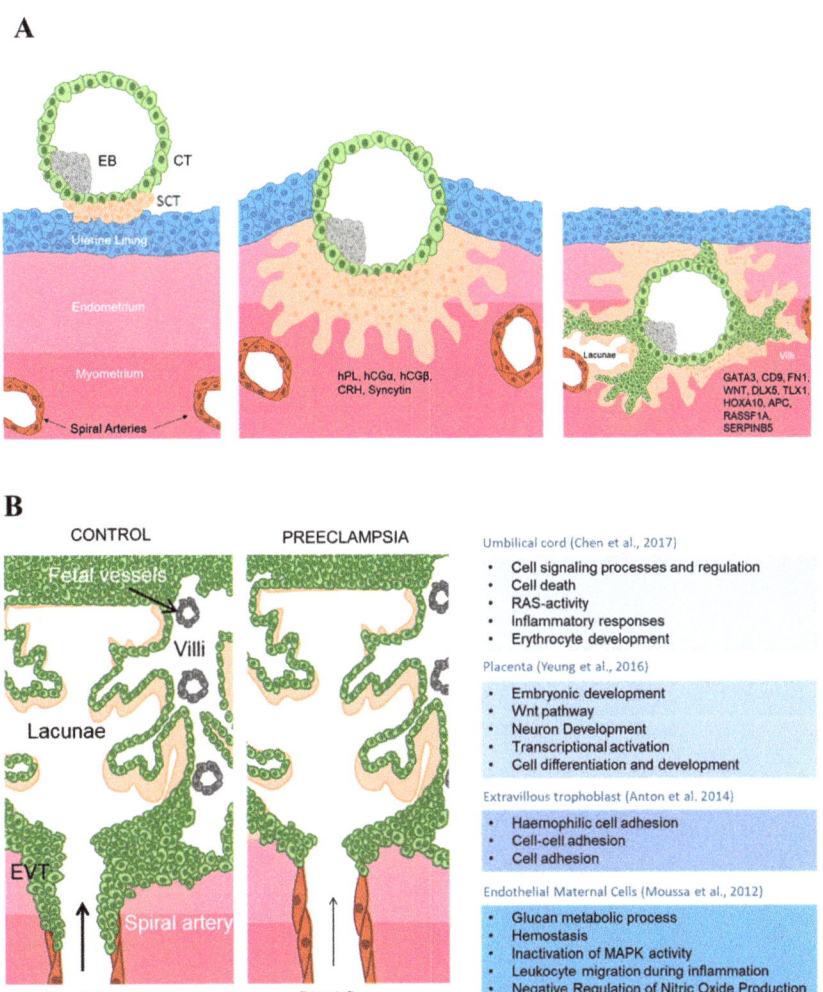

Figure 1. (**A**) Blastocyst implantation and Placenta Development: After recognizing the uterine lining, the blastocyst is formed by the embryoblast (EB) and the cytotrophoblast (CT). The cytotrophoblast starts to differentiate into Synctiotrophoblast (SCT). SCT invades the endometrium towards the maternal spiral arteries located in the myometrium. deregulation of numerous genes is observed [19]. Lacunae develop in the syncytiotrophoblast, which will eventually constitute the intervillous space. Genes upregulated during villi formation are presented on the right figure [20]. Other cytotrophoblasts will invade the maternal spiral arteries by differentiating into Extravillous trophoblast. (**B**) Gene Ontology of genes differentially methylated in PE compared to control samples: (**Left**) in normal pregnancies, extravillous trophoblast (EVT) invades the maternal spiral arteries allowing for an increased blood stream towards the extravillous space. Nutrients cross the placenta, are directed towards the embryonic vessels and collected in the umbilical cord. In PE, decreased invasion of the EVTs induces poor spiral artery remodeling, leading to poor blood flow towards the placenta. Increased amount of microparticles from the syncytiotrophoblast and increased amount of free fetal DNA is observed in the maternal blood. (**Right**) Gene ontology of differentially methylated genes found in PE samples in different tissues affected during pregnancy: Umbilical cord, placenta, EVT, Endothelial Maternal cells (see text for detail).

2.3. Epigenetics Mechanisms in Placental Development

Epigenetic mechanisms are involved in the regulation of gene expression both during development and in differentiated tissues [21,22]. These mechanisms include DNA methylation, histone modifications and biogenesis and action of noncoding RNAs (ncRNAs). They regulate gene expression by modulating the accessibility to DNA of transcription factors and other regulatory proteins. In addition, ncRNAs also regulate gene expression at a post-transcriptional level. Epigenetic mechanisms are essential for cellular differentiation and therefore development, as summarized in Table 1

Table 1. Epigenetic mechanisms in placental development.

Epigenetic Mechanism	Target	Cell Type	Biological Relevance	Reference
H3K9/27me3	MMP-2, MMP-9	Human placenta	Related to trophoblasts motility and invasion	[23]
H3K4 acetylation + H3K9 methylation	Maspin	Human placenta	Negatively correlated with human trophoblasts motility and invasion	[24,25]
Acetylated H3	Pregnancy-Specific Glycoproteins	JEG-3	Inhibition of HDACs in JEG-3 cells up-regulated PSG protein and mRNA expression levels	[26]
HDAC3	GCMa	Cell Line	HDAC3 associates with the proximal GCMa-binding site (pGBS) in the syncytin promoter and inhibits its expression	[27]
Acetylation of H2A and H2B		Murine TSCs	Decreases the EMT and invasiveness of murine TSCs while maintaining their stemness phenotype	[28]
H3K4Me2; H4K20me3	Genome Wide	SCTs	H3K4Me2 co-localizes with active RNAP II in the majority of STB nuclei	[29]
H3K27me3	Genome Wide	vCT	H3K27me3 highly represented in vCT	[30]
lncRNA TUG1	RND3	HTR-8/SVneo, JEG-3	TUG1 epigenetically silences RND3 transcription by interacting with EZH2 involved in cellular proliferation, migration and invasion in trophoblasts	[31]
lncRNA RPAIN	C1q	HTR8/SVneo	Inhibition of proliferation and invasion. Inhibits C1q expression	[32]
lncRNA MALAT1		JEG-3	Regulates proliferation, migration, invasion and apoptosis	[33]
lncRNA MEG3		HTR8/SVneo and JEG-3	Regulates migration and apoptosis	[34]
lncRNA MIR503HG		JEG-3	Regulates migration and invasion	[35]
lncRNA LINC00629		JEG-3	Regulates migration and invasion	[35]
lncRNA SPRY4-IT1	HuR	HTR8/SVneo	Regulates migration and apoptosis/interferes with the β-catenin Wnt signaling	[36,37]
lncRNA H19	Binds small RNAs and proteins	vCT, JAR	Regulates proliferation and apoptosis	[38]
miR-141-3p and miR-200a-3p	Transthyretin (TTR)	syncytitialized BeWo	Inhibits TTR expression by directly binding to the 3′UTR of TTR. Regulate thyroxin uptake by the SCT	[39]
miR-34	Plasminogen activator inhibitor-1 (PAI-1), SERPINA3	JAR	Regulates invasion	[40,41]
miR-155	Cyclin D1	HTR-8/SVneo	attenuates trophoblast proliferation	[42]
miR-17_92, miR-106a_363, miR-106b_25	GCM1		attenuate differentiation of trophoblasts	[43]
miR-675	NOMO1, Igf1R	JEG3 cells	restricts trophoblast proliferation	[44]
C19MC miR cluster		HTR8/SVneo	impaired migration	[45]
methylation of gene body	DAXX	Human placenta	Loss of methylation during both vCT syncytialization to SCT and EVTs differentiation to invasive EVTs	[46]
methylation of gene promoter	APC	Human placenta and choriocarcinoma cells	trophoblast invasiveness	[47]
hypomethylated promoter	MASPIN	Human placenta	inhibits EVTs migration and invasion	[24,25,48]
Hypermethylated promoter	RASSF1A	Human placenta; JAR; JEG3	Possible role in cytotrophoblast development through its effects on ID2	[49]
Genome wide methylation	PMDs (Partially Methylated Domains)	human placenta: Chorionic Villi	genes involved in immune response, Epithelial-mesenchymal transition and inflammation	[50–52]
Genome wide methylation	Genome Wide	human SCTs compared to vCTs	hypomethylated SCTs compared to vCTS	[53]
Genome wide methylation	Genome Wide	BeWo and BeWo + Forskolin	DNA methylation status of numerous genes regulated at the expression level were altered by forskolin-induced fusion	[54]
Methylation	HOX genes: TLX1, HOXA10, DLX5	Human placenta	Increased methylation across gestation correlates with decreased expression. Involved in SCTs differentiation	[46]
Genome wide methylation	Genome Wide	Side-population trophoblasts, vCTs and EVTs	Each cell population has a distinctive methylome	[55,56]
Methylation	Cdx2; Eomes; Plet1; TcFap2c	Mice trophoblast stem cells (TSCs)	methylation regulates the expression of genes involved in the establishment of the TSCs	[57–59]
Methylation	Genome Wide	Blastocyst	hypomethylation of the trophectoderm compared to the inner cell mass	[60]

2.3.1. DNA Methylation

The best studied epigenetic mechanism in the placenta is DNA methylation, the covalent addition of a methyl group to a cytosine, usually in the context of cytosine-phospho-guanine (CpG) dinucleotides. Several reviews have been dedicated to the role of this mechanism in placental development [10,12,61]. Also, several high-throughput analyses have been performed to analyze the methylation epigenetics of the developing placenta (Table 2, Supplementary Table S1 for the details).

Table 2. Summary of DNA methylation studies in developing placenta using genome-wide approaches.

Sample	Method	GEO ID	Findings	Reference
First-trimester and term placenta and maternal blood	Illumina HM450		2944 hypermethylated CpG sites in the first and 5218 in third trimester placenta.	[62]
First-trimester placenta and maternal blood	MeDIP-Seq and Illumina HM450		3759 CpG sites in 2188 regions were differentially methylated	[63]
Placenta (first, second and third trimester)	Illumina HM450 and MethylC-Seq & RNA-Seq	GSE39777	Identification of partially methylated domains (PMDs) and differences between placenta and other tissues	[51]
Placenta (first, second and third trimester)	Illumina HM27		Increase in overall genome methylation observed from first to third trimester.	[64]
Term placenta	MeDIP + custom microarray		Tissue-specific differentially methylated regions in the placenta	[65]
Various human trophoblast populations	Illumina HiSeq 2000	GSE109682	Human trophoblasts are different from somatic cells in terms of global CpG methylation	[56]
Methylation profiles of E18.5 term placenta of WT and Hltf−/− mouse	Illumina HiSeq 2000 (Mus musculus)	GSE114145	Hltf-gene deletion alters the epigenetic landscape of the placenta.	[66]
Fetal placental tissue of both sexes in GR+/+ vs. GR+/− mice	Illumina HiSeq 2000	GSE123188	GR mutation in mice changes the epigenome of placental tissue in a sex-specific manner	[67]
Human placentas	Illumina HM450	GSE108567	Adjusting for batch effects in DNA methylation	[68]
Epigenetic mechanism of mouse embryo development	Illumina HiSeq 2500 (Mus musculus)	GSE104243	H3K27me3 and DNA methylation in extraembryonic and embryonic lineages	[69]
Samples from different normal human tissues	Illumina HM450	GSE103413	Identifying candidate imprinted genes	Database, unpublished
Bisulphite and oxidative bisulphite converted placental DNA	Illumina HM450	GSE93429	Hydroxymethylcytosine and methylcytosine profiles in the human placenta	[70]
Methylation in first and third trimester placental samples	Illumina Genome Analyzer Iix	GSE98752	Complex Association between DNA Methylation and Gene Expression	[71]
DNA Methylation in Human Fetal Tissues and Human IPSC	Illumina HM450	GSE76641	DNA methylation and transcriptional trajectories in human development.	[72]
DNA methylation of fetal membranes, trophoblasts and villi 2nd trimester	Illumina HM450	GSE98938	Genome-scale fluctuations in the cytotrophoblast epigenome	Database, unpublished
Developing mouse placenta	Illumina HiSeq 2000	GSE84350	DNA Methylation Divergence and Tissue Specialization in the Developing Mouse Placenta	[73]
Villous cytotrophoblasts samples	Illumina HM450	GSE93208	DNA methylation profiling of first trimester villous cytotrophoblasts	[52]
Placental tissue collected at term.	Illumina HM450	GSE71719	DNA methylation and hydroxymethylation assessment.	[74]
DNA from chorionic villus from the 1st trimester and maternal blood cell samples	Illumina HiSeq 2000 (Homo sapiens)	GSE58826	DNA Methylation Predictors of Gene Expression in the 1st Trimester Chorionic Villus	Database, unpublished
Methylation patterns of human placenta, blood neutrophils and somatic tissue	Illumina HiSeq 2000 (Homo sapiens)	GSE59988	The human placenta exhibits a dichotomized DNA methylation pattern compared to somatic tissues	[75]
mRNA and DNA methylation profiling of Dnmt3a/3b-null trophoblasts	Illumina HiSeq 2000 (Mus musculus)	GSE66049	Maternal DNA methylation in early trophoblast development	[76]
Imprinted differentially methylated regions in hu-man villous trophoblast and blood samples	Illumina MiSeq (Homo sapiens)	GSE76273	Polymorphic imprinted methylation in the human placenta	[77]
Placental villous explant culture in different growth conditions	Illumina HM450	GSE60885	Genome-wide DNA methylation identifies trophoblast invasion-related genes.	[78]
Trophoblast methylation in NLRP7 knockdown	Illumina HM450	GSE45727	NLRP7 alters CpG methylation	[79]
Bisulphite converted DNA	Illumina HumanMethylation27 BeadChip	GSE36829	Epigenome analysis of placenta samples from newborns	Database, unpublished
First trimester, second trimester and full-term placentas	Illumina HumanMethylation27 BeadChip	GSE31781	Widespread changes in promoter methylation profile in human placentas.	[80]
Chorionic villus and maternal blood cell samples	Illumina HumanMethylation27 BeadChip	GSE23311	DNA Methylation Analysis in Human Chorionic Villus and Maternal Blood Cells	[81]

Differentiation of Stem Cells

Contrary to mice, a Trophoblast Stem Cell (TSC) population has not yet been clearly identified in humans, thus limiting our capacity to study the role of DNA methylation in the early stages of trophoblast differentiation. A recent study has addressed this question using a side-population trophoblasts, a candidate human TSC [55], isolated from first trimester placenta. The comparison of the methylomes of this side-population trophoblasts and the methylomes of vCTs and EVTs all isolated from the same first trimester placenta, showed that each population had a distinctive methylome [56]. In comparison to mature vCTs, side-population trophoblasts, showed differential methylation of genes and miRNAs involved in cell cycle regulation, differentiation and regulation of pluripotency. In addition, the comparison of the methylomes and transcriptomes of vCTs and EVTs revealed the methylation of genes involved in epithelial-mesenchymal transition (EMT) and metastatic cancer pathways, which could be involved in the acquisition of the invasive capacities of the EVTs. However, this study, as many others, failed to establish a systematic correlation between hypermethylation of the genes and downregulated expression. Therefore, the authors conclude that although CpG methylation is involved in the trophoblasts differentiation, it cannot be the only regulatory process.

Regulation of Homeotic Genes

Several studies have identified and established the importance of the transcription factors of the homeobox gene family (HOX) in the development of human placenta [82–86]. Most HOX genes have been found stably hypo-methylated throughout gestation, suggesting that DNA methylation is not the primary mechanism involved in regulating HOX genes expression in the placenta. However, these genes show variable methylation patterns across gestation, with a general trend towards an increase in methylation over gestation. Three genes (*TLX1*, *HOXA10* and *DLX5*) present slightly increased methylation while their mRNA expression decreases throughout pregnancy, supporting a role for DNA methylation in their regulation [46]. Down-regulation of these genes using siRNAs specific for *DLX5*, *HOXA10* and *TLX1* in primary trophoblasts leads to loss of proliferation and to an increase in mRNA expression of differentiation markers, such as *ERVW-1*. This suggests that loss of these proteins is required for proper SCT development [46].

Placental Development and Cancer Pathways

The early steps of placentation are reminiscent of the invasive properties of malignant tumors. Studies on DNA methylation in cancer cells and placental cells have highlighted similarities in their epigenomes, particularly, a widespread hypomethylation throughout the genome and focal hypermethylation at CpG islands. Hypomethylation within the placenta is not uniform but occurs in large domains (>100 kb) called partially methylated domains (PMDs) which are regions of reduced DNA methylation that cover approximately 40% of the placental genome [51]. PMDs are unique to a few different tissue types that include the placenta, cultured and cancer cells [50,51,87]. Placental genes within PMDs tend to be tissue-specific and show higher promoter DNA methylation and reduced expression as compared with somatic tissues [51]. A genome-wide comparison of DNA methylation changes in placental tissues during pregnancy and in 13 types of tumor tissues during neoplastic transformation revealed that megabase-scale patterns of hypomethylation distinguish first from third trimester chorionic villi in the placenta [52]. These patterns mirror those that distinguish many tumors from the corresponding normal tissues. The genomic regions affected by this hypomethylation encompass genes involved in pathways related to EMT, immune response and inflammation, all of them associated to cancer phenotypes. Moreover, the authors observed that hypomethylated blocks distinguish vCTs before 8–10 weeks of gestation and after 12–14 weeks of gestation. The analogy between early placentation and malignant tumors at the epigenetic level is further stressed by studies analyzing the methylation status of the promoters of several tumor suppressor genes (RASSF1A, SERPINB5 also known as APC and Maspin, respectively) in the developing placenta and human choriocarcinoma cell lines (JAR and JEG3) [25,49]. These studies show that promoter DNA-methylation regulates the expression of these tumor suppressor genes which in turn affects the migration and invasive capacities of the trophoblastic cells (As summarized in Table 1).

2.3.2. Non-coding RNAs and Epigenetic Regulation of Placenta Development

Definition

A non-coding RNA (ncRNA) is defined as an RNA molecule that is not translated into a protein. Classes of non-coding RNAs include transfer RNAs (tRNAs) and ribosomal RNAs (rRNAs), small RNAs such as microRNAs (miRNAs), siRNAs, piRNAs, snoRNAs, snRNAs, exRNAs, scaRNAs and the long ncRNAs [88]. The role of these molecules in placental development, physiology and pathology has been recently reviewed in detail [89]. Here we will discuss solely the role of miRNAs and long ncRNAs in the epigenetic control of placental development.

MiRNA and Normal Human Placental Development

The miRNAs are single stranded RNA molecules of 19–24 nucleotides, which act primarily by degrading mRNA transcripts or inhibiting translation of miRNA in to proteins [90]. To date, more than 2000 human miRNAs have been discovered, which appear to regulate 50% of human RNAs [91]. A large number of miRNAs detected in the placenta are expressed from a gene cluster located on chromosome 19 (C19MC) [92,93]. This cluster includes 46 intronic miRNA genes that express 58 miRNA species. These miRNAs are primate-specific, and they are expressed almost exclusively in the placenta (and are thus termed trophomiRs). In the human placenta, the expression of C19MC miRNAs is detected as early as 5 weeks of pregnancy and the expression gradually increases as pregnancy progresses [94]. An imprinted, paternally expressed, CpG-rich domain has a regulatory role in C19MC expression [95]. This DMR, is hypermethylated in cell lines that do not express C19MCs [96]. The C19MC region contains genomic transposable elements called "Alu repeats", which have been implicated in recombination and gene duplication events. Because of their sequence complementarity it has been proposed that several C19MC miRNAs could be responsible of the targeting and degradation of transcribed Alu elements. Also, the C19MC miRNAs are expressed in embryonic and in stem cells but their expression drops considerably when these cells differentiate, which may indicate a role in the maintenance of an undifferentiated state [97–101]. Several members of the C19MC cluster are expressed at much higher levels in vCT compared with EVTs and overexpression of the C19MC cluster results in reduced migration of the extravillous trophoblast line HTR8/SVneo [45]. The chromosome 14 miRNA cluster (C14MC) is another miRNA cluster that is expressed in the placenta [102]. This cluster includes the miRNAs: miR-127, miR-345, miR-370, miR-431 and miR-665. These miRNAs have been involved in the regulation of the immune suppressive, anti-inflammatory response and also in the regulation of the ischemia/hypoxia response [103]. The expression of the C14MC members generally declines during pregnancy [104].

The miR-675 is expressed from the first exon of the H19 long non-coding RNA. Up-regulation of miR-675, which is controlled by the stress-response RNA-binding protein HuR, restricts murine placental growth. Deficiency of H19, promotes placental growth and miR-675 overexpression decreases cell proliferation, likely through targeting Igf1R [105]. Consistent with these findings, the expression of miR-675 rises toward the end of murine pregnancy, when placental growth decelerates. In addition, miR-675 restricts proliferation in JEG3 cells, likely through binding to the nodal modulator 1 (NOMO1) protein [44].

Several other miRNAs are likely involved in placental development by inhibiting genes associated to regulation of trophoblast fate, invasion and proliferation (Let-7a, miR-377, miR-145, members of the miR-17_92 cluster, members of the miR-106a_363 and miR-106b_25 clusters, miR-155, miR-34, miR-141-3p and miR-200a-3p) [106,107]. As additional examples of regulation, mir-431 inhibits invasion of trophoblast cells by targeting the ZEB1 gene [108], miR-106a~303 inhibits trophoblast differentiation by targeting hCYP19A1 and hGCM1 [43], miR-34 targets SERPINA3, a key gene in a variety of biological processes and highly deregulated in placental diseases [41].

These miRNAs regulate diverse processes such as trophoblast physiology, proliferation and invasion (some mentioned in Table 1 and reviewed in Reference [107]).

lncRNA and Normal Human Placental Development

Long non-coding RNAs (lncRNAs) are RNAs greater than 200 nucleotides in length that do not encode a protein product. They are expressed with cellular and temporal specificity and have been involved in many cellular events, including the regulation of gene expression, post-transcriptional modifications and epigenetic modifications, imprinting and X-chromosome inactivation [109]. They act as scaffolds (binding other RNAs or proteins), signals and antisense decoys and engage in transcriptional interference. Usually a single lncRNA has multiple functions. The function of lncRNAs in placental development is poorly understood, mostly inferred from studies on placental pathologies. Nevertheless, lncRNAs have been involved in a number of critical trophoblast functions, from proliferation, invasion and migration, to cell cycle progression [110]. H19 was one of the first lncRNAs to be discovered [111]. H19 is located within a large imprinted domain on chromosome 11, at ~100 kb downstream of IGF2. H19 and IGF2 are reciprocally imprinted that is, for H19 only the maternal allele is expressed, while for IGF2, only the paternal allele is expressed [112]. H19 expression could be regulated by PLAGL1, a zinc finger transcription factor, in the human placenta [113]. Two major functions have been described for H19, specifically as a modulator for binding small RNAs and proteins [114] and as a source of the miRNA mir-675 (see above). H19 has variable levels of biallelic expression in the placenta (reports suggest between 9% and 25% expression occurs from the imprinted allele) until 10 weeks of gestation by which time H19 expression is mostly restricted to the maternal allele [115]. H19 expression is restricted to intermediate and vCT and is not found within SCTs in the human placenta. H19 down-regulation in trophoblast cells leads to inhibition of proliferation and apoptosis [116]. Many other lncRNAs have been involved in placental development, including lincRNA SPRY4-IT1, MIR503HG, LINC00629, MEG3, MALAT1, RPAIN and TUG1 [31–37]. The study of the expression of these lncRNAs during placental development and the manipulation of their expression in vitro in choriocarcinoma cell made it possible to infer their possible function in the context of placental development (Table 1).

2.3.3. Histone Modifications in the Developing Placenta

Histone modification is the process of modification of histone proteins by enzymes, including post-translational modifications, such as methylation, acetylation, phosphorylation and ubiquitination. Histone modifications participate in gene expression regulation by modulating the degree of chromatin compaction [117].

Our knowledge concerning the role of histones modification in human placentation is scarce and refers mostly to studies in mice. Methylation frequently occurs on histones H3 and H4 on specific lysine (K) and arginine (A) residues. Histone lysine methylation can lead to activation or to inhibition, depending on the position in which it is located. For instance, H3K9, H3K27 and H4K20 are considered as important 'inactivation' markers, that is, repressive marks, because of the relationship between these methylations and heterochromatin formation. However, the methylation of H3K4 and H3K36 are considered to be 'activation' marks [118,119].

The heterochromatin methylation marker H3K27me3 was found to be highly active in vCT. That was explained by rapid and transient repression of genes at the time of SCT formation. SCTs nuclei were also found enriched for H4K20me3 [30]. However, this report contrasted with another study reporting that the CTs were enriched with H3K4me3 and that the SCTs were transcriptionally activated by the chromatin marker H3K4me2, which co-localized with active RNAP II in the majority of SCT nuclei [29]. In mouse and other mammals, H3 arginine methylation predisposes blastomeres to contribute to the pluripotent cells of the ICM, which appears to require higher global levels of H3 arginine methylation than the TE/trophoblast lineage [120]. Nevertheless, these lower modification levels in the trophoblast lineage are indispensable for normal placental development.

Acetylation, which in most cases occurs in the N-terminal conserved lysine residues, is also an important way to modify the histone proteins, for example, acetylations of lysine residues 9 and 14 of histone H3 and of lysines 5, 8, 12 and 16 of histone H4 by Histone Acetylases (HATs). Acetylation is generally associated with the activation or opening of the chromatin. On the contrary, de-acetylation of the lysine residues by histone deacetylases (HDACs) leads to chromatin condensation and inactivation of gene transcription. Oxygen (O_2) concentrations strongly influence placental development partially through modifications of the histone methylation codes. Initially, the gestation environment is hypoxic and O_2 concentration increases during development. Hypoxia-inducible factor-1 (HIF-1), consisting of HIF-1α and ARNT subunits, activates many genes involved in the cellular response to O_2 deprivation [121]. HIF-1 is also known to recruit and regulate HDACs [122,123]. Moreover, HIF-1 has been found to bind specific sites on the promoter of the H3K9 demethylases thereby inducing their expression. In particular, it induces JMJD1A and JMJD2A that remove dimethyl marks on H3K9me2, JMJD2B [124,125] which removes trimethyl marks (H3K9me3) and more weakly JMJD2C which converts H3K9me3 to me2 [126]. Studies in rodents have shown that HIFs have important roles in the regulation of TSCs differentiation by integrating physiological, transcriptional and epigenetic inputs. Thus, the crosstalk between HIF and the HDACs is required for normal trophoblast differentiation [123,127].

Another example of histone modification during placentation, is the acetylation of histones H2A and H2B by the CREB-binding protein (CBP). CBP acts as an acetyltransferase that decreases the EMT and invasiveness of murine TSCs while maintaining the properties of stem cells [28].

Trophoblastic fusion depends on the regulation of GCMa activity by HATs and HDACs. Human GCMa transcription factor regulates expression of syncytin, which in turn mediates trophoblastic fusion. It has been demonstrated that CBP-mediated GCMa acetylation underlies the activated cAMP/PKA signaling pathway that stimulates trophoblastic fusion [27]. Human pregnancy-specific glycoproteins (PSG) are the major secreted placental proteins expressed by the SCTs and represent early markers of cytotrophoblast differentiation. Pharmacological inhibition of HDACs in JEG-3 cells up-regulated PSG protein and mRNA expression levels. This correlated with an increase in the amount of acetylated histone H3 associated with PSG promoter [26]. Combined acetylation at H3K9 and H3K4 methylation also activates Maspin, a tumor suppressor gene which is negatively correlated with human trophoblasts motility and invasion [24,25]. The invasive capacity exhibited by EVTs is attributed in part to the extracellular matrix degradation mediated by matrix metalloproteinases (MMPs) such as MMP-2 and MMP-9. Differential expression of these MMPs and their tissue inhibitors (TIMPs) has been associated to histone H3K9/27me3 [23].

2.3.4. Imprinting and Placental Development

Placentation and the Materno-Fetal Conflict

Pregnancy in Eutherian mammals is an immunological challenge as reviewed recently [128]. To note, an ancestral inflammatory response in pregnancy and parturition also exist in marsupials (metatherians), as recently observed [129,130]. Other mechanisms are equally conserved in the formation of the placenta, in particular the fusion mechanisms of cytotrophoblasts into syncytiotrophoblasts that are mediated by retroviruses, in eutherians as well as in metatherians [131].

Once the placenta is formed, it will allow nutrients to transit from the mother circulation to the fetal circulation. In the context of the maternal-fetal conflict hypothesis, tightly regulating the placentation process and limiting placental growth is crucial for the mother survival. The genes controlling this regulation are expected to be found different between viviparous and non-viviparous species. For this, mammals appear as an excellent model as a group of ~4500 species divided into egg-laying animals (prototherians, Platypus and Echidnaes, 5 species), animals with a short-lived placenta (metatherians, Marsupials ~250 species) and viviparous species with a long-lived placenta (eutherians, i.e., all the other mammals, where gestation length can be up to 22 months in the African elephant). One major difference found between the genome of placental species and non-placental species of mammals is the presence of imprinted genes only in the first group.

Definition of Imprinted Genes and Links with Viviparity

Imprinted genes are genes that are expressed from either the maternal or the paternal allele, mainly through differentially methylation mechanisms. Their existence leads to dramatic phenotypic differences in animal hybrids according to the sense of the cross. For instance, interbreeding of lions and tigers results in two morphologically different animals, if the male is the lion or the male is the tiger, leading to a liger or a tigon, respectively [132]. While the tigon has a size like that of its parents, the liger is the largest existing felid (up to >400 kg) and several hypotheses have been raised to explain this fact, mostly connected to the existence of imprinted genes. Experimentally, in the 80s, Solter and Surani carried out nuclear transfer experiments that demonstrated in mice the necessity of a paternal and maternal genome to foster healthy development [133]. Androgenetic embryos lead to the production of a hypertrophic placenta while gynogenetic embryos had a very small placenta and a stunted embryo. Similarly, in humans, development from two paternal genomes leads to hydatiform moles, where the placenta is composed of grapelike vesicles, whereas parthenogenic development leads to the apparition of teratomas [134].

As far as we know today, imprinting is closely associated to viviparity. The sequencing of the platypus genome in 2008 [135] revealed syntenic regions that are relatively well conserved with the eutherian and marsupials, albeit no evidence of imprinted gene can be found in Monotremes. This may be since acquisition of imprinting in a species seems to be associated to the progressive acquisition of CpG islands (besides other mechanisms, such as chromosome translocations or retrotransposons insertions), that appear absent from the platypus genome [136,137]. In marsupials (metatherians), where the placenta is short-lived, the number of imprinted genes is more limited than in eutherian mammals. Two imprinted regions are well conserved between metatherians and eutherians such as the PEG10 and the H19-IGF2 regions [135]. Similarly, an exhaustive analysis of the transcriptome of chicken failed to identify imprinted genes, while allele specific expression does exist [138,139]. The evidence collected therefore strongly links these genes with the placenta presence. Besides, imprinted genes may have a strictly paternal or strictly maternal expression. Series of invalidation experiments in mice indicated that paternal genes tend to increase placental growth while maternal genes tend to limit this growth [140].

Example of the H19-IGF2 Cluster; Cross Species Conservation of Imprinted Genes

A well-known example of this is the H19-IGF2 cluster localized distally at 11p15.5 in humans and 7qF5 in mice. In both species, the structure of the locus is conserved (about 100 kilobases separating the two genes, with differentially methylated regions inside IGF2 and nearby H19). An IMC (Imprinting Control Region), located 3 kb from the starting point of H19 has also been identified, with seven binding sites for the ZNF transcription factor CTCF. H19 is expressed exclusively form the maternal allele, while IGF2 is expressed from the paternal allele. In mice, a placental specific promoter of Igf2 was discovered. The selective invalidation of this promoter [141] leads to a strong decrease of placental development and placental growth. By contrast, the invalidation of H19, leads to placental and fetal overgrowth [142]. Amongst other imprinted genes that affect placental and fetal growth besides H19 and IGF2 are paternally expressed genes, generally identified in mice (Peg1, Peg3, Rasgrf1, Dlk1) and maternally expressed genes (Igf2r, Gnas, Cdkn1c, Grb10).

Interestingly, in mice, the decoy receptor of Igf2, Igf2r is imprinted and with a maternal profile of expression. In humans, surprisingly, the imprinting status of IGF2R seem to be erratic, polymorphically imprinted according to the human individual analyzed. This was first published in 1993 [143] that showed that 2 out of 14 fetuses had an exclusive expression from the maternal allele. Recently it was shown that IGF2R is duly imprinted in macaques [144], showing that even in primates, the imprinting status can vary between relatively close species. Overall, it appears that many placental imprinted mouse genes are biallelic in their expression in humans [145]. Reciprocally, in a study aiming at identifying novel imprinted genes in the human placentas, we compared variants of the placental DNA versus those of cDNAs from the same placentas using SNP microarrays [146,147]. In addition to four known imprinted genes (IPW, GRB10, INPP5F and ZNF597), we could identify 8 novel imprinted genes in the human placentas (ZFAT, ZFAT-AS, GLIS3, NTM, MAGI2, ZC3H12C, LIN28b and DSCAM). Using a mouse cross allowing the following of the allelic origin, we found an astonishing variegation of the imprinting status: only Magi2 was imprinted in the mouse species.

Imprinted genes may have a general impact on the global methylation status of the placenta. For instance, recently a polymorphism located at the IGF2/H19 locus was shown associated to placental DNA methylation and birth weight in association with Assisted Reproductive Technologies usage [148].

Imprinted genes deregulation in the placenta is linked to placental diseases, as reviewed in References [149,150]. In a recent study, Christians and coworkers, analyzed a list of 120 imprinted genes in relation with global expression of 117 placental samples, including PE and Intra Uterine Growth Restriction (IUGR) cases [151]. The authors identified a significant correlation between birth weight and the expression level of imprinted genes but without significant differences between paternally versus maternally expressed genes. Imprinted genes were also more heavily deregulated in preeclampsia than other genes and in this case paternally expressed genes were down-regulated, while maternally expressed genes were up-regulated. The trend was similar for IUGR. Interestingly, the two human-specific microRNA clusters (C19MC and C14MC), both appear to be imprinted (paternally and maternally expressed) for C19MC and C14MC, respectively, clusters that have been duly studied by the team of Yoel Sadovsky [45,89,152]. Recently, we identified duplication in the 19q13.42 imprinted region encompassing the C19MC cluster [153], from a male 26 weeks fetus with severe IUGR, suggesting that a double dose of the miRNA could contribute to the disease. This suggests links between miRNA regulation, imprinting status and the putative consequences for fetal health and growth.

3. Epigenetic Alterations in Preeclampsia

3.1. DNA Methylation Alterations in Preeclampsia

Anomalies of DNA methylation in preeclampsia have been analyzed from different cellular sources. Besides the analysis of placental cells, investigators have analyzed circulating maternal blood cells or cell-free DNA, as well as maternal endothelial cells (much less accessible, though) and cord-blood white blood cells (of fetal origin). A list of genes of which methylation was found altered is presented as Table 3.

A summary of epigenetic mechanisms at work in PE is shown in Figure 2.

3.1.1. Methylation Alterations in the Preeclamptic Placenta

Common Alterations of Gene Expression in PE are Associated to Methylation Alterations

Numerous studies revealed altered expression of various genes in the pathological placentas (as synthesized previously [154]). These alterations of gene expression are partly explained by the existence of epigenetic deregulations. In PE, numerous methylation deregulations have been found in the pathological compared to control placentas, some studies (but not all) taking into account the gestational age, a recurrent issue when normal and pathological placentas are compared, for which there is often a more than 6 weeks difference [155–160]. The different techniques used to analyze methylation globally are presented in a previous review [161]. These epigenetic changes probably originate from the abnormal placental environment in PE (or IUGR), characterized by alternations of low oxygen tension and hyperoxia. As mentioned above, hypoxia *per se* induces the expression of the Hypoxia-Inducible factor (HIF1α), which binds to Hypoxia Responsive Element activating the transcription of various genes related with angiogenesis and metastasis-associated genes [162]. Overall, abnormal oxygen signaling in the placental context leads to increased concentrations of Oxygen Reactive Species (ROS) [163]. Oxidative stress may drive an accelerated ageing of trophoblast cells, which could be key to understand the origin of placental disorders. Indeed, several studies emphasized alterations of telomere length (a mark of ageing) in preeclamptic pregnancies, with a drastic augmentation of short telomeres in PE, especially in Early Onset PE (EOPE) [164–166]. This senescence may be induced by alterations of the management of oxidative stress [167–169]. The accelerated transformation of vCTs into SCTs will lead to a decrease life expectancy of the placenta and an alteration of its capacity to bring the gestation harmoniously to its normal term.

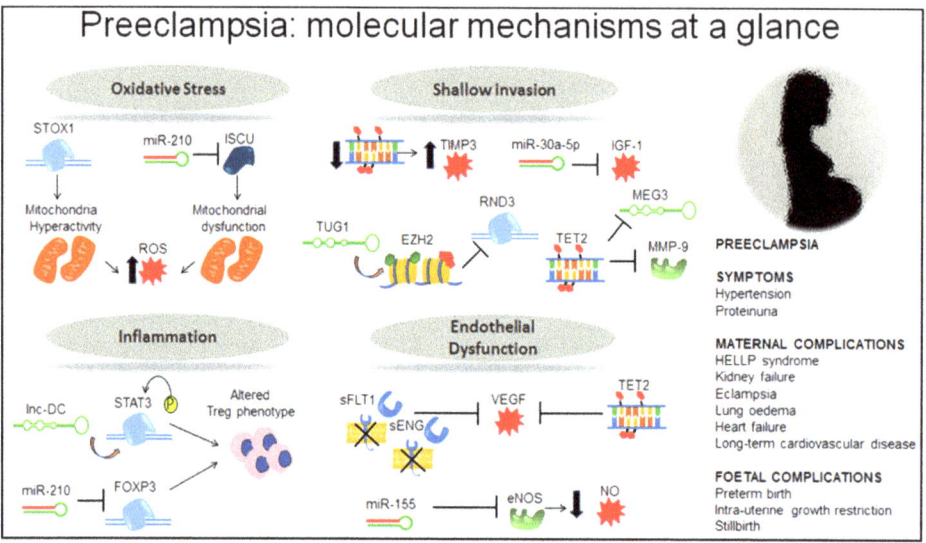

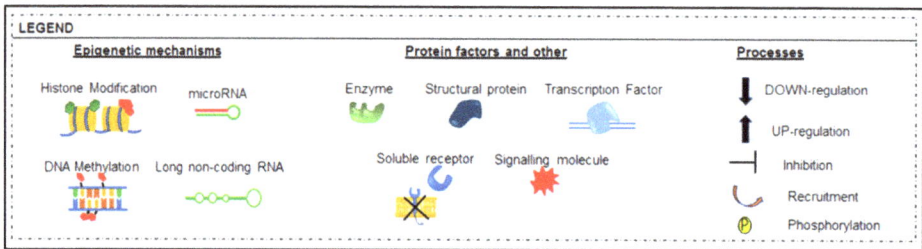

Figure 2. Overview of the molecular mechanisms at play in preeclampsia. Annotations: eNOS = Endothelial Nitric Oxide Synthase; EZH2 = Enhancer of Zeste Homolog 2; FOXP3 = Forkhead box P3; IGF-1 = Insuline-like Growth Factor 1; ISCU = Iron-sulfur cluster; Lnc-DC = Long non-coding RNA DC; miR-30a-5p = microRNA 30a-5p; miR-155 = micro-RNA 155; miR-210 = microRNA 210; MMP-9 = *Matrix Metalloproteinase-9*; NO = Nitric Oxide; RND3 = Rho Family GTPase 3; ROS = Reactive Oxygen Species; sENG = Soluble endoglin; sFLT1 = Soluble fms-like tyrosine kinase *receptor*-1; STAT3 = Signal transducer and activator of transcription 3; STOX1 = Storkhead Box 1; TET2 = Tet methylcytosine dioxygenase 2; TIMP3 = TIMP Metallopeptidase Inhibitor 3; TUG1 = long non-coding RNA taurine-upregulated gene 1; VEGF = Vascular Endothelial Growth Factor.

It is well known that persisting environmental variations induce changes in the epigenetic marks, including DNA methylation. These marks can either be mere biomarkers or participate actively in regulating genes to overcome the changing environmental conditions (although gene expression changes are often disconnected from methylation alterations).

Overall, several of the genome-wide studies showed that the methylation profiles differ between early and late onset of preeclampsia (EOPE and LOPE), suggesting a different etiology between these two types of PE [170–173]. EOPE shows more pronounced genome-wide hypermethylation changes than LOPE, probably since it is caused by earlier alterations allowing the epigenetic reprogramming to install earlier, in reason of the earlier cellular stress [171,174].

Using the Illumina Methylation 450 BeadChip Array, Yeung and coworkers, identified 303 differentially methylated regions in PE, 214 hyper and 89 hypomethylated, after adjusting for gestational age. The genes located nearby or encompassing hypermethylated regions were enriched in gene-ontology (GO) terms such as "ATP transport", in KEGG pathways, such as "steroid hormone biosynthesis", "cellular senescence" and Reactome pathways, such as "Vpr-mediated induction of apoptosis by mitochondrial outer membrane (SLC25A6 and SLC25A4)". The annotation of clusters also revealed an alteration of clusters of homeobox genes, (especially HOXD genes), Wnt2 cell signaling; fertilization and implantation genes; reactive oxygen species signaling (NOX5) and cell adhesion (ALCAM) genes [158]. Amongst the most recent studies, Leavey and coworkers used a novel approach based upon bioinformatics to sort 48 human PE samples through their transcriptome profile before subjecting them to methylation analysis, using the Illumina Human methylation450K array. This made it possible to divide the preeclamptic cases into two groups associated to abnormal methylation marks nearby 'immunological' genes or more 'canonical' EOPE cluster, with for instance abnormally methylated CpG in FLNB, COL17A1, INHBA, SH3PXD2A, as well as in the gene body of FLT1 [160].

In 2015, the study of Zhu and coworkers [175] was the first to analyze simultaneously methylation and hydroxymethylation in the PE placentas. Hydroxymethylation results from the hydroxylation of methyl-Cytosine is a first step towards the active demethylation of DNA through the action of Ten+Eleven Translocation enzyme (TET) proteins, and could play an important role in gene expression regulation [176]. The authors showed that the methylation level is higher in gene promoters and gene bodies in PE versus control placenta. Surprisingly most of the clustering of the genes that were altered, either by methylation or by hydroxymethylation were associated with nervous system development, neurotransmitters, neurogenesis, which are presumably not relevant in a non-neural tissue as the placenta. Nevertheless, positive regulation of vasoconstriction was also enriched as a GO term, as well as regulation of nitrogen compounds, two pathways that have a clear biological sense in terms of placental diseases pathophysiology (association with vascularization and with the modulation of oxidative/nitrosative stresses).

Table 3. Differentially methylated genes in preeclampsia.

Cell Type	Gene	Methylation State in PE	Possible Target	Reference
Placenta and maternal plasma	SERPINB5	Hypomethylated	Trophoblast Invasion	[177]
First-trimester maternal white blood cell and placenta samples	ABCA1	Hypomethylated	Cholesterol transporter in macrophages	[178,179]
First-trimester maternal white blood cell, placenta samples, umbilical cord blood	GNAS	Hypomethylated	Diabetes, hypertension and metabolic diseases	[178,179]
First-trimester maternal white blood cell and placenta samples	TAPBP	Hypomethylated	Peptide loading in the Histocompatibility complex	[178]
First-trimester maternal white blood cell and placenta samples	DYNLL1	Hypomethylated	Phosphate metabolic processing	[178]
First-trimester maternal white blood cell and placenta samples	ORPD1	Hypomethylated	Opioid Receptor	[178]
Placenta	TIMP3	Hypomethylated	Metalloprotease Inhibitor	[180]
Placenta	P2RX4	Hypomethylated	Apoptosis and Inflammation	[170]
Placenta	PAPPA2	Hypomethylated	Insuline-like growth factor regulator	[170]
Placenta	DLX5	Hypomethylated	Trophoblast proliferation and differentiation	[181]
Placenta	KRT15	Hypomethylated	Cytoskeleton	[182]
Placenta	SERPINA3	Hypomethylated	Inhibition of inflammation, pathogen degradation and tissue remodeling	[183]
Placenta	FN1	Hypomethylated	Cell adhesion, trophoblast proliferation, differentiation and apoptosis	[182]
Placenta	TEAD3	Hypomethylated	Cell homeostasis, Inflammation, Coagulation, complement activation	[184]
Placenta	JUNB	Hypomethylated	TNF signaling pathway	[182]
Placenta	PKM2	Hypomethylated	Cellular metabolism	[182]
Placenta	NDRG1	Hypomethylated	Trophoblast invasion	[182]

Table 3. Cont.

Cell Type	Gene	Methylation State in PE	Possible Target	Reference
Placenta	BHLHE40	Hypomethylated	Inhibition of trophoblast differentiation	[171]
Placenta	INHBA	Hypomethylated	Inhibition of trophoblast differentiation	[171]
Placenta	CYP11A1	Hypomethylated	Trophoblast autophagy and steroidogenic pathway	[184]
Placenta	HSD3B1	Hypomethylated	Steroidogenic pathway	[184]
Placenta	TEAD3	Hypomethylated	Steroidogenic pathway	[184]
Placenta	CYP19	Hypomethylated	Steroidogenic pathway	[184]
Placenta	CRH	Hypomethylated	Cortisol bioavailability in the placenta	[184]
Placenta	TFPI-2	Hypomethylated	Block in endothelial dysfunction	[185]
Placenta	VEGF	Hypomethylated	Angiogenesis	[186]
Umbilical cord blood, placenta samples	IGF2	Hypomethylated	Embryonic development and fetal growth	[179,187]
Placenta and Peripheral Blood	GNA12	Hypomethylated	Blood pressure	[188]
Placenta	CAPG	Hypomethylated	Macrophage function	[189]
Placenta	GLI2	Hypomethylated	Embryo development	[189]
Placenta	KRT13	Hypomethylated	Cytoskeleton	[189]
Placenta	LEP	Hypomethylated	Cell homeostasis and metabolism	[190]
Placenta	LP1	Hypomethylated	Lipid metabolism	[191]
Placenta	CEBPα	Hypomethylated	Transcription stimulation of LEP promoter	[191]
Placenta	SH3PXD2A	Hypomethylated	Trophoblast invasion and podosome formation	[191]
Placenta	NCAM1	Hypomethylated	Trophoblast-trophoblast interactions and adhesion	[174]
Cord blood samples	HSD11B2	Hypomethylated	Cortisol transmission from the mother to the fetus	[192]
Placenta	WNT2	Hypermethylated	Placentation and cell signaling	[158,193]
Placenta	SPESP1	Hypermethylated	Fertilization	[158]
Placenta	NOX5	Hypermethylated	Reactive Oxygen Species signaling	[158]
Placenta	ALCAM	Hypermethylated	Cell Adhesion	[158]
Placenta	IGF-1	Hypermethylated	Placentation, trophoblast function, fetal growth.	[194]
Placenta	SOX7	Hypermethylated	Embryonic development and cell fate	[155]
Placenta	CDX1	Hypermethylated	Trophoblast invasion restriction	[155]
Placenta	CXCL1	Hypermethylated	Chemokine inducer of angiogenesis	[155]
Placenta	ADORA2B	Hypermethylated	Placenta impairment and fetal growth restriction	[155]
Placenta	FAM3B	Hypermethylated	Cytokine activity	[182]
Placenta	SYNE1	Hypermethylated	Nuclear organization and structural integrity	[182]
Placenta	AGAP1	Hypermethylated	Cellular development, assembly and function	[182]
Placenta	CRHBP	Hypermethylated	Cortisol bioavailability in the placenta	[190]
Placenta and maternal blood	STAT5A	Hypermethylated	Transcription activation	[195]
Placenta and maternal plasma	RASSF1A	Hypermethylated	Tumor suppressor gene	[177]
Placenta	PTPRN2	Hypermethylated	Phosphate metabolic processing	[173]
Placenta	GATA4	Hypermethylated	Placenta Growth	[173]
	YWHAQ	Hypermethylated	Cellular response to reduce oxygen levels	[196]
Placenta	TNF	Hypermethylated	MMP-9 stimulation, Immune system activation, cell survival, migration and differentiation	[174]
Placenta	COL5A1	Hypermethylated	Extracellular matrix	[174]
Placenta	CDH11	Hypermethylated	Trophoblast anchoring to the decidua, syncytiotrophoblast differentiation	[174]
Placenta	HLA-G	Hypermethylated	Maternal Immune tolerance and immune rejection	[197]

The major modifications of methylation occurring in preeclampsia are presented as Figure 3.

Limits of the Genome-Wide, Multicellular Approach for Preeclampsia Methylation Profiling

As mentioned earlier, a recurrent criticism of genome-wide comparisons between normal and PE placenta is linked to the fact that in general placental samples of PE patients are collected at earlier terms than controls. However, the existence of methylation profiles for control placentas throughout gestation [51] now allows to make the part between the effect of the placental ageing and the effects of the pathology per se. Other limits of these approaches are the complexity of the cell material, the variation between the degree of severity of the disease or the various statistical tests that are used in the different studies. Also, several studies have brought attention to the lack of reproducibility in high-throughput genomic, transcriptomic and epigenomic studies. This has been recently discussed by Komwar and coworkers in a recent study were they analyze the sources of variation in preeclampsia high-throughput studies an propose a methodology to ensure reproducibility and thus facilitate the integration of data across studies [198].

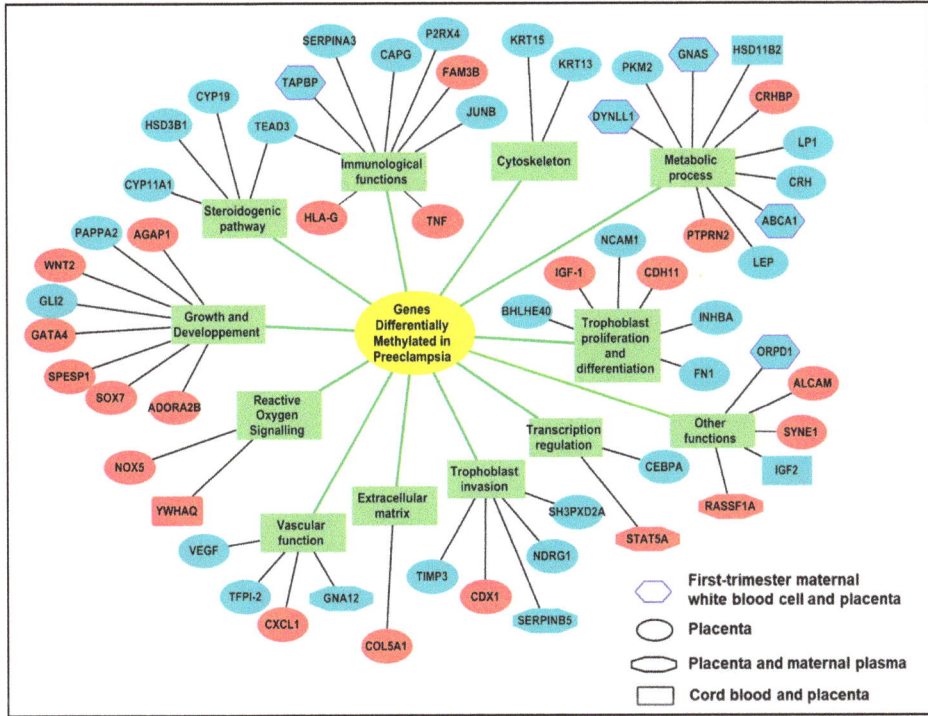

Figure 3. Overview of major methylation alterations in preeclampsia. The main pathways are shown in green boxes. The significant alterations in methylation may be associated either to increased or decreased gene expression (hypermethylated in red and hypomethylated in blue).

Single-Cell Analysis, the Next Frontier to Methylation Epigenomic Approaches

Gene-scale expression studies were recently carried out at the single cell scale [199] and have provided evidence of gene expression shifts during the CT, SCT and EVT differentiation steps, as well as, allowed the reconstructions of differentiation trajectories. This has also been analyzed by genome-scale DNA methylation analysis. Gamage and coworkers have analyzed by RRBS side population trophoblasts, CTs and EVTs from human first trimester placentas [56]. Forty-one genes involved in EMT and metastatic cancer pathways were found methylated between CT and EVTs, possibly contributing to the invasive phenotype of these cells. In the BeWo cell model where fusion can be induced by forskolin, RRBS analysis performed before and after fusion, showed altered methylation of genes involved in cell differentiation and commitment, together with a gain in transcriptionally active histone marks such as H3K4me3 [54]. Such approaches are for the moment difficult to transpose to placenta pathophysiology. Instead, several systems where methylation influences normal placental function have been studied. As an example, we present below the epigenetic regulation of genes involved in placental invasion and PE.

An Example of Specific Gene Alterations of Methylation: Regulation of Invasion

MMPs are well-characterized proteins involved in trophoblast invasion and angiogenesis during pregnancy. They constitute a family of 23 Zn^{2+} and Ca^{2+}-dependent proteases that degrade the extracellular matrix. This family of proteins presents abnormal concentration and behavior in placental diseases such as PE [200], placenta accreta and placenta percreta [201,202]. This has been recently reviewed for preeclampsia [203]. A decreased level of MMP-2 and MMP-9 reduces the remodeling of spiral arteries in early gestation. Besides, other MMPs, such as MMP-1 and MMP-14, may also have a role in this disease. Epigenetic mechanisms are at work for controlling MMP gene expression.

Li and coworkers observed that TET2 is involved in the demethylation of the *MMP-9* promoter, this being associated to the downregulation of the protein and contributing to trophoblast shallow invasion [204].

TIMP3, a MMP inhibitor, shows the highest methylation reduction (over 15%) in EOPE compared to control placentas with an inverse correlation between methylation level and gene expression suggesting an increased transcription of TIMP3 in PE placentas [180,189]. Low levels of TIMP3 lead to poor invasion of the trophoblast and placenta hypoperfusion. Moreover, TIMP3 may be able to inhibit angiogenesis by blocking vascular endothelial growth factor binding to its receptor contributing to impaired placenta blood vessels development. Also, genetic variations of the gene have been associated with cardiovascular disorders and hypertension.

3.1.2. Maternal Blood Epigenetic Marks in Preeclampsia

Alterations in the levels of many plasma and serum proteins have been associated with PE. In 2013, White and coworkers showed that PE was favoring hypermethylation in white blood maternal cells using the methylation-27k arrays from Illumina [205]. GRIN2b. GABRA1. PCDHB7 and BEX1 were found differentially methylated, with an enrichment of the neuropeptide signaling pathway. The re-analysis of methylation of genes known to be involved in PE revealed that in maternal circulating leukocytes, CpG sited from 4 genes associated with PE, POMC, AGT, CALCA and DDAH1, showed differential methylation in PE compared to control, with moderate methylation differences (<6%) [206]. These 4 genes are known to alter immunomodulation and inflammatory response, suggesting that at least alterations of the placental physiology in preeclampsia have epigenomic consequences on maternal circulating cells.

During pregnancy, 3 to 6% of cell-free DNA in the maternal blood plasma is derived from the placenta. Oxidative stress in PE leads to increased trophoblast apoptosis and the release of SCT microparticles and a five to ten-fold increase in circulating fetal DNA in the maternal bloodstream compared with control counterparts [207,208]. These free fetal molecules and their methylation status have been proposed as a non-invasive biomarker of fetal and placental pathologies before the onset of symptoms. This has been shown for Maspin, for which the unmethylated version have a median methylation more than 5.7 fold higher in PE than control pregnancies [209,210]. Another epigenetic marker of preeclampsia is the methylation of RASSF1A (Ras Association domain-containing protein 1) promoter [177,211,212].

3.1.3. Maternal Endothelial Cells

There is limited access to maternal vessels in pregnancy, nevertheless DNA methylation was assessed from this material in 2012 using the 27K methylation array of Illumina [213]. From 14.495 genes interrogated by the array, 65 genes were identified as hypomethylated in PE. Clustering leads to identify biological processes such as smooth muscle contraction, thrombosis, inflammation, redox homeostasis, sugar metabolism and amino acid metabolism. These alterations of the maternal endothelium suggest potential effects on cardiovascular life of the mother after preeclampsia. Focusing on collagen metabolism, the authors revealed an increased expression of MMP1 and MMP8 in vascular smooth muscle cells and infiltrating neutrophils of omental arteries of preeclamptic women, which was associated with reduced methylation in the promoters of both genes in pathological patients compared to control patients [213]. In the same study, several other MMPs, showed reduced hypomethylation in PE patients albeit with lower significance [214,215]. Moreover, pregnant women under dietary supplementation may restore the reduced methylation in the promoters of these genes and be protected against the development of PE. Interestingly, all these MMPs genes are located in chromosome 11, which may be indicative of a specific sensitivity of this chromosome to epigenetic changes caused by oxidative stress during the development of the pathology. The same team reported the reduced methylation in the promoter region of TBXAS1 gene in correlation with increased gene and protein expression of thromboxane synthase in vascular smooth muscle, endothelium and infiltrating neutrophils [215]. Increased levels of thromboxane synthase induce the overproduction of thromboxane A2, a potent vasoconstrictor and platelet activator, contributing to hypertension and coagulation abnormalities classically related to PE.

3.1.4. Cord Blood Cells

In 2014, Nomura and coworkers analyzed the global methylation profile of cord blood cells using the LUMA technique [161] and failed to observe an actual difference but with a limited number of controls samples (5) [216]. Genome-Wide Methylation analysis using the 450K microarray tool on neonatal cord blood DNA showed a significant genome-scale hypomethylation in neonatal cord blood DNA associated with EOPE, with 51,486 hypomethylated and 12,563 hypermethylated CpGs [187]. In this study the most differential methylated genes were associated with inflammatory pathways, cholesterol and lipid metabolism, including IL12B, FAS, PIK31 and IGF1. Deregulation of both metabolic pathways may increase the risk of cardiovascular diseases in the fetus [187]. The same microarray approach allowed to identify 5001 mostly hypermethylated regions in umbilical cord white blood cells and 869 mostly hypomethylated regions in the placenta [217]. In the cord blood cells, the gene networks enriched were involved in cardiovascular system development, cell cycle, cancer, cell morphology, infectious diseases, suggesting specific alterations that could have long-term consequences on the fetal health.

Some studies focused on mitochondrial DNA, showing hypomethylation in PE cord blood cells. The most affected loci are keys in mitochondria functionality: D-loop (control of mitochondrial DNA replication), Cytochrome C oxidase subunit 1 gene (respiratory chain) and TF/RNR1 locus (necessary for protein synthesis) [218]. Increased copy of mitochondria is observed in the placenta and maternal blood during PE suggesting an adaptive response to stress [219,220]. This is also observed in mouse models of PE [221]. Hypomethylation in the D-loop may lead to increased mitochondrial replication explaining the pathological increase of mitochondrial DNA. Methylation assay in endothelial colony-forming cells present in cord blood from PE presents differential methylation level in genes related to RNA metabolic processes, cellular protein modification processes and in positive regulation transcription, as assessed with the EPIC Illumina array, interrogating over 850,000 CpG [222]. However, at later passages, an increased number of genes are abnormally methylated. This suggests that preeclampsia may drive an altered epigenetic program in endothelial cell precursors that will be the building bricks of the newborn vascular system and program later complications.

3.2. Non Coding RNAs

Non-coding RNAs have been found to be differentially expressed in preeclampsia by a number of sources. Some studies have focused on investigating differential expression patterns between PE placental samples of different severities versus control groups looking for miRNAs or lncRNA [223–226], without generally identifying consensual signatures. With the aim of identifying potential biomarkers that could be used diagnostically to predict preeclampsia onset, many groups have set out instead to identify molecules differentially expressed in the plasma of patients, which could potentially be detected by mean of a simple blood test [227]. lncRNA and miRNA are the two classes of non-coding RNAs that have dominated the scene of non-coding molecules in preeclampsia. Other classes of non-coding RNAs have been identified, such as circular RNAs, that appeared recently in the context of PE development and future research will help understand the role of these molecules in the regulation of gene expression and disease [228].

3.2.1. LncRNAs in Preeclampsia

Long non-coding RNAs are RNA molecules longer than 200 nucleotides which are involved in regulation of cell function through a wide range of mechanisms. lncRNAs are expressed in the nucleus as single stranded RNA molecules, which can either function in their native form or undergo maturation through the addition of a 5′cap and polyA tail; however, they are never translated into a protein product [229]. They regulate cell function by a wide range of mechanisms: alteration of the stability of target mRNAs, direct recruitment of chromatin modification enzymes, segregation of transcription factors through specific binding sites contained within the lncRNA sequence, warehousing miRNA as 'miRNA sponges', a function shared with circular RNAs [230]. For a complete overview please see Reference [231].

Transcriptomic analyses of placenta and decidua total RNAs allowed identifying differentially expressed lncRNAs between PE and control patients, often with a difference between EOPE and LOPE [228,232,233]. Most of these lncRNAs had been previously identified in the field of cancer research, often associated with cell proliferation, migration and invasion [234]. As mentioned above, given the parallels between the features of cancer cells and the trophoblasts during placentation such as fast proliferation of the trophoblast, migration and invasion of the maternal tissues, immunotolerance [235–238], this did not come as a surprise and has prompted extensive in vitro research to elucidate the roles of these lncRNAs in trophoblast physiology.

In the present review, we will focus on a few lncRNAs that have been well characterized: MALAT-1, MEG3, RNA-ATB. Finally, we will give a brief overview on how in PE some lncRNAs regulate gene expression by altering chromatin methylation state of their target genes, through direct recruitment of histone methyltransferases, bringing as examples PVT1, TUG1 and DIAPH2-AS1. H19 was discussed above for its important role in placental development and miRNA encoding lncRNA.

MALAT-1

Metastasis associated lung adenocarcinoma transcript-1 (MALAT-1) was firstly identified in lung cancer; it is a lncRNA of over 8 kb [239]. MALAT-1 normally localizes in the nucleus where it forms nuclear aggregates called speckles involved in the regulation of splicing factors availability [240]. MALAT-1 is overexpressed in placental pathologies associated with uncontrolled trophoblast invasion [241], which prompted Chen and coworkers [33] to investigate its expression in PE. Comparing RNA levels in 18 PE placentas with matched controls, MALAT-1 was found significantly downregulated in PE placentas. Overexpression and downregulation of MALAT-1 in JEG-3 regulates cell proliferation and invasion, while inhibiting apoptosis [33]. These findings suggest that MALAT-1 deregulation could lead to poor invasion of the maternal endometrium, affecting the spiral arteries' remodeling and placenta development. Li and coworkers [242] have shown that the role of MALAT-1 is not restricted solely to the trophoblast but has a key role in regulating the angiogenesis and vascularization of the maternal decidua and fetal umbilical vasculature. MALAT-1 is expressed by mesenchymal stem cells (MSCs) in the maternal decidua and in the umbilical cord. These cells are pluripotent progenitors which are able of self-renewal and proliferation, differentiate to promote tissue regeneration, form de novo vasculature, angiogenesis and regulate immune system responses [243]. Li and coworkers (2017) observed a decreased MALAT-1 expression in MSCs from decidua and umbilical cord of preeclamptic pregnancies and set out to investigate its function in these cells. Similarly, MALAT-1 promotes proliferation and protects from apoptosis in isolated MSCs. Interestingly, coculture of MSCs with trophoblast cell line HTR-8/SVneo clearly showed how MALAT-1 overexpression could promote migration and invasion of the trophoblasts towards the MSCs layer. Coculture of the endothelial cell line HUVECs (Human Umbilical Vein Endothelial Cells) in supernatant obtained from MSCs which either expressed or had downregulated MALAT-1 showed how MALAT-1 promotes tube formation this process being dependent on Vascular Endothelial Growth Factor secretion. Finally, MALAT-1 over-expression increased the levels of the IDO protein, which activated macrophage maturation, proving its role in immune system regulation. These findings combined with the work of Chen and coworkers (2015) beautifully illustrates how MALAT-1 has a symmetric regulatory function in placentation: on the one hand, it promotes trophoblast proliferation, invasive and migratory potential and on the other hand, its expression in MSCs cells helps to attract and promote trophoblast invasion, stimulates tube formation, promotes angiogenesis and vascularization. Increase in Reactive Oxygen Species caused MALAT-1 and VEGF downregulation in MSCc exposed to oxidative stress in a dose-dependent manner [242]. MALAT-1 downregulation in preeclampsia could therefore have a huge impact on placentation and further development of the placenta over the course of gestation. It is possible that a first triggering event maybe of immunological nature, causes an increase of oxidative stress during implantation which will then alter the expression level of many targets, including MALAT-1; based on the data, this consequent deregulation would have an impact on both trophoblast and MSCs physiology, culminating in preeclampsia.

MEG3

Maternally Expressed 3 (MEG3) is an imprinted lncRNA which is expressed in many different cell types and tissues and acts as a tumor suppressor and is downregulated in many types of cancer. Physiologically, MEG3 acts by stabilising p53 and activating apoptotic responses [244]. Zhang and coworkers [34] analysed MEG3 RNA levels in 30 placentas from preeclamptic women, compared to 30 control samples and found a statistically significant 80% downregulation. These results were consistent with those of Yu and coworkers [245] studying a cohort of 20 preeclamptic and 20 control placentas, finding that MEG3 RNA was only 28% of the RNA levels of the control group. To elucidate in more detail the function of MEG3 in placenta, Zhang and coworkers (2015) overexpressed MEG3 in two trophoblast cell lines (JEG3 and HTR-8/SVneo), showing enhanced antiapoptotic effects, while downregulation of MEG3 increased the apoptotic cells. Analysis of protein markers showed how MEG3 downregulation increased the levels of pro-apoptotic proteins such as Caspase-3 and Bax. These results contrast with what is observed in cancer, where MEG3 expression is rather associated with the activation of proapototic pathways, possibly suggesting a different mode of action of MEG3 in these cell types. Yu and coworkers [245] focused on the link between MEG3 expression and endothelial-mesenchymal transition (EMT). During implantation and placentation, the trophoblasts undergo EMT in order to be able to migrate and invade the maternal tissues. MEG3 downregulation correlated with increased E-cadherin levels and downregulation of mesenchymal markers such as N-cadherin, vimentin, slug (encoded by the gene SNAI2), in placental RNA and protein extracts, placental sections and in vitro tests (HTR-8/SVneo trophoblast cell line). Changes in MEG3 expression did not influence proliferation but MEG3 overexpression promoted migration and trophoblasts invasion through matrigel matrixes [34,224]. Altogether, MEG3 protects from apoptosis, promotes migration and invasion by regulating endothelial-mesenchymal transition in trophoblast cells and therefore its downregulation possibly affects trophoblast invasion and placentation, playing a key role in preeclampsia. Consistently, the imprinting control region (IG-DMR) of the DLK1-MEG3 cluster was very recently found hypermethylated in human umbilical veins from preeclamptic pregnancies, with an altered expression of both imprinted genes, a lower secretion of nitrite, VEGF and a higher secretion of endothelin 1 (ET1) all factors able to mediate pathological mechanisms in the offspring from preeclampsias [246].

RNA-ATB

As with many other lncRNAs, lncRNA-activated by TGFβ (RNA-ATB) was first discovered in cancer, upregulated in hepatocellular carcinoma, it promotes cell proliferation, migration and invasion [247]. It has been reported that in hepatocells RNA-ATB is expressed in response to TGFβ and in fibroblasts; it can create positive feedback regulation by promoting TGFβ paracrine release. Lnc RNA-ATB was found to be significantly downregulated in placental samples from women with preeclampsia. Moreover patients with EOPE showed an even stronger deregulation [248]. Given the proliferative, invasive and migratory features of trophoblasts and in particular extravillous trophoblast, Liu and coworkers (2017) investigated lncRNA-ATB function in trophoblast cell line HTR-8/SVneo, which is a standard in vitro model of extravillous trophoblast. While overexpression of lncRNA-ATB increased the proliferative, migratory and invasive potential of HTR-8/SVneo cells, the downregulation caused a steep decrease in proliferation, migration and invasion, proving that this gene has an important role on the physiology of the extravillous trophoblast and that its deregulation could explain an aberrant implantation and endometrium invasion in preeclampsia, potentially being linked to incomplete spiral artery remodeling. Whether RNA-ATB regulates trophoblast function through the interaction with members of the miR200 family is yet to be determined. However, increased miR200 has been found to affect the development of endometrium receptivity, negatively impacting implantation [249]. In labor, miR200 is upregulated in the human uterus and has been associated with pre-term labor in murine studies [250]. It seems likely that an interaction between RNA-ATB and miR200 is required for correct placental development, gestation and delivery.

PVT1, TUG1 and DIAPH2-AS1: Regulating Gene Expression through Recruitment of Chromatin Remodeling Complexes

lncRNAs work through different mechanisms, depending on the specific lncRNA, the cell type, the downstream targets [231]. In the past few years a few lncRNAs have been identified in preeclampsia as potential modulators, among which PVT1, TUG1 and DIAPH2-AS1 adopt the same mechanism of action. lncRNA TUG1 is downregulated in preeclamptic placentas. Interference of TUG1 in trophoblast cell lines (JEG3 and HTR-8/SVneo) negatively affected cell proliferation and growth, migration and invasion, network formation, while it increased apoptosis [31]. Transcriptome analysis by RNA-sequencing of HTR-/SVneo cells in which TUG1 was downregulated showed a prevalence of affected genes involved in cell growth, migration and apoptosis. Xu and coworkers (2017) identified RND3 as main downstream factor involved in the phenotypic effects of TUG1 downregulation. RND3 mRNA and protein levels were strongly upregulated in response to TUG1 interference in vitro and RND3 mRNA was upregulated in preeclamptic placenta. RND3 is also known as RhoE, a GTPase that acts as a tumor suppressor, negatively regulating proliferation, migration and invasion [251]. In vitro experiments beautifully elucidated the mechanism by which TUG1 modulates RND3 expression—TUG1 directly interacts with the histone modification factor Enhancer of Zeste Homolog 2 (EZH2) and recruits it to the RND3 promoter, where EZH2 drives the silencing of RND3 by tri-methylating H3K27, resulting in strong RND3 downregulation [31]. A year later, Xu and coworkers [252] identified another lncRNA PVT1, strongly downregulated in preeclamptic placenta, whose downregulation negatively affects proliferation and increases apoptosis of trophoblast cell lines. PVT1 was found to recruit EZH2 to the promoter of the transcription factor ANGPTL4, driving its repression by increase in repressive chromatin markers: this could partially explain the phenotypic effects of PVT1 deregulation. Feng and coworkers [253] uncovered a complicated regulatory network behind PAX3 deregulation in preeclampsia which is linked with decreased proliferation, invasion and migration of trophoblast cells [254]. PAX3 is a transcription factor downregulated in preeclamptic placentas and this correlates with DNA hypermethylation of the promoter region [171,254]. In this study, Feng and coworkers (2019) found that in preeclamptic placentas lncRNA DIAPH2-AS1 is upregulated along with the transcription factor HOXD8. In vitro experiments in HTR-8/SVneo cells clarified the regulatory network: under hypoxia the transcription factor HOXD8 is upregulated and induces expression of the lncRNA DIAPH2-AS1. DIAPH2-AS1 recruits lysine-specific demethylase 1 (LSD1) to the promoter of PAX3 where it alters the chromatin modification state, decreasing methylation of Histone H3. LSD1 can also modify DNA methyl-transferase 1 (DNMT1), stabilizing it. ChIP experiments showed enrichment of LSD1 and DNMT1 at the PAX3 promoter, which correlated with increased DNA methylation and mRNA repression. Interference of DIAPH2-AS1 was enough to reverse the phenotype and increase PAX3 levels [253]. These studies underscore that different epigenetic mechanisms regulate gene expression. It is possible that certain mechanisms are favored in different cell types and future studies will help identify the conserved regulatory networks that plays a role in the etiology of preeclampsia.

3.2.2. micro RNA and Preeclampsia

microRNAs in Preeclampsia

The first study on microRNAs (miRs) in preeclampsia was published in 2007. In this study, the expression levels of a subset of 157 miRNAs expressed in the placenta were tested by qRT-PCR in human placental samples from pregnancies without any complications, with PE, and with PE and small for gestational age (SGA) outcomes. 153 miRNA were detected in the placenta RNA samples and three of them were found to be upregulated in PE: miR-210, miR-155, miR-200b [255]. The first global transcriptomic analysis of microRNAs was performed with 20 PE placental samples and 20 controls, with microarray technology by Zhu and collaborators in 2009. Comparing gene expression profiles of the severe PE group with controls, 11 microRNAs were upregulated and 23 downregulated. Among them, many microRNAs are organized in chromosomal clusters: downregulated clusters are found in 13q31.3, 14q32.31, Xq26.2, Xq26.3, while upregulated clusters are found in 19q13.42 suggesting co-regulation profiles [256]. An integrative analysis was conducted comparing distinct datasets with the aim of identifying microRNAs–transcripts regulatory networks in preeclampsia. resulting in the construction of a map of putative microRNA-gene target interactions in developmental process, response to nutrient levels, cell differentiation, cell junction, membrane components [257].

Although many studies followed, most of them aimed at identifying differentially expressed miRs in placenta and in plasma samples from PE women. Fewer studies have focused in other cell types present in the placenta. For example, in fetal endothelial cells downregulation of miR-29a-3p and miR-29c-3p and upregulation of miR-146a is observed in PE patients [258]. Both miR-29a and miR-29c show proangiogenic functions by stimulating HUVECs proliferation and tube formation through VEGFA-induced and FGF2-induced cell migration pathways [259]. However, other studies suggest an antiangiogenic role of miR-29c through downregulation of the IGF-1 proteins at the post-transcriptional level [260,261]. On the other hand, miR-146a inhibits the de-novo formation of blood vessels in-vitro and reduces tube formation ability in HUVECs [260,261]. The study of the role that miRs may have in the different cell types present in the placenta is indispensable to understand the role of this molecules in the development of the disease. In the long term, it has also been shown that miRNA profiles in the neonate is altered following an hypertensive pregnancy; for instance the level of mir-146a at birth predict microvascular development three months later [262].

Many studies followed, aimed at identifying differentially expressed miRs in placenta and in plasma samples from PE women.

In this review, we will discuss the most well characterized microRNAs miR-210, miR-155 and give an overview of some of the research that has been carried out on circulating microRNAs, given their potential as clinically relevant biomarkers.

miR-210

miR-210 is a microRNA involved in the regulation of mitochondrial function and hypoxia response. It has been well characterized, in placentas as well as in different cancer and tissue types [263]. Most of the knowledge on the regulatory pathways that involve miR-210 comes from oncology research. miR-210 has been soon identified as one of the early hypoxia-response miRs, being directly regulated by the Hypoxia inducible factor 1α (HIF-1α) [264]. Under hypoxic conditions, miR-210 alters mitochondrial function promoting a metabolic switch to glycolysis. This is achieved by negative targeting of genes involved in the electron-transport chain, namely iron-sulfur cluster scaffold homolog (ISCU) and cytochrome C oxidase assembly protein (COX10). As a result, miR-210 also increases the levels of Reactive Oxygen Species (ROS) [265]. Under hypoxia, miR-210 and HIF-1α establish a positive feedback regulation that maintains both expression of both factors. This is achieved by miR-210 downregulation of the mRNA of Glycerol-3-Phosphate Dehydrogenase 1-Like, which would otherwise contribute to targeting HIF1α to the proteasome for degradation. Conversely, stabilized HIF1α directly activates miR-210 expression [266].

In endothelial cells, miR-210 is involved in regulating angiogenesis and vascularization which are fundamental processes in placenta development. Hypoxia causes miR-210 activation which protects endothelial cells from apoptosis and stimulates chemotaxis driven by VEGF, migration and tube formation [267]. In preeclampsia, miR-210 was first identified as upregulated in placenta samples by Pineles and collaborators (2007) using qPCR. In the first comprehensive study carried out with microarray technologies, miR-210 was consistently found upregulated in placenta of severe preeclamptic women, however in mild preeclampsia it was found to be downregulated, which might suggest different mechanisms at play or rather different metabolic states of the placenta, with a more pronounced ischemia in severe preeclamptic placentas [256]. Moreover, subsequent analyses identified significantly upregulated miR-210 in plasma samples from patients with preeclampsia [181]. In the context of PE miR-210 is involved in the mitochondrial dysfunction observed, which causes metabolic imbalance, excessive ROS production and cell damage. Similarly to what happens in cancer, miR-210 negatively regulates ISCU which is downregulated in preeclampsia samples, directly affecting mitochondrial architecture and functionality [268–270]. The deregulation of miR-210 was also found in the placentas of mice from a preeclamptic model [134].

miR-210 is also an important modulator of trophoblast phisiology. In vitro studies using isolated primary trophoblasts and trophoblast cell line JAR, proved how hypoxia induces an increase in miR-210 levels. Artificial overexpression of miR-210 in JAR cells caused a significant downregulation of migration and invasion. In trophoblast cells, hypoxia and ROS can activate HIF1α but more importantly NFκ-B p50—which si found upregulated in preeclamptic placenta tissues. NFκ-B p50 binds a consensus sequence in the miR-210 promoter, activating its expression. In trophoblasts, miR-210 interacts with a perfect match with the 3'-UTR of the transcription factor homeobox-A9 (HOXA9), causing both degradation of the mRNA and downregulation of translation. Another direct target is Ephrin-A3 (EFNA3), a ligand of the Ephrin binding receptors, in this case miR-210 binds the 3'UTR of the gene with an imperfect match, causing only translational downregulation. These two transcription factors activate expression profiles involved in migration, invasion and vascularisation [181]. Therefore, in trophoblast, miR-210 expression correlates with a negative regulation of migration and invasion, mediated by downregulation of EFNA3 and HOXA9, in response to hypoxia, ROS and activated NFκ-B signaling.

Further studies have identified additional downstream targets of miR-210 in preeclampsia, which are downregulated in preeclamptic samples and whose expression is altered upon miR-210 activation in cell models. A few examples are inflammation related molecules STAT6 and IL-4 [271], potassium channel modulatory factor 1 (KCMF1) [272], thrombospondin type I domain containing 7A (THSD7A) [273].

This mounting body of evidence highlights a key role of miR-210 in the development and maintainance of a preeclamptic phenotype. However it is still not clear which is the triggering event. It is possible that complications during implantation trigger an immune response which would create a pro-inflammatory environment, activating NFκ-B signaling, causing aberrant expression of miR-210 and all consequent downstream cascades. Recently, Chen and collaborator (2019) analysed the inflammatory profile of preeclamptic women, compared to patients which experienced healthy pregnancie [274]. The concentrations of proinflammatory cytokines (IL-6, IL-17) were higher in plasma samples from peripheral blood in the preeclampsia group. Moreover, Transforming Growth Factor β1 (TGF β1) levels were higher as well. TGF β1 has the function of promoting the prevalence of a subset of regulatory T cells (Tregs) that maintain immunotolerance, allowing a successful implantation and avoiding an immune response against the foetal tissues. These Tregs are characterised by expression of the fork-head box p3 (Foxp3) transcription factor, which promotes an immunotolerant phenotype [275]. However, proinflammatory signals such as IL-6 cause the activation of T cells at the expense of Foxp3-positive Tregs, causing an activation of inflammatory responses. Zhao and coworkers showed that miR210 was upregulated in preeclamptic placentas and Foxp3 mRNA and protein levels were found downregulated, previous studies had shown evidence of direct regulation of Fox3p by miR210, suggesting a pivotal role of this microRNA in regulating the threshold of immunotolerance by altering the balance of Foxp3+ Tregs/activated Tcells [276].

miR-155

miR-155 is upregulated in preeclamptic placentas [255]. This upregulation correlates inversely with the level of cysteine-rich protein 61(CYR61) [277], which is a factor secreted by different cell types, including trophoblast, involved in promoting migration, invasion, angiogenesis and vascularisation [278,279]. miR-155 directly targets the 3'-UTR of CYR61 mRNA with a perfect match, causing transcriptional and translational repression. In vitro experiments (HTR-8/SVneo trophoblast cell line) showed how miR-155 inhibits CYR61-mediated expression of VEGF, inhibiting trophoblast migration [277]. Decreased trophoblast-mediated secretion of VEGF would negatively affect angiogenesis and vascularisation in the site of placenta development.

miR-155 regulates trophoblast proliferation and migration also by directly targeting the cell cycle gene Cyclin D1 [172]. Cyclin D1 is involved in cell cycle progression, migration and invasion of trophoblast lineages, downregulated in preeclamptic placentas at both mRNA and protein levels [280–282]. In vitro studies have shown how miR-155 through direct targeting of the 3'UTR of CyclinD mRNA downregulates mRNA and protein levels, negatively affecting migration, causing cell cycle arrest and decrease in proliferation in HTR-8/SVneo cells [42]. Exiting cell cycle is a step of terminal differentiation, which suggests how miR-155 overexpression, as found in preeclampsia, could lead to a premature differentiation of cytotrophoblasts, possibly inducing syncytialization. This phenomenon would cause depletion of the cytotrophoblast pool, accelerating placental aging.

In sum, miR-155 modulates proliferation, migration and invasion of trophoblasts and its expression can affect the phenotype of endothelial cells by negatively regulating VEGF release. miR-155 deregulation could have catastrophic consequences in placentation, deeply affecting trophoblast infiltration, vascularization and angiogenesis of the developing placenta.

Circulating miR-155

Maternal plasma from preeclamptic women presented significantly statistically higher levels of miR-155 [283]. In blood, microRNAs are quite stable and can travel through circulation, to be uptaken by different cell types, such as endothelial and immune cells, regulating gene expression [284]. Yang, Zhang and Ding (2017) showed how plasma levels of miR-155 positively correlate with proinflammatory cytokine interleukin-17 (IL-17) and with proteinuria and urine podocytes counts in women with preeclampsia. Similarly to miR-210, miR-155 promoter presents a binding site for NFκ-B and can be activated by this inflammation master regulator, which could suggest a similar pattern of regulation for miR-155 and pro-inflammatory factors, other than a direct interaction between these genes [285].

miR-155 in Endothelial Cells

Endothelial cells play a fundamental role in placentation given the copious vascularisation and angiogenesis that takes place in the maternal endometrium during placentation. In preeclampsia, pro-inflammatory factors and secreted molecules from the preeclamptic placenta produce an excessive activation of the maternal endothelium, resulting in endothelyal dysfunction, culminating in inflammation, blood pressure changes, downstream systemic effects [286]. miR-155 has been found to be downregulated in human umbelical vein endothelial cells (HUVECs) from preeclamptic women, compared to HUVECs from healthy pregnant women [287]. This downregulation correlated with an increase in Angiotensin II Receptor 1 (AT1R) and increased phosphorylation of Extracellular Signal-regulated Kinases1/2 (ERKs), identifying AT1R as direct target of miR-155 [287]. Activation of the Angiotensin II- AT1R through ERK1/2 in endothelial cells causes cell cycle arrest and initiation of senescence pathways; miR-155 depletion-dependent increase in AT1R will render endothelial cells more sensitive to blood level of Angiotensin II, promoting endothelial damage [288].

miR-155 has been implicated in regulating Nitric Oxide (NO) production in endothelial cells. NO is a potent vasodilator and reduced levels of NO have been associated with preeclampsia etiology [289,290]. In vitro studies using HUVECs proved how endothelial Nitric Oxide synthase (eNOS) mRNA is a direct target of miR-155; proinflammatory stimuli upregulate miR-155 expression in these cells in vitro, downregulating eNOS and NO production [290]. As mentioned above, microRNAs can be found in plasma and miR-155 is upregulated in plasma of women with preeclampsia [69]. microRNAs can be free in circulation or travel inside vescicles and exosomes, which can be uptaken by target cells, activating signaling pathways, affecting expression profiles [291]. Shen and collaborators (2018) elegantly showed how exosomes from plasma samples of preeclamptic patients can affect eNOS mRNA and protein levels in HUVECs [292]. In particular, treatment of HUVECs in vitro with isolated exosomes from plasma of preeclamptic patients (compared to exosomes from control group) caused a statistically significant decrease in eNOS mRNA and protein levels, which correlated with decreased NO production. When analysing the composition of the exosomes, miR-155 was found to be upregulated in the preeclamptic group. Follow up in vitro tests proved how miR-155 located in the exosomes affects eNOS regulation in endothelial cells.

miR-155 in Vascular Smooth Muscle Cells

In arteries and arterioles, endothelial cells are interspaced by vascular smooth muscle cells (VSMCs) which thanks to their contractile properties allow vasoconstriction and vasodilation to occur, accomodating for changes in blood pressure. VSMCs generally present a contractile phenotype characterised by elongated spindle-like morphology, high concentration of contractile filaments. In response to external stimuli, they can switch to a synthetic phenotype characterised by loss of contractility markers, rhomboid morphology, increased proliferative and migratory potential; in this state VSMCs cells lose the ability to modulate vascular resistance [293]. Phenotypic regulation of VSMCs is driven by soluble guanylate cyclase (sGC) which increases intracellular levels of guanosine monophosphate (cGMP), key messenger molecule. cGMP is the substrate of cyclic GMP-dependent protein kinase (PKG) which activates downstream signaling pathways promoting VSMCs contractile phenotype. Nitric Oxide produced by endothelial cells positively modulates sGC activity, favouring vasodilation through enhancement of the VSMCs contractile phenotype [294,295].

In the presence of proinflammatory cytokine Transforming Necrosis Factor α (TNFα), miR-155 was found to be directly activated by NFκ-B in in vitro model of VSMCs. The upregulated miR-155 directly interacts with the 3'-UTR of the mRNA of PKG1 [296] and of the β1 subunit of guanylate cyclase (sGCβ1), resulting in translational repression and mRNA degradation [297]. As a consequence of sGCβ1 downregulation, intracellular cGMP levels are strongly decreased and the downregulation of PKG1 inhibits downstream pathways [296,297]. Park and collaborators (2019) co-cultured HUVECs and VSMCs, observing higher cGMP accumulation in VSMCs, which is mediated by Ntric Oxide stimulation, produced by the endothelial cells [297]. This could be countered by ectopic miR-155 expression in VSMCs. miR-155 overexpressing in response to TNFα, mediating inhibition of the sGC/PKG pathway, causes downregulation of contractile protein markers. This results in a shift of VSMCs to a synthetic phenotype, assuming a rhomboid morphology, increasing proliferation and migration rates. Interestingly the pro-contractile effects of Nitric Oxide could be cancelled by miR-155 expression [296,297]. In placental vessels of preeclamptic placenta sGCβ1 mRNA levels are downregulated [297], given the evidence provided on miR-155 repression of the sGC/PKG pathway, we can imagine that PKG1 might be downregulated as well. In response to inflammation, both endothelial and smooth muscle cells are affected and in preeclampsia they overexpress miR-155 which alters their ability to produce and respond to vasodilation stimuli. Taken together, this evidence highlights the pivotal role of inflammation and miR-155 in the etiology of the preeclamptic phenotype.

Potential Biomarkers: microRNAs Circulating in Maternal Plasma

Since the identification of circulating small RNAs in plasma samples, the prospect of their potential use as diagnostic and predictive biomarkers has fueled extensive research [298]. In the context of preeclampsia, the finding that small microRNAs with placental origin can travel in the blood circulation and affect systemically different cell types opens new avenues for the understanding of the mechanisms of this complex disease [299,300].

In Table 4 are listed some of the microRNAs that have been found deregulated in plasma samples of preeclamptic patients. In several studies, groups of microRNAs differentially expressed have been analyzed for their potential as predictive biomarkers of the preeclamptic phenotype [301–305]. These studies show how blood levels elevation of PE-associated microRNAs can be predictive for the preeclamptic phenotype starting from the second trimester. Li and collaborators (2015) evaluated the predictive values of the upregulated micro-RNAs miR-152, miR-183 and miR-210 by plotting the corresponding receiver operating characteristic curves. In the second trimester samples, the Area Under the Curve (AUC) indicated strong predictive values and were respectively 0.93 for miR-210, 0.97 for miR-183 and 0.94 for miR-152. Interestingly, different studies investigated the predictive power of miR-210 and, even though all results highlighted its key role in preeclampsia and potential as diagnostic marker, the AUCs varied in a range between 0.7 and 0.94 [301–303,305]. This variation might be due to differences in patient cohorts, samples collections and handling; however, the fact that miR-210 still emerged as predictive biomarker is encouraging.

Winger and collaborators (2018) collected peripheral blood cells in preeclamptic and control patient group, analysing the expression levels of a subset of 30 microRNAs previously identified altered in preeclampsia. 48 samples were divided in a training and a validation group. Analysis of differentially expressed microRNAs in the training cohort identified a panel of 8 microRNAs with good prediction values (AUC > 0.75) and p value ≤ 0.05: miR-1267, miR-148a, miR-196a, miR-33a, miR-575, miR-582, miR-210, miR-16. The panel was successfully validated and the use of the 8 microRNAs combined increased the prediction power of the tests [305].

From Table 4, it is possible to appreciate the heterogeneity of findings across different studies. These discrepancies in the repertoires of circulating miRNAs complicate the identification of useful biomarkers. This heterogeneity could partly be explained by the fact that preeclampsia is a complex systemic disease that develops over months of gestation; therefore, the panel of circulating molecules in blood samples might vary considerably depending of the time point at which samples are collected. Another possible explanation might reside in the wide range of different methodologies used for the extraction of circulating RNAs which introduce technical variability [306,307]. Moreover, there is mounting evidence on how the current techniques are able to detect only a small fraction of the total bulk of circulating RNAs (WO2009093254A2). Therefore, further research is still required to improve our technical knowledge so to design better, more consistent methodologies for the identification of circulating biomarkers, that might one day allow the design of diagnostic panels for effective early detection and prevention of preeclampsia.

3.2.3. Additional Considerations on the Analysis of lncRNA Functions

Possible Caveats of the Current Trophoblast In Vitro Models

Many of the lncRNAs found to be deregulated in preeclamptic placenta have previously been identified in cancers, where they have a role in regulating proliferation, migration, invasion and apoptosis. Most of these PE-associated lncRNAs have pro-survival and pro-migration properties, therefore downregulation is associated with activation of apoptosis, decreased migratory potential and proliferative rate.

Once they have been found to be downregulated in preeclamptic placenta, the main objective has been to investigate the molecular function of these lncRNAs in the context of placenta physiology and preeclampsia. In vitro studies have seen the use of classical cellular models of trophoblast, either choriocarcinoma cell lines (JEG3 and BeWo) or artificially immortalized cell lines (HTR-8/SVneo). Through these in vitro studies it has been established that most of these lncRNAs regulate proliferation, invasion and migration of the trophoblast.

Table 4. Deregulated miRNA in preeclampsia.

microRNA	PE Placenta	PE Plasma	Function	Gene targets	AUC	References
miR-214	DOWN					[308]
miR-152		DOWN				[300]
miR-218	DOWN					[308]
miR-590	DOWN					[308]
miR-18a	DOWN	DOWN	Promoting trophoblast migration	SMAD2		[225,308]
miR-19a	DOWN					[308]
miR-19b1		DOWN	TGFβ-signaling	SMAD factors		[225]
miR-379	DOWN					[308]
miR-411	DOWN					[308]
miR-195	DOWN					[308]
miR-223	DOWN					[308]
miR-363	DOWN					[308]
miR-542-3p	DOWN					[308]
miR-144		DOWN	Ischemia, hypoxia			[225]
miR-15b		DOWN	Angiotensin-renin system			[225]
miR-181a	UP	UP				[225,308]
miR-584	UP					[308]
miR-30a-3p	UP					[308]
miR-151	UP					[308]
miR-31	UP					[308]
miR-210	UP	UP		PTPN2	0.7 < AUC < 0.9	[225,255,300,302,303,305,308,309]
miR-17-3p	UP					[308]
miR-193b	UP					[308]
miR-638	UP					[308]
miR-525	UP					[308]
miR-515-3p	UP					[308]
miR-519e	UP					[308]
miR-517-5p	UP	UP			AUC = 0.7	[304]
miR-518b	UP	UP				[225,304,308]
miR-524	UP					[308]
miR-296	UP					[308]
miR-362	UP					[308]
miR-574-5p		UP			AUC > 0.7	[302]
miR-1233-3p		UP			AUC > 0.6	[302]
miR-155		UP			AUC > 0.7	[225,303]
miR-1267		UP			AUC > 0.8	[305]
miR-148a		UP	Immune response	HLA-G	AUC > 0.9	[305,310]
miR-196a		UP			AUC = 1	[305]
miR-33a		UP			AUC = 1	[305]
miR-575		UP			AUC > 0.9	[305]
miR-582		UP	Trophoblast invasion, migration	VEGF	1	[305,311]
miR-152	UP	UP	Immune response	HLA-G	AUC > 0.9	[256,301,312]
miR-183	UP	UP	Cell differentiation, apoptosis, invasion		AUC > 0.9	[255,301,313]
miR-215		UP				[225]
miR-650		UP				[225]
miR-21	UP	UP	Apoptosis			[225,314]
miR-29a		UP				[225]
miR-300		UP	Trophoblast differentiation	ETS-1		[315]

Annotations: AUC = Area Under the Curve; SMAD2 = Mothers Against Decapentaplegic Homolog 2; PTPN2 = Tyrosine-protein phosphatase non-receptor type 2; HLA-G = Histocompatibility antigen, alpha chain G; VEGF = Vascular endothelial growth factor; ETS-1 = E26 oncogene homolog 1; TGFβ = Tumor growth factor β.

Have we completely unfolded the role of PE-associated lncRNA in the human placenta? Since lncRNAs have been previously identified in cancers, it is possible that the functions we have attributed them in the placenta are actually a result of the fact that we are analyzing them in cell lines that are cancer-like. Therefore, there is still the possibility that these lncRNAs have additional distinct functions in placenta that could be highlighted using more physiological placenta models. The recent development of placenta organoids from stem cells rises the hope for exciting new avenues, to explore these questions [316].

What about the Syncytiotrophoblast?

Migration, apoptosis, invasiveness and proliferation are functions shared between cancer cells and by cytotrophoblast (CTB) especially by the extravillous trophoblast (EVT) in the placenta, the in vitro investigations into PE associated lncRNAs have so far focused on EVT cell line models (e.g., JEG3, HTR-8/SVneo). However, it is important to highlight how transcriptomic data from placenta samples are a result of overall placenta gene expression levels. The extracted placental RNA comes from all the different cell types present in the tissue and the most abundant cell populations are represented by cytotrophoblasts and syncytiotrophoblasts (SCT). Even though it is true that CTB and EVT cells are fundamental for implantation and correct placental development, the syncytiotrophoblast is the functional core of the placenta itself, constituting the barrier for nutrient exchanges between fetal and maternal vasculatures and acting as secretory organ that hormonally regulates progression of gestation. Liu and coworkers (2017), in their work on RNA-ATB, showed a strong in situ hybridization staining of lncRNA-ATB in the syncytiotrophoblast layer of the placenta, reinforcing the idea that the syncytiotrophoblast might be equally affected by deregulation in the lncRNAs species [248]. Yu and coworkers (2018) work on MEG3 showed how MEG3 downregulation observed in preeclampsia correlates with an increase in adhesion molecule E-cadherin [224]. While it is true that this molecule is important for endothelial-mesenchymal transition, and its alteration would affect trophoblast invasion and EVT migration, E-cadherin downregulation after cytotrophoblast cell-cell interaction has been implicated in CTB syncytialization [317]. Suggesting that MEG3 might affect STB physiology as well.

Therefore, there are still potentially interesting questions to be raised: what are the effects of downregulated lncRNAs on the physiology of the CTB and SCT? Do we see an alteration of the proliferative state of the CTB, does this cause premature placental aging? Does this deregulation affect the differentiation potential of the CTB, affecting the balance between CTB renewal and SCT terminal differentiation? Do these lncRNAs have other functions, exclusive to placenta, other than the ones shared with cancer?

3.3. Histone Modifications

Few studies addressed the question of histone code modifications in PE. Chakraborty and coll. evidenced a HIF-KDM3A-MMP12 signaling cascade that promotes trophoblast invasion and trophoblast-directed uterine spiral artery remodeling in rat placenta and human placental cells. Hypoxia drives HIF activation and KDM3A expression, which in return will alter the histone methylation status of genes promoting development of the invasive trophoblast lineage and tissue remodeling, illustrated with trophoblast-derived MMP12 activation [318]. Hypoxia was also shown to affect the histone demethylase JMJD6 (Jumonji domain containing protein 6) and JMJD6 demethylase activity was shown to be drastically reduced in PE placenta as compared to Control Placenta [319]. Very recently, the expressions of HDACs were investigated in PE placentas and only HDAC9 was found downregulated both at the mRNA and protein levels in syncytiotrophoblast cells. Knock-down of HDAC9 in HTR-8/SVneo cells inhibits trophoblast cell migration and invasion. TIMP3, an inhibitory of MMP involved in invasion and tissue remodeling, is a direct target of HDAC9, identified by ChIP and is upregulated in the absence of HDAC9 [320].

3.4. Imprinting

Overall, preeclampsia cannot be considered an imprinting disease, despite the fact that a recent study showed that imprinted genes are more differentially expressed in PE than other genes, with paternally expressed genes (inducing placental growth) rather down-regulated and maternally expressed genes upregulated [151]. A systematic analysis of preeclampsia placental gene expression and imprinted genes was carried out in 2017 [321], which revealed altered expression of DLX5 in human PE placentas but with a rather mild deregulation (~2 fold). To be mentioned as well, the first gene identified by positional cloning in preeclampsia, STOX1, is imprinted in specific placental cell subtypes [322,323]. The mutation originally found in STOX1 has rather a gain-of-function effect [323] and in fact, overexpression of STOX1 induces a preeclamptic expression profile and a preeclamptic phenotype in cells or in mice, respectively [7,324]. To note, however, we have no evidence that Stox1 is imprinted in mice, therefore it is suspected that the mere ectopic and untimely overexpression of this factor is the cause of the disease. The idea that an imprinted gene is implicated in preeclampsia has been cleverly substantiated by Jennifer Graves as early as 1998 [325] and she gave theoretical reasons why this should be the case. The future will tell us if more examples of imprinted preeclampsia-associated genes exist in the human genome.

4. Perspectives and Conclusions

The recent years have seen the emergence of an increasing number of studies focused on the role of epigenetics in the regulation of placental development and on its potential implication in placental pathologies. However, we still lack a precise picture on how these epigenetic modifications correlate with gene expression. In particular, we have a limited knowledge on how DNA-methylation or Histone modifications impact gene expression in normal and pathological placenta development. In addition, our knowledge on the mechanisms regulating the dynamics of the instauration of the different epigenetic marks across development is very scarce. Nevertheless, recent studies have started to reveal how epigenetics is involved in the regulation of important processes in placental development such as cell fate determination, *syncytialization* or EVT migration and invasion. The emergence of new technologies allowing the study of the epigenetic and transcriptomic profiles of the different cells types of the placenta will certainly greatly contribute to improve our understanding of epigenetics in placenta. Moreover, in the context of PE, to date, the studies analyzing epigenetic modifications have focused on the placenta, however the antiangiogenic and cytotoxic factors released by the PE placenta have the potential to induce epigenetics modifications in maternal target tissues (blood cells, endothelial cells). This could impact the future maternal and fetal health and deserves to be studied in detail. Overall, the comprehension of epigenetic regulation in preeclampsia both at the level of the placenta and other involved organs could provide new biomarkers and therapeutic targets to improve the management of this disease. For the moment, this has not been successfully applied as diagnostic or prognostic of preeclampsia. One explanation of this observation could be that the extraction of circulating RNAs from the plasma is still immature technologically, leading to discrepant results between various laboratories and absence of consensus in defining a panel of diagnostic miRNA. This may evolve in the future, leading to substantial exploitation of these markers in complex diseases, including preeclampsia.

Supplementary Materials: Supplementary materials can be found at http://www.mdpi.com/1422-0067/20/11/2837/s1. Table S1. High-throughput studies analyzing methylation profiles of different relevant tissues in the context of preeclampsia [42,43,47,54–73].

Funding: F.M., C.M. and D.V. are funded by INSERM, C.S.M.R. and C.A. are PhD students, funded by the H2020 European project 'iPLACENTA,' headed by Colin Murdoch.

Conflicts of Interest: The authors declare no conflict of interest. The funders had no role in the design of the study; in the collection, analyses, or interpretation of data; in the writing of the manuscript, or in the decision to publish the results.

References

1. Steegers, E.A.; von Dadelszen, P.; Duvekot, J.J.; Pijnenborg, R. Pre-eclampsia. *Lancet* **2010**, *376*, 631–644. [CrossRef]
2. Roland, C.S.; Hu, J.; Ren, C.E.; Chen, H.; Li, J.; Varvoutis, M.S.; Leaphart, L.W.; Byck, D.B.; Zhu, X.; Jiang, S.W. Morphological changes of placental syncytium and their implications for the pathogenesis of preeclampsia. *Cell. Mol. Life Sci.* **2016**, *73*, 365–376. [CrossRef] [PubMed]
3. Redman, C.W.; Sargent, I.L. Latest advances in understanding preeclampsia. *Science* **2005**, *308*, 1592–1594. [CrossRef] [PubMed]

4. Fisher, S.J. Why is placentation abnormal in preeclampsia? *Am. J. Obstet. Gynecol.* **2015**, *213*, S115–S122. [CrossRef] [PubMed]
5. Huppertz, B. Placental origins of preeclampsia: Challenging the current hypothesis. *Hypertension* **2008**, *51*, 970–975. [CrossRef] [PubMed]
6. Huppertz, B. The Critical Role of Abnormal Trophoblast Development in the Etiology of Preeclampsia. *Curr. Pharm. Biotechnol.* **2018**, *19*, 771–780. [CrossRef] [PubMed]
7. Doridot, L.; Passet, B.; Mehats, C.; Rigourd, V.; Barbaux, S.; Ducat, A.; Mondon, F.; Vilotte, M.; Castille, J.; Breuiller-Fouche, M.; et al. Preeclampsia-like symptoms induced in mice by fetoplacental expression of STOX1 are reversed by aspirin treatment. *Hypertension* **2013**, *61*, 662–668. [CrossRef] [PubMed]
8. Sibley, C.P.; Pardi, G.; Cetin, I.; Todros, T.; Piccoli, E.; Kaufmann, P.; Huppertz, B.; Bulfamante, G.; Cribiu, F.M.; Ayuk, P.; et al. Pathogenesis of intrauterine growth restriction (IUGR)-conclusions derived from a European Union Biomed 2 Concerted Action project 'Importance of Oxygen Supply in Intrauterine Growth Restricted Pregnancies'-a workshop report. *Placenta* **2002**, *23* (Suppl. A), S75–S79. [CrossRef]
9. Possomato-Vieira, J.S.; Khalil, R.A. Mechanisms of Endothelial Dysfunction in Hypertensive Pregnancy and Preeclampsia. *Adv. Pharmacol.* **2016**, *77*, 361–431.
10. Nelissen, E.C.; van Montfoort, A.P.; Dumoulin, J.C.; Evers, J.L. Epigenetics and the placenta. *Hum. Reprod. Update* **2011**, *17*, 397–417. [CrossRef]
11. Vaiman, D. Genes, epigenetics and miRNA regulation in the placenta. *Placenta* **2017**, *52*, 127–133. [CrossRef] [PubMed]
12. Robinson, W.P.; Price, E.M. The human placental methylome. *Cold Spring Harb. Perspect. Med.* **2015**, *5*, a023044. [CrossRef] [PubMed]
13. Januar, V.; Desoye, G.; Novakovic, B.; Cvitic, S.; Saffery, R. Epigenetic regulation of human placental function and pregnancy outcome: Considerations for causal inference. *Am. J. Obstet. Gynecol.* **2015**, *213*, S182–S196. [CrossRef] [PubMed]
14. Fu, G.; Brkic, J.; Hayder, H.; Peng, C. MicroRNAs in Human Placental Development and Pregnancy Complications. *Int. J. Mol. Sci.* **2013**, *14*, 5519–5544. [CrossRef] [PubMed]
15. Burton, G.J.; Fowden, A.L. The placenta: A multifaceted, transient organ. *Philos. Trans. R. Soc. Lond. B Biol. Sci.* **2015**, *370*, 20140066. [CrossRef]
16. James, J.L.; Carter, A.M.; Chamley, L.W. Human placentation from nidation to 5 weeks of gestation. Part I: What do we know about formative placental development following implantation? *Placenta* **2012**, *33*, 327–334. [CrossRef]
17. Knofler, M. Critical growth factors and signalling pathways controlling human trophoblast invasion. *Int. J. Dev. Biol.* **2010**, *54*, 269–280. [CrossRef]
18. Knofler, M.; Pollheimer, J. Human placental trophoblast invasion and differentiation: A particular focus on Wnt signaling. *Front. Genet.* **2013**, *4*, 190. [CrossRef]
19. Rouault, C.; Clement, K.; Guesnon, M.; Henegar, C.; Charles, M.-A.; Heude, B.; Evain-Brion, D.; Degrelle, S.A.; Fournier, T. Transcriptomic signatures of villous cytotrophoblast and syncytiotrophoblast in term human placenta. *Placenta* **2016**, *44*, 83–90. [CrossRef]
20. Khan, M.A.; Manna, S.; Malhotra, N.; Sengupta, J.; Ghosh, D. Expressional regulation of genes linked to immunity & programmed development in human early placental villi. *Indian J. Med. Res.* **2014**, *139*, 125–140.
21. Henikoff, S.; Greally, J.M. Epigenetics, cellular memory and gene regulation. *Curr. Biol.* **2016**, *26*, R644–R648. [CrossRef] [PubMed]
22. Zhang, G.; Pradhan, S. Mammalian epigenetic mechanisms. *IUBMB Life* **2014**, *66*, 240–256. [CrossRef] [PubMed]
23. Rahat, B.; Sharma, R.; Bagga, R.; Hamid, A.; Kaur, J. Imbalance between matrix metalloproteinases and their tissue inhibitors in preeclampsia and gestational trophoblastic diseases. *Reproduction* **2016**, *152*, 11–22. [CrossRef] [PubMed]
24. Dokras, A.; Gardner, L.M.; Kirschmann, D.A.; Seftor, E.A.; Hendrix, M.J. The tumour suppressor gene maspin is differentially regulated in cytotrophoblasts during human placental development. *Placenta* **2002**, *23*, 274–280. [CrossRef] [PubMed]
25. Dokras, A.; Coffin, J.; Field, L.; Frakes, A.; Lee, H.; Madan, A.; Nelson, T.; Ryu, G.Y.; Yoon, J.G.; Madan, A. Epigenetic regulation of maspin expression in the human placenta. *Mol. Hum. Reprod.* **2006**, *12*, 611–617. [CrossRef] [PubMed]

26. Camolotto, S.A.; Racca, A.C.; Ridano, M.E.; Genti-Raimondi, S.; Panzetta-Dutari, G.M. PSG gene expression is up-regulated by lysine acetylation involving histone and nonhistone proteins. *PLoS ONE* **2013**, *8*, e55992. [CrossRef] [PubMed]
27. Chuang, H.C.; Chang, C.W.; Chang, G.D.; Yao, T.P.; Chen, H. Histone deacetylase 3 binds to and regulates the GCMa transcription factor. *Nucleic Acids Res.* **2006**, *34*, 1459–1469. [CrossRef] [PubMed]
28. Abell, A.N.; Jordan, N.V.; Huang, W.; Prat, A.; Midland, A.A.; Johnson, N.L.; Granger, D.A.; Mieczkowski, P.A.; Perou, C.M.; Gomez, S.M.; et al. MAP3K4/CBP-regulated H2B acetylation controls epithelial-mesenchymal transition in trophoblast stem cells. *Cell Stem Cell* **2011**, *8*, 525–537. [CrossRef]
29. Ellery, P.M.; Cindrova-Davies, T.; Jauniaux, E.; Ferguson-Smith, A.C.; Burton, G.J. Evidence for transcriptional activity in the syncytiotrophoblast of the human placenta. *Placenta* **2009**, *30*, 329–334. [CrossRef]
30. Fogarty, N.M.; Burton, G.J.; Ferguson-Smith, A.C. Different epigenetic states define syncytiotrophoblast and cytotrophoblast nuclei in the trophoblast of the human placenta. *Placenta* **2015**, *36*, 796–802. [CrossRef]
31. Xu, Y.; Ge, Z.; Zhang, E.; Zuo, Q.; Huang, S.; Yang, N.; Wu, D.; Zhang, Y.; Chen, Y.; Xu, H.; et al. The lncRNA TUG1 modulates proliferation in trophoblast cells via epigenetic suppression of RND3. *Cell Death Dis.* **2017**, *8*, e3104. [CrossRef] [PubMed]
32. Song, X.; Rui, C.; Meng, L.; Zhang, R.; Shen, R.; Ding, H.; Li, J.; Li, J.; Long, W. Long non-coding RNA RPAIN regulates the invasion and apoptosis of trophoblast cell lines via complement protein C1q. *Oncotarget* **2017**, *8*, 7637–7646. [CrossRef] [PubMed]
33. Chen, H.; Meng, T.; Liu, X.; Sun, M.; Tong, C.; Liu, J.; Wang, H.; Du, J. Long non-coding RNA MALAT-1 is downregulated in preeclampsia and regulates proliferation, apoptosis, migration and invasion of JEG-3 trophoblast cells. *Int. J. Clin. Exp. Pathol.* **2015**, *8*, 12718–12727. [PubMed]
34. Zhang, Y.; Zou, Y.; Wang, W.; Zuo, Q.; Jiang, Z.; Sun, M.; De, W.; Sun, L. Down-regulated long non-coding RNA MEG3 and its effect on promoting apoptosis and suppressing migration of trophoblast cells. *J. Cell. Biochem.* **2015**, *116*, 542–550. [CrossRef] [PubMed]
35. Muys, B.R.; Lorenzi, J.C.; Zanette, D.L.; Lima e Bueno Rde, B.; de Araujo, L.F.; Dinarte-Santos, A.R.; Alves, C.P.; Ramao, A.; de Molfetta, G.A.; Vidal, D.O.; et al. Placenta-Enriched LincRNAs MIR503HG and LINC00629 Decrease Migration and Invasion Potential of JEG-3 Cell Line. *PLoS ONE* **2016**, *11*, e0151560. [CrossRef] [PubMed]
36. Zou, Y.; Jiang, Z.; Yu, X.; Sun, M.; Zhang, Y.; Zuo, Q.; Zhou, J.; Yang, N.; Han, P.; Ge, Z.; et al. Upregulation of long noncoding RNA SPRY4-IT1 modulates proliferation, migration, apoptosis, and network formation in trophoblast cells HTR-8SV/neo. *PLoS ONE* **2013**, *8*, e79598. [CrossRef] [PubMed]
37. Zuo, Q.; Huang, S.; Zou, Y.; Xu, Y.; Jiang, Z.; Zou, S.; Xu, H.; Sun, L. The Lnc RNA SPRY4-IT1 Modulates Trophoblast Cell Invasion and Migration by Affecting the Epithelial-Mesenchymal Transition. *Sci. Rep.* **2016**, *6*, 37183. [CrossRef] [PubMed]
38. Yu, L.L.; Chang, K.; Lu, L.S.; Zhao, D.; Han, J.; Zheng, Y.R.; Yan, Y.H.; Yi, P.; Guo, J.X.; Zhou, Y.G.; et al. Lentivirus-mediated RNA interference targeting the H19 gene inhibits cell proliferation and apoptosis in human choriocarcinoma cell line JAR. *BMC Cell Biol.* **2013**, *14*, 26. [CrossRef] [PubMed]
39. Saha, S.; Chakraborty, S.; Bhattacharya, A.; Biswas, A.; Ain, R. MicroRNA regulation of Transthyretin in trophoblast differentiation and Intra-Uterine Growth Restriction. *Sci. Rep.* **2017**, *7*, 16548. [CrossRef]
40. Umemura, K.; Ishioka, S.; Endo, T.; Ezaka, Y.; Takahashi, M.; Saito, T. Roles of microRNA-34a in the pathogenesis of placenta accreta. *J. Obstet. Gynaecol. Res.* **2013**, *39*, 67–74. [CrossRef]
41. Doridot, L.; Houry, D.; Gaillard, H.; Chelbi, S.T.; Barbaux, S.; Vaiman, D. miR-34a expression, epigenetic regulation, and function in human placental diseases. *Epigenetics* **2014**, *9*, 142–151. [CrossRef] [PubMed]
42. Dai, Y.; Qiu, Z.; Diao, Z.; Shen, L.; Xue, P.; Sun, H.; Hu, Y. MicroRNA-155 inhibits proliferation and migration of human extravillous trophoblast derived HTR-8/SVneo cells via down-regulating cyclin D1. *Placenta* **2012**, *33*, 824–829. [CrossRef]
43. Kumar, P.; Luo, Y.; Tudela, C.; Alexander, J.M.; Mendelson, C.R. The c-Myc-regulated microRNA-17~92 (miR-17~92) and miR-106a~363 clusters target hCYP19A1 and hGCM1 to inhibit human trophoblast differentiation. *Mol. Cell. Biol.* **2013**, *33*, 1782–1796. [CrossRef] [PubMed]
44. Gao, W.L.; Liu, M.; Yang, Y.; Yang, H.; Liao, Q.; Bai, Y.; Li, Y.X.; Li, D.; Peng, C.; Wang, Y.L. The imprinted H19 gene regulates human placental trophoblast cell proliferation via encoding miR-675 that targets Nodal Modulator 1 (NOMO1). *RNA Biol.* **2012**, *9*, 1002–1010. [CrossRef] [PubMed]

45. Xie, L.; Mouillet, J.F.; Chu, T.; Parks, W.T.; Sadovsky, E.; Knofler, M.; Sadovsky, Y. C19MC microRNAs regulate the migration of human trophoblasts. *Endocrinology* **2014**, *155*, 4975–4985. [CrossRef] [PubMed]
46. Novakovic, B.; Fournier, T.; Harris, L.K.; James, J.; Roberts, C.T.; Yong, H.E.J.; Kalionis, B.; Evain-Brion, D.; Ebeling, P.R.; Wallace, E.M.; et al. Increased methylation and decreased expression of homeobox genes TLX1, HOXA10 and DLX5 in human placenta are associated with trophoblast differentiation. *Sci. Rep.* **2017**, *7*, 4523. [CrossRef] [PubMed]
47. Wong, N.C.; Novakovic, B.; Weinrich, B.; Dewi, C.; Andronikos, R.; Sibson, M.; Macrae, F.; Morley, R.; Pertile, M.D.; Craig, J.M.; et al. Methylation of the adenomatous polyposis coli (APC) gene in human placenta and hypermethylation in choriocarcinoma cells. *Cancer Lett.* **2008**, *268*, 56–62. [CrossRef] [PubMed]
48. Shi, X.; Liu, H.; Cao, J.; Liu, Q.; Tang, G.; Liu, W.; Liu, H.; Deng, D.; Qiao, F.; Wu, Y. Promoter Hypomethylation of Maspin Inhibits Migration and Invasion of Extravillous Trophoblast Cells during Placentation. *PLoS ONE* **2015**, *10*, e0135359. [CrossRef] [PubMed]
49. Chiu, R.W.; Chim, S.S.; Wong, I.H.; Wong, C.S.; Lee, W.S.; To, K.F.; Tong, J.H.; Yuen, R.K.; Shum, A.S.; Chan, J.K.; et al. Hypermethylation of RASSF1A in human and rhesus placentas. *Am. J. Pathol.* **2007**, *170*, 941–950. [CrossRef] [PubMed]
50. Lister, R.; Pelizzola, M.; Kida, Y.S.; Hawkins, R.D.; Nery, J.R.; Hon, G.; Antosiewicz-Bourget, J.; O'Malley, R.; Castanon, R.; Klugman, S.; et al. Hotspots of aberrant epigenomic reprogramming in human induced pluripotent stem cells. *Nature* **2011**, *471*, 68–73. [CrossRef] [PubMed]
51. Schroeder, D.I.; Blair, J.D.; Lott, P.; Yu, H.O.; Hong, D.; Crary, F.; Ashwood, P.; Walker, C.; Korf, I.; Robinson, W.P.; et al. The human placenta methylome. *Proc. Natl. Acad. Sci. USA* **2013**, *110*, 6037–6042. [CrossRef] [PubMed]
52. Nordor, A.V.; Nehar-Belaid, D.; Richon, S.; Klatzmann, D.; Bellet, D.; Dangles-Marie, V.; Fournier, T.; Aryee, M.J. The early pregnancy placenta foreshadows DNA methylation alterations of solid tumors. *Epigenetics* **2017**, *12*, 793–803. [CrossRef] [PubMed]
53. Yuen, R.K.; Chen, B.; Blair, J.D.; Robinson, W.P.; Nelson, D.M. Hypoxia alters the epigenetic profile in cultured human placental trophoblasts. *Epigenetics* **2013**, *8*, 192–202. [CrossRef] [PubMed]
54. Shankar, K.; Kang, P.; Zhong, Y.; Borengasser, S.J.; Wingfield, C.; Saben, J.; Gomez-Acevedo, H.; Thakali, K.M. Transcriptomic and epigenomic landscapes during cell fusion in BeWo trophoblast cells. *Placenta* **2015**, *36*, 1342–1351. [CrossRef] [PubMed]
55. James, J.L.; Hurley, D.G.; Gamage, T.K.; Zhang, T.; Vather, R.; Pantham, P.; Murthi, P.; Chamley, L.W. Isolation and characterisation of a novel trophoblast side-population from first trimester placentae. *Reproduction* **2015**, *150*, 449–462. [CrossRef] [PubMed]
56. Gamage, T.K.; Schierding, W.; Hurley, D.; Tsai, P.; Ludgate, J.L.; Bhoothpur, C.; Chamley, L.W.; Weeks, R.J.; Macaulay, E.C.; James, J.L. The role of DNA methylation in human trophoblast differentiation. *Epigenetics* **2018**. [CrossRef] [PubMed]
57. Ng, R.K.; Dean, W.; Dawson, C.; Lucifero, D.; Madeja, Z.; Reik, W.; Hemberger, M. Epigenetic restriction of embryonic cell lineage fate by methylation of Elf5. *Nat. Cell Biol.* **2008**, *10*, 1280–1290. [CrossRef] [PubMed]
58. Senner, C.E.; Krueger, F.; Oxley, D.; Andrews, S.; Hemberger, M. DNA methylation profiles define stem cell identity and reveal a tight embryonic-extraembryonic lineage boundary. *Stem Cells* **2012**, *30*, 2732–2745. [CrossRef]
59. Murray, R.; Bryant, J.; Titcombe, P.; Barton, S.J.; Inskip, H.; Harvey, N.C.; Cooper, C.; Lillycrop, K.; Hanson, M.; Godfrey, K.M. DNA methylation at birth within the promoter of ANRIL predicts markers of cardiovascular risk at 9 years. *Clin. Epigenet.* **2016**, *8*, 90. [CrossRef]
60. Santos, J.; Pereira, C.F.; Di-Gregorio, A.; Spruce, T.; Alder, O.; Rodriguez, T.; Azuara, V.; Merkenschlager, M.; Fisher, A.G. Differences in the epigenetic and reprogramming properties of pluripotent and extra-embryonic stem cells implicate chromatin remodelling as an important early event in the developing mouse embryo. *Epigenet. Chromatin* **2010**, *3*, 1. [CrossRef]
61. Bianco-Miotto, T.; Mayne, B.T.; Buckberry, S.; Breen, J.; Rodriguez Lopez, C.M.; Roberts, C.T. Recent progress towards understanding the role of DNA methylation in human placental development. *Reproduction* **2016**, *152*, R23–R30. [CrossRef] [PubMed]
62. Ou, X.; Wang, H.; Qu, D.; Chen, Y.; Gao, J.; Sun, H. Epigenome-wide DNA methylation assay reveals placental epigenetic markers for noninvasive fetal single-nucleotide polymorphism genotyping in maternal plasma. *Transfusion* **2014**, *54*, 2523–2533. [CrossRef] [PubMed]

63. Xiang, Y.; Zhang, J.; Li, Q.; Zhou, X.; Wang, T.; Xu, M.; Xia, S.; Xing, Q.; Wang, L.; He, L.; et al. DNA methylome profiling of maternal peripheral blood and placentas reveal potential fetal DNA markers for non-invasive prenatal testing. *Mol. Hum. Reprod.* **2014**, *20*, 875–884. [CrossRef] [PubMed]
64. Novakovic, B.; Yuen, R.K.; Gordon, L.; Penaherrera, M.S.; Sharkey, A.; Moffett, A.; Craig, J.M.; Robinson, W.P.; Saffery, R. Evidence for widespread changes in promoter methylation profile in human placenta in response to increasing gestational age and environmental/stochastic factors. *BMC Genom.* **2011**, *12*, 529. [CrossRef] [PubMed]
65. Rakyan, V.K.; Down, T.A.; Thorne, N.P.; Flicek, P.; Kulesha, E.; Graf, S.; Tomazou, E.M.; Backdahl, L.; Johnson, N.; Herberth, M.; et al. An integrated resource for genome-wide identification and analysis of human tissue-specific differentially methylated regions (tDMRs). *Genome Res.* **2008**, *18*, 1518–1529. [CrossRef] [PubMed]
66. Kaur, G.; Helmer, R.A.; Smith, L.A.; Martinez-Zaguilan, R.; Dufour, J.M.; Chilton, B.S. Alternative splicing of helicase-like transcription factor (Hltf): Intron retention-dependent activation of immune tolerance at the feto-maternal interface. *PLoS ONE* **2018**, *13*, e0200211. [CrossRef] [PubMed]
67. Schmidt, M.; Lax, E.; Zhou, R.; Cheishvili, D.; Ruder, A.M.; Ludiro, A.; Lapert, F.; Macedo da Cruz, A.; Sandrini, P.; Calzoni, T.; et al. Fetal glucocorticoid receptor (Nr3c1) deficiency alters the landscape of DNA methylation of murine placenta in a sex-dependent manner and is associated to anxiety-like behavior in adulthood. *Transl. Psychiatry* **2019**, *9*, 23. [CrossRef]
68. Price, E.M.; Cotton, A.M.; Penaherrera, M.S.; McFadden, D.E.; Kobor, M.S.; Robinson, W. Different measures of "genome-wide" DNA methylation exhibit unique properties in placental and somatic tissues. *Epigenetics* **2012**, *7*, 652–663. [CrossRef] [PubMed]
69. Yang, A.; Sun, Y.; Mao, C.; Yang, S.; Huang, M.; Deng, M.; Ding, N.; Yang, X.; Zhang, M.; Jin, S.; et al. Folate Protects Hepatocytes of Hyperhomocysteinemia Mice From Apoptosis via Cystic Fibrosis Transmembrane Conductance Regulator (CFTR)-Activated Endoplasmic Reticulum Stress. *J. Cell. Biochem.* **2017**, *118*, 2921–2932. [CrossRef] [PubMed]
70. Hernandez Mora, J.R.; Sanchez-Delgado, M.; Petazzi, P.; Moran, S.; Esteller, M.; Iglesias-Platas, I.; Monk, D. Profiling of oxBS-450K 5-hydroxymethylcytosine in human placenta and brain reveals enrichment at imprinted loci. *Epigenetics* **2018**, *13*, 182–191. [CrossRef]
71. Lim, Y.C.; Li, J.; Ni, Y.; Liang, Q.; Zhang, J.; Yeo, G.S.H.; Lyu, J.; Jin, S.; Ding, C. A complex association between DNA methylation and gene expression in human placenta at first and third trimesters. *PLoS ONE* **2017**, *12*, e0181155. [CrossRef] [PubMed]
72. Roost, M.S.; Slieker, R.C.; Bialecka, M.; van Iperen, L.; Gomes Fernandes, M.M.; He, N.; Suchiman, H.E.D.; Szuhai, K.; Carlotti, F.; de Koning, E.J.P.; et al. DNA methylation and transcriptional trajectories during human development and reprogramming of isogenic pluripotent stem cells. *Nat. Commun.* **2017**, *8*, 908. [CrossRef] [PubMed]
73. Decato, B.E.; Lopez-Tello, J.; Sferruzzi-Perri, A.N.; Smith, A.D.; Dean, M.D. DNA Methylation Divergence and Tissue Specialization in the Developing Mouse Placenta. *Mol. Biol. Evol.* **2017**, *34*, 1702–1712. [CrossRef] [PubMed]
74. Green, B.B.; Houseman, E.A.; Johnson, K.C.; Guerin, D.J.; Armstrong, D.A.; Christensen, B.C.; Marsit, C.J. Hydroxymethylation is uniquely distributed within term placenta, and is associated with gene expression. *FASEB J.* **2016**, *30*, 2874–2884. [CrossRef] [PubMed]
75. Chatterjee, A.; Macaulay, E.C.; Rodger, E.J.; Stockwell, P.A.; Parry, M.F.; Roberts, H.E.; Slatter, T.L.; Hung, N.A.; Devenish, C.J.; Morison, I.M. Placental Hypomethylation Is More Pronounced in Genomic Loci Devoid of Retroelements. *G3 (Bethesda)* **2016**, *6*, 1911–1921. [CrossRef] [PubMed]
76. Branco, M.R.; King, M.; Perez-Garcia, V.; Bogutz, A.B.; Caley, M.; Fineberg, E.; Lefebvre, L.; Cook, S.J.; Dean, W.; Hemberger, M.; et al. Maternal DNA Methylation Regulates Early Trophoblast Development. *Dev. Cell* **2016**, *36*, 152–163. [CrossRef] [PubMed]
77. Hanna, C.W.; Penaherrera, M.S.; Saadeh, H.; Andrews, S.; McFadden, D.E.; Kelsey, G.; Robinson, W.P. Pervasive polymorphic imprinted methylation in the human placenta. *Genome Res.* **2016**, *26*, 756–767. [CrossRef] [PubMed]
78. Hu, Y.; Blair, J.D.; Yuen, R.K.; Robinson, W.P.; von Dadelszen, P. Genome-wide DNA methylation identifies trophoblast invasion-related genes: Claudin-4 and Fucosyltransferase IV control mobility via altering matrix metalloproteinase activity. *Mol. Hum. Reprod.* **2015**, *21*, 452–465. [CrossRef]

79. Mahadevan, S.; Wen, S.; Wan, Y.W.; Peng, H.H.; Otta, S.; Liu, Z.; Iacovino, M.; Mahen, E.M.; Kyba, M.; Sadikovic, B.; et al. NLRP7 affects trophoblast lineage differentiation, binds to overexpressed YY1 and alters CpG methylation. *Hum. Mol. Genet.* **2014**, *23*, 706–716. [CrossRef] [PubMed]
80. Novakovic, B.; Gordon, L.; Wong, N.C.; Moffett, A.; Manuelpillai, U.; Craig, J.M.; Sharkey, A.; Saffery, R. Wide-ranging DNA methylation differences of primary trophoblast cell populations and derived cell lines: Implications and opportunities for understanding trophoblast function. *Mol. Hum. Reprod.* **2011**, *17*, 344–353. [CrossRef] [PubMed]
81. Amorim, R.P.; Araujo, M.G.L.; Valero, J.; Lopes-Cendes, I.; Pascoal, V.D.B.; Malva, J.O.; da Silva Fernandes, M.J. Silencing of P2X7R by RNA interference in the hippocampus can attenuate morphological and behavioral impact of pilocarpine-induced epilepsy. *Purinergic Signal.* **2017**, *13*, 467–478. [CrossRef] [PubMed]
82. Oudejans, C.B.; Pannese, M.; Simeone, A.; Meijer, C.J.; Boncinelli, E. The three most downstream genes of the Hox-3 cluster are expressed in human extraembryonic tissues including trophoblast of androgenetic origin. *Development* **1990**, *108*, 471–477. [PubMed]
83. Chui, A.; Pathirage, N.A.; Johnson, B.; Cocquebert, M.; Fournier, T.; Evain-Brion, D.; Roald, B.; Manuelpillai, U.; Brennecke, S.P.; Kalionis, B.; et al. Homeobox gene distal-less 3 is expressed in proliferating and differentiating cells of the human placenta. *Placenta* **2010**, *31*, 691–697. [CrossRef] [PubMed]
84. Grati, F.R.; Sirchia, S.M.; Gentilin, B.; Rossella, F.; Ramoscelli, L.; Antonazzo, P.; Cavallari, U.; Bulfamante, G.; Cetin, I.; Simoni, G.; et al. Biparental expression of ESX1L gene in placentas from normal and intrauterine growth-restricted pregnancies. *Eur. J. Hum. Genet.* **2004**, *12*, 272–278. [CrossRef] [PubMed]
85. Quinn, L.M.; Johnson, B.V.; Nicholl, J.; Sutherland, G.R.; Kalionis, B. Isolation and identification of homeobox genes from the human placenta including a novel member of the Distal-less family, DLX4. *Gene* **1997**, *187*, 55–61. [CrossRef]
86. Rajaraman, G.; Murthi, P.; Quinn, L.; Brennecke, S.P.; Kalionis, B. Homeodomain protein HLX is expressed primarily in cytotrophoblast cell types in the early pregnancy human placenta. *Reprod. Fertil. Dev.* **2008**, *20*, 357–367. [CrossRef] [PubMed]
87. Schroeder, D.I.; LaSalle, J.M. How has the study of the human placenta aided our understanding of partially methylated genes? *Epigenomics* **2013**, *5*, 645–654. [CrossRef] [PubMed]
88. Hombach, S.; Kretz, M. Non-coding RNAs: Classification, Biology and Functioning. *Adv. Exp. Med. Biol.* **2016**, *937*, 3–17. [PubMed]
89. Sadovsky, Y.; Mouillet, J.F.; Ouyang, Y.; Bayer, A.; Coyne, C.B. The Function of TrophomiRs and Other MicroRNAs in the Human Placenta. *Cold Spring Harb. Perspect. Med.* **2015**, *5*, a023036. [CrossRef] [PubMed]
90. Guo, H.; Ingolia, N.T.; Weissman, J.S.; Bartel, D.P. Mammalian microRNAs predominantly act to decrease target mRNA levels. *Nature* **2010**, *466*, 835–840. [CrossRef]
91. Krol, J.; Loedige, I.; Filipowicz, W. The widespread regulation of microRNA biogenesis, function and decay. *Nat. Rev. Genet.* **2010**, *11*, 597–610. [CrossRef] [PubMed]
92. Bentwich, I.; Avniel, A.; Karov, Y.; Aharonov, R.; Gilad, S.; Barad, O.; Barzilai, A.; Einat, P.; Einav, U.; Meiri, E.; et al. Identification of hundreds of conserved and nonconserved human microRNAs. *Nat. Genet.* **2005**, *37*, 766–770. [CrossRef] [PubMed]
93. Donker, R.B.; Mouillet, J.F.; Chu, T.; Hubel, C.A.; Stolz, D.B.; Morelli, A.E.; Sadovsky, Y. The expression profile of C19MC microRNAs in primary human trophoblast cells and exosomes. *Mol. Hum. Reprod.* **2012**, *18*, 417–424. [CrossRef] [PubMed]
94. Zhang, R.; Wang, Y.Q.; Su, B. Molecular evolution of a primate-specific microRNA family. *Mol. Biol. Evol.* **2008**, *25*, 1493–1502. [CrossRef] [PubMed]
95. Noguer-Dance, M.; Abu-Amero, S.; Al-Khtib, M.; Lefevre, A.; Coullin, P.; Moore, G.E.; Cavaille, J. The primate-specific microRNA gene cluster (C19MC) is imprinted in the placenta. *Hum. Mol. Genet.* **2010**, *19*, 3566–3582. [CrossRef] [PubMed]
96. Tsai, K.W.; Kao, H.W.; Chen, H.C.; Chen, S.J.; Lin, W.C. Epigenetic control of the expression of a primate-specific microRNA cluster in human cancer cells. *Epigenetics* **2009**, *4*, 587–592. [CrossRef]
97. Bar, M.; Wyman, S.K.; Fritz, B.R.; Qi, J.; Garg, K.S.; Parkin, R.K.; Kroh, E.M.; Bendoraite, A.; Mitchell, P.S.; Nelson, A.M.; et al. MicroRNA discovery and profiling in human embryonic stem cells by deep sequencing of small RNA libraries. *Stem Cells* **2008**, *26*, 2496–2505. [CrossRef] [PubMed]

98. Laurent, L.C.; Chen, J.; Ulitsky, I.; Mueller, F.J.; Lu, C.; Shamir, R.; Fan, J.B.; Loring, J.F. Comprehensive microRNA profiling reveals a unique human embryonic stem cell signature dominated by a single seed sequence. *Stem Cells* **2008**, *26*, 1506–1516. [CrossRef] [PubMed]
99. Morin, R.D.; O'Connor, M.D.; Griffith, M.; Kuchenbauer, F.; Delaney, A.; Prabhu, A.L.; Zhao, Y.; McDonald, H.; Zeng, T.; Hirst, M.; et al. Application of massively parallel sequencing to microRNA profiling and discovery in human embryonic stem cells. *Genome Res.* **2008**, *18*, 610–621. [CrossRef] [PubMed]
100. Ren, J.; Jin, P.; Wang, E.; Marincola, F.M.; Stroncek, D.F. MicroRNA and gene expression patterns in the differentiation of human embryonic stem cells. *J. Transl. Med.* **2009**, *7*, 20. [CrossRef] [PubMed]
101. Stadler, B.; Ivanovska, I.; Mehta, K.; Song, S.; Nelson, A.; Tan, Y.; Mathieu, J.; Darby, C.; Blau, C.A.; Ware, C.; et al. Characterization of microRNAs involved in embryonic stem cell states. *Stem Cells Dev.* **2010**, *19*, 935–950. [CrossRef]
102. Morales-Prieto, D.M.; Ospina-Prieto, S.; Chaiwangyen, W.; Schoenleben, M.; Markert, U.R. Pregnancy-associated miRNA-clusters. *J. Reprod. Immunol.* **2013**, *97*, 51–61. [CrossRef] [PubMed]
103. Gu, Y.; Sun, J.; Groome, L.J.; Wang, Y. Differential miRNA expression profiles between the first and third trimester human placentas. *Am. J. Physiol. Endocrinol. Metab.* **2013**, *304*, E836–E843. [CrossRef] [PubMed]
104. Liang, Y.; Ridzon, D.; Wong, L.; Chen, C. Characterization of microRNA expression profiles in normal human tissues. *BMC Genom.* **2007**, *8*, 166. [CrossRef] [PubMed]
105. Keniry, A.; Oxley, D.; Monnier, P.; Kyba, M.; Dandolo, L.; Smits, G.; Reik, W. The H19 lincRNA is a developmental reservoir of miR-675 that suppresses growth and Igf1r. *Nat. Cell Biol.* **2012**, *14*, 659–665. [CrossRef] [PubMed]
106. Forbes, K.; Farrokhnia, F.; Aplin, J.D.; Westwood, M. Dicer-dependent miRNAs provide an endogenous restraint on cytotrophoblast proliferation. *Placenta* **2012**, *33*, 581–585. [CrossRef] [PubMed]
107. Doridot, L.; Miralles, F.; Barbaux, S.; Vaiman, D. Trophoblasts, invasion, and microRNA. *Front. Genet.* **2013**, *4*, 248. [CrossRef] [PubMed]
108. Yang, X.; Meng, T. MicroRNA-431 affects trophoblast migration and invasion by targeting ZEB1 in preeclampsia. *Gene* **2019**, *683*, 225–232. [CrossRef] [PubMed]
109. Ransohoff, J.D.; Wei, Y.; Khavari, P.A. The functions and unique features of long intergenic non-coding RNA. *Nat. Rev. Mol. Cell Biol.* **2018**, *19*, 143–157. [CrossRef] [PubMed]
110. McAninch, D.; Roberts, C.T.; Bianco-Miotto, T. Mechanistic Insight into Long Noncoding RNAs and the Placenta. *Int. J. Mol. Sci.* **2017**, *18*, 1371. [CrossRef]
111. Brannan, C.I.; Dees, E.C.; Ingram, R.S.; Tilghman, S.M. The product of the H19 gene may function as an RNA. *Mol. Cell. Biol.* **1990**, *10*, 28–36. [CrossRef] [PubMed]
112. Gabory, A.; Jammes, H.; Dandolo, L. The H19 locus: Role of an imprinted non-coding RNA in growth and development. *Bioessays* **2010**, *32*, 473–480. [CrossRef] [PubMed]
113. Iglesias-Platas, I.; Martin-Trujillo, A.; Petazzi, P.; Guillaumet-Adkins, A.; Esteller, M.; Monk, D. Altered expression of the imprinted transcription factor PLAGL1 deregulates a network of genes in the human IUGR placenta. *Hum. Mol. Genet.* **2014**, *23*, 6275–6285. [CrossRef] [PubMed]
114. Kallen, A.N.; Zhou, X.B.; Xu, J.; Qiao, C.; Ma, J.; Yan, L.; Lu, L.; Liu, C.; Yi, J.S.; Zhang, H.; et al. The imprinted H19 lncRNA antagonizes let-7 microRNAs. *Mol. Cell* **2013**, *52*, 101–112. [CrossRef] [PubMed]
115. Jinno, Y.; Ikeda, Y.; Yun, K.; Maw, M.; Masuzaki, H.; Fukuda, H.; Inuzuka, K.; Fujishita, A.; Ohtani, Y.; Okimoto, T.; et al. Establishment of functional imprinting of the H19 gene in human developing placentae. *Nat. Genet.* **1995**, *10*, 318–324. [CrossRef]
116. Yu, L.; Chen, M.; Zhao, D.; Yi, P.; Lu, L.; Han, J.; Zheng, X.; Zhou, Y.; Li, L. The H19 gene imprinting in normal pregnancy and pre-eclampsia. *Placenta* **2009**, *30*, 443–447. [CrossRef]
117. Jenuwein, T.; Allis, C.D. Translating the histone code. *Science* **2001**, *293*, 1074–1080. [CrossRef]
118. Mellor, J.; Dudek, P.; Clynes, D. A glimpse into the epigenetic landscape of gene regulation. *Curr. Opin. Genet. Dev.* **2008**, *18*, 116–122. [CrossRef]
119. Grewal, S.I.; Jia, S. Heterochromatin revisited. *Nat. Rev. Genet.* **2007**, *8*, 35–46. [CrossRef]
120. Torres-Padilla, M.E.; Parfitt, D.E.; Kouzarides, T.; Zernicka-Goetz, M. Histone arginine methylation regulates pluripotency in the early mouse embryo. *Nature* **2007**, *445*, 214–218. [CrossRef]
121. Semenza, G.L. HIF-1 and mechanisms of hypoxia sensing. *Curr. Opin. Cell Biol.* **2001**, *13*, 167–171. [CrossRef]

122. Charron, C.E.; Chou, P.C.; Coutts, D.J.; Kumar, V.; To, M.; Akashi, K.; Pinhu, L.; Griffiths, M.; Adcock, I.M.; Barnes, P.J.; et al. Hypoxia-inducible factor 1alpha induces corticosteroid-insensitive inflammation via reduction of histone deacetylase-2 transcription. *J. Biol. Chem.* **2009**, *284*, 36047–36054. [CrossRef] [PubMed]
123. Maltepe, E.; Krampitz, G.W.; Okazaki, K.M.; Red-Horse, K.; Mak, W.; Simon, M.C.; Fisher, S.J. Hypoxia-inducible factor-dependent histone deacetylase activity determines stem cell fate in the placenta. *Development* **2005**, *132*, 3393–3403. [CrossRef] [PubMed]
124. Pollard, P.J.; Loenarz, C.; Mole, D.R.; McDonough, M.A.; Gleadle, J.M.; Schofield, C.J.; Ratcliffe, P.J. Regulation of Jumonji-domain-containing histone demethylases by hypoxia-inducible factor (HIF)-1alpha. *Biochem. J.* **2008**, *416*, 387–394. [CrossRef] [PubMed]
125. Wellmann, S.; Bettkober, M.; Zelmer, A.; Seeger, K.; Faigle, M.; Eltzschig, H.K.; Buhrer, C. Hypoxia upregulates the histone demethylase JMJD1A via HIF-1. *Biochem. Biophys. Res. Commun.* **2008**, *372*, 892–897. [CrossRef] [PubMed]
126. Xia, M.; Yao, L.; Zhang, Q.; Wang, F.; Mei, H.; Guo, X.; Huang, W. Long noncoding RNA HOTAIR promotes metastasis of renal cell carcinoma by up-regulating histone H3K27 demethylase JMJD3. *Oncotarget* **2017**, *8*, 19795–19802. [CrossRef] [PubMed]
127. Maltepe, E.; Bakardjiev, A.I.; Fisher, S.J. The placenta: Transcriptional, epigenetic, and physiological integration during development. *J. Clin. Investig.* **2010**, *120*, 1016–1025. [CrossRef] [PubMed]
128. Franasiak, J.M.; Scott, R.T. Contribution of immunology to implantation failure of euploid embryos. *Fertil. Steril.* **2017**, *107*, 1279–1283. [CrossRef] [PubMed]
129. Griffith, O.W.; Chavan, A.R.; Protopapas, S.; Maziarz, J.; Romero, R.; Wagner, G.P. Embryo implantation evolved from an ancestral inflammatory attachment reaction. *Proc. Natl. Acad. Sci. USA* **2017**, *114*, E6566–E6575. [CrossRef] [PubMed]
130. Hansen, V.L.; Faber, L.S.; Salehpoor, A.A.; Miller, R.D. A pronounced uterine pro-inflammatory response at parturition is an ancient feature in mammals. *Proc. Biol. Sci.* **2017**, *284*, 20171694. [CrossRef] [PubMed]
131. Cornelis, G.; Funk, M.; Vernochet, C.; Leal, F.; Tarazona, O.A.; Meurice, G.; Heidmann, O.; Dupressoir, A.; Miralles, A.; Ramirez-Pinilla, M.P.; et al. An endogenous retroviral envelope syncytin and its cognate receptor identified in the viviparous placental Mabuya lizard. *Proc. Natl. Acad. Sci. USA* **2017**, *114*, E10991–E11000. [CrossRef] [PubMed]
132. McKinnell, Z.; Wessel, G. Ligers and tigons and.....what?....oh my! *Mol. Reprod. Dev.* **2012**, *79*, Fm i. [CrossRef] [PubMed]
133. Surani, M.A.; Barton, S.C.; Norris, M.L. Development of reconstituted mouse eggs suggests imprinting of the genome during gametogenesis. *Nature* **1984**, *308*, 548–550. [CrossRef] [PubMed]
134. Wake, N.; Arima, T.; Matsuda, T. Involvement of IGF2 and H19 imprinting in choriocarcinoma development. *Int. J. Gynaecol. Obstet.* **1998**, *60* (Suppl. 1), S1–S8. [CrossRef]
135. Warren, W.C.; Hillier, L.W.; Marshall Graves, J.A.; Birney, E.; Ponting, C.P.; Grutzner, F.; Belov, K.; Miller, W.; Clarke, L.; Chinwalla, A.T.; et al. Genome analysis of the platypus reveals unique signatures of evolution. *Nature* **2008**, *453*, 175–183. [CrossRef] [PubMed]
136. Suzuki, S.; Shaw, G.; Kaneko-Ishino, T.; Ishino, F.; Renfree, M.B. The evolution of mammalian genomic imprinting was accompanied by the acquisition of novel CpG islands. *Genome Biol. Evol.* **2011**, *3*, 1276–1283. [CrossRef] [PubMed]
137. Renfree, M.B.; Suzuki, S.; Kaneko-Ishino, T. The origin and evolution of genomic imprinting and viviparity in mammals. *Philos. Trans. R. Soc. Lond. B Biol. Sci.* **2013**, *368*, 20120151. [CrossRef] [PubMed]
138. Fresard, L.; Leroux, S.; Servin, B.; Gourichon, D.; Dehais, P.; Cristobal, M.S.; Marsaud, N.; Vignoles, F.; Bed'hom, B.; Coville, J.L.; et al. Transcriptome-wide investigation of genomic imprinting in chicken. *Nucleic Acids Res.* **2014**, *42*, 3768–3782. [CrossRef] [PubMed]
139. Zhuo, Z.; Lamont, S.J.; Abasht, B. RNA-Seq Analyses Identify Frequent Allele Specific Expression and No Evidence of Genomic Imprinting in Specific Embryonic Tissues of Chicken. *Sci. Rep.* **2017**, *7*, 11944. [CrossRef] [PubMed]
140. Piedrahita, J.A. The role of imprinted genes in fetal growth abnormalities. *Birth Defects Res. A Clin. Mol. Teratol.* **2011**, *91*, 682–692. [CrossRef] [PubMed]
141. Constancia, M.; Hemberger, M.; Hughes, J.; Dean, W.; Ferguson-Smith, A.; Fundele, R.; Stewart, F.; Kelsey, G.; Fowden, A.; Sibley, C.; et al. Placental-specific IGF-II is a major modulator of placental and fetal growth. *Nature* **2002**, *417*, 945–948. [CrossRef] [PubMed]

142. Ripoche, M.A.; Kress, C.; Poirier, F.; Dandolo, L. Deletion of the H19 transcription unit reveals the existence of a putative imprinting control element. *Genes Dev.* **1997**, *11*, 1596–1604. [CrossRef] [PubMed]
143. Xu, Y.; Goodyer, C.G.; Deal, C.; Polychronakos, C. Functional polymorphism in the parental imprinting of the human IGF2R gene. *Biochem. Biophys. Res. Commun.* **1993**, *197*, 747–754. [CrossRef] [PubMed]
144. Cheong, C.Y.; Chng, K.; Ng, S.; Chew, S.B.; Chan, L.; Ferguson-Smith, A.C. Germline and somatic imprinting in the nonhuman primate highlights species differences in oocyte methylation. *Genome Res.* **2015**, *25*, 611–623. [CrossRef] [PubMed]
145. Monk, D.; Arnaud, P.; Apostolidou, S.; Hills, F.A.; Kelsey, G.; Stanier, P.; Feil, R.; Moore, G.E. Limited evolutionary conservation of imprinting in the human placenta. *Proc. Natl. Acad. Sci. USA* **2006**, *103*, 6623–6628. [CrossRef]
146. Barbaux, S.; Gascoin-Lachambre, G.; Buffat, C.; Monnier, P.; Mondon, F.; Tonanny, M.B.; Pinard, A.; Auer, J.; Bessieres, B.; Barlier, A.; et al. A genome-wide approach reveals novel imprinted genes expressed in the human placenta. *Epigenetics* **2012**, *7*, 1079–1090. [CrossRef]
147. Allach El Khattabi, L.; Backer, S.; Pinard, A.; Dieudonne, M.N.; Tsatsaris, V.; Vaiman, D.; Dandolo, L.; Bloch-Gallego, E.; Jammes, H.; Barbaux, S. A genome-wide search for new imprinted genes in the human placenta identifies DSCAM as the first imprinted gene on chromosome 21. *Eur. J. Hum. Genet.* **2019**, *27*, 49–60. [CrossRef]
148. Marjonen, H.; Auvinen, P.; Kahila, H.; Tsuiko, O.; Koks, S.; Tiirats, A.; Viltrop, T.; Tuuri, T.; Soderstrom-Anttila, V.; Suikkari, A.M.; et al. rs10732516 polymorphism at the IGF2/H19 locus associates with genotype-specific effects on placental DNA methylation and birth weight of newborns conceived by assisted reproductive technology. *Clin. Epigenet.* **2018**, *10*, 80. [CrossRef]
149. Peters, J. The role of genomic imprinting in biology and disease: An expanding view. *Nat. Rev. Genet.* **2014**, *15*, 517–530. [CrossRef]
150. Monk, D. Genomic imprinting in the human placenta. *Am. J. Obstet. Gynecol.* **2015**, *213*, S152–S162. [CrossRef]
151. Christians, J.K.; Leavey, K.; Cox, B.J. Associations between imprinted gene expression in the placenta, human fetal growth and preeclampsia. *Biol. Lett.* **2017**, *13*, 20170643. [CrossRef] [PubMed]
152. Xie, L.; Sadovsky, Y. The function of miR-519d in cell migration, invasion, and proliferation suggests a role in early placentation. *Placenta* **2016**, *48*, 34–37. [CrossRef] [PubMed]
153. Petre, G.; Lores, P.; Sartelet, H.; Truffot, A.; Poreau, B.; Brandeis, S.; Martinez, G.; Satre, V.; Harbuz, R.; Ray, P.F.; et al. Genomic duplication in the 19q13.42 imprinted region identified as a new genetic cause of intrauterine growth restriction. *Clin. Genet.* **2018**. [CrossRef] [PubMed]
154. Vaiman, D.; Calicchio, R.; Miralles, F. Landscape of transcriptional deregulations in the preeclamptic placenta. *PLoS ONE* **2013**, *8*, e65498. [CrossRef] [PubMed]
155. Jia, R.Z.; Zhang, X.; Hu, P.; Liu, X.M.; Hua, X.D.; Wang, X.; Ding, H.J. Screening for differential methylation status in human placenta in preeclampsia using a CpG island plus promoter microarray. *Int. J. Mol. Med.* **2012**, *30*, 133–141.
156. Anton, L.; Olarerin-George, A.O.; Schwartz, N.; Srinivas, S.; Bastek, J.; Hogenesch, J.B.; Elovitz, M.A. miR-210 inhibits trophoblast invasion and is a serum biomarker for preeclampsia. *Am. J. Pathol.* **2013**, *183*, 1437–1445. [CrossRef]
157. Liu, L.; Zhang, X.; Rong, C.; Rui, C.; Ji, H.; Qian, Y.J.; Jia, R.; Sun, L. Distinct DNA methylomes of human placentas between pre-eclampsia and gestational diabetes mellitus. *Cell. Physiol. Biochem.* **2014**, *34*, 1877–1889. [CrossRef]
158. Yeung, K.R.; Chiu, C.L.; Pidsley, R.; Makris, A.; Hennessy, A.; Lind, J.M. DNA methylation profiles in preeclampsia and healthy control placentas. *Am. J. Physiol. Heart Circ. Physiol.* **2016**, *310*, H1295–H1303. [CrossRef]
159. Zhu, Y.; Song, X.; Wang, J.; Li, Y.; Yang, Y.; Yang, T.; Ma, H.; Wang, L.; Zhang, G.; Cho, W.C.; et al. Placental mesenchymal stem cells of fetal origin deposit epigenetic alterations during long-term culture under serum-free condition. *Expert Opin. Biol. Ther.* **2015**, *15*, 163–180. [CrossRef]
160. Leavey, K.; Wilson, S.L.; Bainbridge, S.A.; Robinson, W.P.; Cox, B.J. Epigenetic regulation of placental gene expression in transcriptional subtypes of preeclampsia. *Clin. Epigenet.* **2018**, *10*, 28. [CrossRef]
161. Calicchio, R.; Doridot, L.; Miralles, F.; Mehats, C.; Vaiman, D. DNA methylation, an epigenetic mode of gene expression regulation in reproductive science. *Curr. Pharm. Des.* **2014**, *20*, 1726–1750. [CrossRef] [PubMed]

162. Horiuchi, A.; Hayashi, T.; Kikuchi, N.; Hayashi, A.; Fuseya, C.; Shiozawa, T.; Konishi, I. Hypoxia upregulates ovarian cancer invasiveness via the binding of HIF-1alpha to a hypoxia-induced, methylation-free hypoxia response element of S100A4 gene. *Int. J. Cancer* **2012**, *131*, 1755–1767. [CrossRef] [PubMed]
163. Aouache, R.; Biquard, L.; Vaiman, D.; Miralles, F. Oxidative Stress in Preeclampsia and Placental Diseases. *Int. J. Mol. Sci.* **2018**, *19*, 1496. [CrossRef] [PubMed]
164. Biron-Shental, T.; Sukenik Halevy, R.; Goldberg-Bittman, L.; Kidron, D.; Fejgin, M.D.; Amiel, A. Telomeres are shorter in placental trophoblasts of pregnancies complicated with intrauterine growth restriction (IUGR). *Early Hum. Dev.* **2010**, *86*, 451–456. [CrossRef] [PubMed]
165. Sukenik-Halevy, R.; Amiel, A.; Kidron, D.; Liberman, M.; Ganor-Paz, Y.; Biron-Shental, T. Telomere homeostasis in trophoblasts and in cord blood cells from pregnancies complicated with preeclampsia. *Am. J. Obstet. Gynecol.* **2016**, *214*, 283.e1–283.e7. [CrossRef]
166. Farladansky-Gershnabel, S.; Gal, H.; Kidron, D.; Krizhanovsky, V.; Amiel, A.; Sukenik-Halevy, R.; Biron-Shental, T. Telomere Homeostasis and Senescence Markers Are Differently Expressed in Placentas From Pregnancies With Early- Versus Late-Onset Preeclampsia. *Reprod. Sci.* **2018**, 1933719118811644. [CrossRef]
167. Cindrova-Davies, T.; Fogarty, N.M.E.; Jones, C.J.P.; Kingdom, J.; Burton, G.J. Evidence of oxidative stress-induced senescence in mature, post-mature and pathological human placentas. *Placenta* **2018**, *68*, 15–22. [CrossRef]
168. Londero, A.P.; Orsaria, M.; Marzinotto, S.; Grassi, T.; Fruscalzo, A.; Calcagno, A.; Bertozzi, S.; Nardini, N.; Stella, E.; Lelle, R.J.; et al. Placental aging and oxidation damage in a tissue micro-array model: An immunohistochemistry study. *Histochem. Cell Biol.* **2016**, *146*, 191–204. [CrossRef]
169. Burton, G.J.; Yung, H.W.; Murray, A.J. Mitochondrial—Endoplasmic reticulum interactions in the trophoblast: Stress and senescence. *Placenta* **2017**, *52*, 146–155. [CrossRef]
170. Chu, T.; Bunce, K.; Shaw, P.; Shridhar, V.; Althouse, A.; Hubel, C.; Peters, D. Comprehensive analysis of preeclampsia-associated DNA methylation in the placenta. *PLoS ONE* **2014**, *9*, e107318. [CrossRef]
171. Blair, J.D.; Yuen, R.K.; Lim, B.K.; McFadden, D.E.; von Dadelszen, P.; Robinson, W.P. Widespread DNA hypomethylation at gene enhancer regions in placentas associated with early-onset pre-eclampsia. *Mol. Hum. Reprod.* **2013**, *19*, 697–708. [CrossRef] [PubMed]
172. Yung, H.W.; Atkinson, D.; Campion-Smith, T.; Olovsson, M.; Charnock-Jones, D.S.; Burton, G.J. Differential activation of placental unfolded protein response pathways implies heterogeneity in causation of early- and late-onset pre-eclampsia. *J. Pathol.* **2014**, *234*, 262–276. [CrossRef] [PubMed]
173. Zhu, L.; Lv, R.; Kong, L.; Cheng, H.; Lan, F.; Li, X. Genome-Wide Mapping of 5mC and 5hmC Identified Differentially Modified Genomic Regions in Late-Onset Severe Preeclampsia: A Pilot Study. *PLoS ONE* **2015**, *10*, e0134119. [CrossRef] [PubMed]
174. Anton, L.; Brown, A.G.; Bartolomei, M.S.; Elovitz, M.A. Differential methylation of genes associated with cell adhesion in preeclamptic placentas. *PLoS ONE* **2014**, *9*, e100148. [CrossRef] [PubMed]
175. Nie, X.; Zhang, K.; Wang, L.; Ou, G.; Zhu, H.; Gao, W.Q. Transcription factor STOX1 regulates proliferation of inner ear epithelial cells via the AKT pathway. *Cell Prolif.* **2015**, *48*, 209–220. [CrossRef] [PubMed]
176. Guibert, S.; Weber, M. Functions of DNA methylation and hydroxymethylation in mammalian development. *Curr. Top. Dev. Biol.* **2013**, *104*, 47–83. [PubMed]
177. Bellido, M.L.; Radpour, R.; Lapaire, O.; De Bie, I.; Hosli, I.; Bitzer, J.; Hmadcha, A.; Zhong, X.Y.; Holzgreve, W. MALDI-TOF mass array analysis of RASSF1A and SERPINB5 methylation patterns in human placenta and plasma. *Biol. Reprod.* **2010**, *82*, 745–750. [CrossRef] [PubMed]
178. Anderson, C.M.; Ralph, J.L.; Wright, M.L.; Linggi, B.; Ohm, J.E. DNA methylation as a biomarker for preeclampsia. *Biol. Res. Nurs.* **2014**, *16*, 409–420. [CrossRef] [PubMed]
179. He, J.; Zhang, A.; Fang, M.; Fang, R.; Ge, J.; Jiang, Y.; Zhang, H.; Han, C.; Ye, X.; Yu, D.; et al. Methylation levels at IGF2 and GNAS DMRs in infants born to preeclamptic pregnancies. *BMC Genom.* **2013**, *14*, 472. [CrossRef]
180. Xiang, Y.; Zhang, X.; Li, Q.; Xu, J.; Zhou, X.; Wang, T.; Xing, Q.; Liu, Y.; Wang, L.; He, L.; et al. Promoter hypomethylation of TIMP3 is associated with pre-eclampsia in a Chinese population. *Mol. Hum. Reprod.* **2013**, *19*, 153–159. [CrossRef]
181. Zhang, Y.; Fei, M.; Xue, G.; Zhou, Q.; Jia, Y.; Li, L.; Xin, H.; Sun, S. Elevated levels of hypoxia-inducible microRNA-210 in pre-eclampsia: New insights into molecular mechanisms for the disease. *J. Cell. Mol. Med.* **2012**, *16*, 249–259. [CrossRef] [PubMed]

182. Wilson, S.L.; Leavey, K.; Cox, B.; Robinson, W.P. Mining DNA methylation alterations towards a classification of placental pathologies. *Hum. Mol. Genet.* **2018**, *27*, 135–146. [CrossRef] [PubMed]
183. Chelbi, S.T.; Wilson, M.L.; Veillard, A.C.; Ingles, S.A.; Zhang, J.; Mondon, F.; Gascoin-Lachambre, G.; Doridot, L.; Mignot, T.M.; Rebourcet, R.; et al. Genetic and epigenetic mechanisms collaborate to control SERPINA3 expression and its association with placental diseases. *Hum. Mol. Genet.* **2012**, *21*, 1968–1978. [CrossRef] [PubMed]
184. Hogg, K.; Blair, J.D.; McFadden, D.E.; von Dadelszen, P.; Robinson, W.P. Early onset pre-eclampsia is associated with altered DNA methylation of cortisol-signalling and steroidogenic genes in the placenta. *PLoS ONE* **2013**, *8*, e62969. [CrossRef] [PubMed]
185. Xirong, X.; Tao, X.; Wang, Y.; Zhu, L.; Ye, Y.; Liu, H.; Zhou, Q.; Li, X.; Xiong, Y. Hypomethylation of tissue factor pathway inhibitor 2 in human placenta of preeclampsia. *Thrombosis Res.* **2017**, *152*, 7–13.
186. Sundrani, D.P.; Reddy, U.S.; Joshi, A.A.; Mehendale, S.S.; Chavan-Gautam, P.M.; Hardikar, A.A. Differential placental methylation and expression of VEGF, FLT-1 and KDR genes in human term and preterm preeclampsia. *Clin. Epigenet.* **2013**, *5*. [CrossRef]
187. Ching, T.; Ha, J.; Song, M.A.; Tiirikainen, M.; Molnar, J.; Berry, M.J.; Towner, D.; Garmire, L.X. Genome-scale hypomethylation in the cord blood DNAs associated with early onset preeclampsia. *Clin. Epigenet.* **2015**, *7*, 21. [CrossRef]
188. Ye, W.; Shen, L.; Xiong, Y.; Zhou, Y.; Gu, H.; Yang, Z. Preeclampsia is Associated with Decreased Methylation of the GNA12 Promoter. *Ann. Hum. Genet.* **2016**, *80*, 7–10. [CrossRef]
189. Yuen, R.K.; Penaherrera, M.S.; von Dadelszen, P.; McFadden, D.E.; Robinson, W.P. DNA methylation profiling of human placentas reveals promoter hypomethylation of multiple genes in early-onset preeclampsia. *Eur. J. Hum. Genet.* **2010**, *18*, 1006–1012. [CrossRef]
190. Hogg, K.; Blair, J.D.; von Dadelszen, P.; Robinson, W.P. Hypomethylation of the LEP gene in placenta and elevated maternal leptin concentration in early onset pre-eclampsia. *Mol. Cell. Endocrinol.* **2013**, *367*, 64–73. [CrossRef]
191. Xiang, Y.; Cheng, Y.; Li, X.; Li, Q.; Xu, J.; Zhang, J.; Liu, Y.; Xing, Q.; Wang, L.; He, L.; et al. Up-regulated expression and aberrant DNA methylation of LEP and SH3PXD2A in pre-eclampsia. *PLoS ONE* **2013**, *8*, e59753. [CrossRef] [PubMed]
192. Hu, W.; Weng, X.; Dong, M.; Liu, Y.; Li, W.; Huang, H. Alteration in methylation level at 11β-hydroxysteroid dehydrogenase type 2 gene promoter in infants born to preeclamptic women. *BMC Genet.* **2014**, *15*, 96. [CrossRef] [PubMed]
193. Liu, Y.; Ma, Y. Promoter Methylation Status of WNT2 in Placenta from Patients with Preeclampsia. *Med. Sci. Monit. Int. Med. J. Exp. Clin. Res.* **2017**, *23*, 5294–5301. [CrossRef] [PubMed]
194. Ma, M.; Zhou, Q.-J.; Xiong, Y.; Li, B.; Li, X.-T. Preeclampsia is associated with hypermethylation of IGF-1 promoter mediated by DNMT1. *Am. J. Transl. Res.* **2018**, *10*, 16–39. [PubMed]
195. Rahat, B.; Thakur, S.; Bagga, R.; Kaur, J. Epigenetic regulation of STAT5A and its role as fetal DNA epigenetic marker during placental development and dysfunction. *Placenta* **2016**, *44*, 46–53. [CrossRef]
196. Choux, C.; Carmignac, V.; Bruno, C.; Sagot, P.; Vaiman, D.; Fauque, P. The placenta: Phenotypic and epigenetic modifications induced by Assisted Reproductive Technologies throughout pregnancy. *Clin. Epigenet.* **2015**, *7*, 87. [CrossRef] [PubMed]
197. Tang, Y.; Liu, H.; Li, H.; Peng, T.; Gu, W.; Li, X. Hypermethylation of the HLA-G promoter is associated with preeclampsia. *Mol. Hum. Reprod.* **2015**, *21*, 736–744. [CrossRef]
198. Konwar, C.; Del Gobbo, G.; Yuan, V.; Robinson, W.P. Considerations when processing and interpreting genomics data of the placenta. *Placenta* **2019**. [CrossRef]
199. Tsang, J.C.H.; Vong, J.S.L.; Ji, L.; Poon, L.C.Y.; Jiang, P.; Lui, K.O.; Ni, Y.B.; To, K.F.; Cheng, Y.K.Y.; Chiu, R.W.K.; et al. Integrative single-cell and cell-free plasma RNA transcriptomics elucidates placental cellular dynamics. *Proc. Natl. Acad. Sci. USA* **2017**, *114*, E7786–E7795. [CrossRef]
200. Anacker, J.; Segerer, S.E.; Hagemann, C.; Feix, S.; Kapp, M.; Bausch, R.; Kammerer, U. Human decidua and invasive trophoblasts are rich sources of nearly all human matrix metalloproteinases. *Mol. Hum. Reprod.* **2011**, *17*, 637–652. [CrossRef]
201. Vettraino, I.M.; Roby, J.; Tolley, T.; Parks, W.C. Collagenase-I, stromelysin-I, and matrilysin are expressed within the placenta during multiple stages of human pregnancy. *Placenta* **1996**, *17*, 557–563. [CrossRef]

202. Kocarslan, S.; Incebiyik, A.; Guldur, M.E.; Ekinci, T.; Ozardali, H.I. What is the role of matrix metalloproteinase-2 in placenta percreta? *J. Obstet. Gynaecol. Res.* **2015**, *41*, 1018–1022. [CrossRef] [PubMed]
203. Espino, Y.S.S.; Flores-Pliego, A.; Espejel-Nunez, A.; Medina-Bastidas, D.; Vadillo-Ortega, F.; Zaga-Clavellina, V.; Estrada-Gutierrez, G. New Insights into the Role of Matrix Metalloproteinases in Preeclampsia. *Int. J. Mol. Sci.* **2017**, *18*, 1448. [CrossRef] [PubMed]
204. Li, X.; Wu, C.; Shen, Y.; Wang, K.; Tang, L.; Zhou, M.; Yang, M.; Pan, T.; Liu, X.; Xu, W. Ten-eleven translocation 2 demethylates the MMP9 promoter, and its down-regulation in preeclampsia impairs trophoblast migration and invasion. *J. Biol. Chem.* **2018**, *293*, 10059–10070. [CrossRef] [PubMed]
205. White, W.M.; Brost, B.; Sun, Z.; Rose, C.; Craici, I.; Wagner, S.J.; Turner, S.T.; Garovic, V.D. Genome-wide methylation profiling demonstrates hypermethylation in maternal leukocyte DNA in preeclamptic compared to normotensive pregnancies. *Hypertens. Pregnancy* **2013**, *32*, 257–269. [CrossRef] [PubMed]
206. White, W.M.; Sun, Z.; Borowski, K.S.; Brost, B.C.; Davies, N.P.; Rose, C.H.; Garovic, V.D. Preeclampsia/Eclampsia candidate genes show altered methylation in maternal leukocytes of preeclamptic women at the time of delivery. *Hypertens. Pregnancy* **2016**, *35*, 394–404. [CrossRef] [PubMed]
207. Levine, R.J.; Maynard, S.E.; Qian, C.; Lim, K.H.; England, L.J.; Yu, K.F.; Schisterman, E.F.; Thadhani, R.; Sachs, B.P.; Epstein, F.H.; et al. Circulating angiogenic factors and the risk of preeclampsia. *N. Engl. J. Med.* **2004**, *350*, 672–683. [CrossRef] [PubMed]
208. Taglauer, E.S.; Wilkins-Haug, L.; Bianchi, D.W. Review: Cell-free fetal DNA in the maternal circulation as an indication of placental health and disease. *Placenta* **2014**, *35* (Suppl.), S64–S68. [CrossRef]
209. Chim, S.S.; Tong, Y.K.; Chiu, R.W.; Lau, T.K.; Leung, T.N.; Chan, L.Y.; Oudejans, C.B.; Ding, C.; Lo, Y.M. Detection of the placental epigenetic signature of the maspin gene in maternal plasma. *Proc. Natl. Acad. Sci. USA* **2005**, *102*, 14753–14758. [CrossRef]
210. Qi, Y.H.; Teng, F.; Zhou, Q.; Liu, Y.X.; Wu, J.F.; Yu, S.S.; Zhang, X.; Ma, M.Y.; Zhou, N.; Chen, L.J. Unmethylated-maspin DNA in maternal plasma is associated with severe preeclampsia. *Acta Obstet. Gynecol. Scand.* **2015**, *94*, 983–988. [CrossRef]
211. Tsui, D.W.; Chan, K.C.; Chim, S.S.; Chan, L.W.; Leung, T.Y.; Lau, T.K.; Lo, Y.M.; Chiu, R.W. Quantitative aberrations of hypermethylated RASSF1A gene sequences in maternal plasma in pre-eclampsia. *Prenat. Diagn.* **2007**, *27*, 1212–1218. [CrossRef] [PubMed]
212. Salvianti, F.; Inversetti, A.; Smid, M.; Valsecchi, L.; Candiani, M.; Pazzagli, M.; Cremonesi, L.; Ferrari, M.; Pinzani, P.; Galbiati, S. Prospective evaluation of RASSF1A cell-free DNA as a biomarker of pre-eclampsia. *Placenta* **2015**, *36*, 996–1001. [CrossRef] [PubMed]
213. Mousa, A.A.; Archer, K.J.; Cappello, R.; Estrada-Gutierrez, G.; Isaacs, C.R.; Strauss, J.F., 3rd; Walsh, S.W. DNA methylation is altered in maternal blood vessels of women with preeclampsia. *Reprod. Sci.* **2012**, *19*, 1332–1342. [CrossRef] [PubMed]
214. Mousa, A.A.; Cappello, R.E.; Estrada-Gutierrez, G.; Shukla, J.; Romero, R.; Strauss, J.F., 3rd; Walsh, S.W. Preeclampsia is associated with alterations in DNA methylation of genes involved in collagen metabolism. *Am. J. Pathol.* **2012**, *181*, 1455–1463. [CrossRef] [PubMed]
215. Mousa, A.A.; Strauss, J.F., 3rd; Walsh, S.W. Reduced methylation of the thromboxane synthase gene is correlated with its increased vascular expression in preeclampsia. *Hypertension* **2012**, *59*, 1249–1255.
216. Nomura, Y.; Lambertini, L.; Rialdi, A.; Lee, M.; Mystal, E.Y.; Grabie, M.; Manaster, I.; Huynh, N.; Finik, J.; Davey, M.; et al. Global methylation in the placenta and umbilical cord blood from pregnancies with maternal gestational diabetes, preeclampsia, and obesity. *Reprod. Sci.* **2014**, *21*, 131–137. [CrossRef]
217. Chen, J.; Steegers-Theunissen, R.P.M.; van Meurs, J.B.; Felix, J.F.; Eggink, A.J.; Herzog, E.M.; Wijnands, K.P.J.; Stubbs, A.; Slieker, R.C.; van der Spek, P.J.; et al. Early- and late-onset preeclampsia and the tissue-specific epigenome of the placenta and newborn. *Placenta* **2017**, *58*, 122–132.
218. Novielli, C.; Mando, C.; Tabano, S.; Anelli, G.M.; Fontana, L.; Antonazzo, P.; Miozzo, M.; Cetin, I. Mitochondrial DNA content and methylation in fetal cord blood of pregnancies with placental insufficiency. *Placenta* **2017**, *55*, 63–70. [CrossRef]
219. Qiu, C.; Hevner, K.; Enquobahrie, D.A.; Williams, M.A. A case-control study of maternal blood mitochondrial DNA copy number and preeclampsia risk. *Int. J. Mol. Epidemiol. Genet.* **2012**, *3*, 237–244.

220. Vishnyakova, P.A.; Volodina, M.A.; Tarasova, N.V.; Marey, M.V.; Tsvirkun, D.V.; Vavina, O.V.; Khodzhaeva, Z.S.; Kan, N.E.; Menon, R.; Vysokikh, M.Y.; et al. Mitochondrial role in adaptive response to stress conditions in preeclampsia. *Sci. Rep.* **2016**, *6*, 32410. [CrossRef]
221. Doridot, L.; Chatre, L.; Ducat, A.; Vilotte, J.L.; Lombes, A.; Mehats, C.; Barbaux, S.; Calicchio, R.; Ricchetti, M.; Vaiman, D. Nitroso-redox balance and mitochondrial homeostasis are regulated by STOX1, a pre-eclampsia-associated gene. *Antioxid. Redox Signal.* **2014**, *21*, 819–834. [CrossRef] [PubMed]
222. Brodowski, L.; Zindler, T.; von Hardenberg, S.; Schroder-Heurich, B.; von Kaisenberg, C.S.; Frieling, H.; Hubel, C.A.; Dork, T.; von Versen-Hoynck, F. Preeclampsia-Associated Alteration of DNA Methylation in Fetal Endothelial Progenitor Cells. *Front. Cell Dev. Biol.* **2019**, *7*, 32. [CrossRef] [PubMed]
223. Wang, X.; Chen, Y.; Du, L.; Li, X.; Li, X.; Chen, D. Evaluation of circulating placenta-related long noncoding RNAs as potential biomarkers for preeclampsia. *Exp. Ther. Med.* **2018**, *15*, 4309–4317. [CrossRef] [PubMed]
224. Yu, L.; Kuang, L.Y.; He, F.; Du, L.L.; Li, Q.L.; Sun, W.; Zhou, Y.M.; Li, X.M.; Li, X.Y.; Chen, D.J. The Role and Molecular Mechanism of Long Nocoding RNA-MEG3 in the Pathogenesis of Preeclampsia. *Reprod. Sci.* **2018**, *25*, 1619–1628. [CrossRef] [PubMed]
225. Jairajpuri, D.S.; Malalla, Z.H.; Mahmood, N.; Almawi, W.Y. Circulating microRNA expression as predictor of preeclampsia and its severity. *Gene* **2017**, *627*, 543–548. [CrossRef] [PubMed]
226. Lykoudi, A.; Kolialexi, A.; Lambrou, G.I.; Braoudaki, M.; Siristatidis, C.; Papaioanou, G.K.; Tzetis, M.; Mavrou, A.; Papantoniou, N. Dysregulated placental microRNAs in Early and Late onset Preeclampsia. *Placenta* **2018**, *61*, 24–32. [CrossRef] [PubMed]
227. Purwosunu, Y.; Sekizawa, A.; Okazaki, S.; Farina, A.; Wibowo, N.; Nakamura, M.; Rizzo, N.; Saito, H.; Okai, T. Prediction of preeclampsia by analysis of cell-free messenger RNA in maternal plasma. *Am. J. Obstet. Gynecol.* **2009**, *200*, 386.e1–386.e7. [CrossRef] [PubMed]
228. Tong, J.; Zhao, W.; Lv, H.; Li, W.P.; Chen, Z.J.; Zhang, C. Transcriptomic Profiling in Human Decidua of Severe Preeclampsia Detected by RNA Sequencing. *J. Cell. Biochem.* **2018**, *119*, 607–615. [CrossRef] [PubMed]
229. Zhang, Y.; Yang, L.; Chen, L.L. Life without A tail: New formats of long noncoding RNAs. *Int. J. Biochem. Cell Biol.* **2014**, *54*, 338–349. [CrossRef] [PubMed]
230. Hansen, T.B.; Jensen, T.I.; Clausen, B.H.; Bramsen, J.B.; Finsen, B.; Damgaard, C.K.; Kjems, J. Natural RNA circles function as efficient microRNA sponges. *Nature* **2013**, *495*, 384–388. [CrossRef] [PubMed]
231. Marchese, F.P.; Raimondi, I.; Huarte, M. The multidimensional mechanisms of long noncoding RNA function. *Genome Biol.* **2017**, *18*, 206. [CrossRef] [PubMed]
232. He, X.; He, Y.; Xi, B.; Zheng, J.; Zeng, X.; Cai, Q.; OuYang, Y.; Wang, C.; Zhou, X.; Huang, H.; et al. LncRNAs expression in preeclampsia placenta reveals the potential role of LncRNAs contributing to preeclampsia pathogenesis. *PLoS ONE* **2013**, *8*, e81437. [CrossRef] [PubMed]
233. Long, W.; Rui, C.; Song, X.; Dai, X.; Xue, X.; Lu, Y.; Shen, R.; Li, J.; Li, J.; Ding, H. Distinct expression profiles of lncRNAs between early-onset preeclampsia and preterm controls. *Clin. Chim. Acta* **2016**, *463*, 193–199. [CrossRef] [PubMed]
234. Hosseini, E.S.; Meryet-Figuiere, M.; Sabzalipoor, H.; Kashani, H.H.; Nikzad, H.; Asemi, Z. Dysregulated expression of long noncoding RNAs in gynecologic cancers. *Mol. Cancer* **2017**, *16*, 107. [CrossRef] [PubMed]
235. Amigorena, S. © 1998 Nature Publishing Group. *Nature Medicine*. 1998. Available online: http://www.nature.com/naturemedicine (accessed on 3 May 2019).
236. Mullen, C.A. Review: Analogies between trophoblastic and malignant cells. *Am. J. Reprod. Immunol.* **1998**, *39*, 41–49. [CrossRef] [PubMed]
237. Ferretti, C.; Bruni, L.; Dangles-Marie, V.; Pecking, A.P.; Bellet, D. Molecular circuits shared by placental and cancer cells, and their implications in the proliferative, invasive and migratory capacities of trophoblasts. *Hum. Reprod. Update* **2007**, *13*, 121–141. [CrossRef] [PubMed]
238. Genbacev, O.; Zhou, Y.; Ludlow, J.W.; Fisher, S.J. Regulation of human placental development by oxygen tension. *Science* **1997**, *277*, 1669–1672. [CrossRef] [PubMed]
239. Ji, P.; Diederichs, S.; Wang, W.; Böing, S.; Metzger, R.; Schneider, P.M.; Tidow, N.; Brandt, B.; Buerger, H.; Bulk, E.; et al. MALAT-1, a novel noncoding RNA, and thymosin β4 predict metastasis and survival in early-stage non-small cell lung cancer. *Oncogene* **2003**, *22*, 8031–8041. [CrossRef] [PubMed]
240. Miyagawa, R.; Tano, K.; Mizuno, R.; Nakamura, Y.; Ijiri, K.; Rakwal, R.; Shibato, J.; Masuo, Y.; Mayeda, A.; Hirose, T.; et al. Identification of cis- and trans-acting factors involved in the localization of MALAT-1 noncoding RNA to nuclear speckles. *RNA* **2012**, *18*, 738–751. [CrossRef]

241. Tseng, J.-J.; Hsieh, Y.-T.; Hsu, S.-L.; Chou, M.-M. Metastasis associated lung adenocarcinoma transcript 1 is up-regulated in placenta previa increta/percreta and strongly associated with trophoblast-like cell invasion in vitro. *Mol. Hum. Reprod.* **2009**, *15*, 725–731. [CrossRef]
242. Li, X.; Song, Y.; Liu, F.; Liu, D.; Miao, H.; Ren, J.; Xu, J.; Ding, L.; Hu, Y.; Wang, Z.; et al. Long Non-Coding RNA MALAT1 Promotes Proliferation, Angiogenesis, and Immunosuppressive Properties of Mesenchymal Stem Cells by Inducing VEGF and IDO. *J. Cell. Biochem.* **2017**, *118*, 2780–2791. [CrossRef] [PubMed]
243. Hass, R.; Kasper, C.; Böhm, S.; Jacobs, R. Different populations and sources of human mesenchymal stem cells (MSC): A comparison of adult and neonatal tissue-derived MSC. *Cell Commun. Signal.* **2011**, *9*, 12. [CrossRef] [PubMed]
244. Zhou, Y.; Zhang, X.; Klibanski, A. MEG3 noncoding RNA: A tumor suppressor. *J. Mol. Endocinol.* **2012**, *48*, 45–53. [CrossRef] [PubMed]
245. Davatzikos, C.; Rathore, S.; Bakas, S.; Pati, S.; Bergman, M.; Kalarot, R.; Sridharan, P.; Gastounioti, A.; Jahani, N.; Cohen, E.; et al. Cancer imaging phenomics toolkit: Quantitative imaging analytics for precision diagnostics and predictive modeling of clinical outcome. *J. Med. Imaging* **2018**, *5*, 011018. [CrossRef] [PubMed]
246. Yu, Y.C.; Jiang, Y.; Yang, M.M.; He, S.N.; Xi, X.; Xu, Y.T.; Hu, W.S.; Luo, Q. Hypermethylation of delta-like homolog 1/maternally expressed gene 3 loci in human umbilical veins: Insights into offspring vascular dysfunction born after preeclampsia. *J. Hypertens.* **2019**, *37*, 581–589. [CrossRef] [PubMed]
247. Yuan, J.H.; Yang, F.; Wang, F.; Ma, J.Z.; Guo, Y.J.; Tao, Q.F.; Liu, F.; Pan, W.; Wang, T.T.; Zhou, C.C.; et al. A Long Noncoding RNA Activated by TGF-β promotes the invasion-metastasis cascade in hepatocellular carcinoma. *Cancer Cell* **2014**, *25*, 666–681. [CrossRef] [PubMed]
248. Liu, X.; Chen, H.; Kong, W.; Zhang, Y.; Cao, L.; Gao, L.; Zhou, R. Down-regulated long non-coding RNA-ATB in preeclampsia and its effect on suppressing migration, proliferation, and tube formation of trophoblast cells. *Placenta* **2017**, *49*, 80–87. [CrossRef] [PubMed]
249. Zheng, Q.; Zhang, D.; Yang, Y.U.; Cui, X.; Sun, J.; Liang, C.; Qin, H.; Yang, X.; Liu, S.; Yan, Q. MicroRNA-200c impairs uterine receptivity formation by targeting FUT4 and α1,3-fucosylation. *Cell Death Differ.* **2017**, *24*, 2161–2172. [CrossRef] [PubMed]
250. Renthal, N.E.; Chen, C.-C.; Williams, K.C.; Gerard, R.D.; Prange-Kiel, J.; Mendelson, C.R. miR-200 family and targets, ZEB1 and ZEB2, modulate uterine quiescence and contractility during pregnancy and labor. *Proc. Natl. Acad. Sci. USA* **2010**, *107*, 20828–20833. [CrossRef]
251. Paysan, L.; Piquet, L.; Saltel, F.; Moreau, V. Rnd3 in Cancer: A Review of the Evidence for Tumor Promoter or Suppressor. *Mol. Cancer Res.* **2016**, *14*, 1033–1044. [CrossRef]
252. Xu, Y.; Lian, Y.; Zhang, Y.; Huang, S.; Zuo, Q.; Yang, N.; Chen, Y.; Wu, D.; Sun, L. The long non-coding RNA PVT1 represses ANGPTL4 transcription through binding with EZH2 in trophoblast cell. *J. Cell. Mol. Med.* **2018**, *22*, 1272–1282. [CrossRef] [PubMed]
253. Feng, Y.; Wang, J.; He, Y.; Zhang, H.; Jiang, M.; Cao, D.; Wang, A. HOXD8/DIAPH2-AS1 epigenetically regulates PAX3 and impairs HTR-8/SVneo cell function under hypoxia. *Biosci. Rep.* **2019**, *39*, BSR20182022. [CrossRef] [PubMed]
254. Loupe, J.M.; Miller, P.J.; Bonner, B.P.; Maggi, E.C.; Vijayaraghavan, J.; Crabtree, J.S.; Taylor, C.M.; Zabaleta, J.; Hollenbach, A.D. Comparative transcriptomic analysis reveals the oncogenic fusion protein PAX3-FOXO1 globally alters mRNA and miRNA to enhance myoblast invasion. *Oncogenesis* **2016**, *5*, e246. [CrossRef] [PubMed]
255. Pineles, B.L.; Romero, R.; Montenegro, D.; Tarca, A.L.; Han, Y.M.; Kim, Y.M.; Draghici, S.; Espinoza, J.; Kusanovic, J.P.; Mittal, P.; et al. Distinct subsets of microRNAs are expressed differentially in the human placentas of patients with preeclampsia. *Am. J. Obstet. Gynecol.* **2007**, *196*, e261. [CrossRef] [PubMed]
256. Zhu, X.m.; Han, T.; Sargent, I.L.; Yin, G.w.; Yao, Y.q. Differential expression profile of microRNAs in human placentas from preeclamptic pregnancies vs normal pregnancies. *Am. J. Obstet. Gynecol.* **2009**, *200*, e661. [CrossRef]
257. Biró, O.; Nagy, B.; Rigó, J. Identifying miRNA regulatory mechanisms in preeclampsia by systems biology approaches. *Hypertens. Pregnancy* **2017**, *36*, 90–99. [CrossRef]
258. Zhou, C.; Zou, Q.Y.; Li, H.; Wang, R.F.; Liu, A.X.; Magness, R.R.; Zheng, J. Preeclampsia Downregulates MicroRNAs in Fetal Endothelial Cells: Roles of miR-29a/c-3p in Endothelial Function. *J. Clin. Endocrinol. Metab.* **2017**, *102*, 3470–3479. [CrossRef] [PubMed]

259. Yang, Z.; Wu, L.; Zhu, X.; Xu, J.; Jin, R.; Li, G.; Wu, F. MiR-29a modulates the angiogenic properties of human endothelial cells. *Biochem. Biophys. Res. Commun.* **2013**, *434*, 143–149. [CrossRef]
260. Davis, E.F.; Newton, L.; Lewandowski, A.J.; Lazdam, M.; Kelly, B.A.; Kyriakou, T.; Leeson, P. Pre-eclampsia and offspring cardiovascular health: Mechanistic insights from experimental studies. *Clin. Sci. (Lond.)* **2012**, *123*, 53–72. [CrossRef]
261. Butalia, S.; Audibert, F.; Cote, A.M.; Firoz, T.; Logan, A.G.; Magee, L.A.; Mundle, W.; Rey, E.; Rabi, D.M.; Daskalopoulou, S.S.; et al. Hypertension Canada's 2018 Guidelines for the Management of Hypertension in Pregnancy. *Can. J. Cardiol.* **2018**, *34*, 526–531. [CrossRef]
262. Yu, G.Z.; Reilly, S.; Lewandowski, A.J.; Aye, C.Y.L.; Simpson, L.J.; Newton, L.; Davis, E.F.; Zhu, S.J.; Fox, W.R.; Goel, A.; et al. Neonatal Micro-RNA Profile Determines Endothelial Function in Offspring of Hypertensive Pregnancies. *Hypertension* **2018**, *72*, 937–945. [CrossRef] [PubMed]
263. BAVELLONI, A.; Ramazzotti, G.; Poli, A.; Piazzi, M.; Focaccia, E.; Blalock, W.; Faenza, I. MiRNA-210: A Current Overview. *Anticancer Res.* **2017**, *37*, 6511–6521. [PubMed]
264. Kulshreshtha, R.; Ferracin, M.; Wojcik, S.E.; Garzon, R.; Alder, H.; Agosto-Perez, F.J.; Davuluri, R.; Liu, C.-G.; Croce, C.M.; Negrini, M.; et al. A MicroRNA Signature of Hypoxia. *Mol. Cell. Biol.* **2006**, *27*, 1859–1867. [CrossRef] [PubMed]
265. Chen, Z.; Li, Y.; Zhang, H.; Huang, P.; Luthra, R. Hypoxia-regulated microRNA-210 modulates mitochondrial function and decreases ISCU and COX10 expression. *Oncogene* **2010**, *29*, 4362–4368. [CrossRef] [PubMed]
266. Kelly, T.J.; Souza, A.L.; Clish, C.B.; Puigserver, P. A Hypoxia-Induced Positive Feedback Loop Promotes Hypoxia-Inducible Factor 1 Stability through miR-210 Suppression of Glycerol-3-Phosphate Dehydrogenase 1-Like. *Mol. Cell. Biol.* **2012**, *32*, 898. [CrossRef]
267. Fasanaro, P.; Di Stefano, V.; Melchionna, R.; Romani, S.; Pompilio, G.; Capogrossi, M.C.; Martelli, F. MicroRNA-210 Modulates Endothelial Cell Response to Hypoxia and Inhibits the Receptor Tyrosine Kinase Ligand Ephrin-A3. *J. Biol. Chem.* **2008**, *283*, 15878–15883. [CrossRef] [PubMed]
268. Cabello, C.M.; Bair, W.B.; Lamore, S.D.; Ley, S.; Alexandra, S.; Azimian, S.; Wondrak, G.T. The cinnamon-derived Michael acceptor cinnamic aldehyde impairs melanoma cell proliferation, invasiveness, and tumor growth. *Free Radic. Biol. Med.* **2009**, *46*, 220–231.
269. Lee, D.-C.; Romero, R.; Kim, J.-S.; Tarca, A.L.; Montenegro, D.; Pineles, B.L.; Kim, E.; Lee, J.; Kim, S.Y.; Draghici, S.; et al. miR-210 Targets Iron-Sulfur Cluster Scaffold Homologue in Human Trophoblast Cell Lines. *Am. J. Pathol.* **2011**, *179*, 590–602. [CrossRef]
270. Muralimanoharan, S.; Maloyan, A.; Mele, J.; Guo, C.; Myatt, L.G.; Myatt, L. MIR-210 modulates mitochondrial respiration in placenta with preeclampsia. *Placenta* **2012**, *33*, 816–823. [CrossRef]
271. Kopriva, S.E.; Chiasson, V.L.; Mitchell, B.M.; Chatterjee, P. TLR3-Induced Placental miR-210 Down-Regulates the STAT6/Interleukin-4 Pathway. *PLoS ONE* **2013**, *8*, e67760. [CrossRef]
272. Luo, R.; Shao, X.; Xu, P.; Liu, Y.; Wang, Y.; Zhao, Y.; Liu, M.; Ji, L.; Li, Y.X.; Chang, C.; et al. MicroRNA-210 contributes to preeclampsia by downregulating potassium channel modulatory factor 1. *Hypertension* **2014**, *64*, 839–845. [CrossRef] [PubMed]
273. Luo, R.; Wang, Y.; Xu, P.; Cao, G.; Zhao, Y.; Shao, X.; Li, Y.X.; Chang, C.; Peng, C.; Wang, Y.L. Hypoxia-inducible miR-210 contributes to preeclampsia via targeting thrombospondin type I domain containing 7A. *Sci. Rep.* **2016**, *6*, 19588. [CrossRef] [PubMed]
274. Chen, J.; Zhao, L.; Wang, D.; Xu, Y.; Gao, H.; Tan, W.; Wang, C. Contribution of regulatory T cells to immune tolerance and association of microRNA-210 and Foxp3 in preeclampsia. *Mol. Med. Rep.* **2019**, *19*, 1150–1158. [CrossRef]
275. Rudensky, A.Y. Regulatory T Cells and Foxp3. *Immunol. Rev.* **2011**, *241*, 260–268. [CrossRef] [PubMed]
276. Zhao, M.; Wang, L.T.; Liang, G.P.; Zhang, P.; Deng, X.J.; Tang, Q.; Zhai, H.Y.; Chang, C.C.; Su, Y.W.; Lu, Q.J. Up-regulation of microRNA-210 induces immune dysfunction via targeting FOXP3 in CD4(+) T cells of psoriasis vulgaris. *Clin. Immunol.* **2014**, *150*, 22–30. [CrossRef]
277. Zhang, Y.; Diao, Z.; Su, L.; Sun, H.; Li, R.; Cui, H.; Hu, Y. MicroRNA-155 contributes to preeclampsia by down-regulating CYR61. *Am. J. Obstet. Gynecol.* **2010**, *202*, e461–e466. [CrossRef] [PubMed]
278. Mo, F.-E.; Muntean, A.G.; Chen, C.-C.; Stolz, D.B.; Watkins, S.C.; Lau, L.F. CYR61 (CCN1) Is Essential for Placental Development and Vascular Integrity. *Mol. Cell. Biol.* **2002**, *22*, 8709–8720. [CrossRef] [PubMed]
279. Holbourn, K.; Ravi Acharya, K.; Perbal, B. The CCN family of proteins: Structure–function relationships. *Trends Biochem. Sci.* **2008**, *33*, 561–573. [CrossRef]

280. Deloia, J.A.; Burlingame, J.M.; Krasnow, J.S. Differential Expression of G1 Cyclins During Human Placentogenesis. *Placenta* **1997**, *18*, 9–16. [CrossRef]
281. Baldin, V.; Marcote, M.J.; Lukas, J.; Draetta, G.; Pagano, M. Cyclin D1 is a nuclear protein required for cell cycle progression in G1. *Genes Dev.* **2007**, *7*, 812–821. [CrossRef] [PubMed]
282. Yung, H.-w.; Calabrese, S.; Hynx, D.; Hemmings, B.A.; Cetin, I.; Charnock-Jones, D.S.; Burton, G.J. Evidence of Placental Translation Inhibition and Endoplasmic Reticulum Stress in the Etiology of Human Intrauterine Growth Restriction. *Am. J. Pathol.* **2008**, *173*, 451–462. [CrossRef] [PubMed]
283. Yang, X.; Zhang, J.; Ding, Y. Association of microRNA-155, interleukin 17A, and proteinuria in preeclampsia. *Medicine* **2017**, *96*, e6509. [CrossRef] [PubMed]
284. Martin, D.B.; Nelson, P.S.; Knudsen, B.S.; Parkin, R.K.; Noteboom, J.; Kroh, E.M.; O'Briant, K.C.; Drescher, C.W.; Vessella, R.L.; Gentleman, R.; et al. Circulating microRNAs as stable blood-based markers for cancer detection. *Proc. Natl. Acad. Sci. USA* **2008**, *105*, 10513–10518.
285. Dai, Y.; Diao, Z.; Sun, H.; Li, R.; Qiu, Z.; Hu, Y. MicroRNA-155 is involved in the remodelling of human-trophoblast-derived HTR-8/SVneo cells induced by lipopolysaccharides. *Hum. Reprod.* **2011**, *26*, 1882–1891. [CrossRef] [PubMed]
286. Chambers, J.C.; Fusi, L.; Haskard, D.O.; Swiet, M.D.; Page, P. Association of Maternal Endothelial Dysfunction With Preeclampsia. *JAMA J. Am. Med. Assoc.* **2014**, *28*, 1607–1612.
287. Cheng, W.; Liu, T.; Jiang, F.; Liu, C.; Zhao, X.; Gao, Y.; Wang, H.; Liu, Z. microRNA-155 regulates angiotensin II type 1 receptor expression in umbilical vein endothelial cells from severely pre-eclamptic pregnant women. *Int. J. Mol. Med.* **2011**, *27*, 393–399. [PubMed]
288. Shan, H.Y.; Bai, X.J.; Chen, X.M. Angiotensin II induces endothelial cell senescence via the activation of mitogen-activated protein kinases. *Cell Biochem. Funct.* **2008**, *26*, 459–466. [CrossRef]
289. Seligman, S.P.; Buyon, J.P.; Clancy, R.M.; Young, B.K.; Abramson, S.B. The role of nitric oxide in the pathogenesis of preeclampsia. *Am. J. Obstet. Gynecol.* **1994**, *171*, 944–948. [CrossRef]
290. Sun, H.X.; Zeng, D.Y.; Li, R.T.; Pang, R.P.; Yang, H.; Hu, Y.L.; Zhang, Q.; Jiang, Y.; Huang, L.Y.; Tang, Y.B.; et al. Essential role of microRNA-155 in regulating endothelium-dependent vasorelaxation by targeting endothelial nitric oxide synthase. *Hypertension* **2012**, *60*, 1407–1414. [CrossRef]
291. Théry, C.; Zitvogel, L.; Amigorena, S. Exosomes: Composition, biogenesis and function. *Nat. Rev. Immunol.* **2002**, *2*, 569–579. [CrossRef]
292. Shen, L.; Li, Y.; Li, R.; Diao, Z.; Yany, M.; Wu, M.; Sun, H.; Yan, G.; Hu, Y. Placenta-associated serum exosomal miR-155 derived from patients with preeclampsia inhibits eNOS expression in human umbilical vein endothelial cells. *Int. J. Mol. Med.* **2018**, *41*, 1731–1739. [CrossRef] [PubMed]
293. Rensen, S.S.M.; Doevendans, P.A.F.M.; Van Eys, G.J.J.M. Regulation and characteristics of vascular smooth muscle cell phenotypic diversity. *Neth. Heart J.* **2007**, *15*, 100–108. [CrossRef] [PubMed]
294. Boerth, N.J.; Dey, N.B.; Cornwell, T.L.; Lincoln, T.M. Cyclic GMP-Dependent Protein Kinase Regulates Vascular Smooth Muscle Cell Phenotype. *J. Vasc. Res.* **1997**, *34*, 245–259. [CrossRef] [PubMed]
295. Lincoln, T.M.; Dey, N.B.; Boerth, N.J.; Cornwell, T.L.; Soff, G.A. Nitric oxide—Cyclic GMP pathway regulates vascular smooth muscle cell phenotypic modulation: Implications in vascular diseases. *Acta Physiol. Scand.* **1998**, *164*, 507–515. [CrossRef] [PubMed]
296. Choi, S.; Park, M.; Kim, J.; Park, W.; Kim, S.; Lee, D.K.; Hwang, J.Y.; Choe, J.; Won, M.H.; Ryoo, S.; et al. TNF-α elicits phenotypic and functional alterations of vascular smooth muscle cells by miR-155-5p–dependent down-regulation of cGMP-dependent kinase 1. *J. Biol. Chem.* **2018**, *293*, 14812–14822. [CrossRef] [PubMed]
297. Park, M.; Choi, S.; Kim, S.; Kim, J.; Lee, D.K.; Park, W.; Kim, T.; Jung, J.; Hwang, J.Y.; Won, M.H.; et al. NF-κB-responsive miR-155 induces functional impairment of vascular smooth muscle cells by downregulating soluble guanylyl cyclase. *Exp. Mol. Med.* **2019**, *51*, 17. [CrossRef]
298. Lo, Y.M.; Chiu, R.W. Prenatal diagnosis: Progress through plasma nucleic acids. *Nat. Rev. Genet.* **2007**, *8*, 71–77.
299. Chim, S.S.; Shing, T.K.; Hung, E.C.; Leung, T.Y.; Lau, T.K.; Chiu, R.W.; Lo, Y.M. Detection and characterization of placental microRNAs in maternal plasma. *Clin. Chem.* **2008**, *54*, 482–490. [CrossRef]
300. Gunel, T.; Zeybek, Y.G.; Akcakaya, P.; Kalelioglu, I.; Benian, A.; Ermis, H.; Aydinli, K. Serum microRNA expression in pregnancies with preeclampsia. *Genet. Mol. Res.* **2011**, *10*, 4034–4040. [CrossRef]
301. Li, Q.; Long, A.; Jiang, L.; Cai, L.; Xie, L.I.; Gu, J.; Chen, X.; Tan, L. Quantification of preeclampsia-related microRNAs in maternal serum. *Biomed. Rep.* **2015**, *3*, 792–796. [CrossRef]

302. Munaut, C.; Tebache, L.; Blacher, S.; Noel, A.; Nisolle, M.; Chantraine, F. Dysregulated circulating miRNAs in preeclampsia. *Biomed. Rep.* **2016**, *5*, 686–692. [CrossRef] [PubMed]
303. Gan, L.; Liu, Z.; Wei, M.; Chen, Y.; Yang, X.; Chen, L.; Xiao, X. MIR-210 and miR-155 as potential diagnostic markers for pre-eclampsia pregnancies. *Medicine* **2017**, *96*, e7515. [CrossRef] [PubMed]
304. Hromadnikova, I.; Kotlabova, K.; Ivankova, K.; Krofta, L. First trimester screening of circulating C19MC microRNAs and the evaluation of their potential to predict the onset of preeclampsia and IUGR. *PLoS ONE* **2017**, *12*, e0171756. [CrossRef] [PubMed]
305. Winger, E.E.; Reed, J.L.; Ji, X.; Nicolaides, K. Peripheral blood cell microRNA quantification during the first trimester predicts preeclampsia: Proof of concept. *PLoS ONE* **2018**, *13*, e0190654. [CrossRef] [PubMed]
306. Moldovan, L.; Batte, K.E.; Trgovcich, J.; Wisler, J.; Marsh, C.B.; Piper, M. Methodological challenges in utilizing miRNAs as circulating biomarkers. *J. Cell. Mol. Med.* **2014**, *18*, 371–390. [CrossRef] [PubMed]
307. El-Khoury, V.; Pierson, S.; Kaoma, T.; Bernardin, F.; Berchem, G. Assessing cellular and circulating miRNA recovery: The impact of the RNA isolation method and the quantity of input material. *Sci. Rep.* **2016**, *6*, 19529. [CrossRef] [PubMed]
308. Xu, P.; Zhao, Y.; Liu, M.; Wang, Y.; Wang, H.; Li, Y.X.; Zhu, X.; Yao, Y.; Wang, H.; Qiao, J.; et al. Variations of microRNAs in human placentas and plasma from preeclamptic pregnancy. *Hypertension* **2014**, *63*, 1276–1284. [CrossRef]
309. Adel, S.; Mansour, A.; Louka, M.; Matboli, M.; Elmekkawi, S.F.; Swelam, N. Evaluation of MicroRNA-210 and Protein tyrosine phosphatase, non-receptor type 2 in Pre-eclampsia. *Gene* **2017**, *596*, 105–109. [CrossRef]
310. Manaster, I.; Goldman-Wohl, D.; Greenfield, C.; Nachmani, D.; Tsukerman, P.; Hamani, Y.; Yagel, S.; Mandelboim, O. MiRNA-Mediated Control of HLA-G Expression and Function. *PLoS ONE* **2012**, *7*, e33395. [CrossRef]
311. Su, M.-T.; Tsai, P.-Y.; Tsai, H.-L.; Chen, Y.-C.; Kuo, P.-L. miR-346 and miR-582-3p-regulated EG-VEGF expression and trophoblast invasion via matrix metalloproteinases 2 and 9. *BioFactors* **2017**, *43*, 210–219. [CrossRef]
312. Tan, Z.; Randall, G.; Fan, J.; Camoretti-Mercado, B.; Brockman-Schneider, R.; Pan, L.; Solway, J.; Gern, J.E.; Lemanske, R.F.; Nicolae, D.; et al. Allele-Specific Targeting of microRNAs to HLA-G and Risk of Asthma. *Am. J. Hum. Genet.* **2007**, *81*, 829–834. [CrossRef] [PubMed]
313. Zhang, Q.-H.; Sun, H.-M.; Zheng, R.-Z.; Li, Y.-C.; Zhang, Q.; Cheng, P.; Tang, Z.-H.; Huang, F. Meta-analysis of microRNA-183 family expression in human cancer studies comparing cancer tissues with noncancerous tissues. *Gene* **2013**, *527*, 26–32. [CrossRef] [PubMed]
314. Lasabova, Z.; Vazan, M.; Zibolenova, J.; Svecova, I. Overexpression of miR-21 and miR-122 in preeclamptic placentas. *Neuro Endocrinol. Lett.* **2015**, *36*, 695–699. [PubMed]
315. Gao, S.; Wang, Y.; Han, S.; Zhang, Q. Up-regulated microRNA-300 in maternal whole peripheral blood and placenta associated with pregnancy-induced hypertension and preeclampsia. *Int. J. Clin. Exp. Pathol.* **2017**, *10*, 4232–4242.
316. Turco, M.Y.; Gardner, L.; Kay, R.G.; Hamilton, R.S.; Prater, M.; Hollinshead, M.S.; McWhinnie, A.; Esposito, L.; Fernando, R.; Skelton, H.; et al. Trophoblast organoids as a model for maternal-fetal interactions during human placentation. *Nature* **2018**, *564*, 263–267. [CrossRef]
317. Coutifaris, C.; Kao, L.C.; Sehdev, H.M.; Chin, U.; Babalola, G.O.; Blaschuk, O.W.; Strauss, J.F. E-cadherin expression during the differentiation of human trophoblasts. *Development (Camb. Engl.)* **1991**, *113*, 767–777.
318. Chakraborty, D.; Cui, W.; Rosario, G.X.; Scott, R.L.; Dhakal, P.; Renaud, S.J.; Tachibana, M.; Rumi, M.A.; Mason, C.W.; Krieg, A.J.; et al. HIF-KDM3A-MMP12 regulatory circuit ensures trophoblast plasticity and placental adaptations to hypoxia. *Proc. Natl. Acad. Sci. USA* **2016**, *113*, E7212–E7221. [CrossRef]
319. Alahari, S.; Post, M.; Rolfo, A.; Weksberg, R.; Caniggia, I. Compromised JMJD6 Histone Demethylase Activity Affects VHL Gene Repression in Preeclampsia. *J. Clin. Endocrinol. Metab.* **2018**, *103*, 1545–1557. [CrossRef]
320. Xie, D.; Zhu, J.; Liu, Q.; Li, J.; Song, M.; Wang, K.; Zhou, Q.; Jia, Y.; Li, T. Dysregulation of HDAC9 Represses Trophoblast Cell Migration and Invasion Through TIMP3 Activation in Preeclampsia. *Am. J. Hypertens.* **2019**, *32*, 515–523. [CrossRef]
321. Zadora, J.; Singh, M.; Herse, F.; Przybyl, L.; Haase, N.; Golic, M.; Yung, H.W.; Huppertz, B.; Cartwright, J.E.; Whitley, G.; et al. Disturbed Placental Imprinting in Preeclampsia Leads to Altered Expression of DLX5, a Human-Specific Early Trophoblast Marker. *Circulation* **2017**, *136*, 1824–1839. [CrossRef]

322. Van Dijk, M.; Mulders, J.; Poutsma, A.; Konst, A.A.; Lachmeijer, A.M.; Dekker, G.A.; Blankenstein, M.A.; Oudejans, C.B. Maternal segregation of the Dutch preeclampsia locus at 10q22 with a new member of the winged helix gene family. *Nat. Genet.* **2005**, *37*, 514–519. [CrossRef] [PubMed]
323. Van Dijk, M.; van Bezu, J.; van Abel, D.; Dunk, C.; Blankenstein, M.A.; Oudejans, C.B.; Lye, S.J. The STOX1 genotype associated with pre-eclampsia leads to a reduction of trophoblast invasion by alpha-T-catenin upregulation. *Hum. Mol. Genet.* **2010**, *19*, 2658–2667. [CrossRef] [PubMed]
324. Rigourd, V.; Chauvet, C.; Chelbi, S.T.; Rebourcet, R.; Mondon, F.; Letourneur, F.; Mignot, T.M.; Barbaux, S.; Vaiman, D. STOX1 overexpression in choriocarcinoma cells mimics transcriptional alterations observed in preeclamptic placentas. *PLoS ONE* **2008**, *3*, e3905. [CrossRef] [PubMed]
325. Graves, J.A. Genomic imprinting, development and disease–is pre-eclampsia caused by a maternally imprinted gene? *Reprod. Fertil. Dev.* **1998**, *10*, 23–29. [CrossRef] [PubMed]

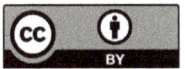

© 2019 by the authors. Licensee MDPI, Basel, Switzerland. This article is an open access article distributed under the terms and conditions of the Creative Commons Attribution (CC BY) license (http://creativecommons.org/licenses/by/4.0/).

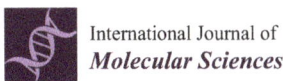

Review

The Role of Nitric Oxide, ADMA, and Homocysteine in The Etiopathogenesis of Preeclampsia—Review

Weronika Dymara-Konopka * and Marzena Laskowska

Department of Obstetrics and Perinatology, Medical University of Lublin, Poland, 20-950 Lublin, Jaczewskiego 8, Poland; weronika.dymara@gmail.com
* Correspondence: melaskowska@go2.pl

Received: 19 May 2019; Accepted: 28 May 2019; Published: 5 June 2019

Abstract: Preeclampsia is a serious, pregnancy-specific, multi-organ disease process of compound aetiology. It affects 3–6% of expecting mothers worldwide and it persists as a leading cause of maternal and foetal morbidity and mortality. In fact, hallmark features of preeclampsia (PE) result from vessel involvement and demonstrate maternal endothelium as a target tissue. Growing evidence suggests that chronic placental hypoperfusion triggers the production and release of certain agents that are responsible for endothelial activation and injury. In this review, we will present the latest findings on the role of nitric oxide, asymmetric dimethylarginine (ADMA), and homocysteine in the etiopathogenesis of preeclampsia and their possible clinical implications.

Keywords: preeclampsia; asymmetric dimethylarginine; nitric oxide; homocysteine

1. Preeclampsia—Background

Preeclampsia (PE) is a serious, pregnancy-specific, multi-organ disease process of compound aetiology. It affects 3–6% of expecting mothers worldwide and it persists as a leading cause of maternal and foetal morbidity and mortality [1]. The diagnosis of PE is clinical. The diagnostic criteria were revised in 2013 and 2014: it is defined as new onset hypertension developing after 20 weeks of gestation and the coexistence of a minimum of one of the following new onset conditions: proteinuria, maternal end- organ dysfunction (including renal, hepatic, haematological, or neurological complications), or uteroplacental dysfunction reflected in foetal growth restriction (FGR) [2,3]. The disease can be further clinically classified as PE with or without severe features, as well as early-onset syndrome (presenting before 34 weeks of gestation, versus late-onset after completed 34 weeks), preterm PE (occurring from 34 + 1 but before 37 + 0 weeks), and term PE (after completed 37 weeks) [4]. The current management of the disease mainly depends on gestational age and assessment of PE severity, focusing on blood pressure control, maternal and foetal surveillance, and it aims to deliver the baby in optimal condition prolongating the pregnancy without worsening state of the mother [3]. It requires individualized calculations of risks and benefits, but unfortunately delivery still remains the only definitive treatment.

In recent times, a huge progress has been made in understanding the disease, getting scientist and doctors closer to explain biological mechanisms underlying the development of PE that possibly can be used to create new therapeutic strategies targeting them.

Within the last decade, subsequent studies confirmed the hypothesis of Roberts and colleagues from 1989, who suggested that PE clinical manifestations might be due to maternal endothelium dysfunction [5]. In fact, the hallmark features of PE result from vessel involvement and demonstrate maternal endothelium as a target tissue. However, the placenta, as the interface between mother and fetus, is also regarded a key and causative player in pathogenesis of PE. Growing evidence suggests that chronic placental hypoperfusion triggers the production and release of certain agents that are responsible for endothelial activation and injury. (Figure 1)

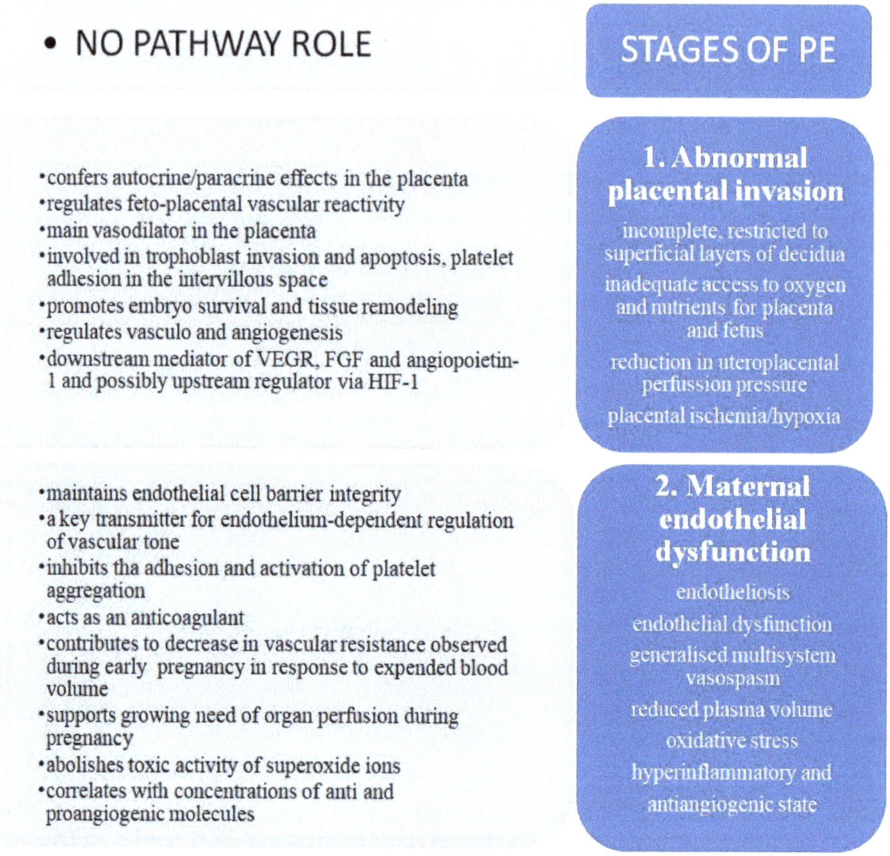

- **NO PATHWAY ROLE**

- confers autocrine/paracrine effects in the placenta
- regulates feto-placental vascular reactivity
- main vasodilator in the placenta
- involved in trophoblast invasion and apoptosis, platelet adhesion in the intervillous space
- promotes embryo survival and tissue remodeling
- regulates vasculo and angiogenesis
- downstream mediator of VEGR, FGF and angiopoietin-1 and possibly upstream regulator via HIF-1

- maintains endothelial cell barrier integrity
- a key transmitter for endothelium-dependent regulation of vascular tone
- inhibits tha adhesion and activation of platelet aggregation
- acts as an anticoagulant
- contributes to decrease in vascular resistance observed during early pregnancy in response to expended blood volume
- supports growing need of organ perfusion during pregnancy
- abolishes toxic activity of superoxide ions
- correlates with concentrations of anti and proangiogenic molecules

STAGES OF PE

1. Abnormal placental invasion

incomplete, restricted to superficial layers of decidua

inadequate access to oxygen and nutrients for placenta and fetus

reduction in uteroplacental perfussion pressure

placental ischemia/hypoxia

2. Maternal endothelial dysfunction

endotheliosis

endothelial dysfunction

generalised multisystem vasospasm

reduced plasma volume

oxidative stress

hyperinflammatory and antiangiogenic state

Figure 1. Physiological roles of NO pathway in pregnancy and their possible influence on preeclampsia (PE) development in two-stage model of disease. NO PATHWAY ROLE: Nitric oxide (NO) pathway role; STAGES OF PE: Stages of preeclampsia (PE).

The development of PE involves a two-stage process [6]. The first, crucially important step is asymptomatic and it takes place during placental invasion and differentiation. While, during normal placentation, the embryo-derived cytotrophoblast properly invades the uterine wall, including the myometrium and spiral arterioles and it leads to transformation of maternal spiral arteries into large capacitance and low resistance vessels; this process is defective in preeclampsia [7–9]. The invasion of cytotrophoblast is incomplete, restricted to superficial layers of decidua that provides inadequate access to maternal oxygen and nutrients for the placenta and growing foetus. Poor placental invasion leads to diminished uteroplacental perfusion pressure and ischemia.

Abnormalities of placental invasion anticipate maternal disorder. Clinical manifestations that define PE represent the second stage of disease. Chronic placental hypoperfusion triggers abnormal production and the release of numerous bioactive factors into the maternal circulation. These circulating substances target endothelial cells resulting in widespread endotheliosis, endothelial dysfunction, generalized multi-system vasospasm, reduced plasma volume, oxidative stress, and hyperinflammatory state. Excessive expression of antiangiogenic proteins, like soluble fms-like tyrosine kinase 1 (sFlt-1) and soluble Endoglin (sEng), which catch circulating, decreased proangiogenic substances, like vascular endothelial growth factor (VEGF), placental growth factor (PlGF), and transforming growth factor β (TGFβ) result in an understanding of PE as an antiangiogenic state [10–13].

Defective trophoblast invasion is an early event in preeclampsia development. However, it has not been resolved whether it is the reason or result of another underlying problem. It remains unclear why trophoblast invasion is interrupted, but an altered immunological response at maternal-foetal interphase, genetics, and environmental factors are believed to contribute, although their role may vary between patients [14,15]. Furthermore, it is suggested that maternal susceptibility and response to placental derangements determines the onset, severity, clinical manifestations, and progression of the disease [16]. The most recent theory identifies PE as a complex disease with two distinct clinical presentations. The first, placental phenotype is associated with shallow trophoblastic invasion and restricted foetal growth, as opposed to PE associated with maternal metabolic syndrome. The second phenotype is associated with normal fetal growth and maternal low-grade inflammation, mainly due to placental oxidative stress, placental villi overcrowding, and decidual lesions [17,18].

Nitric oxide (NO) is one of the key players in the regulation of placental blood flow. It is actively engaged in cytotrophoblast endovascular invasion and development of the placenta, through its unique angiogenic and vasculogenic properties [19]. Current evidence supports altered NO production in the feto-placental unit in preeclampsia, which, by reduced bioavailability, may contribute to vasoconstriction of the placental bed, abnormal placental perfusion, and its maternal consequences, like increased blood pressure, systemic vascular resistance, and sensitivity to the pressors [20–25].

Asymmetric dimethylarginine (ADMA), which is an endogenous inhibitor of NO synthase (NOS), has also been associated with impaired endothelial function and with uterine artery flow disturbances that are characteristic for preeclampsia [24,26,27].

Homocysteine (Hcy) elevated concentrations in preeclamptic women lead to elevated ADMA levels, since Hcy has an inhibitory effect on ADMA metabolism. Hyperhomocysteinemia (HHcy) is also associated with endothelial cells lesions due to vascular fibrosis, which results in alterations in the coagulation system, enhanced platelet activation, and thrombogenesis—changes that are noted in preeclampsia [28–30].

In this review, we will present the latest findings on the role of nitric oxide, ADMA, and homocysteine in the etiopathogenesis of preeclampsia and their possible clinical implications.

2. Metabolism and Biological Role of NO, ADMA, and Homocysteine

Furchgott initially described nitric oxide as an endothelium-derived relaxant factor (EDRF) in 1980 after attributing a vasodilatory effect on vascular smooth muscle by stimulation of cholinergic nerves to the endothelium [31]. The identification of EDRF as NO was reported seven years later and was awarded a Nobel Prize in Physiology or Medicine for Furchgott, Ignarro, and Murad in 1998 for their discoveries concerning nitric oxide as key transmitter in the cardiovascular system. NO is produced through L-arginine-NO synthase pathway by converting L-arginine to L-citrulline in the presence of oxygen and the cofactor tetrahydrobiopterin or alternative enzymatic and non-enzymatic nitrate-nitrite-NO pathways [32,33].

Nitric oxide synthase (NOS) possess three different isoforms, namely neuronal NOS (nNOS) or type 1, inducible NOS (iNOS) or type 2 and endothelial NOS (eNOS) or type 3 [32]. NOS1 and NOS3 are considered as constitutive NOS. Endothelial NOS is stored in plasma membrane caveolae and its distribution and activity are regulated by numerous mechanisms [34]. Being released from endothelial cells, NO is quickly transported to the closest vascular smooth muscle cells, where it exerts its role by inducing the production of cyclic guanosine monophosphate (cGMP) as a second messenger. It may be neutralized by reactive oxygen species on the way to its target cells [35].

NO is the key transmitter for the endothelium-dependent regulation of the vascular tone that is controlled by humoral, metabolic and mechanical factors, for example, in response to increased blood flow [36]. Furthermore, NO inhibits the adhesion and activation of platelet aggregation, abolishes the toxic activity of superoxide ions, and acts as an anticoagulant and antiatherogenic substance [22,32].

It is also considered to have major effects on the gestational endothelial function as well as to play a supportive role in promoting embryo survival, tissue remodelling, immunosuppression, and vasoregulation critical for placental nutrient transport [37–39]. The human foeto-placental vasculature lacks autonomic innervation and, therefore, NO confers autocrine and/or paracrine effects, influencing different aspects of physiological pregnancy. In particular, NO is the main vasodilator that is involved in foeto-placental vascular reactivity regulation, placental bed vascular resistance, trophoblast invasion and apoptosis, and platelet adhesion and aggregation in the intervillous space [40].

Further, the role of NO is also established in vasculogenesis, which results from the de novo formation of vessels derived from pluripotent precursor cells and angiogenesis, the formation of functional capillaries from pre-existing vasculature. Vascular endothelial growth factor (VEGF) is a key particle in these processes. Its expression is mediated by NO release and was required for initiation of vasculogenesis [41]. NO is also a critical downstream mediator of other than VEGF potent angiogenic substances, like basic fibroblast growth factor (FGF), and angiopoietin-1 [42]. The critical role of NO in angiogenesis has been shown in eNOS knockout mice [43]. NOS inhibition is accompanied by defective angiogenesis, as exemplified by deficient vascular sprouting. Interestingly, NO may also act upstream of angiogenic growth factors, because hypoxia-inducible factor-1 (HIF-1) perhaps mediated the effect of NO on VEGF production [44].

Asymmetric dimethylarginine (ADMA), which is an analogue of L-arginine, constitutes a natural metabolite that is found in human plasma. Dimethylarginines are formed as a result of the degradation of methylated arginine residues in proteins [45]. Approximately 80% of ADMA undergoes enzymatic transformation by two dimethylarginine dimethylaminohydrolases (DDAH-1 and -2) to L-citrulline and dimethylamine, whereas kidneys excrete the rest. ADMA is endogenous competitive inhibitor of L-arginine for all three isoforms of NOS. Elevated levels of ADMA block NO synthesis and limit the cellular uptake of L-arginine, thereby contributing to oxidative stress and disrupting further NO biogenesis. In this way, ADMA impairs the endothelial function and thus promotes atherosclerosis. Therefore, it is recognized as a biomarker of endothelial disorders. The ADMA levels are found to be elevated in patients with various cardiovascular and metabolic conditions, such as hypercholesterolemia, atherosclerosis, hypertension, chronic heart or renal failure, diabetes mellitus, stroke, and hyperhomocysteinemia [29,45–47]. ADMA has been shown to increase systemic vascular resistance in humans, as an endogenous inhibitor of NOS [45].

Homocysteine (Hcy) is a sulfur-containing amino acid that is produced during the conversion of essential amino acid methionine (Met) to cysteine (Cys) [48]. Its synthesis occurs in the transsulfuration of dietary methionine, which is abundant in animal protein, but it can also occur in demethylation that is related to fasting conditions. Hcy is metabolized by one of the two following pathways: remethylation to methionine, which requires the addition of a methyl group from 5-methyltetrahydrofolate (5-methyl THF) and the cofactor vitamin B12 (or betaine in an alternative reaction, restricted to the liver and independent of vitamin B12); and, transsulfuration to cystathionine; and finally, to cysteine, which requires vitamin B6 as a cofactor [49]. Methionine derivative, S-adenosyl methionine, is a cofactor that serves as a most important methyl donor of the body, whereas cysteine is used for glutathione synthesis or it is metabolised into taurine.

5-methyltetrahydrofolate (5-MTHF), which is the predominant circulating form of folate is the result of a reduction of 5,10-methylenetetrahydrofolate (5,10-MTHF) catalysed by the MTHFR (methylenetetrahydrofolate reductase) enzyme, coded by MTHFR gene, whose locus is on chromosome 1 at the end of the short arm (1p36.6) [50,51]. Polymorphisms of the MTHFR gene play a significant role in the pathogenesis of hyperhomocysteinemia.

The definition of hyperhomocysteinemia (HHcy), generally understood as increased homocysteine in the blood, differs between authors [52]. The total fasting concentration of Hcy in plasma of healthy patients is low and its level is 5.0–12.0 µmol/l when the immunoassay methods are used or between 5.0 and 15.0 µmol/L when assessed with the use of HPLC (high-performance liquid chromatography) [53]. Modarate HHcy is diagnosed if the levels are within the range of 16 to 30 µmol/L, 31–100 µmol/L is considered to be intermediate and a value above 100 µmol/L is classified as severe hyperhomocysteinemia [54].

The main causes of elevations in homocysteine levels are vitamin deficiency (B6,B12,folate), aforementioned genetic defects in enzymes that are involved in its metabolism (cystathionine β-synthase deficiency and MTHFR), and disease conditions that interfere in the metabolism of cofactor levels, disturbing the transsulphuration and remethylation processes. In the general population, higher values of Hcy are observed in men then in women, although the discrepancy diminishes with age and in postmenopausal patients who tend to have higher Hcy levels [55].

In general, we can divide HHcys in two types: severe, but rare forms due to major genetic defects (individuals with the rare homocystinuria typically have levels of >100 μmol/L) and more common, moderately elevated homocysteine levels that are related to a pathogenesis, such as genetic and environmental factors, which is observed in up to 5% to 12% of the general population [52,56].

The most common cause of severe hyperhomocysteinemia and classic homocystinuria (congenital homocystinuria) is considered to be the homozygous deficiency of CβS (cystathione-β-synthase). This defect is responsible for an increase as much as up to 40-fold in fasting total homocysteine. Other not often observed genetically conditioned states of HHcy are the homozygous deficiency of MTHFR, deficiency of methionine synthase, and impaired activity of methionine synthase due to impaired vitamin B12 metabolism [54].

However, the most common genetic deficiency, which occurs at large rates in various populations, is single nucleotide polymorphism of MTHFR that has been associated with mild and moderate (25–60 μmol/L) hyperhomocysteinemia [57]. A point mutation C-to-Tsubstitution at nucleotide 677 (677C→T) in the gene for MTHFR causes a thermolabile variant of the enzyme and has half-reduced activity, whereas in people who are homozygousfor MTHFR C677T, there is only 30% of normal enzyme function [54]. Another point mutation, called MTHFR A1298C, leads to 60% of normal enzyme function. Double heterozygous (1 abnormal MTHFR C677T gene plus 1 abnormal MTHFR A1298C gene) results in decreased reductase activity as those homozygous for the C677Tpolymorphism [58].

However, the leading cause of HHcy is folate, vitamin B12, and less commonly, B6 deficiency due to low supply, malabsorption, and treatment with substances, such as cyclosporin, methotrexate, fibrates, Levodopa (L-DOPA), and carbamazepine that interfere with the metabolic paths of these vitamins [59,60]. High Hcy levels have been also associated with impaired renal function, high plasma creatinine, smoking, coffee consumption, and alcoholism [52].

HHcy is generally recognized as an independent risk factor for coronary, cerebral, and peripheral atherosclerosis, which was first reported by McCully in 1969 and later confirmed in a meta-analysis of numerous additional studies [61–63]. An extend meta-analysis suggested that an increment of homocysteine of 5 mmol/L is comparable to the increase in the risk of coronary artery disease caused by cholesterol elevation of 0.5 mmol/L [62]. An association between HHcys and cardiovascular disease, as well as some age-related pathologies, like stroke, Alzheimer's disease, Parkinson's disease, chronic renal failure, and osteoporosis is widely described [61–72]. There are ongoing efforts to understand if HHcy observed in vascular diseases is a causative factor or a consequence of endothelial activation [73].

3. NO, ADMA and Homocysteine in Pregnancy

During uncomplicated pregnancy, increased NOS activity in human uterine artery leads to higher NO levels [74]. NOS3 expression raises primarily in the syncytiotrophoblasts and NOS2 activity grows throughout pregnancy, with a peak around mid-gestation [38,39,75,76]. Physiological reduction of blood pressure during pregnancy may greatly rely on the vasodilatory action of NO. NO contributes to the vasodilatation of blood vessels and the decrease in vascular resistance observed during early pregnancy, when maternal blood volume expands, while systemic vascular resistance and systemic blood pressure both decline [22,25,75–77].

In normal pregnancy, also levels of cGMP, a second messenger of NO signalling is particularly increased during the first trimester in plasma and urine [78]. Furthermore, a NO-cGMP pathway is present in the human uterus and it may be responsible for maintaining its relaxation. Spontaneous contractility in vitro was enhanced by the NOS inhibitor L-NAME (nitro-L-arginine methyl ester) and decreased by NO. Thus, uterine reduced the responsiveness to nitric oxide at term may play a role in the initiation of labour [79].

Different studies on total NO in pregnancy gave conflicting results. The measurement of its relatively stable metabolites, nitrate, and nitrite (NOx) is often employed as an indicator of NO production and as a marker of NOS enzyme activity because NO is highly labile molecule [80]. Still, the plasma level is influenced, not only by the production, but also by the clearance of NO derivatives [79]. Some studies found that NO production increases with gestational age during normal pregnancy, especially in the second trimester, and it peaks in the third trimester [81–83]. However, contrary results were also published reporting that maternal circulating nitrite level decreased with advancing gestation [84], or even that there were no changes in NO production when compared to the nonpregnant state [85,86].

Likewise, studies investigating the circulating levels of NO in preeclampsia have also reported conflicting results [87]. These observations suggest that the status of NO biosynthesis in women during normal pregnancy and preeclampsia remains to be defined.

3.1. ADMA in Pregnancy

In normotensive pregnancy, the maternal plasma ADMA levels are generally reduced when comparing to non-pregnant group. The lowest concentration of ADMA is described during the first trimester, when the early fall in blood pressure is accompanied by a significant fall in ADMA concentration. The ADMA levels increase with gestational age in the second and third trimester [24,26]. These findings lead to a conclusion that, in early pregnancy, the reduction in ADMA and concomitant increase in NO are responsible for previously described hemodynamic adaptation, a higher need of organ perfusion in pregnancy, and uterine relaxation. In advanced pregnancy, physiologically increased ADMA levels thus help to prepare the uterine muscle fibers for the higher contractile activity before the labour. This is reflected by the higher ADMA concentrations after caesarean birth when compared with vaginal delivery and it may contribute to decreased nitric oxide production and bioavailability in neonatal vascular beds [88].

3.2. Homocysteine and Pregnancy

The homocysteine plasma levels fall in normal pregnancy [89,90]. An increase in plasma volume and associated haemodilution, glomerular hyperfiltration and postulated raised foetal need for methionine are mechanisms considered to contribute to this effect [91]. The importance of homocysteine to early foetal metabolism is demonstrated in a number of studies [92].

The reference values for HHcys in pregnancy that are proposed in one study were established as: higher than 7.7 mmol/L in the second trimester, and 10.5 mmol/L in the third trimester [93], although different authors usually defined their own cut-off values.

In the pathology of pregnancy, the disturbance of maternal homocysteine metabolism has been linked with recurrent pregnancy loss, deep venous thrombosis, foetal neural tube defects, and various conditions characterized by placental vasculopathy, such as preeclampsia, foetal growth restriction, and abruption [94–98].

4. NO, ADMA, and Homocysteine in Preeclampsia

4.1. NO Pathway Dysfunction in PE

In preeclamptic patients, like in normotensive pregnancies, the measurements of total NO concentration have shown variable results, ranging from decreased [81,99,100], unchanged [101], and increased [102,103] levels of circulating NO metabolites. The dietary intake of these substances could also influence the disparity, although a study that was conducted on women with PE, subjected to a reduced nitrate/nitrite diet, did not show decreased endogenous NO production [78]. In fact, NO measurements may be difficult to interpret, since they reflect the total activity of all three isoforms of

NOS, not just endothelial. While the whole body NO may not change in PE, in view of the evidence for reduced endothelial NO signalling and decrease in vascular relaxation in PE, tissue-specific differences in NOS expression and NO bioavailability could be expected. For instance, in late pregnant rats, renal eNOS decreases by 39%, while iNOS and nNOS increase by 31% and 25%, respectively [104].

PE is associated with abnormalities eNOS-NO pathway that probably exists at different stages of signal transduction process. There is not one particular defect, but multiple changes in key regulatory aspects in NO signaling. In studies where serum from PE women was placed on isolated vessels, nitric oxide-mediated vasorelaxation appeared to be absent [105].

Some studies have indicated that measuring plasma nitrite levels may reflect endogenous NO formation because NO is rapidly oxidized to nitrite. This is because 70% of plasma nitrites derive from NO synthase activity in the endothelium and its inhibition was associated with corresponding decreases in plasma nitrite concentrations [106,107]. By only using nitrite levels (which may be a better measure than total nitrite + nitrate), a reduction from 40 to 60% of total whole blood or plasma nitrite concentration was reported in PE women [108–110].

There is clinical evidence for the link between impaired NO formation and antiangiogenic factors overexpression in preeclampsia. Significant negative correlation between two antiangiogenic factors: sEng and sFlt-1, and nitrite concentrations was described [110], which suggested a possible inhibitory effect caused by these substances on the production of NO in patients with preeclampsia. Experimental studies have shown that NO increases proangiogenic VEGF and PlGF and it decreases sFlt-1 in hypoxic human trophoblast cells [111].

Using the nitrate reductase assay to measure NO, also a correlation between reductions in plasma NO with disease severity was identified, such that the levels were about 30% lower in severe PE vs. healthy pregnant controls [112].

Attempts to assess eNOS activity in PE led to the conclusion that it is still unknown whether eNOS deficiency plays a causal role there. In the murine model, chronic NOS inhibition reversed systemic vasodilation and glomerular hyperfiltration in pregnancy, which suggested its role for endothelial damage and decreased NO in the pathogenesis of preeclampsia [113]. However, different study with the use of eNOS knockout mice showed reduced uterine artery diameter, spiral artery length, and, as a consequence, diminished uteroplacental blood flow, resulting in elevated markers of placental hypoxia in the junctional zone. Even so, interestingly, sFlt-1concentration was not elevated in the eNOS knockout mice [43].

Data from PE women is quite limited and without consensus on eNOS expression, as higher, lower, and unchanged levels of mRNA or enzyme have been reported. Several human studies failed to detect any significant differences in the circulating levels of eNOS [114,115]. One of the earliest studies on eNOS activity found an increase in eNOS expression in syncytiotrophoblast, foetal terminal villous capillary, and stem villous vessel endothelium, whereas the lack of eNOS expression in vascular terminal villi and weak expression in endothelial cells of villous vessels in placenta from normal pregnancy was noted [116]. These results are supported with a recent finding that caveolar eNOS expression is increased in PE placentas [117]. However, this stays in contrast to the observed similar placental levels of eNOS activity in PE patients [118], and to a more recent study in which placental syncytiotrophoblast eNOS expression was even decreased [119]. Apart from these confusing findings, altered placental eNOS levels may not directly relate to peripheral vascular endothelial function.

The reduced availability of eNOS substrate (L-Arginine) or the competitive inhibition by ADMA constitute other factors that may contribute to dysfunctional endothelial NO signalling in PE. One of proposed animal PE models involves administering the aforementioned L-NAME, a competitive inhibitor of arginine, which leads to maternal hypertension and proteinuria, and reduced foetal weight in a dose-dependent way [120]. L-NAME-induced hypertension and high circulating levels of sFlt-1 could be attenuated by the administration of exogenous sodium nitrite, and in this way restoring NO bioavailability [121].

In pregnancies that are complicated by PE, the ADMA levels are significantly higher than in both normotensive gestational age-matched and the nonpregnant control group [24,115,122–124]. Even higher concentration of ADMA in patients with early-onset PE may suggest a relationship between disease severity and determining the time of PE clinical manifestation [125,126]. Moreover, ADMA may have a predictive value in PE, since its modestly (+26%) elevated concentrations were observed as early as in the first trimester [127] and significantly elevated during second trimester in pregnancies that developed PE in more advanced gestational age [128]. Another hypothesis is that increased ADMA concentration may contribute to development of PE in early pregnancy, leading to impaired placentation and its consequences [126]. The association of abnormal uterine artery Doppler waveforms with elevated ADMA levels [129,130] supports the role of endogenous NOS inhibitors adversely affecting maternal vasodilation and blood pressure.

It has been postulated that hyperhomocysteinemia (HHcy) may contribute to the development of PE, as it leads to endothelial dysfunction and accumulation af ADMA [29,30].

4.2. Homocysteine in PE

The association of hyperhomocysteinemia and preeclampsia has initially been suggested by Decker et al. [131], and all authors have not confirmed it. However, the majority of evidence suggests a positive correlation.

Higher maternal plasma homocysteine concentrations in preeclamptic pregnancies as compared to normotensive were widely reported [93,125,130,132–137]. Overall, these differences seem to be present at all of the investigated time points across the gestation, starting from early pregnancy before 20 weeks [138–142] and in both severe and non-severe forms of PE. Comprehensively, this finding led to a conclusion that high homocysteine in early pregnancy constitutes a risk factor for PE. Therefore, attempts to introduce Hcy measurement into a screening test for PE to improve the prediction model, for example, by combining it with uterine artery Doppler test in the second trimester, resulted in being valuable [140]. However, there are also studies that rejected an association between elevated Hcy in early second trimester and subsequent PE [143–145]. This could result from differences in study designs, laboratory techniques, and disease definitions, among other reasons, which may be further investigated in a systematic review.

Still, most of the papers focus on the third trimester [93,130,132–135,137], where the differences between HHcys in severe and non-severe PE are marked. Pregnant women complicated with severe preeclampsia displayed significantly higher serum Hcy levels than with non-severe form [93,112,132,134,136,146]. Thus, homocysteine concentrations positively correlating with the clinical presentation of disease may constitute a marker of severity of preeclampsia.

Besides elevated Hcy concentrations in maternal plasma, the majority of authors analyse the possible association with either folate or vitamin B12 deficiencies, as well as NO pathways in preeclamptic patients. Here, contrary results are presented. Folate and vitamin B12 serum levels were described as unchanged [132,134,135] in PE when comparing to normotensive healthy women with uncomplicated pregnancies. However, opposite results indicating these vitamins deficiencies were also reported [135,146]. Nevertheless, further studies are needed to confirm whether the prescription of these vitamins could decrease serum homocysteine, thereby possibly reducing the risk of preeclampsia or (if it occurs) its severity.

Interesting association between HHcy and NO signalling pathway was reported. Homocysteine inhibits the expression and activity of dimethylamino dimethyl hydrolase (DDAH), which is the enzyme degrading ADMA to citrulline and dimethylamine [22,147–149]. It has been suggested that elevated ADMA is a mediator of endothelial dysfunction in hyperhomocysteinemia due to this metabolic relation [148,150]. HHcy, leading to accumulation of ADMA, may contribute to eNOS blockade and NO deficiency in the presence of general appropriate concentration of its synthase. The reduced release of NO by endothelial cells in HHcy was observed, suggesting the impairment of the eNOS pathway by DDAH inhibition [29].

The hypothesized mechanisms of disease linking homocysteine to preeclampsia are complex and still incompletely understood.

To date, vascular endothelial cell dysfunction that is provoked by an elevated level of homocysteine (Hcy) is suggested to be the most important connection. However, some authors questioned whether mild HHcy observed in PE, with Hcy values that are similar to those found in normotensive non-pregnant women, can provoke damage of the vascular endothelium. They postulate that this damage can be mediated rather by oxidative stress, as endothelium of pregnant women might be more vulnerable to oxidative injury [151]. Hyperhomocysteinemia is also associated with lesions in endothelial cells, due to vascular fibrosis, which results in alterations in coagulation system, enhanced platelet activation, and thrombogenesis—changes that are noted in preeclampsia [28–30].

On the other hand, metabolism in the kidney is the major route by which homocysteine is cleared from plasma. The association between Hcy and glomerular filtration rate (GFR) seems linear and it is present, even in the hyperfiltrating range [152,153]. Thus, this route of elimination may be affected by the already established preeclamptic changes in the kidney and secondarily lead to increased Hcy concentrations in plasma [154].

5. Therapeutic Potential of NO Pathway during Pregnancy

Enhancing the NO signalling in pregnancy is still thought to be an attractive option in both preeclampsia prevention in high-risk groups of women and treatment. There are attempts to prolong the pregnancy with the use of NOS substrates (L-arginine and L-citrulline), as well as NO-donors (glyceryl trinitrate, S-nitrosoglutathione, isosorbide mononitrate), natural derivatives, or vasodilators, such as sildenafil citrate [155–158]. NO donors and substrates have been also used for the management of other pregnancy disorders, like recurrent abortions, treatment of preterm labour, and dysmenorrhea [155]. Unfortunately, the analysis of use of these substances in PE gives conflicting results.

In vitro, nitric oxide synthase activity is inhibited by intracellular ADMA and is rescued by L-arginine [159]. Therefore, L-arginine supplementation in pregnancy could possibly overcome NOS blockage and its consequences. A study of intravenous infusion of L-arginine in pregnant women showed a significant reduction in blood pressure—an effect that was greater in women with preeclampsia [157,160]. Additionally, a significant reduction in PE incidence was described in high risk women who received L-arginine and vitamins C and E (as antioxidants reducing oxidative stress implicated in the pathophysiology of PE) before 24 weeks of gestation, when comparing to placebo and only vitamin group, although the effects of L-arginine alone were not studied [161]. However, last year, meta-analysis showed that combined vitamin C and E supplementation has no influences on the occurrence of preeclampsia [162], although an interaction between these vitamins and L-arginine is not well explained. Supplementation of L-arginine for pregnant women with chronic hypertension showed less need for antihypertensive drugs use, but no reduction in the incidence of superimposed preeclampsia [163]. Interestingly, women who go on to develop PE have been found to have higher, not lower, plasma L-arginine concentrations [129], which can counteract the raised ADMA values, but other vasoconstrictor effects may persist in women who are vulnerable to preeclampsia.

The Cochrane database systematic review, including six trials demonstrates, that there is insufficient evidence to draw reliable conclusions about whether NO donors and precursors prevent PE or its complications. Another 13 papers are still waiting to be assessed [164]. Conclusions from the review are limited mainly due to the fact that too few women have been studied. Adverse effects that were described during supplementation of NO donors included mainly headaches, often sufficiently severe to stop medication. However, more recent studies clearly show that isosorbid mononitrate and L-arginine are both effective in prevention of PE [165,166]. Besides the significant reduction of PE incidence in the treatment groups, there was also a reduction in FGR and improvement in foetal outcome, including less neonatal admissions to the intensive care unit.

An inorganic nitrate, NO3, with a capacity to increase the bioavailability of NO has been recently implemented in a clinical trial with beetroot juice as a norganic nitrate ($NO3^-$) rich dietary supplement [167]. It was the first trial to investigate effects of nitrate supplementation on blood pressure in human pregnancy, according to the authors. The treatment group consisted of pregnant women with chronic hypertension. In this group, the administration of NO_3^- donors significantly increased plasma and salivary nitrate/nitrite when compared with placebo, but there was no overall reduction in blood pressure. However, there was a highly significant correlation between changes in plasma nitrite and only lowering diastolic blood pressure in the nitrate-treated arm [168]

Sildenafil exerts its role by inducing vasodilatation, via inhibiting phosphodiesterase and thereby maintaining the availability of cGMP, the effector of NO activity within the cell [169]. In vivo studies of sildenafil citrate in rat models of preeclampsia have shown a significant reduction in the production of antiangiogenic molecules sFlt-1 and sEng [170], as well as an improvement in blood pressure, proteinuria, uteroplacental and foetal perfusion after treatment [171]. Lately, a randomized controlled trial to evaluate PE therapy with sildenafil showed that, when compared to controls (receiving a placebo), therapy with sildenafil resulted in four days prolongation of pregnancy [158].

Glyceryl trinitrate (GTN), which is commonly known as nitroglycerin, is a widely used organic nitrate in clinical practice, particularly for the treatment of angina pectoris. Transdermal nitroglycerin patches have been the focus of various studies, for both the prevention and management of PE and related disorders. Studies of both forms: transdermal [172,173] and sublingual GTN [156] in preeclamptic patients consistently showed a significant reduction in blood pressure and resistance in the uterine artery without an adverse effect on the foetal Doppler parameters. Nonetheless, these studies have highlighted the potential use of GTN as an antihypertensive agent in PE. However, it remains to be established whether GTN offers any competitive advantage over already existing treatment options. Certainly, the major disadvantage of organic nitrates, in general, and GTN, in particular, is the development of tolerance upon continuous dosing, necessitating the requirement of regular 'nitrate-free' intervals.

6. Conclusions

New therapeutic options emerge as our understanding of preeclampsia improves. Enhancing NO pathway, by overcoming eNOS block and neutralizing raised ADMA values and by homocysteine reduction, may be a perspective goal in the treatment and prevention of PE.

Still new, prospective clinical trials are needed to safely develop effective management strategies with the use of pharmacological modulators of the NO system, which seem to hold promise for the treatment of preeclampsia.

Funding: This research received no external funding.

Conflicts of Interest: The authors declare no conflict of interest.

References

1. Abalos, E.; Cuesta, C.; Grosso, A.L.; Chou, D.; Say, L. Global and regional estimates of preeclampsia and eclampsia: A systematic review. *Eur. J. Obstet. Gynecol. Reprod. Biol.* **2013**, *170*, 1–7. [CrossRef] [PubMed]
2. Tranquilli, A.L.; Dekker, G.; Magee, L.; Roberts, J.; Sibai, B.M.; Steyn, W.; Zeeman, G.G.; Brown, M.A. The classification, diagnosis and management of the hypertensive disorders of pregnancy: A revised statement from the ISSHP. *Pregnancy Hypertens* **2014**, *4*, 97–104. [CrossRef] [PubMed]
3. American College of Obstetricians and Gynecologists; Task Force on Hypertension in Pregnancy. Hypertension in Pregnancy. Report of the American College of Obstetricians and Gynecologists' Task Force on Hypertension in Pregnancy. *Obstet. Gynecol.* **2013**, *122*, 1122–1131.
4. Tranquilli, A.L.; Brown, M.A.; Zeeman, G.G.; Dekker, G.; Sibai, B.M. The definition of severe and early-onset preeclampsia. Statements from the International Society for the Study of Hypertension in Pregnancy (ISSHP). *Pregnancy Hypertens.* **2013**, *3*, 44–47. [CrossRef] [PubMed]
5. Roberts, J.M.; Taylor, R.N.; Musci, T.J.; Rodgers, G.M.; Hubel, C.A.; McLaughlin, M.K. Preeclampsia: An endothelial cell disorder. *Am. J. Obstet. Gynecol.* **1989**, *161*, 1200–1204. [CrossRef]

6. Roberts, J.M.; Hubel, C.A. The two stage model of preeclampsia: Variations on the theme. *Placenta* **2009**, *30*, S32–S37. [CrossRef] [PubMed]
7. Cross, J.C.; Werb, Z.; Fisher, S.K. Implantation and the placenta: Key pieces of the development puzzle. *Science* **1994**, *266*, 1508–1518. [CrossRef] [PubMed]
8. Brosens, I.A.; Robertson, W.B.; Dixon, H.G. The role of the spiral arteries in the pathogenesis of preeclampsia. *Obstet. Gynecol. Annu.* **1972**, *1*, 177–191. [CrossRef]
9. Huppertz, B. Placental origins of preeclampsia: Challenging the current hypothesis. *Hypertension* **2008**, *51*, 970–975. [CrossRef]
10. Maynard, S.E.; Min, J.Y.; Merchan, J.; Lim, K.H.; Li, J.; Mondal, S.; Libermann, T.A.; Morgan, J.P.; Sellke, F.W.; Stillman, I.E.; et al. Excess placental soluble fms-like tyrosine kinase 1 (sFlt-1) may contribute to endothelial dysfunction, hypertension, and proteinuria in preeclampsia. *J. Clin. Invest.* **2003**, *111*, 649–658. [CrossRef]
11. Chaiworapongsa, T.; Romero, R.; Kim, Y.M.; Kim, G.J.; Kim, M.R.; Espinoza, J.; Bujold, E.; Goncalves, L.; Gomez, R.; Edwin, S.; et al. Plasma soluble vascular endothelial growth factor receptor -1 concentration is elevated prior to the cinical diagnosis of preeclampsia. *J. Matern. Fetal Neonatal Med.* **2005**, *17*, 3–18. [CrossRef] [PubMed]
12. Venkatesha, S.; Toporsian, M.; Lam, C.; Hanai, J.; Mammoto, T.; Kim, Y.M.; Bdolah, Y.; Lim, K.H.; Yuan, H.T.; Libermann, T.A.; et al. Soluble endoglin contributes to the pathogenesis of preeclampsia. *Nat. Med.* **2006**, *12*, 642–649. [CrossRef] [PubMed]
13. Dymara-Konopka, W.; Laskowska, M.; Blazewicz, A. Angiogenic Imbalance as a Contributor of Preeclampsia. *Curr. Pharm. Biotechnol.* **2018**, *19*, 797–815. [CrossRef] [PubMed]
14. Harihana, N.; Shoemker, A.; Wagner, S. Pathophysiology of hypertension in preeclampsia. *Clin. Pract.* **2016**, *13*, 33–37.
15. Karumanchi, S.A.; Maynard, S.E.; Stillman, I.E.; Epstein, F.H.; Sukhatme, V.P. Preeclampsia: A renal perspective. *Kidney Int.* **2005**, *67*, 2101–2113. [CrossRef] [PubMed]
16. Roberts, J.M.; Escudero, C. The Placenta in Preeclampsia. *Pregnancy Hypertens* **2012**, *2*, 72–83. [CrossRef] [PubMed]
17. Ferrazzi, E.; Zullino, S.; Stampalija, T.; Vener, C.; Cavoretto, P.; Gervasi, M.T.; Vergani, P.; Mecacci, F.; Marozio, L.; Oggè, G.; et al. Bedside diagnosis of two major clinical phenotypes of hypertensive disorders of pregnancy. *Ultrasound Obstet. Gynecol.* **2016**, *48*, 224–231. [CrossRef]
18. Redman, C.W.; Sargent, I.L.; Staff, A.C. IFPA Senior Award Lecture: Making sense of pre-eclampsia. *Placenta* **2014**, *35*, S20–S25. [CrossRef]
19. Huang, L.T.; Hsieh, C.S.; Chang, K.A.; Tain, Y.L. Roles of nitric oxide and asymmetric dimethylarginine in pregnancy and fetal programming. *Int. J. Mol. Sci.* **2012**, *13*, 14606–14622. [CrossRef]
20. Baylis, C.; Beinder, E.; Suto, T.; August, P. Recent insights into the roles of nitric oxide and renin-angiotensin in the pathophysiology of preeclamptic pregnancy. *Semin. Nephrol.* **1998**, *18*, 208–230.
21. Lowe, D.T. Nitric oxide dysfunction in the pathophysiology of preeclampsia. *Nitric Oxide* **2000**, *4*, 441–458. [CrossRef] [PubMed]
22. Demir, B.; Demir, S.; Pasa, S. The role of homocysteine, asymmetric dimethylarginine and nitric oxide in preeclampsia. *J. Obstet. Gynaecol.* **2012**, *32*, 525–528. [CrossRef] [PubMed]
23. Khalil, R.A.; Granger, J.P. Vascular mechanisms of increased arterial pressure in preeclampsia: Lessons from animal models. *Am. J. Physiol. Regul. Integr. Comp. Physiol.* **2002**, *283*, R29–R45. [CrossRef] [PubMed]
24. Fickling, S.A.; Williams, D.; Vallance, P.; Nussey, S.S.; Whitley, G.S. Plasma concentrations of endogenous inhibitor of nitric oxide synthesis in normal pregnancy and preeclampsia. *Lancet* **1993**, *342*, 242–243. [CrossRef]
25. Speer, P.D.; Powers, R.W.; Frank, M.P.; Harger, G.; Markovic, N.; Roberts, J.M. Elevated asymmetric dimethylarginine concentrations precede clinical preeclampsia, but not pregnancies with small-for-gestational-age infants. *Am. J. Obstet. Gynecol.* **2008**, *198*, 112 e111–112 e117. [CrossRef]
26. Holden, D.P.; Fickling, S.A.; Whitley, G.S.; Nussey, S.S. Plasma concentrations of asymmetric dimethylarginine, a natural inhibitor of nitric oxide synthase, in normal pregnancy and preeclampsia. *Am. J. Obstet. Gynecol.* **1998**, *178*, 551–556. [CrossRef]
27. Pettersson, A.; Hedner, T.; Milsom, I. Increased circulating concentrations of asymmetric dimethylarginine (ADMA), an endogenous inhibitor of nitric oxide synthesis, in preeclampsia. *Acta Obstet. Gynecol. Scand.* **1998**, *77*, 808–813. [CrossRef]

28. Aubard, Y.; Darodes, N.; Cantaloube, M. Hyperhomocysteinemia and pregnancy—Review of our present understanding and therapeutic implications. *Eur. J. Obstet. Gynecol. Reprod. Biol.* **2000**, *93*, 157–165. [CrossRef]
29. Stühlinger, M.C.; Tsao, P.S.; Her, J.H.; Kimoto, M.; Balint, R.F.; Cooke, J.P. Homocysteine impairs the nitric oxide synthase pathway: Role of asymmetric dimethylarginine. *Circulation* **2001**, *104*, 2569–2575. [CrossRef]
30. Herrmann, W.; Isber, S.; Obeid, R.; Herrmann, M.; Jouma, M. Concentrations of homocysteine, related metabolites and asymmetric dimethylarginine in preeclamptic women with poor nutritional status. *Clin. Chem. Lab. Med.* **2005**, *43*, 1139–1146. [CrossRef]
31. Furchgott, R.F.; Zawadzk, J.V. The obligatory role of endothelial cells in the relaxation of arterial smooth muscle by acetylcholine. *Nature* **1980**, *288*, 373–376. [CrossRef] [PubMed]
32. Ignarro, L.J. Nitric oxide. A novel signal transduction mechanism for transcellular communication. *Hypertension* **1990**, *16*, 477–483. [CrossRef] [PubMed]
33. Lundberg, J.O.; Weitzberg, E.; Gladwin, M.T. The nitrate-nitrite-nitric oxide pathway in physiology and therapeutics. *Nat. Rev. Drug. Discovery* **2008**, *7*, 156–167. [CrossRef] [PubMed]
34. Ramadoss, J.; Pastore, M.B.; Magness, R.R. Endothelial caveolar subcellular domain regulation of endothelial nitric oxide synthase. *Clin. Exp. Pharmacol. Physiol.* **2013**, *40*, 753–764. [CrossRef] [PubMed]
35. Gielen, S.; Sandri, M.; Erbs, S.; Adams, V. Exercise-induced modulation of endothelial nitric oxide production. *Curr. Pharm. Biotechnol.* **2011**, *12*, 1375–1384. [CrossRef] [PubMed]
36. Quillon, A.; Fromy, B.; Debret, R. Endothelium microenvironment sensing leading to nitric oxide mediated vasodilation: A review of nervous and biomechanical signals. *Nitric Oxide* **2015**, *45*, 20–26. [CrossRef] [PubMed]
37. Sladek, S.M.; Magness, R.R.; Conrad, K.P. Nitric oxide and pregnancy. *Am. J. Physiol.* **1997**, *272*, R441–R463. [CrossRef] [PubMed]
38. Suzuki, T.; Mori, C.; Yoshikawa, H.; Miyazaki, Y.; Kansaku, N.; Tanaka, K.; Morita, H.; Takizawa, T. Changes in nitric oxide production levels and expression of nitric oxide synthase isoforms in the rat uterus during pregnancy. *Biosci. Biotechnol. Biochem.* **2009**, *73*, 2163–2166. [CrossRef]
39. Purcell, T.L.; Given, R.; Chwalisz, K.; Garfield, R.E. Nitric oxide synthase distribution during implantation in the mouse. *Mol. Hum. Reprod.* **1999**, *5*, 467–475. [CrossRef]
40. Myatt, L. Placental adaptive responses and fetal programming. *J. Physiol.* **2006**, *572*, 25–30. [CrossRef]
41. Shizukuda, Y.; Tang, S.; Yokota, R.; Ware, J.A. Vascular endothelial growth factor-induced endothelial cell migration and proliferation depend on a nitric oxide-mediated decrease in protein kinase C activity. *Circ. Res.* **1999**, *85*, 247–256. [CrossRef] [PubMed]
42. Frank, S.; Stallmeyer, B.; Kampfer, H.; Schaffner, C.; Pfeilschifter, J. Differential regulation of vascular endothelial growth factor and its receptor fms-like-tyrosine kinase is mediated by nitric oxide in rat renal mesangial cells. *Biochem. J.* **1999**, *338*, 367–374. [CrossRef] [PubMed]
43. Kulandavelu, S.; Whiteley, K.J.; Qu, D.; Mu, J.; Bainbridge, S.A.; Adamson, S.L. Endothelial nitric oxide synthase deficiency reduces uterine blood flow, spiral artery elongation, and placental oxygenation in pregnant mice. *Hypertension* **2012**, *60*, 231–238. [CrossRef] [PubMed]
44. Dulak, A.; Jozkowicz, J. Regulation of vascular endothelial growth factor synthesis by nitric oxide: Facts and controversies. *Antioxid. Redox. Signal.* **2003**, *5*, 123–132. [CrossRef] [PubMed]
45. Vallance, P.; Leiper, J. Cardiovascular biology of the asymmetric dimethylarginine:dimethylarginine dimethylaminohydrolase pathway. *Arterioscler. Thromb. Vasc. Biol.* **2004**, *24*, 1023–1030. [CrossRef] [PubMed]
46. Teerlink, T.; Luo, Z.; Palm, F.; Wilcox, C.S. Cellular ADMA: Regulation and action. *Pharmacol. Res.* **2009**, *60*, 448–460. [CrossRef]
47. Sibal, L.; Agarwal, S.C.; Home, P.D.; Boger, R.H. The role of asymmetric dimethylarginine (ADMA) in endothelial dysfunction and cardiovascular disease. *Curr. Cardiol. Rev.* **2010**, *6*, 82–90. [CrossRef]
48. Brustolin, S.; Giugliani, R.; Félix, T.M. Genetics of homocysteine metabolism and associated disorders. *Braz. J. Med. Biol. Res.* **2010**, *43*, 1–7. [CrossRef]
49. Walker, M.; Smith, G.; Perkins, S.; Keely, E.; Garner, P. Changes in homocysteine levels during normal pregnancy. *Am. J. Obstet. Gynecol.* **1999**, *180*, 660–664. [CrossRef]
50. Bailey, L.; Gregory, J. Polymorphisms of methylenetetrahydrofolate reductase and other enzymes: Metabolic significance, risks and impact on folate requirement. *J. Nutr.* **1999**, *129*, 919–922. [CrossRef]

51. Goyette, P.; Sumner, J.; Milos, R.; Duncan, A.; Rosenblatt, D.; Matthews, R.; Rozen, R. Human methylenetetrahydrofolate reductase: Isolation of cDNA, mapping, and mutation identification. *Nat. Genet.* **1994**, *7*, 195–200. [CrossRef] [PubMed]
52. Faeh, D.; Chiolero, A.; Paccaud, F. Homocysteine as a risk factor for cardiovascular disease: Should we (still) worry about it? *Swiss Med. Wkly.* **2006**, *136*, 745–756. [PubMed]
53. Baszczuk, A.; Kopczynski, Z. Hyperhomocysteinemia in patients with cardiovascular disease. *Postepy Hig. Med. Dosw.* **2014**, *68*, 579. [CrossRef] [PubMed]
54. Hankey, G.J.; Eikelboom, J.W. Homocysteine and vascular disease. *Lancet* **1999**, *354*, 407–413. [CrossRef]
55. Clarke, R.; Woodhouse, P.; Ulvik, A.; Frost, C.; Sherliker, P.; Refsum, H. Variability and determinants of total homocysteine concentrations in plasma in an elderly population. *Clin. Chem.* **2010**, *44*, 102–107.
56. Thrombosis Interest Group of Canada. Thrombophilia: Homocysteinemia and Methylene Tetrahydrofolate Reductase. Available online: http://thrombosiscanada.ca/?page_id=18# (accessed on 17 June 2015).
57. Curro, M.; Gugliandolo, A.; Gangemi, C.; Risitano, R.; Ientile, R.; Caccamo, D. Toxic effects of mildly elevated homocysteine concentrations in neuronal-like cells. *Neurochem. Res.* **2014**, *39*, 1485–1495. [CrossRef] [PubMed]
58. Weisberg, I.S.; Jacques, P.F.; Selhub, J.; Bostom, A.G.; Chen, Z.; Curtis Ellison, R.; Eckfeldt, J.H.; Rozen, R. The 1298A→C polymorphism in methylenetetrahydrofolate reductase (MTHFR): In vitro expression and association with homocysteine. *Atherosclerosis* **2001**, *156*, 409–415. [CrossRef]
59. Stanger, O.; Herrmann, W.; Pietrzik, K.; Fowler, B.; Geisel, J.; Dierkes, J.; Weger, M. Clinical use and rational management of homocysteine, folic acid, and B vitamins in cardiovascular and thrombotic diseases. *Z. Kardiol.* **2004**, *93*, 439–453. [CrossRef]
60. Ntaios, G.; Savopoulos, C.; Grekas, P.; Hatzitolios, A. The controversial role of B-vitamins in cardiovascular risk: An update. *Arch. Cardiovasc. Dis.* **2009**, *102*, 847–854. [CrossRef]
61. McCully, K.S. Vascular pathology of homocysteinemia: Implications for the pathogenesis of arteriosclerosis. *Am. J. Pathol.* **1969**, *56*, 111.
62. Boushey, C.J.; Beresford, S.A.; Omenn, G.S.; Motulsky, A.G. A quantitative assessment of plasma homocysteine as a risk factor for vascular disease. Probable benefits of increasing folic acid intakes. *JAMA* **1995**, *274*, 1049–1057. [CrossRef] [PubMed]
63. Refsum, H.; Ueland, P.M.; Nygard, O.; Vollset, S.E. Homocysteine and cardiovascular disease. *Annu. Rev. Med.* **1998**, *49*, 31–62. [CrossRef] [PubMed]
64. Guilland, J.; Favier, A.; Potier de Courcy, G.; Galan, P.; Hercberg, S. Hyperhomocysteinemia: An independent risk factor or a simple marker of vascular disease?. 1. Basic data. *Pathol. Biol.* **2003**, *51*, 101–110. [CrossRef]
65. Wong, Y.Y.; Golledge, J.; Flicker, L.; McCaul, K.A.; Hankey, G.J.; van Bockxmeer, F.M.; Yeap, B.B.; Norman, P.E. Plasma total homocysteine is associated with abdominal aortic aneurysm and aortic diameter in older men. *J. Vasc. Surg.* **2013**, *58*, 364–370. [CrossRef] [PubMed]
66. Fu, Y.; Wang, X.; Kong, W. Hyperhomocysteinaemia and vascular injury: Advances in mechanisms and drug targets. *Br. J. Pharmacol.* **2017**, *175*, 1173–1189. [CrossRef] [PubMed]
67. Morris, M.S. Homocysteine and Alzheimer's disease. *Lancet Neurol.* **2003**, *2*, 425–428. [CrossRef]
68. Seshadri, S.; Beiser, A.; Selhub, J.; Jacques, P.F.; Rosenberg, I.H.; D'Agostino, R.B.; Wilson, P.W.F.; Wolf, P.A. Plasma Homocysteine as a risk factor for dementia and Alzheimer's disease. *N. Engl. J. Med.* **2002**, *346*, 476–483. [CrossRef]
69. McIlroy, S.P.; Dynan, K.B.; Lawson, J.T.; Patterson, C.C.; Passmore, A.P. Moderately elevated plasma homocysteine, methylenetetrahydrofolate reductase genotype, and risk for stroke, vascular dementia, and Alzheimer disease in Northern Ireland. *Stroke* **2002**, *33*, 2351–2356. [CrossRef] [PubMed]
70. Rueda-Clausen, C.; Córdoba-Porras, A.; Bedoya, G.; Silva, F.; Zarruk, J.; López-Jaramillo, P.; Villa, L. Increased plasma levels of total homocysteine but not asymmetric dimethylarginine in Hispanic subjects with ischemic stroke FREC-VI sub-study. *Eur. J. Neurol.* **2012**, *19*, 417–425. [CrossRef]
71. Herrmann, M.; Widmann, T.; Herrmann, W. Homocysteine–a newly recognised risk factor for osteoporosis. *Clin. Chem. Lab. Med.* **2005**, *43*, 1111–1117. [CrossRef]
72. Perna, A.F.; Sepe, I.; Lanza, D.; Pollastro, R.M.; De Santo, N.G.; Ingrosso, D. Hyperhomocysteinemia in chronic renal failure: Alternative therapeutic strategies. *J. Ren. Nutr.* **2012**, *22*, 191–194. [CrossRef] [PubMed]
73. Brattström, L.; Wilcken, D.E. Homocysteine and cardiovascular disease: Cause or effect? *Am. J. Clin. Nutr.* **2000**, *72*, 315–323. [CrossRef] [PubMed]

74. Nelson, S.H.; Steinsland, O.S.; Wang, Y.; Yallampalli, C.; Dong, Y.L.; Sanchez, J.M. Increased nitric oxide synthase activity and expression in the human uterine artery during pregnancy. *Circ. Res.* **2000**, *87*, 406–411. [CrossRef] [PubMed]
75. Stefano, G.B.; Kream, R.M. Reciprocal regulation of cellular nitric oxide formation by nitric oxide synthase and nitrite reductases. *Med. Sci. Monit.* **2011**, *17*, RA221–RA226. [CrossRef] [PubMed]
76. Sanghavi, M.; Rutherford, J.D. Cardiovascular physiology of pregnancy. *Circulation* **2014**, *130*, 1003–1008. [CrossRef] [PubMed]
77. Leiva, A.; Fuenzalida, B.; Barros, E.; Sobrevia, B.; Salsoso, R.; Sáez, T.; Villalobos, R.; Silva, L.; Chiarello, I.; Toledo, F.; et al. Nitric oxide is a central common metabolite in vascular dysfunction associated with diseases of human pregnancy. *Curr. Vasc. Pharmacol.* **2016**, *14*, 237–259. [CrossRef]
78. Conrad, K.P.; Kerchner, L.J.; Mosher, M.D. Plasma and 24-h NO(x) and cGMP during normal pregnancy and preeclampsia in women on a reduced NO(x) diet. *Am. J. Physiol.* **1999**, *277*, F48–F57.
79. Buhimschi, I.; et al. Involvement of a nitric oxide-cyclic guanosine monophosphate pathway in control of human uterine contractility during pregnancy. *Am. J. Obstet. Gynecol.* **1995**, *172*, 1577–1584. [CrossRef]
80. Baylis, C.; Vallance, P. Measurement of nitrite and nitrate levels in plasma and urine: What does this measure tell us about the activity of the endogenous nitric oxide system? *Curr. Opin. Nephrol. Hypertens.* **1998**, *7*, 59–62. [CrossRef]
81. Choi, J.W.; Im, M.W.; Pai, S.H. Nitric oxide production increases during normal pregnancy and decreases in preeclampsia. *Ann. Clin. Lab. Sci.* **2002**, *32*, 257–263.
82. Jo, T.; Takauchi, Y.; Nakajima, Y.; Fukami, K.; Kosaka, H.; Terada, N. Maternal or umbilical venous levels of nitrite/nitrate during pregnancy and at delivery. *In Vivo* **1998**, *12*, 523–526. [PubMed]
83. Shaamash, A.H.; Elsnosy, E.D.; Makhlouf, A.M.; Zakhari, M.M.; Ibrahim, O.A.; EL-dien, H.M. Maternal and fetal serum nitric oxide (NO) concentrations in normal pregnancy, pre-eclampsia and eclampsia. *Int. J. Gynaecol. Obstet.* **2000**, *68*, 207–214. [CrossRef]
84. Hata, T.; Hashimoto, M.; Kanenishi, K.; Akiyama, M.; Yanagihara, T.; Masumura, S. Maternal circulation nitrite levels are decreased in both normal normotensive pregnancies and pregnancies with preeclampsia. *Gynecol. Obstet. Invest.* **1999**, *48*, 93–97. [CrossRef] [PubMed]
85. Brown, M.A.; Tibben, E.; Zammit, V.C.; Cario, G.M.; Carlton, M.A. Nitric oxide excretion in normal and hypertensive pregnancies. *Hyperten. Pregnancy* **1995**, *14*, 319–326. [CrossRef]
86. Smarason, A.K.; Allman, K.G.; Young, D.; Redman, C.W.G. Elevated levels of serum nitrate, a stable end product of nitric oxide, in women with preeclampsia. *Br. J. Obstet. Gynecol.* **1997**, *104*, 538–543. [CrossRef]
87. Shah, D.A.; Khalil, R.A. Bioactive factors in uteroplacental and systemic circulation link placental ischemia to generalized vascular dysfunction in hypertensive pregnancy and preeclampsia. *Biochem. Pharmacol.* **2015**, *95*, 211–226. [CrossRef]
88. Vida, G.; Sulyok, E.; Ertl, T.; Martens-Lobenhoffer, J.; Bode-Böger, S.M. Birth by cesarean section is associated with elevated neonatal plasma levels of dimethylarginines. *Pediatr. Int.* **2012**, *54*, 476–479. [CrossRef] [PubMed]
89. Andersson, A.; Hultberg, B.; Brattström, L.; Isaksson, A. Decreased serum homocysteine in pregnancy. *Eur. J. Clin. Chem. Clin. Biochem.* **1992**, *30*, 377–379.
90. Hague, B.; Whiting, M.; Tallis, G. South Australian experience with hyperhomocysteinaemia as a risk factor in obstetrics. Time for a trial? *Neth. J. Med.* **1997**, *52*, S24.
91. Malinow, M.R.; Rajkovic, A.; Duell, P.B.; Hess, D.L.; Upson, B.M. The relationship between maternal and neonatal umbilical cord plasma homocysteine suggests a potential role for maternal homocysteine in fetal metabolism. *Obstet. Gynecol.* **1998**, *178*, 228–233.
92. Steegers-Theunissen, R.; Wathen, N.; Eskes, T.; Van Raaij-Selten, B.; Chard, T. Maternal and fetal levels of methionine and homocysteine in early human pregnancy. *Br. J. Obstet. Gynecol.* **1997**, *104*, 20–24. [CrossRef]
93. Lopez-Quesada, E.; Vilaseca, M.A.; Lailla, J.M. Plasma total homocysteine in uncomplicated pregnancy and in preeclampsia. *Eur. J. Obstet. Gynecol. Reprod. Biol.* **2003**, *108*, 45–49. [CrossRef]
94. Bergen, N.E.; Jaddoe, V.W.; Timmermans, S.; Hofman, A.; Lindemans, J.; Russcher, H.; Raat, H.; SteegersTheunissen, R.P.; Steegers, E.A. Homocysteine and folate concentrations in early pregnancy and the risk of adverse pregnancy outcomes: The Generation R Study. *BJOG* **2012**, *119*, 739–751. [CrossRef] [PubMed]

95. Mills, J.L.; McPartlin, J.M.; Kirke, P.N.; Lee, Y.J.; Conley, M.R.; Weir, D.G.; Scott, J.M. Homocysteine metabolism in pregnancies complicated by neuraltube defects. *Lancet* **1995**, *345*, 149–151. [CrossRef]
96. Chen, H.; Yang, X.; Lu, M. Methylenetetrahydrofolate reductase gene polymorphisms and recurrent pregnancy loss in China: A systematic review and meta-analysis. *Arch. Gynecol. Obstet.* **2016**, *293*, 283–290. [CrossRef] [PubMed]
97. De Falco, M.; Pollio, F.; Scaramelino, M.; Pontillo, M.; Lieto, A.D. Homocysteinemia during pregnancy and placental disease. *Clin. Exp. Obstet. Gynecol.* **2000**, *27*, 188–190. [PubMed]
98. Steegers-Theunissen, R.P.; Van Iersel, C.A.; Peer, P.G.; Nelen, W.L.; Steegers, E.A. Hyperhomocysteinemia, pregnancy complications, and the timing of investigation. *Obstet. Gynecol.* **2004**, *104*, 336–343. [CrossRef] [PubMed]
99. Seligman, S.P.; et al. The role of nitric oxide in the pathogenesis of preeclampsia. *Am. J. Obstet. Gynecol.* **1994**, *171*, 944–948. [CrossRef]
100. Mutlu-Turkoglu, U.; Aykac-Toker, G.; Ibrahimoglu, L.; Ademoglu, E.; Uysal, M. Plasma nitric oxide metabolites and lipid peroxide levels in preeclamptic pregnant women before and after delivery. *Gynecol. Obstet. Invest.* **1999**, *48*, 247–250. [CrossRef] [PubMed]
101. Silver, R.K.; et al. Evaluation of nitric oxide as a mediator of severe preeclampsia. *Am. J. Obstet. Gynecol.* **1996**, *175*, 1013–1017. [CrossRef]
102. Schiessl, B.; Strasburger, C.; Bidlingmaier, M.; Mylonas, I.; Jeschke, U.; Kainer, F.; Friese, K. Plasma- and urine concentrations of nitrite/nitrate and cyclic Guanosinemono phosphate in intrauterine growth restricted and preeclamptic pregnancies. *Arch. Gynecol. Obstet.* **2006**, *274*, 150–154. [CrossRef]
103. Pathak, N.; et al. Estimation of oxidative products of nitric oxide (nitrates, nitrites) in preeclampsia. *Aust. N. Z. J. Obstet. Gynaecol.* **1999**, *39*, 484–487. [PubMed]
104. Alexander, B.T.; Miller, M.T.; Kassab, S.; Novak, J.; Reckelhoff, J.F.; Kruckeberg, W.C.; Granger, J.P. Differential expression of renal nitric oxide synthase isoforms during pregnancy in rats. *Hypertension* **1999**, *33*, 435–439. [CrossRef] [PubMed]
105. Walsh, S.K.; English, F.A.; Johns, E.J.; Kenny, L.C. Plasma-Mediated Vascular Dysfunction in the Reduced Uterine Perfusion Pressure Model of Preeclampsia: A Microvascular Characterization. *Hypertension* **2009**, *54*, 345–351. [CrossRef]
106. Kleinbongard, P.; Dejam, A.; Lauer, T.; Rassaf, T.; Schindler, A.; Picker, O.; Scheeren, T.; Godecke, A.; Schrader, J.; Schulz, R.; et al. Plasma nitrite reflects constitutive nitric oxide synthase activity in mammals. *Free Radic. Biol. Med.* **2003**, *35*, 790–796. [CrossRef]
107. Kelm, M.; Preik-Steinhoff, H.; Preik, M.; Strauer, B.E. Serum nitrite sensitively reflects endothelial NO formation in human forearm vasculature: Evidence for biochemical assessment of the endothelial L-arginine-NO pathway. *Cardiovasc. Res.* **1999**, *41*, 765–772. [CrossRef]
108. Pimentel, A.M.; Pereira, N.R.; Costa, C.A.; Mann, G.E.; Cordeiro, V.S.; de Moura, R.S.; Brunini, T.M.C.; Mendes-Ribeiro, A.C.; Resende, Â.C. L-arginine-nitric oxide pathway and oxidative stress in plasma and platelets of patients with pre-eclampsia. *Hypertens. Res.* **2013**, *36*, 783–788. [CrossRef]
109. Eleuterio, N.M.; Palei, A.C.; Machado, J.S.R.; Tanus-Santos, J.E.; Cavalli, R.C.; Sandrim, V.C. Relationship between adiponectin and nitrite in healthy and preeclampsia pregnancies. *Clin. Chim. Acta.* **2013**, *423*, 112–115. [CrossRef] [PubMed]
110. Sandrim, V.C.; Palei, A.C.; Metzger, I.F.; Gomes, V.A.; Cavalli, R.C.; Tanus-Santos, J.E. Nitric oxide formation is inversely related to serum levels of antiangiogenic factors soluble fms-like tyrosine kinase-1 and soluble endoglin in preeclampsia. *Hypertension* **2008**, *52*, 402–407. [CrossRef] [PubMed]
111. Groesch, K.A.; Torry, R.J.; Wilber, A.C.; Abrams, R.; Bieniarz, A.; Guilbert, L.J.; Torry, D.S. Nitric oxide generation affects pro- and anti-angiogenic growth factor expression in primary human trophoblast. *Placenta* **2011**, *32*, 926–931. [CrossRef] [PubMed]
112. Zeng, Y.; Li, M.; Chen, Y.; Wang, S. Homocysteine, endothelin-1 and nitric oxide in patients with hypertensive disorders complicating pregnancy. *Int. J. Clin. Exp. Pathol.* **2015**, *8*, 15275–15279.
113. Cadnapaphornchai, M.A.; Ohara, M.; Morris, K.G.; Knotek, M.; Rogachev, B.; Ladtkow, T.; Carter, E.P.; Schrier, R.W. Chronic NOS inhibition reverses systemic vasodi- lation and glomerular hyperfiltration in pregnancy. *Am. J. Physiol. Ren. Physiol.* **2001**, *280*, 592–598. [CrossRef]

114. Laskowska, M.; Laskowska, K.; Oleszczuk, J. The relation of maternalserum eNOS, NOSTRIN and ADMA levels with aetiopathogenesis of preeclampsia and/or intrauterine fetal growth restriction. *J. Matern. Fetal. Neonatal. Med.* **2015**, *28*, 26–32. [CrossRef]
115. Laskowska, M.; Laskowska, K.; Oleszczuk, J. PP135. Maternal serum levels of endothelial nitric oxide synthase and ADMA, an endogenous ENOS inhibitor in pregnancies complicated by severe preeclampsia. *Pregnancy Hypertens.* **2012**, *2*, 312. [CrossRef]
116. Myatt, L.; Eis, A.L.; Brockman, D.E.; Greer, I.A.; Lyall, F. Endothelial nitric oxide synthase in placental villous tissue from normal, pre-eclamptic and intrauterine growth restricted pregnancies. *Hum. Reprod.* **1997**, *12*, 167–172. [CrossRef]
117. Smith-Jackson, K.; Hentschke, M.R.; Poli-de-Figueiredo, C.E.; da Costa, B.P.; Kurlak, L.O.; Pipkin, F.B.; Czajkad, A.; Mistry, H. D. Placental expression of eNOS, iNOS and the major protein components of caveolae in women with preeclampsia. *Placenta* **2015**, *36*, 607–610. [CrossRef]
118. Beinder, E.; Mohaupt, M.G.; Schlembach, D.; Fischer, T.; Sterzel, R.B.; Lang, N.; Baylis, C. Nitric oxide synthase activity and Doppler parameters in the fetoplacental and uteroplacental circulation in preeclampsia. *Hypertens. Pregnancy* **1999**, *18*, 115–127. [CrossRef]
119. Orange, S.J.; et al. Placental endothelial nitric oxide synthase localization and expression in normal human pregnancy and preeclampsia. *Clin. Exp. Pharmacol. Physiol.* **2003**, *30*, 376–381. [CrossRef]
120. Marshall, S.A.; Hannan, N.J.; Jelinic, M.; Nguyen, T.P.; Girling, J.E.; Parry, L.J. Animal models of preeclampsia: Translational failings and why. *Am. J. Physiol. Regul. Integr. Comp. Physiol.* **2018**, *314*, R499–R508. [CrossRef]
121. Gonçalves-Rizzi, V.H.; Possomato-Vieira, J.S.; Graça, T.U.S.; Nascimento, R.A.; Dias-Junior, C.A. Sodium nitrite attenuates hypertension- in-pregnancy and blunts increases in soluble fms-like tyrosine kinase-1 and in vascular endothelial growth factor. *Nitric Oxide* **2016**, *57*, 71–78.
122. Khalil, A.A.; Tsikas, D.; Akolekar, R.; Jordan, J.; Nicolaides, K.H. Asymmetric dimethylarginine, arginine and homoarginine at 11-13 weeks' gestation and preeclampsia: A case-control study. *J. Hum. Hypertens.* **2013**, *27*, 38–43. [CrossRef] [PubMed]
123. López-Alarcón, M.; Montalvo-Velarde, I.; Vital-Reyes, V.S.; Hinojosa-Cruz, J.C.; Leaños-Miranda, A.; Martínez-Basila, A. Serial determinations of asymmetric dimethylarginine and homocysteine during pregnancy to predict pre-eclampsia: A longitudinal study. *BJOG* **2015**, *122*, 1586–1592.
124. Zheng, J.J.; Wang, H.O.; Huang, M.; Zheng, F.Y. Assessment of ADMA, estradiol, and progesterone in severe preeclampsia. *Clin. Exp. Hypertens.* **2016**, *38*, 347–351. [CrossRef] [PubMed]
125. Laskowska, M.; Laskowska, K.; Terbosh, M.; Oleszczuk, J. A comparison of maternal serum levels of endothelial nitric oxide synthase, asymmetric dimethylarginine, and homocysteine in normal and preeclamptic pregnancies. *Med. Sci. Monit.* **2013**, *19*, 430–437.
126. Alpoim, P.N.; Godoi, L.C.; Freitas, L.G.; Gomes, K.B.; Dusse, L.M. Assessment of L-arginine asymmetric 1 dimethyl (ADMA) in early-onset and late-onset (severe) preeclampsia. *Nitric Oxide* **2013**, *33*, 81–82. [CrossRef]
127. Bian, Z.; Shixia, C.; Duan, T. First-trimester maternal serum levels of sFLT1, PGF and ADMA predict preeclampsia. *PLoS One* **2015**, *10*, e0124684. [CrossRef]
128. Rizos, D.; Eleftheriades, M.; Batakis, E.; Rizou, M.; Halisassos, A.; Hassiakos, D.; Botsis, D. Levels of asymmetric dimethylarginine throughout normal pregnancy and in pregnancies complicated by preeclampsia or had a small for gestational age baby. *J. Matern. Fetal. Neonatal. Med.* **2012**, *25*, 1311–1315. [CrossRef]
129. Savvidou, M.D.; Hingorani, A.D.; Tsikas, D.; Frolich, J.C.; Vallance, P.; Nicolaides, K.H. Endothelial dysfunction and raised plasma concentrations of asymmetric dimethylarginine in pregnant women who subsequently develop pre-eclampsia. *Lancet* **2003**, *361*, 1511–1517. [CrossRef]
130. Kim, M.W.; Hong, S.C.; Choi, J.S.; Han, J.Y.; Oh, M.J.; Kim, H.J.; Nava-Ocampo, A.; Koren, G. Homocysteine, folate and pregnancy outcomes. *J. Obstet. Gynaecol.* **2012**, *32*, 520–524. [CrossRef]
131. Dekker, A.G.; DeVries, J.I.P.; Doelitzsch, P.M.; Huijgens, P.C.; von Blomberg, B.M.; Jakobs, C.; van Geijn, H.P. Underlying disorders associated with severe early onset preeclampsia. *Am. J. Obstet. Gynecol.* **1995**, *173*, 1042–1048. [CrossRef]
132. Acilmis, Y.G.; Dikensoy, E.; Kutlar, A.I.; Balat, O.; Cebesoy, F.B.; Ozturk, E.; Cicek, H.; Pence, S. Homocysteine, folic acid and vitamin B12 levels in maternal and umbilical cord plasma and homocysteine levels in placenta in pregnant women with preeclampsia. *J. Obstet. Gynaecol. Res.* **2011**, *37*, 45–50. [CrossRef] [PubMed]

133. Mujawar, S.A.; Patil, V.W.; Daver, R.G. Study of serum homocysteine, folic Acid and vitamin B(12) in patients with preeclampsia. *Indian J. Clin. Biochem.* **2011**, *26*, 257–260. [CrossRef] [PubMed]
134. Guven, M.A.; Coskun, A.; Ertas, I.E.; Aral, M.; Zencirci, B.; Oksuz, H. Association of maternal serum CRP, IL-6, TNF-alpha, homocysteine, folic acid and vitamin B12 levels with the severity of preeclampsia and fetal birth weight. *Hypertens. Pregnancy* **2009**, *28*, 190–200. [CrossRef] [PubMed]
135. Makedos, G.; Papanicolaou, A.; Hitoglou, A.; Kalogiannidis, I.; Makedos, A.; Vrazioti, V.; Goutzioulis, M. Homocysteine, folic acid and B12 serum levels in pregnancy complicated with preeclampsia. *Arch. Gynecol. Obstet.* **2007**, *275*, 121–124. [CrossRef]
136. Patrick, T.E.; Powers, R.W.; Daftary, A.R.; Ness, R.B.; Roberts, J.M. Homocysteine and folic acid are inversely related in black women with preeclampsia. *Hypertension* **2004**, *43*, 1279–1282. [CrossRef] [PubMed]
137. Sanchez, S.E.; Zhang, C.; Rene Malinow, M.; Ware-Jauregui, S.; Larrabure, G.; Williams, M.A. Plasma folate, vitamin B(12), and homocyst(e)ine concentrations in preeclamptic and normotensive Peruvian women. *Am. J. Epidemiol.* **2001**, *153*, 474–480. [CrossRef] [PubMed]
138. Wadhwani, N.S.; Patil, V.V.; Mehendale, S.S.; Wagh, G.N.; Gupte, S.A.; Joshi, S.R. Increased homocysteine levels exist in women with preeclampsia from early pregnancy. *J. Matern. Fetal. Neonatal. Med.* **2016**, *29*, 2719–2725. [CrossRef] [PubMed]
139. Dodds, L.; Fell, D.B.; Dooley, K.C.; Armson, B.A.; Allen, A.C.; Nassar, B.A.; Joseph, K.S. Effect of Homocysteine Concentration in Early Pregnancy on Gestational Hypertensive Disorders and Other Pregnancy Outcomes. *Clin. Chem.* **2008**, *54*, 326–334. [CrossRef]
140. Maged, A.M.; Saad, H.; Meshaal, H.; Salah, E.; Abdelaziz, S.; Omran, E.; Katta, M. Maternal serum homocysteine and uterine artery Doppler as predictors of preeclampsia and poor placentation. *Arch. Gynecol. Obstet.* **2017**, *296*, 475–482. [CrossRef]
141. Cotter, A.M.; Molloy, A.M.; Scott, J.M.; Daly, S.F. Elevated plasma homocysteine in early pregnancy: A risk factor for the development of severe preeclampsia. *Am. J. Obstet. Gynecol.* **2001**, *185*, 781–785. [CrossRef]
142. Cotter, A.M.; Molloy, M.; Scott, J.M.; Daly, S. Elevated plasma homocysteine in early pregnancy: A risk factor for the development of nonsevere preeclampsia. *Am. J. Obstet. Gynecol.* **2003**, *189*, 391–396. [CrossRef]
143. Raijmakers, M.T.; Zusterzeel, P.L.; Steegers, E.A.; Peters, W.H. Hyperhomocysteinaemia: A risk factor for preeclampsia? *Eur. J. Obstet. Gynecol. Reprod. Biol.* **2001**, *95*, 226–228. [CrossRef]
144. Hietala, R.; Turpeinen, U.; Laatikainen, T. Serum homocysteine at 16 weeks and subsequent preeclampsia. *Obstet. Gynecol.* **2001**, *97*, 527–529. [PubMed]
145. Hogg, B.B.; Tamura, T.; Johnston, K.E.; Dubard, M.B.; Goldenberg, R.L. Second-trimester plasma homocysteine levels and pregnancy-induced hypertension, preeclampsia, and intrauterine growth restriction. *Am. J. Obstet. Gynecol.* **2000**, *183*, 805–809. [CrossRef] [PubMed]
146. Shahbazian, N.; Mohammad Jafari, R.; Haghnia, S. The evaluation of serum homocysteine, folic acid, and vitamin B12 in patients complicated with preeclampsia. *Electron. Physician* **2016**, *8*, 3057–3061. [CrossRef] [PubMed]
147. Stuhlinger, M.C.; Oka, R.K.; Graf, E.E.; Schmölzer, I.; Upson, B.M.; Kapoor, O.; Szuba, A.; Malinow, M.R.; Wascher, T.C.; Pachinger, O.; et al. Endothelial dysfunction induced by hyperhomocyst(e)inemia: Role of asymmetric dimethylarginine. *Circulation* **2003**, *108*, 933–938. [CrossRef]
148. Ray, J.G.; Laskin, C.A. Folic acid and homocysteine metabolic defects and the risk of placental abruption, preeclampsia and spontaneous pregnancy loss: A systematic review. *Placenta* **1999**, *20*, 519–529. [CrossRef]
149. Lentz, S.R. Mechanisms of homocysteinee-induced atherothrombosis. *J. Thromb. Haemost.* **2005**, *3*, 1646–1654. [CrossRef]
150. Mao, D.; Che, J.; Li, K.; Han, S.; Yue, Q.; Zhu, L.; Li, L. Association of homocysteine, asymmetric dimethylarginine, and nitric oxide with preeclampsia. *Arch. Gynecol. Obstet.* **2010**, *282*, 371–375. [CrossRef]
151. Powers, R.; Evans, R.; Majors, A.; Ojimba, J.; Ness, R.; Crombleholme, W.R.; Roberts, J.M. Plasma homocysteine concentration is increased in preeclampsia and is associated with evidence of endothelial activation. *Am. J. Obstet. Gynecol.* **1998**, *179*, 1605–1611. [CrossRef]
152. Wollesen, F.; Brattstrom, L.; Refsum, H.; Ueland, P.M.; Berglund, L.; Berne, C. Plasma total homocysteine and cysteine in relation to glomerular filtration rate in diabetes mellitus. *Kidney Int.* **1999**, *55*, 1028–1035. [CrossRef] [PubMed]

153. Veldman, B.A.; Vervoort, G.; Blom, H.; Smits, P. Reduced plasma total homocysteine concentrations in Type 1 diabetes mellitus is determined by increased renal clearance. *Diabet. Med.* **2005**, *22*, 301–305. [CrossRef] [PubMed]
154. Bostom, A.G.; Lathrop, L. Hyperhomocysteinemia in end-stage renal disease: Prevalence, etiology, and potential relationship to arteriosclerotic outcomes. *Kidney Int.* **1997**, *52*, 10–20. [CrossRef] [PubMed]
155. Maul, H.; Longo, M.; Saade, G.R.; Garfield, R.E. Nitric oxide and its role duringpregnancy: From ovulation to delivery. *Curr. Pharm. Des.* **2003**, *9*, 359–380. [CrossRef] [PubMed]
156. Luzi, G.; Caserta, G.; Iammarino, G.; Clerici, G.; Di Renzo, G.C. Nitric oxide donors in pregnancy: Fetomaternal hemodynamic effects induced in mild pre-eclampsia and threatened preterm labor. *Ultrasound Obstetrics Gynecol.* **1999**, *14*, 101–109. [CrossRef] [PubMed]
157. Ledingham, M.-A.; Denison, F.C.; Kelly, R.W.; Young, A.; Norman, J.E. Nitric oxide donors stimulate prostaglandin F2α and inhibit thromboxane B2 production in the human cervix during the first trimester of pregnancy. *Mol. Hum. Reprod.* **1999**, *5*, 973–982. [CrossRef] [PubMed]
158. Trapani, A., Jr.; Goncalves, L.F.; Trapani, T.F.; Vieira, S.; Pires, M.; Pires, M.M. Perinatal and hemodynamic evaluation of Sildenafil citrate for preeclampsia treatment: A randomized controlled trial. *Obstet. Gynecol.* **2016**, *128*, 253e9. [CrossRef] [PubMed]
159. Cardounel, A.J.; Cui, H.; Samouilov, A.; Johnson, W.; Kearns, P.; Tsai, A.L.; Berka, V.; Zweier, J.L. Evidence for the pathophysiological role of endogenous methylarginines in regulation of endothelial NO production and vascular function. *J. Biol. Chem.* **2007**, *282*, 879–887. [CrossRef] [PubMed]
160. Facchinetti, F.; Longo, M.; Piccinini, F.; Neri, I.; Volpe, A. L-arginine infusion reduces blood pressure in preeclamptic women through nitric oxide release. *J. Soc. Gynecol. Investig.* **1999**, *6*, 202–207.
161. Vadillo-Ortega, F.; Perichart-Perera, O.; Espino, S.; Avila-Vergara, M.A.; Ibarra, I.; Ahued, R.; Strauss, J.F. Effect of supplementation during pregnancy with L-arginine and antioxidant vitamins in medical food on pre-eclampsia in high risk population: Randomised controlled trial. *BMJ* **2011**, *342*, d2901. [CrossRef]
162. Fu, Z.; Ma, Z.; Liu, G.; Wang, L.; Guo, Y. Vitamins supplementation affects the onset of preeclampsia. *J. Formos. Med. Assoc.* **2018**, *117*, 6–13. [CrossRef] [PubMed]
163. Neri, I.; Monari, F.; Sgarbi, L.; Berardi, A.; Masellis, G.; Facchinetti, F. L-arginine supplementation in women with chronic hypertension: Impact on blood pressure and maternal and neonatal complications. *J. Matern. Fetal. Neonatal. Med.* **2010**, *23*, 1456–1460. [CrossRef] [PubMed]
164. Meher, S.; Duley, L. Nitric oxide for preventing pre-eclampsia and its complications. *Cochrane Database Syst. Rev.* **2007**, *2*, CD006490. [CrossRef] [PubMed]
165. Camarena Pulido, E.E.; García Benavides, L.; Panduro Baron, J.G.; Pascoe Gonzalez, S.; Madrigal Saray, A.J.; García Padilla, F.E.; Totsuka Sutto, S.E. Efficacy of L-arginine for preventing preeclampsia in high risk pregnancies: A double-blind randomized clinical trial. *Hypertens. Pregnancy* **2016**, *35*, 217–225. [CrossRef] [PubMed]
166. Abdelrazik, M.; ElBerry, S.; Abosereah, M.; Edris, Y.; Sharafeldeen, A. Prophylactic treatment for preeclampsia in high risk teenage primigravida with nitricoxide donors: A pilot study. *J. Matern. Fetal. Neonatal. Med.* **2016**, *29*, 2617e20.
167. Coles, L.T.; Clifton, P.M. Effect of beetroot juice on lowering blood pressure in freeliving, disease-free adults: A randomized, placebo-controlled trial. *Nutr. J.* **2012**, *11*, 106. [CrossRef]
168. Ormesher, L.; Myers, J.E.; Chmiel, C.; Wareing, M.; Greenwood, S.L.; Tropea, T.; Cottrell, E.C. Effects of dietary nitrate supplementation, from beetroot juice, on blood pressure in hypertensive pregnant women: A randomised, double-blind, placebo-controlled feasibility trial. *Nitric Oxide* **2018**, *80*, 37–44. [CrossRef]
169. Moreland, R.B.; Goldstein, I.I.; Kim, N.N.; Traish, A. Sildenafil Citrate, a Selective Phosphodiesterase Type 5 Inhibitor. *Trends Endocrinol. Metab.* **1999**, *10*, 97–104. [CrossRef]
170. Ramesar, S.V.; Mackraj, I.; Gathiram, P.; Moodley, J. Sildenafil citrate decreases sFlt-1 and sEng in pregnant l-NAME treated Sprague-Dawley rats. *Eur. J. Obstet. Gynecol. Reprod. Biol.* **2011**, *157*, 136–140. [CrossRef]
171. Herraiz, S.; Pellicer, B.; Serra, V.; Cauli, O.; Cortijo, J.; Felipo, V.; Pellicer, A. Sildenafil citrate improves perinatal outcome in fetuses from pre-eclamptic rats. *BJOG* **2012**, *119*, 1394–1402. [CrossRef]

172. Cacciatore, B.; Halmesmäki, E.; Kaaja, R.; Teramo, K.; Ylikorkala, O. Effects of transdermal nitroglycerin on impedance to flow in the uterine, umbilical, and fetal middle cerebral arteries in pregnancies complicated by preeclampsia and intrauterine growth retardation. *Am. J. Obstet. Gynecol.* **1998**, *179*, 140–145. [CrossRef]
173. Trapani, A., Jr.; Gonçalves, L.F.; Pires, M.M. Transdermal nitroglycerin in patients with severe pre-eclampsia with placental insufficiency: Effect on uterine, umbilical and fetal middle cerebral artery resistance indices. *Ultrasound Obstet. Gynecol.* **2011**, *38*, 389–394. [CrossRef] [PubMed]

© 2019 by the authors. Licensee MDPI, Basel, Switzerland. This article is an open access article distributed under the terms and conditions of the Creative Commons Attribution (CC BY) license (http://creativecommons.org/licenses/by/4.0/).

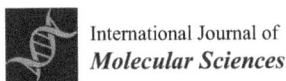

Review

Molecular Targets of Aspirin and Prevention of Preeclampsia and Their Potential Association with Circulating Extracellular Vesicles during Pregnancy

Suchismita Dutta [1], Sathish Kumar [2], Jon Hyett [3] and Carlos Salomon [1,4,5,*]

[1] Exosome Biology Laboratory, Centre for Clinical Diagnostics, University of Queensland Centre for Clinical Research, Royal Brisbane and Women's Hospital, The University of Queensland, Brisbane, QLD 4029, Australia
[2] Departments of Comparative Biosciences and Obstetrics and Gynecology, University of Wisconsin, Madison, WI 53792, USA
[3] Royal Prince Alfred Hospital Sydney, University of Sydney, Camperdown, NSW 2050, Australia
[4] Maternal-Fetal Medicine, Department of Obstetrics and Gynecology, Ochsner Clinic Foundation, New Orleans, LA 70124, USA
[5] Department of Clinical Biochemistry and Immunology, Faculty of Pharmacy, University of Concepción, Concepción, Region Bio-Bio 4070386, Chile
* Correspondence: c.salomongallo@uq.edu.au; Tel.: +61-7-3346-5500; Fax: +61-7-3346-5509

Received: 19 May 2019; Accepted: 26 August 2019; Published: 5 September 2019

Abstract: Uncomplicated healthy pregnancy is the outcome of successful fertilization, implantation of embryos, trophoblast development and adequate placentation. Any deviation in these cascades of events may lead to complicated pregnancies such as preeclampsia (PE). The current incidence of PE is 2–8% in all pregnancies worldwide, leading to high maternal as well as perinatal mortality and morbidity rates. A number of randomized controlled clinical trials observed the association between low dose aspirin (LDA) treatment in early gestational age and significant reduction of early onset of PE in high-risk pregnant women. However, a substantial knowledge gap exists in identifying the particular mechanism of action of aspirin on placental function. It is already established that the placental-derived exosomes (PdE) are present in the maternal circulation from 6 weeks of gestation, and exosomes contain bioactive molecules such as proteins, lipids and RNA that are a "fingerprint" of their originating cells. Interestingly, levels of exosomes are higher in PE compared to normal pregnancies, and changes in the level of PdE during the first trimester may be used to classify women at risk for developing PE. The aim of this review is to discuss the mechanisms of action of LDA on placental and maternal physiological systems including the role of PdE in these phenomena. This review article will contribute to the in-depth understanding of LDA-induced PE prevention.

Keywords: pregnancy; placentation; preeclampsia; low dose aspirin; exosomes

1. Introduction

Pregnancy is an important event that leads to significant changes in maternal physiology. Successful pregnancy requires involvement of a series of processes commencing from fertilization to establishment of placental and maternal vascular connection with the fetus in correct order. Adequate placentation is one of the prerequisites for maintaining a normal healthy pregnancy. New insights into the placentation process involve migration, invasion, adherence, proliferation and differentiation of the placental principal cellular component, i.e., extravillous trophoblasts (EVTs), followed by their interaction with the pre-decasualized maternal uterine blood vessels, glands and lymphatics [1]. Placentation further evolves by digestion of the extracellular matrix where the EVTs tolerate surrounding maternal circulatory oxidative stress and the effects of soluble cytokines [1]. Nonetheless, the allogenic

EVTs also interact with maternal decidual immune cells to provide immune competence [2]. Any deviation in these events may lead to pathological pregnancies, i.e., preeclampsia (PE). The broad concept of PE pathophysiology includes defective trophoblast invasion and inadequate uterine spiral arterial remodeling in the first trimester that follows with reduced uteroplacental perfusion [3]. This subsequently leads to poorly perfused and stressed placental syncytiotrophoblasts that release a range of mediators causing endothelial dysfunction and PE clinical manifestations [3]. Moreover, such abnormal placentation leads to the secretion of abnormal levels of anti-angiogenic and inflammatory proteins that enter the systemic maternal circulation and impair maternal systemic vascular function, resulting in the clinical manifestations of PE. Since PE and its clinical symptoms rapidly abate after delivery (removal of the placenta), the placenta must play a central or initiating role in this pregnancy disorder.

Novel pharmacological interventions for the prevention of PE have not been developed for many years, as the complex pathophysiology, diversified clinical presentation of the disease and difficulties associated with conducting drug discovery research in pregnant women have hampered their development. Low dose aspirin (LDA) is considered to be the most effective prophylactic therapy for reducing disease prevalence in women at high risk for developing early-onset PE. The use of LDA in pregnant women is generally considered to be safe as it does not affect the pregnant mothers and/or their unborn fetuses inadvertently. It has been suggested that the principal mechanism of action by which LDA exerts its effect is via the inhibition of thromboxane production that leads to the inhibition of platelet aggregation. Additionally, LDA has a direct positive effect on the villous trophoblasts [4]. However, recent evidence suggests that LDA prevents the development of PE by promoting trophoblast invasion and migration into the uterine arteries, interfering with cytokine production and stimulating the production of proangiogenic protein placental growth factor (PlGF); thereby, inhibiting apoptosis and premature uterine arterial remodeling [5].

Recent meta-analysis suggest that LDA (≥100 mg/day) in early gestation (before 16 weeks) is beneficial in preventing common pregnancy complications; i.e., PE, fetal growth restriction, preterm birth [6–9], suggesting that aspirin may have effect on implantation and early placentation [10]. Low-dose aspirin has been utilized for many years to prevent PE [11–13]. A recent individual patient data meta-analysis observed that LDA can reduce the risk of PE development by 10% and small for gestational age (SGA) births by 24% [14] without posing a major safety risk to mothers or fetuses other than placental abruption in some cases [15]. Other studies reported that low dose aspirin is generally well tolerated within both preconception and early pregnancy periods [16].

In normal healthy pregnancy, placental syncytiotrophoblast release extracellular vesicles (EVs) including exosomes into the maternal bloodstream that contain some information (i.e., micro RNA, mRNA, proteins) to convey from the originating cells to their distant target cells such as maternal immune cells in order to adapt to the pregnancy associated physiological changes [17]. This EV release is further increased from the preeclamptic placenta due to oxidative stress, causing widespread systemic endothelial dysfunction, giving rise to maternal hypertension, feto-placental circulatory compromise and damaging various maternal organs [17]. Some recently published reports have suggested that LDA could influence platelet derived EV release; however, the effect of LDA on the regulation of placental EV release is not known. Therefore, in this review, we will discuss the potential mechanisms of action of aspirin in the context of PE prevention and the potential role of extracellular vesicles released from the placenta in this phenomenon (Figure 1).

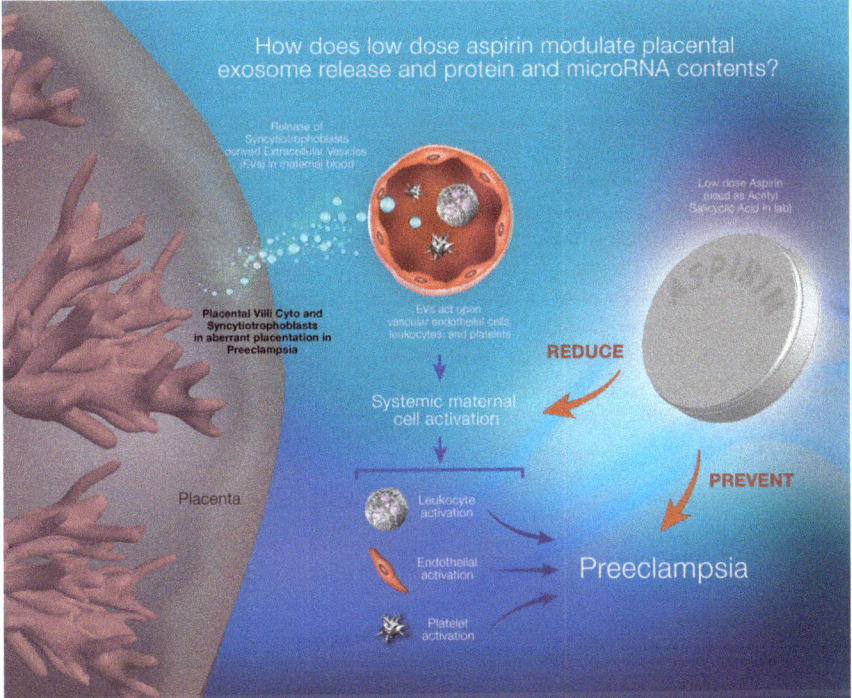

Figure 1. Diagrammatic representation of preeclampsia (PE) development pathogenesis and mechanism of prevention by low dose aspirin (LDA). In PE, syncytiotrophoblast-derived extracellular vesicles (EVs), including exosomes, are released into the maternal circulation in increased amounts due to inadequate placental vascular remodeling. These EVs activate the vascular endothelial cells, leukocytes and platelets and cause dysfunction. LDA prevents the development of PE by reducingendothelial cell dysfunction. The proposed mechanism that was investigated; acetylsalicylic acid, the crude form of aspirin, modulates trophoblast derived exosome release and changes their proteomic and microRNA contents.

2. Physiology of Pregnancy

Pregnancy induces a number of alterations to maternal physiology for maintaining the correct course of pregnancy and it involves a cascade of processes commencing from fertilization to the establishment of feto-maternal communication and cross-talk mediated via the placenta. Preimplantation conditions, vascularisation, invasion of the embryonic cells to the maternal uterine wall and oxidative stress are the essential regulators in the function of pregnancy events [18]. Prior to implantation, there is a postovulatory surge of circulatory progesterone level that inhibits the proliferation of estrogen-dependent uterine epithelium and induces secretory transformation of uterine glands. In the early stages of development, i.e., ~day 6 of fertilization, the microvilli of the blastocyst interact with the pinopodes of the uterine endometrial luminal epithelium in order to establish apposition, which becomes stable through the increased adherence of the trophectoderm and the uterine luminal epithelium. During this interaction, a range of molecules are secreted from the immune activated cells including mucin, selectin, integrin and cadherin [18,19]. Shortly thereafter, invasion begins and trophectoderm penetrates the uterine epithelium, invading the wall of the uterine arteries where they interact with the cells of the maternal circulatory immune system and mediate the remodeling of the uterine spiral arteries that supply the placenta. This is followed by deportation of aggregates containing transcriptive materials.

There is direct evidence that platelets are involved in the placentation process. During placentation, trophoblasts invade the decidual stroma including the uterine glands and migrate into the maternal uterine spiral arteries replacing the vascular smooth muscle cells to remodel the arteries as low resistance, large caliber vessels [20]. This process ensures adequate placental perfusion by the remodeling of maternal uterine vessels. Histological examination shows deposition of maternal platelets in the trophoblast aggregates formed in the uterine spiral arteries. A number of studies discovered that these platelets are activated, releasing soluble factors enhancing the invasive capacity of trophoblast cells [21]. The trophoblasts produce a range of vasoconstrictors and vasodialators that are in balance to maintain the placental blood flow for proper fetal development during pregnancy [22].

During pregnancy, the viscosity and coagulability of maternal blood upsurges due to the increase in pro-coagulant agents, such as plasminogen activator inhibitor-1, fibrinogen, factor VII, VIII, von Willebrand factor and to the reduced fibrinolysis. The hypercoagulable state is attributed to the activation of platelets [23]. Maternal serum biochemical markers of pregnancy, namely alpha fetoprotein (AFP), human chorionic gonadotrophin (hCG), unconjugated estriol [24] and inhibin-A [25], are produced and found in higher concentration in the maternal peripheral circulation due to the implantation and placentation processes of pregnancy.

3. Pathogenesis of Preeclampsia

Preeclampsia (PE) is defined as new onset of hypertension after 20 weeks' gestation with renal, hepatic, hematologic, neurological, pulmonary or fetal involvement. Physical signs of preeclampsia are hypertension, proteinuria, renal insufficiency, hemolysis, reduced platelet count and/or increased platelet activation [26]. It is a serious complication of pregnancy affecting ~7.6% pregnancies globally and is associated with high morbidity and mortality in affected mothers and children [27]. It is a lifelong disorder with increased risks of neonatal and child morbidity and mortality including health risks in adulthood [27]. Pregnancy induced hypertension is one of the most prevalent risk factors for the development of PE. The consequences of PE include intrauterine fetal growth restriction (IUGR) and preterm birth [28].

In PE, there is widespread systemic endothelial dysfunction that leads to hypertension and concomitant proteinuria [29]. Clinical risk factors for developing PE assessed before 16 weeks of gestation include prior history of hypertension, chronic hypertension, pre-gestational diabetes, pre-pregnancy BMI > 30 and use of assisted reproductive technology [30]. The most commonly used screening test for early prediction of PE involves analysis of maternal characteristics, maternal mean arterial pressure, uterine arterial Doppler pulsatility index and serum biochemistry (PaPP-A and/or PlGF). This test is performed at 11–13 weeks of gestation [31]. The present management of patients with PE depends on symptom severity. Currently, some drugs are available to treat mild to severe PE (e.g., methyldopa, hydralazine, magnesium sulphate) [32]. However, the best treatment currently available for PE is delivery of the newborn and placenta as all the signs and symptoms of PE abolish when the placenta is separated from the mother.

In early-onset PE, there is defective implantation and placentation due to inadequate extravillous trophoblast invasion and partial failure of uterine arterial remodeling, resulting in high resistance and low capacitance vascular supply to the placenta and fetus [33]; however, this phenomenon is not evident in late-onset PE. Some research studies showed that during normal healthy pregnancy, the invasive trophoblast cells replace the smooth muscle and elastic lamina of the maternal uterine vessels, causing dilation and funneling at the vessel mouth and facilitating further migration of trophoblasts. In the absence of conversion of the maternal uterine vessels, there is retention of smooth muscle cells contributing to increased resistance to maternal blood flow. Nonetheless, maternal blood enters into the intervillous space as a turbulent jet that increases the risk of spontaneous vasoconstriction and ischemia-reperfusion injury, generating oxidative stress within the maternal circulation [34]. This in turn gives rise to placental villous infarcts, constriction of spiral arteries due to the mural hypertrophy and fibrin deposition, leading to the abnormal ultrasound indices and biochemical markers seen in the maternal circulation. This failure in vascular dilation has a direct impact on placental blood flow and is the primary determinant of pregnancy pathology [34]. In addition to the general concept of PE pathogenesis, where there is defective EVT invasion and uterine arterial remodeling, there is also an imbalance of angiogenic and antiangiogenic factors. These factors include vascular endothelial growth factor (VEGF), soluble endoglin, soluble fms-like tyrosine kinase-1 receptors (sFlt-1) and placental growth factor (PlGF). Abnormal production of these factors is closely associated with PE and intrauterine growth restriction [35]. At the end of the first trimester of pregnancy, the extravillous trophoblasts (EVT) invade the uterine spiral arteries and replace the vascular smooth muscle and the endothelium to remodel the arteries, which lead to the formation of low resistance and high capacitance vessels that facilitates increased placental perfusion. When there is perturbation of this process, there is reduced placental perfusion causing placental stress where platelets aggregate and accumulate in the partially damaged placenta [36]. In PE, there are interactions between maternal characteristics and risk factors and placental pathophysiological factors leading to a vicious cycle of maternal inflammation, vascular dysfunction and the activation of pro-coagulation pathways [33].

Current research on PE is focused on the role of extracellular vesicles released from the placenta [33]. Following placentation, the residual syncytiotrophoblastic material generated from placental shedding or by placental microparticles releases various vessel constricting factors that cause systemic endothelial dysfunction [37,38]. These microparticles contain a set of proteins including some pro-inflammatory and pro-coagulatory molecules that contribute to the development of PE [39–41] A recent article on PE stated that there was interaction between fetal Human Leukocyte Antigen-C (HLA-C) molecule and maternal natural killer cells' killer-cell immunoglobulin-like receptor (KIR) in severe PE; these molecules are carried by the EVs released from the placenta and maternal circulatory cells [42]. Inadequate placentation causes the development of pregnancy-induced hypertension (PIH) and preeclampsia (PE) [43,44], leading to focal regions of hypoxia that are responsible for modifying the production of growth factors, cytokines [45], lipid peroxides [46] and prostaglandins by placental trophoblasts [45]. Elevated placental levels of inflammatory cytokines, such as tumor necrosis factor-α, interleukin (IL)-1α, IL-1β and IL-6, are generally considered unfavorable to pregnancy [47]. Moreover, clinical studies have shown changes in the levels of cytokines and prostaglandins in women with PE [48,49]. Maternal circulatory neutrophils are activated in pregnancy and further activated in PE, which are the source of oxidative stress by generating reactive oxygen species such as hydrogen peroxide and superoxide anion and these molecules cause damage to the proteins, lipids and nucleic acids [50]. Neutrophil activation is initiated in the intervillous space by increased secretion of lipid peroxides by the placenta, which is abnormally increased in PE. This stimulates phospholipase A2 and cyclooxygenase enzymes to increase the production of thromboxane. Thromboxane is implicated in monocyte activation responses and plays role in mediating tumor necrosis factor alpha (TNF-α) production by neutrophils in response to oxidative stress [50].

In PE, the production of thromboxane A2 and prostaglandin I2 is altered with excessive accumulation of THXA2 metabolite in the maternal systemic circulation [51,52]. This results to the increased activation and aggregation of platelets and vasoconstriction causing impaired placental perfusion and oxidative stress [53–57]. The platelet count is reduced in PE due to platelet activation and aggregation under the effect of elevated levels of ThXA2 Synthase [28]. In addition [36], PE contributes to some biochemical changes in maternal circulatory system, such as, increase in phosphodiesterase-5 [58], thromboxane synthase [28] and an elevated hCG level [59]. Nonetheless, immunological changes also take place in PE. There is rise in anti β_2-glycoprotein I antibodies that are related with aberrant implantation [60]. many predictive biomarkers for PE have been described including placental biomarkers (PAPP-A, PLGF, s-FLT-1, placental protein 13 (PP 13)), Free HbF, Alpha 1 Macroglobulin and Uterine Artery Doppler Pulsatility Index [61,62]. Not all studies have consistently shown value of these markers, for example changes in PP13 have not been consistently replicated [63]. Measurements of total cell free DNA and fetal fraction in maternal plasma at 11–13 and 20–24 weeks are not predictive of PE [64].

4. Pharmacology of Aspirin and Basis for Its Use in PE

The chemical name of aspirin is acetylsalicylic acid (ASA) [65–69]. It is a nonsteroidal anti-inflammatory drug (NSAID). It is typically used in two dose regimens—high dose (600 mg) and low dose (60–150 mg). It has anti-inflammatory, analgesic, antipyretic and antiplatelet effects [70]. The endothelial dysfunction in PE involves increased lipid peroxidation, which activates COX and inhibits prostacyclin synthase, thus inducing rapid imbalance in the TXA2/prostacyclin (PGI2) ratio in favor of TXA2 [51]. TXA2 favors systemic vasoconstriction, and increasing platelet aggregation and adhesion, which is compensated in this context by the vasodilator effect of prostacyclins, levels of which drop sharply. This imbalance is present from 13 weeks of gestation in high-risk PE patients [71]. LDA treatment for 2 weeks reverses TXA2/PGI2 imbalance by inhibiting THXA2 production [72,73]. Some studies observed that LDA can reduce the release of sFLT-1 from trophoblast cells and induce the production of vascular endothelial growth factor thereby promoting angiogenesis [74]. LDA also modulates cytokine production, reduces apoptosis and alters cell aggregation and fusion thereby improving defective trophoblast implantation [5]. LDA improves EVT migration and invasion into the maternal uterine spiral arteries and reduces placental cell apoptosis [75]. PE is associated with some augmented anti-angiogenic, oxidative and pro-inflammatory markers, as well as increasing human polymorphonuclear neutrophil (PMN)-endothelial cell adhesion [76]. LDA reduces the circulatory levels of these factors and improves the cytokine profile [5]. LDA causes retardation in leukocyte-endothelial cell adhesion and interaction and thus it prevents the endothelial cell dysfunction in PE [76]. Several reports have suggested that few biomarkers can be identified in maternal blood to be monitored for assessing treatment response after initiation of LDA treatment in pregnant women at high risk for preeclampsia; i.e., placental growth factor, placental protein 13, alpha fetoprotein [77].

The mechanism of action of aspirin involves a cascade of events. Aspirin irreversibly acetylates the platelet enzyme cyclooxygenase (COX), modifying the production of different prostaglandins and also acts as an analgesic, anti-inflammatory agent. There are three isoforms of COX enzyme upon which aspirin acts; the sources of these enzymes are mainly platelets, but they are also found in other immune cells namely leukocytes, monocytes and macrophages. Aspirin inhibits COX-1 irreversibly and COX-2 reversibly to a lesser extent. The resultant inhibition of COX-dependent generation of thromboxane A2 prevents platelet aggregation. This effect is maintained for the entire platelet lifespan of 8–9 days [78].

5. Low Dose Aspirin (LDA) and Pregnancy

Low dose aspirin reduces the mortality and morbidity in pregnant women at high risk for PE [79–82]. National guidelines typically suggest that women considered to be at high risk of developing pre-eclampsia should be treated with prophylactic low dose aspirin to reduce the prevalence of disease, although there are differences in how "high risk" is defined (NICE guidelines and ACOG recommendations (2017)). Acetylsalicylic Acid (ASA) is considered a highly attractive pharmacological agent to use in pregnancy for the prevention of maternal and perinatal mortality and morbidity worldwide due to its low cost, widespread availability, ease of administration and safety profile [83]. Aspirin is listed as a US Food and Drug Administration (FDA) category C drug during the first and second trimester and a category D drug in the third trimester of pregnancy [70]. Although some recent evidence has suggested that aspirin can affect the fetus adversely causing congenital anomaly, the FDA has assigned this drug as pregnancy category C, and treatment is relatively safe [84]. Although aspirin can cross the placenta, it is safe in low doses [85].

Low dose aspirin is a very effective treatment. Meta-analysis of a series of >30 randomized controlled trials have shown that low dose aspirin prophylaxis (any dose, any gestation) reduces the incidence of PE by 10% [11,12,14,86]. If analysis is restricted to assessment of outcomes for PE leading to delivery before 34 weeks in women who commence aspirin <16 weeks gestation and have a higher dose (>100 mg/day), then the data show a 90% reduction in early PE [87]. Aspirin also appears to be effective at reducing the prevalence of intrauterine growth restriction (IUGR); once again, this meta-analysis shows that treatment is more effective if a higher dose (>100 mg/day) is given and treatment is started before 16 weeks [88]. Other meta-analyses have also shown that low dose aspirin may be effective in preventing spontaneous preterm birth [6–9]. Other studies have demonstrated that low dose aspirin is generally well tolerated in both preconception and early pregnancy periods [16].

To date, several studies have attempted to assess the beneficial effects of aspirin treatment in gestational hypertensive disorders, in particular PE. In spite of different conflicting results on the effects of aspirin in pregnancy, one study found that aspirin administered early i.e., from the eighth week of gestation has in fact a positive effect on the pregnancy outcome without the manifestation of teratogenicity or fetotoxicity [29]. Recent studies on PE found that in high risk pregnancies, any preventative treatment should be aimed at or before 16 gestational weeks to be effective as placentation and uterine spiral arterial remodeling is completed by 20 gestational weeks [11]. Additionally, to prevent perinatal death and to improve perinatal outcomes, low dose aspirin should be prescribed before 16 gestational weeks [89]. Cost benefit analysis in a US based research study showed that aspirin prophylaxis through pregnancy would reduce morbidity and mortality, leading to a reduction in health care costs [90].

Following the preparation of a systematic review, the US Preventive Service Task Force recommended the use of low-dose aspirin (81 mg/d) as preventive medication after 12 weeks of gestation in women who are at high risk for PE [91–93]. The US Preventive Service Task Force also found that LDA prophylaxis in early pregnancy does not increase the chances of placental abruption, postpartum hemorrhage, fetal intracranial hemorrhage or perinatal mortality [94].

Other authors have suggested that the dose and timing of aspirin prophylaxis is also important. Ayala et al., 2013, identified that (i) 100 mg/d ASA should be the recommended minimum dose for prevention of complications in pregnancy; (ii) ingestion of low-dose ASA should be started at ≤16 weeks of gestation and (iii) low-dose ASA should be ingested at bedtime, not during the morning. Aspirin prescribed in this way significantly regulates ambulatory blood pressure (BP) and reduces the incidence of PE, gestational hypertension, preterm delivery and intrauterine growth restriction (IUGR) [95].

Other agents have been used for prophylaxis against PE in high risk women, either alone or in combination with LDA. There is a significant body of literature investigating whether low molecular weight (LMWH) or unfractionated heparin can reduce rates of PE, preterm birth, perinatal mortality and small for gestational age babies when prescribed to high risk women [96,97]. Heparin is safe from a fetal perspective and does not cross the placental barrier due to its high molecular weight [85,98]. While some observational studies that have combined the use of aspirin and LMWH show significant reduction in rates of PE in very high risk groups [99,100], an individual patient meta-analysis did not show significant benefit to this intervention [101]. Calcium (1 g/day) has also been widely investigated and appears to be particularly useful in low and middle income settings where dietary calcium intake is poor [102]. Vitamin C, D, E [103–105], fish oil/omega 3, statins [35], L-arginine [106] and antihypertensive drugs such as calcium channel blockers [107] have also been investigated, although there is a paucity of randomized controlled trial-based data for these investigations. The most significant ongoing research issues are to establish why aspirin is less effective in some groups of women; for example, those that have chronic hypertension and to determine whether additional agents can impact rates of term pre-eclampsia, which are not as significantly reduced using aspirin therapy.

A table on recent studies involving aspirin and pregnancy has been presented in the Table 1.

Table 1. Recent Studies on Aspirin and Pregnancy.

Study Design	Mode of Treatment	Outcome of Study	Reference
Randomized controlled trial (RCT)	Low dose aspirin (LDA) and/or Low Molecular Weight Heparin (LMWH)	Improved pregnancy outcomes (Less PE and IUGR incidence)	[108]
Prospective case-control study	LDA and LMWH in first trimester	Reduced incidence of unexplained recurrent spontaneous abortion	[109]
Database searching for RCTs involving LDA and placebo in PE	LDA or Placebo	LDA reduces PE risk	[110]
Literature searching on LDA and PE	LDA at 100 mg/day <16 gestational weeks	Reduced PE incidence due to LDA prophylaxis	[111]
Systematic literature searches about aspirin and PE	LDA	LDA prophylaxis in at risk patients to develop PE have higher advantages compared to negligible disadvantages i.e., feto-maternal bleeding, aspirin resistance etc.	[112]
Systematic review and an individual participant data meta-analysis	Antiplatelet aspirin therapy in early pregnancy	10–15% reduction in the risk of PE	[113]
A systematic review and meta-analysis of randomized controlled trials	50–150 mg/day aspirin or no treatment at <16 or >16 gestational weeks	LDA at <16 weeks, there was a significant reduction and a dose-response effect for the prevention of preeclampsia	[87]
A systematic review and meta-analysis through electronic database searches (PubMed, Cochrane, Embase).	LDA or placebo at <16 or >16 gestational weeks	<16 weeks, significant reduction of PE. >16 weeks, negligible impact on PE and related disorders	[11]
Databases searching involving keywords 'aspirin' and 'pregnancy'	RCTs that evaluated the prophylactic use of LDA (50–150 mg/day) during pregnancy were included.	LDA initiated at ≤16 weeks of gestation is associated with a greater reduction of perinatal death and other adverse perinatal outcomes than when initiated at >16 weeks.	[114]
Meta-analysis of individual patient data recruited to 31 RCTs of PE primary prevention.	One or more antiplatelet agents (e.g., LDA or dipyridamole) versus a placebo or no antiplatelet agent.	Antiplatelet agents were associated with a significant 10% reduction in the relative risk of both PE ($p = 0.004$) and preterm birth before 34 weeks' gestation ($p = 0.011$) compared to control cases.	[86]
Women at high risk for preterm PE were recruited to RCTs	150 mg/day of aspirin was used to reduce the incidence of aspirin resistance and maximize the effect.	LDA reduced the incidence of preterm PE	[115]

Table 1. *Cont.*

Study Design	Mode of Treatment	Outcome of Study	Reference
A planned secondary analysis of the Effects of Aspirin in Gestation and Reproduction (EAGeR) trial, a multicenter, block-randomized, double-blind, placebo-controlled trial investigating the effects of LDA on the incidence of live birth.	Daily LDA (81 mg, n = 615) or placebo (n = 613) and were followed for up to six menstrual cycles or through gestation if they became pregnant.	Preconception LDA appears to be well tolerated by women trying to conceive, women who become pregnant, and by their fetuses and neonates.	[16]
Chronological, cumulative meta-analyses of two recently published meta-analyses of RCTs examining the effects of antioxidant or LDA on the rates of PE.	Antioxidant or Low Dose Acetylsalicylic Acid (LDAA) therapy	Studies with smaller sample sizes are more likely to be biased against the null hypothesis. As such, cumulative meta-analysis is an effective tool in predicting potential bias against the null hypothesis and the need for additional studies.	[116]
Prospective cohort study involving 533 pregnant women in their first trimester	LDAA and LMWH	The use of ASA may be associated with an increased risk of developing a sub-chorionic hematoma (SCH) during the first trimester.	[117]
Multicentre RCTs involving 32 women with a previous delivery <34 weeks gestation with HD and/or SGA and aPLA were included before 12 weeks gestation.	The intervention was daily LMWH with aspirin or aspirin alone.	Combined LMWH and aspirin treatment started before 12 weeks gestation in a subsequent pregnancy did not show reduction of onset of recurrent HD either <34 weeks gestation or irrespective of gestational age, compared with aspirin alone.	[118]
Prospective randomized, placebo-controlled, double-blinded, multinational clinical trial	Daily administration of LDA (81 mg/day) initiated between 6 and 13 weeks of pregnancy and continued upto 36 weeks.	PTB, PE, SGA, perinatal mortality were reduced.	[119]
Prospective RCTs	Preconception LDA daily	It is not associated with reduction of pregnancy loss	[120]
Multicenter, double blind, placebo-controlled trial involving women at high risk for preterm PE	Some of them received 150 mg/day aspirin and some of them received placebo at 11–14 gestational weeks until 36 weeks of gestation	Primary outcome was delivery with PE before 37 weeks of gestation. Treatment with aspirin reduced the incidence of preterm preeclampsia.	[121]

6. Effects of LDA on Placental and Maternal Body System Function

To date, a number of studies have attempted to elucidate the role of aspirin in the prevention of adverse pregnancy outcomes. However, the particular function of LDA in preventing PE and other pregnancy-induced hypertension is not clearly understood. Some in-vitro studies found that there is no specific effect of LDA or LMWH on BeWo choriocarcinoma cells when treated with forskolin except cell fusion due to the placental protein level 13 increase [122]. Some studies reported that thromboxane has been found to be involved with vasoconstriction leading to placental ischemia, thrombosis and platelet aggregation [123]. Other research studies reported that aspirin can negatively act on COX2 enzyme, thereby inhibiting thromboxane A2 production from arachidonic acid [124,125]. Interestingly, there are also data suggesting that aspirin can reduce the release of thromboxane from the trophoblasts [22].

Low-dose aspirin, which selectively inhibits TXA2 production, is used to prevent high-risk PE [28]. Low-dose aspirin, a common antiplatelet agent, usually restores prostacyclin and thromboxane levels that prevent vasoconstriction, and therefore, has been targeted as an intervention to reduce PE in at-risk women [124,126]. LDA increases the production of prostaglandin I_2 by blocking the synthesis of thromboxane A2 [73]. This PGI_2 increases vasodilatation and prevent thromboxane mediated damage [127]. Some studies have shown that TXA2 analogues cause hypertension in pregnancy and TXAS depletion prevents hypertension and IUGR [128]. Urine specimens of PE women show the presence of thromboxane B2, which is the metabolite of thromboxane A2 and LDA shifts the balance between THXA2 and PGI2 favoring the production of PGI2 that increases the blood flow to the placenta [129].

In normal, healthy pregnancies, uterine spiral arterial remodeling occurs at around 8 weeks of gestation and is complete by 16–20 weeks [130]. However, in PE, placentation is inadequate and under stress due to impaired uterine spiral arterial remodeling [131]. Some randomized controlled clinical trials observed that LDA is associated with improvement in uterine arterial pulsatility index when started in the first trimester of pregnancy [132,133]. Another study observed that low dose aspirin reduces the UtA Doppler pulsatility index, indicating improved blood flow [134].

In-vitro studies found an association of LDA treated trophoblast cells and an improvement in cytokine profile that prevents trophoblast apoptosis and promotes angiogenesis by increasing the production of placental growth factor (PlGF) [75]. Another similar study by Panagodage, et al. identified a number of factors that are involved in preeclampsia prevention with low dose aspirin (LDA) treatment. The authors observed that placental growth factor is significantly decreased in preeclamptic women's sera compared to normotensive women's sera; LDA increases trophoblast secretion of PlGF and restores abnormal cytokine (Activated Leukocyte cell adhesion molecule ALCAM, CXCL-16 and ErbB3) production by trophoblasts in PE [5]. Soluble fms-like tyrosine kinase-1 (sFLT1) is an antiangiogenic factor and its expression is increased in preeclamptic placentas and in cytotrophoblast exposed to hypoxia. Aspirin inhibits the production of sFLT1 in CTBs and this effect is mediated by the inhibition of COX-1 [74].

Preeclampsia is associated with some augmented anti-angiogenic, oxidative and pro-inflammatory markers, as well as increasing human polymorphonuclear neutrophil (PMN)-endothelial cell adhesion. This cell adhesion is reduced when human PMN are incubated with ATL (aspirin triggered lipoxin A4) [76]. This aspirin triggered lipoxin is similar to endogenously produced lipoxins but the duration of action is prolonged [135]. ATL acts as an anti-inflammatory agent; it promotes angiogenesis and causes immunosuppression and it also blocks the generation of reactive oxygen species in the endothelial cells, inhibits chemotaxis of polymorphonuclear neutrophil and the leukocyte-endothelial interaction [136–140] causes nuclear factor kappa B activation [137,141] and secretion of tumor necrosis factor alpha (TNF-α) in activated T cells [142]. Additionally, ATL can increase nitric oxide synthesis where the heme oxygenase-1 enzyme is also involved [143] and this effect is responsible for resolving inflammation [143]. Heme oxygenase enzyme-1 degrades heme to generate bilirubin, carbon monoxide and iron, exerting their anti-oxidant, antiapoptotic and cytoprotective actions [144]. Additionally, another recently conducted study identified that aspirin prevents TNF-alpha-induced endothelial cell dysfunction by regulating the NF-kappa B-dependent miR-155/eNOS pathway in preeclampsia [145].

The pathophysiology of PE also involves the genetic expression of the STOX1 transcription factor by extravillous trophoblasts that modulate trophoblast proliferation [146,147]. The STOX1 gene is overexpressed in human placental extravillous trophoblasts and is associated with PE pathogenesis [147–149]. Founds et al. [150] showed, in transcriptomic analysis, that STOX1 is overexpressed during the first trimester of pregnancies that had a preeclamptic outcome. Other studies have performed functional assays to determine the function of the STOX1 gene; using an in-vivo mouse model, this gene was found to cause severe gestational hypertension, proteinuria, an increased circulatory level of antiangiogenic factors and histological alterations in the kidney as well as the placenta [151]. These researchers also demonstrated that low dose aspirin improved maternal PE-like symptoms [152]. LDA improves uterine perfusion and favourably affects aspects of reproduction [153]. In addition, empirical introduction of LDA during in vitro fertilization (IVF) treatment improves the quality of oocytes and embryos [154]. Low dose aspirin and heparin in combination improve the live birth rate in IVF for unexplained implantation failure [155]. Low-dose aspirin effectively improves perifollicular artery blood flow and enhances oocyte quality and clinical pregnancy rates [156].

7. Complications of LDA for Fetuses and Mothers

A systematic evidence review by the US Preventive Services Task Force (USPSTF) identified no adverse impact on the mother or offspring during the perinatal period following aspirin use for prevention of preeclampsia [157] including no documented adverse effect on neonatal platelets [158]. However, some studies have identified adverse effects with the antenatal and perinatal use of aspirin, albeit taken at a higher dose. Potential risks associated with aspirin therapy during the third trimester include premature closure of the ductus arteriosus and hemorrhagic complications [159], subchorionic hematoma if administered in first trimester of pregnancy [117], fetal loss [160], endocrine disturbances in the human fetal testis and interference in the testicular descent [161], childhood asthma [162] and fetal complications [110]. Some research studies observed that high doses of aspirin may affect fertility, increases the risk of miscarriages and may cause fetal cryptorchidism [163–165]. Additionally, LDA therapy in the late gestational age has on rare occasion been reported to cause renal injury, cardiovascular abnormality such as closure of the ductus arteriosus, necrotizing enterocolitis and intracranial hemorrhage in the fetus as well as reduced breast milk supply in the mother, likely due to the inhibition of cyclooxygenase enzyme pathways [164]. The common adverse effects of aspirin in adults are significantly associated with gastrointestinal or cerebral bleeding episodes [166]. Given the risks of aspirin therapy, it is better to reserve treatment for women deemed high-risk of deep placentation related disorders rather than to prescribe it universally.

8. Predictive Biomarkers for Preeclampsia Cases Treated with Low Dose Aspirin

Few biomarkers have been identified in maternal blood as candidates for monitoring treatment response after initiation of low dose aspirin treatment in pregnant women at high risk for preeclampsia:

(i) Maternal serum concentrations of placental growth factor (PlGF) level are generally low in preeclampsia.
(ii) Low-dose aspirin reduces adverse pregnancy outcome such as PE and delivery before 34 weeks of gestation in pregnant women with unexplained elevated levels of alpha-fetoprotein (AFP) [167,168].
(iii) Normotension in the first trimester is associated with reduced risk of PE [169].
(iv) In a randomized controlled clinical trial conducted by Asemi Z. et al., low dose aspirin (80 mg) was administered with calcium supplementation (500 mg) in pregnant women who were at risk for PE. The treatment was continued for nine consecutive weeks before measuring high

sensitivity C-reactive protein (hs-CRP), total antioxidant capacity (TAC), total glutathione (GSH) in plasma and serum glucose and insulin level. The study showed a significant difference in serum hs-CRP level and increased levels of plasma TAC and total GSH in pregnant women at risk for preeclampsia as compared to those that took placebo (did not receive any treatment), but serum insulin levels were not affected at all [170].

9. Extracellular Vesicles (EVs)

Extracellular vesicles (EVs) are mediators that can modify the function of target cells by transferring proteins and genomic materials to other cells; thus, EVs have an active participation in cell-to-cell communication [171]. EVs shred from a variety of cells and have a number of important physiological as well as pathological functions as they are capable of trafficking and transfecting the genetic material from cell to cell. The biogenesis and contents of EVs predominantly depends on the originating cell type and their surrounding microenvironment [172]. Several studies using electron microscopy analysis to characterize the morphology of EVs demonstrate that are spherical with lipid bilayer membrane [173,174]. The correct classification of EVs still a manner of debate and the majority of the information in the literature classify them according to their size and the different biogenesis pathways. Typically, EVs are categorized as exosomes (~40–100 nm), microvesicles (~100–1000 nm) and apoptotic bodies (~1000–5000 nm) based on their size and origin. Microvesicles and apoptotic bodies are formed directly via budding of the plasma membrane, whereas exosomes are produced via an endocytic pathway [174]. Distinction between different EVs subgroups is difficult, due to the minimal physical and morphological differences, to the lack of specific markers, and to the fact that the same cellular source may dynamically produce different class of EVs in response to different conditions [175]. Recently, the international society of extracellular vesicles has recommended classifying the vesicles according to the their size in small EVs (<100–200 nm) and medium/large EVs (>200 nm), or density (low, middle, high, with each range will defined) or their biochemical composition (e.g., $CD63^{+ve}$) [176]. Currently, there is no single method allowing for accurate characterization and discrimination of the different EVs classes [175]. EVs can be ordinarily isolated from different biological fluids using the differential and buoyant density centrifugation methods followed by ultrafiltration/size exclusion chromatography or flow cytometry or precipitation using polymers or antibodies to enrich the pure EVs population [177]. EVs play an important role in cell-to-cell communication and influence a variety of cellular functions, including cytokine production modulation, cell proliferation, apoptosis and metabolism, by transferring their protein, lipid or messenger RNA and micro RNA molecules [173,178]. EVs can be isolated both biological fluids (e.g., plasma/serum, urine, cerebrospinal fluid, saliva, etc.) and in vitro from cell-conditioned media. Moreover, as EVs are natural carriers of bioactive molecules, different research studies are addressing the therapeutic potential of EVs due to their specific genetic material packaging capabilities [175]. Several groups have identified EVs in maternal biofluids during normal and complication of pregnancies and the potential role of EV during pregnancy have been reviewed in details by our group previously [179–182].

10. Extracellular Vesicles/Exosomes in Normal and Preeclamptic Pregnancies

Different research studies utilized a variety of experimental models (i.e., biological fluids, primary placental trophoblasts, trophoblast cell line, placental explant, placental perfusate etc.) to isolate different subpopulations (exosomes, microvesicles) of EVs and studied their role in the context of healthy as well as in pathological pregnancies. Small and large EVs originating from the placenta have been identified in maternal plasma. Concentrations of both total and placenta-derived exosomes present in maternal circulation increase across gestation [183] and are higher in complicated pregnancies (such as those affected by PE) as compared to normal pregnancies [184,185]. Interestingly, the global miRNA profile within small vesicles such as exosomes differs between normal and PE pregnancies across gestation and it is likely that PE is not only associated with changes in the circulating levels of exosomes, but also in their miRNA content [186]. Recently, Biro et al. identified that hsa-miR-210 level increased in the circulating exosomes isolated from PE pregnancies [187]. Poor placentation is associated with hypoxia and oxidative stress, which are features of PE and affects the invasion of extravillous trophoblast (EVT) and the uterine spiral arterial remodeling. Truong et al. studied whether low oxygen tension alters exosome release and the exosomal miRNA profile from HTR-8/SVneo cell line and examined their interaction with endothelial cells [188]. HTR-8/SVneo cells are commonly used as a model for EVT cells, although they are not ideal, as they contain a heterogenous population of trophoblast and stromal cells [189]. In this study, low oxygen tension to exosomes from EVTs cultured under normoxic conditions. Moreover, a specific set of miRNAs within exosomes from EVTs cultured under hypoxia were identified, and these miRNAs are present in circulating exosomes at early gestation from women who develop PE later in pregnancy. This data suggests that aberrant extracellular vesicle signaling is one of the common factors in the development of PE. In normal healthy pregnancy, syncytiotrophoblast derived EVs release into the maternal blood stream where they act upon their target endothelial cells and circulating immune cells [33,190–192]. Placental EVs carry different proteins, lipids and nucleic acids that play a crucial role in feto-maternal communication to maintain pregnancy [193]. Interestingly, concentrations of large EVs gradually increase through pregnancy irrespective of their origin [186] and these EVs convey pro-inflammatory and pro-thrombotic antigens that might contribute to the hypercoagulable state observed in the last trimester of pregnancy [186]. Chang et al. identified that high levels of preeclamptic exosomes contain abundant sFlt-1 and sEng that can induce vascular dysfunction as these proteins were captured by vascular endothelial cells [194]. Tannetta et al. investigated the level of expression of placental protein 13 in syncytiotrophoblast derived extracellular vesicles (STBEVs) isolated from PE and normal pregnancy placental perfusate and found it was low in PE placenta [195]. Tong et al. described a novel mechanism by which placental EVs can attenuate PE pathogenesis in the presence of antiphospholipid antibody (aPL), which can induce the synthesis of toll-like receptors on placental EVs to increase the level of expression of mitochondrial DNA in these vesicles [196]. Thus, placenta-derived EVs are involved in gene regulation, placental homeostasis and cellular function that overall reflect the placental-maternal crosstalk [197]. Placental exosomes were also observed in fetal blood and their concentration correlated with fetal growth [198]. The concentration of placental exosomes in the fetal circulation was higher than that found in the maternal circulation and was also higher in pregnancies affected by PE [199]. Interestingly, not only the concentration of circulation exosomes in PE is different compared with normal pregnancies, and specific changes in the protein cargo of exosomes in PE have been identified [200].

Another recent study measured the level of different biomarkers including copeptin, annexin V and placental growth factor in maternal serum derived microparticles at 10–14 gestational weeks in women with PE and compared with that of normal healthy pregnancy [201]. Interestingly, the levels of nitric oxide synthase enzyme in the STBEVs were lower in STBEVs from PE compared to normal pregnancies [202]. In this regard, in a similar study, the levels of the protein neprilysin were increased in EVs of PE placenta [203].

Kohli et al. identified a novel pathway by which the placental EVs interact and causes release of EVs from endothelial cells and platelets that further activate the inflammasome in the trophoblast resulting in the development of PE [204]. The role of EVs in relation to PE pathophysiology including their different contents has been summarized in Table 2.

Table 2. Updated Research Studies on EVs in PE Pathophysiology.

EVs	Sample Type	Gestational Age	Isolation Method	Pregnancy Condition	Biological Process/Results	Reference
Maternal Blood Stream and other Body Fluids						
Trophoblast derived exosomal micro RNA (has-miR-210)	Plasma and HTR-8 cell culture conditioned media	Third trimester	Membrane affinity spin column method	Normal and PE	This micro RNA is responsible for PE pathogenesis	[187]
Exosomes	Plasma	Third trimester (before cesarean section)	Commercial kit (ExoQuick)	Normal and PE	Vascular dysfunction	[194]
Exosomal micro RNAs	Placental mesenchymal stem cells culture conditioned media and peripheral blood	During cesarean section delivery	Ultracentrifugation followed by Real Time PCR	Normal Pregnancy (NP) and PE	High level of exosomal miRNA-136, 494, 495 in PE	[205]
Urinary Exosomal proteins	Urine	After 20 weeks	Centrifugation	Healthy non-pregnant, Normal pregnancy, PE	Phosphorylation of renal tubular sodium transporter proteins that enhance sodium reabsorption in PE compared to NP	[206]
Exosomes	Human umbilical cord mesenchymal stem cells (MSC)	After delivery	Flow cytometry based detection of MSC surface markers	PE	Effect on placental tissue morphology and angiogenesis in rat PE placenta	[207,208]
Placental syncytiotrophoblast derived extracellular vesicles (STBEVs)	Placental perfusate	Following cesarean section delivery	Centrifugation	Normal and PE pregnancy	Lower level of placental protein 13 was found in STBEVs of PE placenta	[195]
Placental extracellular vesicles	Cultured human placental villi explant and Maternal serum	First trimester placenta	Sequential centrifugation and ultracentrifugation	Normal pregnancy	Presence of antiphospholipid antibody increases the level of mitochondrial DNA in the placental EVs and increases the risk to develop PE	[196]
Microparticles	Maternal serum	10–14 weeks	Centrifugation	Normal, PE, IUGR	Serum copeptin, annexin V were higher and placental growth factor was low in PE	[201]

Table 2. Cont.

EVs	Sample Type	Gestational Age	Isolation Method	Pregnancy Condition	Biological Process/Results	Reference
Macovesicles/placental debris	Placental explant and maternal serum	First trimester (8-10 weeks)	Centrifugation	PE	Melatonin is secreted from placental explant that reduce PE sera induced production of endothelial cell activating placental EVs	[209]
Nanovesicles	Placenta	First trimester and term placenta	Differential centrifugation	PE	Transthyretin is increased in amount and incorporated in placental nanovesicles	[210]
EVs	Urine	Maternal urine	EVs were stained for annexin, nephrin and podocin proteins	PE and Normotensive pregnant women	Nephrin protein was packaged in increased amount in urinary EVs of PE women	[211]
Syncytiotrophoblast derived extracellular vesicles (STBEV)	Placental perfusion and maternal plasma	Gestational age matched	Differential centrifugation	Normal and PE	Less nitric oxide synthase in STBEVs of PE women	[202]
EVs	Placental explant	First and second trimester	Sequential centrifugation	Normal and PE	Endothelial dysfunction in severe early onset PE is via soluble angiogenic factors, not by EVs	[212]
Exosomes	Maternal plasma	First, second and third trimester	Differential centrifugation, ultracentrifugation followed by density gradient centrifugation	Normal and PE	The concentration of exosomes is higher and miRNA content is different in PE compared to normal pregnancy	[184]
Microparticles	Placental trophoblasts	At term (>37 weeks)	Two-step centrifugation	Uncomplicated and preeclamptic	Increase MP shedding from PE placenta; upregulation of caveolin-1 and downregulation of eNOS in these MPs which is modulated by vitamin-D	[213]
EVs	Endothelial cells and Platelets	Not mentioned	Differential centrifugation	Normal and PE	Inflammasome activation in placental trophoblasts results in PE development	[204]

Table 2. Cont.

EVs	Sample Type	Gestational Age	Isolation Method	Pregnancy Condition	Biological Process/Results	Reference
Fetal Circulation						
Exosomes	Umbilical cord blood	At delivery	Differential Centrifugation + Density gradient centrifugation	Normal	No difference in concentration of exosomes in term, small for gestational age, fetal growth restricted neonates	[198]
Microparticle (MPs)	Umbilical cord blood	At delivery	MPs were identified by size and annexin V fluorescein isothiocyanate (FITC) labelling	Normal and PE	MP levels is higher compared to maternal blood in PE	[199]
Exosomes	Umbilical cord blood	At delivery	Differential centrifugation + Filtration	Normal and PE	Altered protein expression profile that are involved with PE etiology	[200]

A number of drugs that can be used to treat PE appear to modulate EV expression. Some studies also addressed the mode of action of different antihypertensives, including thiazide diuretics that are used to treat the hypertension in PE. Hu et al. identified some changes in the sodium transporters in the renal tubule that were incorporated in the urinary exosomes isolated from PE women [206]. Another very interesting study by Chamley L. et al. identified melatonin as an effective agent that can reduce the endothelial cell activating placental EVs release in PE [209]. In a similar study, transthyretin which is the thyroxin binding protein, was found in aggregated form and packaged in the small placental EVs in PE [210]. Xu et al. identified potential molecular mechanisms by which vitamin-D can reduce oxidative-stress induced PE [213]. Among the different therapeutic agents, the efficacy of aspirin was evaluated due to its availability and cost-effectiveness. However, there is lack of understanding in the mechanism of action of aspirin in the context of EV secretion regulation.

11. Effects of LDA on Exosomal Secretion

Up until now, there has been very limited evidence on the potential effect of aspirin on the release and content of EVs. Goetzl E.J. et al., discovered that in the presence of some coagulation factors (e.g., thrombin/ collagen) induces changes in the plasmatic levels of platelet-derived exosomes and their protein content (i.e., α-granule chemokines CXCL4 and CXCL7 and cytoplasmic high-mobility group box 1 (HMGB1)) [214]. Incubation of normal platelets with aspirin significantly inhibits arachidonic acid (AA)-induced platelet reactivity, EV formation and pro-coagulant activity [215]. Interestingly, aspirin therapy can significantly reduce microparticle (MP) shredding from erythrocytes, monocytes and vascular smooth muscle cells, reversing the effects of diabetes-induced stress on these cells [216]. Other studies have identified that aspirin changes the miRNA profile and EV release from platelet [217]. Syncytiotropholast-derived extracellular vesicles that are placental alkaline phosphatase (PLAP) positive inhibit the aggregation of platelets that were treated with aspirin [218]. Tannetta et al. observed that STBEV that are placental alkaline phosphatase (PLAP) positive inhibit the aggregation of platelets that were treated with aspirin [218]. On the contrary, platelets were activated and thrombus formation was increased by the STBEV isolated from preeclamptic placentas. Another study observed the effect of anticoagulant therapy (treatment with either unfractionated heparin (UFH) or low molecular weight heparin (LMWH), and/or LDA) on cell derived microparticles and outcome of pregnancy [219]. These findings indicate that placenta-derived extracellular vesicles may provide understanding in their potential role in low dose aspirin induced placental functions. Although there is significant evidence for dysregulation of both concentrations and bioactivity of circulating placental EVs in PE compared to normal pregnancies, no studies have described the potential effect of aspirin on EVs released from placental cells and their bioactivity.

12. Summary

Several studies focused on EVs (mainly small EVs called exosomes) highlighting their extraordinary characteristics as natural carriers of bioactive molecules, which can be used as biomarker for several pathological conditions including PE. These vesicles are unique in terms of their cell trafficking and transfecting capabilities. These nanovesicles are released from almost all types of cells into different human body fluids. Their release and contents are dependent on the microenvironment where the cells are exposed and the origin of the cells [172]. Therefore, EVs can be used as a diagnostic tool as well as prognostic marker for several pathologies, and we have proposed that the analysis of placental vesicles in maternal plasma can function as a liquid biopsy to establish placental function during pregnancy. During pregnancy, placenta and other cells, such as platelets and immune cells, secrete exosomes into the maternal circulation; this process is exaggerated in pathological pregnancies (i.e., PE, PIH, IUGR) in an attempt to modulate the pathology [43,190,191]. Very few studies [218,219] have been conducted to identify the particular mechanism of action that exosomes can produce on the placenta and overall maternal physiological system when treated with low dose aspirin and other antithrombotic medication. An avenue is open to explore the placental and other cell derived exosomal functions in placental dysfunctional disorders when treated with antithrombotic medications including low dose aspirin. A better understanding of these processes may lead to the development of novel prognostic markers utilizing placenta specific exosomes or for monitoring the response to aspirin treatment for placental pathologies.

Funding: Carlos Salomon is supported by The Lions Medical Research Foundation, National Health and Medical Research Council (NHMRC; 1114013) and the Fondo Nacional de Desarrollo Científico y Tecnológico (FONDECYT 1170809). Suchismita Dutta received the Australian postgraduate award scholarship.

Conflicts of Interest: The authors declare no conflict of interest.

References

1. Mendes, S. New Insights into the Process of Placentation and the Role of Oxidative Uterine Microenvironment. *Oxid. Med. Cell. Longev.* **2019**, *2019*, 9174521. [CrossRef]
2. Solano, M.E. Decidual immune cells: Guardians of human pregnancies. *Best Pr. Res. Clin. Obs. Gynaecol.* **2019**. [CrossRef]
3. Burton, G.J. Pre-eclampsia: Pathophysiology and clinical implications. *BMJ* **2019**, *366*, 12381. [CrossRef]
4. Bose, P. Heparin and aspirin attenuate placental apoptosis in vitro: Implications for early pregnancy failure. *Am. J. Obstet. Gynecol.* **2005**, *192*, 23–30. [CrossRef]
5. Panagodage, S. Low-Dose Acetylsalicylic Acid Treatment Modulates the Production of Cytokines and Improves Trophoblast Function in an in Vitro Model of Early-Onset Preeclampsia. *Am. J. Pathol.* **2016**, *186*, 3217–3224. [CrossRef]
6. Villa, P.M.; Kajantie, E.; Laivuori, H. Acetylsalicylic acid and prevention of preeclampsia. *Duodecim* **2014**, *130*, 243–250.
7. Oyola, S.; Kirley, K. Another good reason to recommend Low-Dose Aspirin. *J. Fam. Pract.* **2015**, *64*, 301–303.
8. Yao, S.; Wu, H.; Yu, Y. Early intervention with aspirin for preventing preeclampsia in high-risk women: A meta-analysis. *Nan Fang Yi Ke Da Xue Xue Bao* **2015**, *35*, 868–873.
9. Andreoli, L.; Bertsias, G.K.; Agmon-Levin, N.; Brown, S.; Cervera, R.; Costedoat-Chalumeau, N.; Doria, A.; Fischer-Betz, R.; Forger, F.; Moraes-Fontes, M.F.; et al. EULAR recommendations for women's health and the management of family planning, assisted reproduction, pregnancy and menopause in patients with systemic lupus erythematosus and/or antiphospholipid syndrome. *Ann. Rheum. Dis.* **2016**, *76*, 476–485. [CrossRef]
10. Wang, L. Efficacy evaluation of low-dose aspirin in IVF/ICSI patients evidence from 13 RCTs: A systematic review and meta-analysis. *Medicine (Baltimore)* **2017**, *96*, e7720. [CrossRef]
11. Bujold, E. Prevention of preeclampsia and intrauterine growth restriction with aspirin started in early pregnancy: A meta-analysis. *Obstet. Gynecol.* **2010**, *116*, 402–414. [CrossRef]
12. Villa, P.M. Aspirin in the prevention of pre-eclampsia in high-risk women: A randomised placebo-controlled PREDO Trial and a meta-analysis of randomised trials. *Bjog* **2013**, *120*, 64–74. [CrossRef]
13. Fantasia, H.C. Low-Dose Aspirin for the Prevention of Preeclampsia. *Nurs. Womens Health* **2018**, *22*, 87–92. [CrossRef]
14. Roberge, S. Early administration of low-dose aspirin for the prevention of severe and mild preeclampsia: A systematic review and meta-analysis. *Am. J. Perinatol.* **2012**, *29*, 551–556. [CrossRef]
15. Xu, T.T.; Zhou, F.; Deng, C.Y.; Huang, G.Q.; Li, J.K.; Wang, X.D. Low-Dose Aspirin for Preventing Preeclampsia and Its Complications: A Meta-Analysis. *J. Clin. Hypertens (Greenwich)* **2015**, *17*, 567–573. [CrossRef]
16. Ahrens, K.A. Complications and Safety of Preconception Low-Dose Aspirin Among Women WITH Prior Pregnancy Losses. *Obstet. Gynecol.* **2016**, *127*, 689–698. [CrossRef]
17. Cronqvist, T. Syncytiotrophoblast derived extracellular vesicles transfer functional placental miRNAs to primary human endothelial cells. *Sci. Rep.* **2017**, *7*, 4558. [CrossRef]
18. Holcberg, G. Implantation, Physiology of Placentation. In *Recurrent Pregnancy Loss*; Springer International Publishing: Basel, Switzerland, 2016.
19. Haller-Kikkatalo, K. Autoimmune activation toward embryo implantation is rare in immune-privileged human endometrium. *Semin. Reprod. Med.* **2014**, *32*, 376–384. [CrossRef]
20. Moser, G.; Huppertz, B. Implantation and extravillous trophoblast invasion: From rare archival specimens to modern biobanking. *Placenta* **2017**, *56*, 19–26. [CrossRef]

21. Sato, Y.; Fujiwara, H.; Konishi, I. Role of platelets in placentation. *Med. Mol. Morphol.* **2010**, *43*, 129–133. [CrossRef]
22. Zhao, S. Predominant basal directional release of thromboxane, but not prostacyclin, by placental trophoblasts from normal and preeclamptic pregnancies. *Placenta* **2008**, *29*, 81–88. [CrossRef]
23. Mierzynski, R. Anticoagulant therapy in pregnant patients with metabolic syndrome: A review. *Curr. Pharm. Biotechnol.* **2014**, *15*, 47–63. [CrossRef]
24. Graves, J.C.; Miller, K.E.; Sellers, A.D. Maternal serum triple analyte screening in pregnancy. *Am. Fam. Physician* **2002**, *65*, 915–920.
25. Maternal Serum Marker Screening. In *Understanding Genetics*; Genetic Alliance: Washington, DC, USA, 2010.
26. Nwanodi, O.B. Preeclampsia-Eclampsia Adverse Outcomes Reduction: The Preeclampsia-Eclampsia Checklist. *Healthcare* **2016**, *4*, 26. [CrossRef]
27. Helou, A. Management of pregnancies complicated by hypertensive disorders of pregnancy: Could we do better? *Aust. N. Z. J. Obstet. Gynaecol.* **2016**, *57*, 253–269. [CrossRef]
28. Pai, C.H. Lack of Thromboxane Synthase Prevents Hypertension and Fetal Growth Restriction after High Salt Treatment during Pregnancy. *PLoS ONE* **2016**, *11*, e0151617. [CrossRef]
29. Bakhti, A.; Vaiman, D. Prevention of gravidic endothelial hypertension by aspirin treatment administered from the 8th week of gestation. *Hypertens Res.* **2011**, *34*, 1116–1120. [CrossRef]
30. Bartsch, E. Clinical risk factors for pre-eclampsia determined in early pregnancy: Systematic review and meta-analysis of large cohort studies. *BMJ* **2016**, *353*, 1753. [CrossRef]
31. Nicolaides, K.H. A model for a new pyramid of prenatal care based on the 11 to 13 weeks' assessment. *Prenat. Diagn.* **2011**, *31*, 3–6. [CrossRef]
32. McCoy, S.; Baldwin, K. Pharmacotherapeutic options for the treatment of preeclampsia. *Am. J. Health Syst. Pharm.* **2009**, *66*, 337–344. [CrossRef]
33. Gilani, S.I. Preeclampsia and Extracellular Vesicles. *Curr. Hypertens. Rep.* **2016**, *18*, 1–11. [CrossRef]
34. Burton, G.J. Rheological and physiological consequences of conversion of the maternal spiral arteries for uteroplacental blood flow during human pregnancy. *Placenta* **2009**, *30*, 473–482. [CrossRef]
35. Friedman, A.M.; Cleary, K.L. Prediction and prevention of ischemic placental disease. *Semin. Perinatol.* **2014**, *38*, 177–182. [CrossRef]
36. Cuckle, H.; von Dadelszen, P.; Ghidini, A. Current controversies in prenatal diagnosis 4: Pregnancy complications due to placental vascular disease (pre-eclampsia, FGR): Are we ready for prevention? *Prenat. Diagn.* **2013**, *33*, 17–20. [CrossRef]
37. Armant, D.R. Human trophoblast survival at low oxygen concentrations requires metalloproteinase-mediated shedding of heparin-binding EGF-like growth factor. *Development* **2006**, *133*, 751–759. [CrossRef]
38. Redman, C.W.; Sargent, I.L. Placental stress and pre-eclampsia: A revised view. *Placenta* **2009**, *30*, S38–S42. [CrossRef]
39. Blumenstein, M. A proteomic approach identifies early pregnancy biomarkers for preeclampsia: Novel linkages between a predisposition to preeclampsia and cardiovascular disease. *Proteomics* **2009**, *9*, 2929–2945. [CrossRef]
40. Auer, J. Serum profile in preeclampsia and intra-uterine growth restriction revealed by iTRAQ technology. *J. Proteom.* **2010**, *73*, 1004–1017. [CrossRef]
41. Chelbi, S.T. Expressional and epigenetic alterations of placental serine protease inhibitors: SERPINA3 is a potential marker of preeclampsia. *Hypertension* **2007**, *49*, 76–83. [CrossRef]
42. Larsen, T.G. Fetal human leukocyte antigen-C and maternal killer-cell immunoglobulin-like receptors in cases of severe preeclampsia. *Placenta* **2019**, *75*, 27–33. [CrossRef]
43. Redman, C.W.; Sargent, I.L. Placental debris, oxidative stress and pre-eclampsia. *Placenta* **2000**, *21*, 597–602. [CrossRef]
44. Furuya, M. Pathophysiology of placentation abnormalities in pregnancy-induced hypertension. *Vasc. Health Risk Manag.* **2008**, *4*, 1301–1313. [CrossRef]
45. Granger, J.P. Pathophysiology of preeclampsia: Linking placental ischemia/hypoxia with microvascular dysfunction. *Microcirculation* **2002**, *9*, 147–160. [CrossRef]
46. Lyall, F.; Myatt, L. The role of the placenta in pre-eclampsia–a workshop report. *Placenta* **2002**, *23*, 142–145. [CrossRef]

47. Lockwood, C.J. Preeclampsia-related inflammatory cytokines regulate interleukin-6 expression in human decidual cells. *Am. J. Pathol.* **2008**, *172*, 1571–1579. [CrossRef]
48. Benyo, D.F. Expression of inflammatory cytokines in placentas from women with preeclampsia. *J. Clin. Endocrinol. Metab.* **2001**, *86*, 2505–2512.
49. Raghupathy, R. Cytokines as key players in the pathophysiology of preeclampsia. *Med. Princ. Pr.* **2013**, *22*, 8–19. [CrossRef]
50. Vaughan, J.E.; Walsh, S.W.; Ford, G.D. Thromboxane mediates neutrophil superoxide production in pregnancy. *Am. J. Obstet. Gynecol.* **2006**, *195*, 1415–1420. [CrossRef]
51. Walsh, S.W. Eicosanoids in preeclampsia. *Prostaglandins Leukot. Essent. Fat. Acids* **2004**, *70*, 223–232. [CrossRef]
52. Walsh, S.W. Preeclampsia: An imbalance in placental prostacyclin and thromboxane Production. *Am. J. Obstet. Gynecol.* **1985**, *152*, 335–340. [CrossRef]
53. Reslan, O.M.; Khalil, R.A. Molecular and vascular targets in the pathogenesis and management of the hypertension associated with preeclampsia. *Cardiovasc. Hematol. Agents Med. Chem.* **2010**, *8*, 204–226. [CrossRef]
54. Yusuf, K. Thromboxane A2 Limits Differentiation and Enhances Apoptosis of Cultured Human Trophoblasts. *Pediatr. Res.* **2001**, *50*, 203–209. [CrossRef]
55. Ally, A.I.; Horrobin, D.F. Thromboxane A2 in blood vessel walls and its physiological significance: Relevance to thrombosis and hypertension. *Prostaglandins Med.* **1980**, *4*, 431–438. [CrossRef]
56. Sellers, M.M.; Stallone, J.N. Sympathy for the devil: The role of thromboxane in the regulation of vascular tone and blood pressure. *Am. J. Physiol. Heart Circ. Physiol.* **2008**, *294*, H1978–H1986. [CrossRef]
57. Gilbert, J.S. Pathophysiology of hypertension during preeclampsia: Linking placental ischemia with endothelial dysfunction. *Am. J. Physiol. Heart Circ. Physiol.* **2008**, *294*, H541–H550. [CrossRef]
58. Downing, J.W. Hypothesis: Selective phosphodiesterase-5 inhibition improves outcome in preeclampsia. *Med. Hypotheses* **2004**, *63*, 1057–1064. [CrossRef]
59. Euser, A.G. Low-dose aspirin for pre-eclampsia prevention in twins with elevated human chorionic gonadotropin. *J. Perinatol.* **2016**, *36*, 601–605. [CrossRef]
60. Di Simone, N. Pathogenic role of anti-beta2-glycoprotein I antibodies on human placenta: Functional effects related to implantation and roles of heparin. *Hum. Reprod. Update* **2007**, *13*, 189–196. [CrossRef]
61. Anderson, U.D. First trimester prediction of preeclampsia. *Curr. Hypertens Rep.* **2015**, *17*, 584. [CrossRef]
62. Meiri, H. Prediction of preeclampsia by placental protein 13 and background risk factors and its prevention by aspirin. *J. Perinat. Med.* **2014**, *42*, 591–601. [CrossRef]
63. Seravalli, V. Relationship between first-trimester serum placental protein-13 and maternal characteristics, placental Doppler studies and pregnancy outcome. *J. Perinat. Med.* **2016**, *44*, 543–549. [CrossRef]
64. Rolnik, D.L. Maternal plasma cell-free DNA in the prediction of pre-eclampsia. *Ultrasound Obstet Gynecol.* **2015**, *45*, 106–111. [CrossRef]
65. Schrör, K. Acetylsalicylic Acid. In *Acetylsalicylic Acid*; John Wiley and Sons: Weinheim, Germany, 2010.
66. Cadavid, A.P. Aspirin: The Mechanism of Action Revisited in the Context of Pregnancy Complications. *Front. Immunol.* **2017**, *8*, 261.
67. Lafont, O. From the willow to aspirin. *Rev. Hist. Pharm. (Paris)* **2007**, *55*, 209–216. [CrossRef]
68. Botting, R.M. Vane's discovery of the mechanism of action of aspirin changed our understanding of its clinical pharmacology. *Pharm. Rep.* **2010**, *62*, 518–525. [CrossRef]
69. West, G.B. Aspirin and the prostaglandins. *Chem. Drug* **1972**, *198*, 196–197.
70. Finkel, R.M.A.C.; Luigi, X. (Eds.) *Antiinflammatory Drugs and Autacoids in Lippincott's Illustrated Reviews: Pharmacology*, 4th ed.; Lippincott Williams & Wilkins: Philadelphia, PA, USA, 2009; p. 499.
71. Walsh, S.W. Low-dose aspirin: Treatment for the imbalance of increased thromboxane and decreased prostacyclin in preeclampsia. *Am. J. Perinatol.* **1989**, *6*, 124–132. [CrossRef]
72. Perneby, C. Thromboxane Metab. Excretion Dur. Pregnancy–Influ. Preeclampsia Aspirin Treat. *Thromb. Res.* **2011**, *127*, 605–606. [CrossRef]
73. Sibai, B.M. Low-dose aspirin in pregnancy. *Obstet. Gynecol.* **1989**, *74*, 551–557. [CrossRef]
74. Li, C. Aspirin inhibits expression of sFLT1 from human cytotrophoblasts induced by hypoxia, via cyclo-oxygenase 1. *Placenta* **2015**, *36*, 446–453. [CrossRef]

75. Da Silva Costa, F. 274: Low-dose aspirin improves trophoblastic function in early-onset pre-eclampsia. *Am. J. Obstet. Gynecol.* **2014**, *210*, S145. [CrossRef]
76. Gil-Villa, A.M. Aspirin triggered-lipoxin A4 reduces the adhesion of human polymorphonuclear neutrophils to endothelial cells initiated by preeclamptic plasma. *Prostaglandins Leukot. Essent. Fat. Acids* **2012**, *87*, 127–134. [CrossRef]
77. Sentilhes, L.; Azria, E.; Schmitz, T. Aspirin versus Placebo in Pregnancies at High Risk for Preterm Preeclampsia. *N. Engl. J. Med.* **2017**, *377*, 2399–2400.
78. Navaratnam, K.; Alfirevic, A.; Alfirevic, Z. Low dose aspirin and pregnancy: How important is aspirin resistance? *Bjog* **2016**, *123*, 1481–1487. [CrossRef]
79. Bujold, E. Low-dose aspirin reduces morbidity and mortality in pregnant women at high-risk for preeclampsia. *Evid. Based Nurs.* **2015**, *18*, 71. [CrossRef]
80. Sibai, B.M. Therapy: Low-dose aspirin to reduce the risk of pre-eclampsia? *Nat. Rev. Endocrinol.* **2015**, *11*, 6–8. [CrossRef]
81. Henderson, J.T.; Whitlock, E.P.; O'Connor, E. Low-dose aspirin for prevention of morbidity and mortality from preeclampsia. *Ann. Intern. Med.* **2014**, *160*, 695–703. [CrossRef]
82. Roberge, S.; Demers, S.; Bujold, E. Low-dose aspirin for prevention of morbidity and mortality from preeclampsia. *Ann. Intern. Med.* **2014**, *161*, 613. [CrossRef]
83. Bartsch, E. Risk threshold for starting low dose aspirin in pregnancy to prevent preeclampsia: An opportunity at a low cost. *PLoS ONE* **2015**, *10*, e0116296. [CrossRef]
84. Toyoda, K. Antithrombotic therapy for pregnant women. *Neurol. Med. Chir. (Tokyo)* **2013**, *53*, 526–530. [CrossRef]
85. Yurdakok, M. Fetal and neonatal effects of anticoagulants used in pregnancy: A review. *Turk. J. Pediatr.* **2012**, *54*, 207–215.
86. Askie, L.M. Antiplatelet agents for prevention of pre-eclampsia: A meta-analysis of individual patient data. *Lancet* **2007**, *369*, 1791–1798. [CrossRef]
87. Roberge, S. The role of aspirin dose on the prevention of preeclampsia and fetal growth restriction: Systematic review and meta-analysis. *Am. J. Obstet. Gynecol.* **2017**, *216*, 110–120. [CrossRef]
88. Summaries for patients: Aspirin to prevent preeclampsia-related complications and death: U.S. Preventive Services Task Force recommendation statement. *Ann. Intern. Med.* **2014**, *161*, I28. [CrossRef]
89. Roberge, S.; Demers, S.; Bujold, E. Initiation of aspirin in early gestation for the prevention of pre-eclampsia. *Bjog* **2013**, *120*, 773–774. [CrossRef]
90. Ortved, D. Cost-effectiveness of first-trimester screening with early preventative use of aspirin in women at high risk of early-onset pre-eclampsia. *Ultrasound Obstet. Gynecol.* **2019**, *53*, 239–244. [CrossRef]
91. LeFevre, M.L. Low-dose aspirin use for the prevention of morbidity and mortality from preeclampsia: U.S. Preventive Services Task Force recommendation statement. *Ann. Intern. Med.* **2014**, *161*, 819–826. [CrossRef]
92. Bond, S. US Preventive Services Task Force guideline supports low-dose aspirin for prevention of preeclampsia. *J. Midwifery Womens Health* **2015**, *60*, 222–223. [CrossRef]
93. Sidaway, P. Pre-eclampsia: Low-dose aspirin for pre-eclampsia. *Nat. Rev. Nephrol.* **2014**, *10*, 613.
94. Voelker, R. USPSTF: Low-dose aspirin may help reduce risk of preeclampsia. *JAMA* **2014**, *311*, 2055. [CrossRef]
95. Ayala, D.E.; Ucieda, R.; Hermida, R.C. Chronotherapy with low-dose aspirin for prevention of complications in pregnancy. *Chronobiol. Int.* **2013**, *30*, 260–279. [CrossRef]
96. Mutlu, I. Effects of anticoagulant therapy on pregnancy outcomes in patients with thrombophilia and previous poor obstetric history. *Blood Coagul. Fibrinolysis* **2015**, *26*, 267–273. [CrossRef]
97. Dodd, J.M. Antithrombotic therapy for improving maternal or infant health outcomes in women considered at risk of placental dysfunction. *Cochrane Database Syst. Rev.* **2013**, *24*, Cd006780. [CrossRef]
98. Chauleur, C. News on antithrombotic therapy and pregnancy. *Therapie* **2011**, *66*, 437–443. [CrossRef]
99. De Vries, J.I. Low-molecular-weight heparin added to aspirin in the prevention of recurrent early-onset pre-eclampsia in women with inheritable thrombophilia: The FRUIT-RCT. *J. Thromb. Haemost.* **2012**, *10*, 64–72. [CrossRef]
100. Gris, J.C. Addition of enoxaparin to aspirin for the secondary prevention of placental vascular complications in women with severe pre-eclampsia. The pilot randomised controlled NOH-PE trial. *Thromb. Haemost.* **2011**, *106*, 1053–1061.

101. Rodger, M.A. Low-molecular-weight heparin and recurrent placenta-mediated pregnancy complications: A meta-analysis of individual patient data from randomised controlled trials. *Lancet* **2016**, *388*, 2629–2641. [CrossRef]
102. Souza, E.V. Aspirin plus calcium supplementation to prevent superimposed preeclampsia: A randomized trial. *Braz. J. Med. Biol. Res.* **2014**, *47*, 419–425. [CrossRef]
103. Browne, J.L. Prevention of Hypertensive Disorders of Pregnancy: A Novel Application of the Polypill Concept. *Curr. Cardiol. Rep.* **2016**, *18*, 1–11. [CrossRef]
104. Grandone, E.; Villani, M.; Tiscia, G.L. Aspirin and heparin in pregnancy. *Expert Opin. Pharm.* **2015**, *16*, 1793–1803. [CrossRef]
105. Ghesquiere, L. Can we prevent preeclampsia? *Presse. Med.* **2016**, *45*, 403–413.
106. Kane, S.C.; Da Silva Costa, F.; Brennecke, S.P. New directions in the prediction of pre-eclampsia. *Aust. N. Z. J. Obstet. Gynaecol.* **2014**, *54*, 101–107. [CrossRef]
107. Jiang, N. The effect of calcium channel blockers on prevention of preeclampsia in pregnant women with chronic hypertension. *Clin. Exp. Obstet. Gynecol.* **2015**, *42*, 79–81.
108. Neykova, K. Antithrombotic Medication in Pregnant Women with Previous Intrauterine Growth Restriction. *Akush Ginekol. (Sofiia)* **2016**, *55*, 3–9.
109. Maged, A.M. The role of prophylactic use of low dose aspirin and calheparin in patients with unexplained recurrent abortion. *Gynecol. Endocrinol.* **2016**, *32*, 970–972. [CrossRef]
110. Gan, J.; He, H.; Qi, H. Preventing preeclampsia and its fetal complications with low-dose aspirin in East Asians and non-East Asians: A systematic review and meta-analysis. *Hypertens Pregnancy* **2016**, *35*, 426–435. [CrossRef]
111. Tong, S.; Mol, B.W.; Walker, S.P. Preventing preeclampsia with aspirin: Does dose or timing matter? *Am. J. Obstet. Gynecol.* **2017**, *216*, 95–97. [CrossRef]
112. Mone, F. Should we recommend universal aspirin for all pregnant women? *Am. J. Obstet. Gynecol.* **2017**, *216*, e1–e141. [CrossRef]
113. Meher, S. Antiplatelet therapy before or after 16 weeks' gestation for preventing preeclampsia: An individual participant data meta-analysis. *Am. J. Obstet. Gynecol.* **2017**, *216*, 121–128. [CrossRef]
114. Roberge, S. Prevention of perinatal death and adverse perinatal outcome using low-dose aspirin: A meta-analysis. *Ultrasound Obstet. Gynecol.* **2013**, *41*, 491–499. [CrossRef]
115. O'Gorman, N. Study protocol for the randomised controlled trial: Combined multimarker screening and randomised patient treatment with ASpirin for evidence-based PREeclampsia prevention (ASPRE). *BMJ Open* **2016**, *6*, e011801. [CrossRef]
116. Etwel, F.; Koren, G. When positive studies of novel therapies are subsequently nullified: Cumulative meta-analyses in preeclampsia. *Clin. Investig. Med.* **2015**, *38*, 274–283. [CrossRef]
117. Truong, A. Subchorionic hematomas are increased in early pregnancy in women taking low-dose aspirin. *Fertil. Steril.* **2016**, *105*, 1241–1246. [CrossRef]
118. Van Hoorn, M.E. Low-molecular-weight heparin and aspirin in the prevention of recurrent early-onset pre-eclampsia in women with antiphospholipid antibodies: The FRUIT-RCT. *Eur. J. Obstet. Gynecol. Reprod. Biol.* **2016**, *197*, 168–173. [CrossRef]
119. Hoffman, M.K. A description of the methods of the aspirin supplementation for pregnancy indicated risk reduction in nulliparas (ASPIRIN) study. *BMC Pregnancy Childbirth* **2017**, *17*, 135. [CrossRef]
120. Mumford, S.L. Expanded findings from a randomized controlled trial of preconception low-dose aspirin and pregnancy loss. *Hum. Reprod.* **2016**, *31*, 657–665. [CrossRef]
121. Rolnik, D.L.; Wright, D.; Poon, L.C.; O'Gorman, N.; Syngelaki, A.; de Paco Matallana, C.; Akolekar, R.; Cicero, S.; Janga, D.; Singh, M.; et al. Aspirin versus Placebo in Pregnancies at High Risk for Preterm Preeclampsia. *N. Engl. J. Med.* **2017**, *377*, 613–622. [CrossRef]
122. Orendi, K. Effects of vitamins C and E, acetylsalicylic acid and heparin on fusion, beta-hCG and PP13 expression in BeWo cells. *Placenta* **2010**, *31*, 431–438. [CrossRef]
123. Rigourd, V. Re-evaluation of the role of STOX1 transcription factor in placental development and preeclampsia. *J. Reprod. Immunol.* **2009**, *82*, 174–181. [CrossRef]
124. Benigni, A. Effect of low-dose aspirin on fetal and maternal generation of thromboxane by platelets in women at risk for pregnancy-induced hypertension. *N. Engl. J. Med.* **1989**, *321*, 357–362. [CrossRef]

125. Schiff, E. The use of aspirin to prevent pregnancy-induced hypertension and lower the ratio of thromboxane A2 to prostacyclin in relatively high risk pregnancies. *N. Engl. J. Med.* **1989**, *321*, 351–356. [CrossRef]
126. Sibai, B.M. Prevention of preeclampsia with low-dose aspirin in healthy, nulliparous pregnant women. The National Institute of Child Health and Human Development Network of Maternal-Fetal Medicine Units. *N. Engl. J. Med.* **1993**, *329*, 1213–1218. [CrossRef]
127. Knight, M. Antiplatelet agents for preventing and treating pre-eclampsia. *Cochrane Database Syst. Rev.* **2000**, Cd000492. [CrossRef]
128. Woodworth, S.H. Eicosanoid biosynthetic enzymes in placental and decidual tissues from preeclamptic pregnancies: Increased expression of thromboxane-A2 synthase gene. *J. Clin. Endocrinol. Metab.* **1994**, *78*, 1225–1231.
129. Katsi, V. Aspirin vs Heparin for the Prevention of Preeclampsia. *Curr. Hypertens Rep.* **2016**, *18*, 57. [CrossRef]
130. Pijnenborg, R. Trophoblastic invasion of human decidua from 8 to 18 weeks of pregnancy. *Placenta* **1980**, *1*, 3–19. [CrossRef]
131. Brosens, I. The "Great Obstetrical Syndromes" are associated with disorders of deep placentation. *Am. J. Obstet. Gynecol.* **2011**, *204*, 193–201. [CrossRef]
132. Jamal, A.; Milani, F.; Al-Yasin, A. Evaluation of the effect of metformin and aspirin on utero placental circulation of pregnant women with PCOS. *Iran. J. Reprod. Med.* **2012**, *10*, 265–270.
133. Turan, O. 284: Starting aspirin (ASA) in the first trimester (T1) promotes placental invasion in low-risk pregnancy. *Am. J. Obstet. Gynecol.* **2014**, *210*, S149–S150. [CrossRef]
134. Haapsamo, M.; Martikainen, H.; Rasanen, J. Low-dose aspirin reduces uteroplacental vascular impedance in early and mid gestation in IVF and ICSI patients: A randomized, placebo-controlled double-blind study. *Ultrasound Obstet. Gynecol.* **2008**, *32*, 687–693. [CrossRef]
135. Serhan, C.N.; Yacoubian, S.; Yang, R. Anti-inflammatory and proresolving lipid mediators. *Annu. Rev. Pathol.* **2008**, *3*, 279–312. [CrossRef]
136. Nascimento-Silva, V. Aspirin-triggered lipoxin A4 blocks reactive oxygen species generation in endothelial cells: A novel antioxidative mechanism. *Thromb. Haemost.* **2007**, *97*, 88–98.
137. Cezar-de-Mello, P.F. ATL-1, an analogue of aspirin-triggered lipoxin A4, is a potent inhibitor of several steps in angiogenesis induced by vascular endothelial growth factor. *Br. J. Pharmcol.* **2008**, *153*, 956–965. [CrossRef]
138. Fiorucci, S. Evidence that 5-lipoxygenase and acetylated cyclooxygenase 2-derived eicosanoids regulate leukocyte-endothelial adherence in response to aspirin. *Br. J. Pharmacol.* **2003**, *139*, 1351–1359. [CrossRef]
139. Morris, T. Effects of low-dose aspirin on acute inflammatory responses in humans. *J. Immunol.* **2009**, *183*, 2089–2096. [CrossRef]
140. Morris, T. Dichotomy in duration and severity of acute inflammatory responses in humans arising from differentially expressed proresolution pathways. *Proc. Natl. Acad. Sci. USA* **2010**, *107*, 8842–8847. [CrossRef]
141. Jozsef, L. Lipoxin A4 and aspirin-triggered 15-epi-lipoxin A4 inhibit peroxynitrite formation, NF-kappa B and AP-1 activation, and IL-8 gene expression in human leukocytes. *Proc. Natl. Acad. Sci. USA* **2002**, *99*, 13266–13271. [CrossRef]
142. Ariel, A. Aspirin-triggered lipoxin A4 and B4 analogs block extracellular signal-regulated kinase-dependent TNF-alpha secretion from human T cells. *J. Immunol.* **2003**, *170*, 6266–6272. [CrossRef]
143. Levy, B.D. Lipid mediator class switching during acute inflammation: Signals in resolution. *Nat. Immunol.* **2001**, *2*, 612–619. [CrossRef]
144. Nascimento-Silva, V. Novel lipid mediator aspirin-triggered lipoxin A4 induces heme oxygenase-1 in endothelial cells. *Am. J. Physiol. Cell Physiol.* **2005**, *289*, C557–C563. [CrossRef]
145. Kim, J. Aspirin prevents TNF-alpha-induced endothelial cell dysfunction by regulating the NF-kappaB-dependent miR-155/eNOS pathway: Role of a miR-155/eNOS axis in preeclampsia. *Free Radic. Biol. Med.* **2017**, *104*, 185–198. [CrossRef]
146. Van Dijk, M. The STOX1 genotype associated with pre-eclampsia leads to a reduction of trophoblast invasion by alpha-T-catenin upregulation. *Hum. Mol. Genet.* **2010**, *19*, 2658–2667. [CrossRef]
147. Van Dijk, M.; Drewlo, S.; Oudejans, C.B.M. Differential methylation of STOX1 in human placenta. *Epigenetics* **2010**, *5*, 736–742. [CrossRef]
148. Fenstad, M.H. STOX2 but not STOX1 is differentially expressed in decidua from pre-eclamptic women: Data from the Second Nord-Trondelag Health Study. *Mol. Hum. Reprod.* **2010**, *16*, 960–968. [CrossRef]

149. Van Dijk, M.; Oudejans, C.B. STOX1: Key player in trophoblast dysfunction underlying early onset preeclampsia with growth retardation. *J. Pregnancy* **2011**, *2011*, 521826. [CrossRef]
150. Founds, S.A. Altered global gene expression in first trimester placentas of women destined to develop preeclampsia. *Placenta* **2009**, *30*, 15–24. [CrossRef]
151. Erlandsson, L. Alpha-1 microglobulin as a potential therapeutic candidate for treatment of hypertension and oxidative stress in the STOX1 preeclampsia mouse model. *Sci. Rep.* **2019**, *9*, 8561. [CrossRef]
152. Doridot, L. Preeclampsia-like symptoms induced in mice by fetoplacental expression of STOX1 are reversed by aspirin treatment. *Hypertension* **2013**, *61*, 662–668. [CrossRef]
153. Schisterman, E.F. A randomised trial to evaluate the effects of low-dose aspirin in gestation and reproduction: Design and baseline characteristics. *Paediatr Perinat Epidemiol.* **2013**, *27*, 598–609. [CrossRef]
154. Gizzo, S. Could empirical low-dose-aspirin administration during IVF cycle affect both the oocytes and embryos quality via COX 1-2 activity inhibition? *J. Assist. Reprod. Genet.* **2014**, *31*, 261–268. [CrossRef]
155. Clark, D.A. Aspirin and heparin to improve live birth rate in IVF for unexplained implantation failure? *Reprod. Biomed. Online* **2013**, *26*, 538–541. [CrossRef]
156. Zhao, Y. Effects of combining lowdose aspirin with a Chinese patent medicine on follicular blood flow and pregnancy outcome. *Mol. Med. Rep.* **2014**, *10*, 2372–2376. [CrossRef]
157. Leeson, P. Updated review identifies no adverse impact on mother or offspring during the perinatal period of aspirin use for prevention of preeclampsia. *Evid. Based Med.* **2015**, *20*, 11. [CrossRef]
158. Dasari, R. Effect of maternal low dose aspirin on neonatal platelet function. *Indian Pediatr.* **1998**, *35*, 507–511.
159. Levy, G.; Garrettson, L.K. Kinetics of salicylate elimination by newborn infants of mothers who ingested aspirin before delivery. *Pediatrics* **1974**, *53*, 201–210.
160. Zarek, S.M. Antimullerian hormone and pregnancy loss from the Effects of Aspirin in Gestation and Reproduction trial. *Fertil. Steril.* **2016**, *105*, 946–952. [CrossRef]
161. Mazaud-Guittot, S. Paracetamol, aspirin, and indomethacin induce endocrine disturbances in the human fetal testis capable of interfering with testicular descent. *J. Clin. Endocrinol. Metab.* **2013**, *98*, E1757–E1767. [CrossRef]
162. Chu, S. In Utero Exposure to Aspirin and Risk of Asthma in Childhood. *Epidemiology* **2016**, *27*, 726–731. [CrossRef]
163. Kristensen, D.M. Paracetamol (acetaminophen), aspirin (acetylsalicylic acid) and indomethacin are anti-androgenic in the rat foetal testis. *Int. J. Androl.* **2012**, *35*, 377–384. [CrossRef]
164. Bloor, M.; Paech, M. Nonsteroidal anti-inflammatory drugs during pregnancy and the initiation of lactation. *Anesth. Analg.* **2013**, *116*, 1063–1075. [CrossRef]
165. Jensen, M.S. Analgesics during pregnancy and cryptorchidism: Additional analyses. *Epidemiology* **2011**, *22*, 610–612. [CrossRef]
166. De Berardis, G. Association of aspirin use with major bleeding in patients with and without diabetes. *JAMA* **2012**, *307*, 2286–2294. [CrossRef]
167. Khazardoost, S. Effect of aspirin in prevention of adverse pregnancy outcome in women with elevated alpha-fetoprotein. *J. Matern. Fetal. Neonatal. Med.* **2014**, *27*, 561–565. [CrossRef]
168. Demers, S.; Roberge, S.; Bujold, E. Low-dose aspirin for the prevention of adverse pregnancy outcomes in women with elevated alpha-fetoprotein. *J. Matern. Fetal. Neonatal. Med.* **2015**, *28*, 726. [CrossRef]
169. Block-Abraham, D.M. First-trimester risk factors for preeclampsia development in women initiating aspirin by 16 weeks of gestation. *Obs. Gynecol.* **2014**, *123*, 611–617. [CrossRef]
170. Asemi, Z. A randomized controlled clinical trial investigating the effect of calcium supplement plus low-dose aspirin on hs-CRP, oxidative stress and insulin resistance in pregnant women at risk for pre-eclampsia. *Pak. J. Biol. Sci.* **2012**, *15*, 469–476.
171. Durcin, M. Characterisation of adipocyte-derived extracellular vesicle subtypes identifies distinct protein and lipid signatures for large and small extracellular vesicles. *J. Extracell. Vesicles* **2017**, *6*, 1305677. [CrossRef]
172. Morel, O. Microparticles: A critical component in the nexus between inflammation, immunity, and thrombosis. *Semin. Immunopathol.* **2011**, *33*, 469–486. [CrossRef]
173. Gho, Y.S.; Lee, C. Emergent properties of extracellular vesicles: A holistic approach to decode the complexity of intercellular communication networks. *Mol. Biosyst.* **2017**, *13*, 1291–1296. [CrossRef]
174. Borges, F.T.; Reis, L.A.; Schor, N. Extracellular vesicles: Structure, function, and potential clinical uses in renal diseases. *Braz. J. Med. Biol. Res.* **2013**, *46*, 824–830. [CrossRef]

175. Di Rocco, G.; Baldari, S.; Toietta, G. Towards Therapeutic Delivery of Extracellular Vesicles: Strategies for In Vivo Tracking and Biodistribution Analysis. *Stem Cells Int.* **2016**, *2016*, 5029619. [CrossRef]
176. Thery, C. Minimal information for studies of extracellular vesicles 2018 (MISEV2018): A position statement of the International Society for Extracellular Vesicles and update of the MISEV2014 guidelines. *J. Extracell. Vesicles* **2018**, *7*, 1535750. [CrossRef]
177. Momen-Heravi, F. Current methods for the isolation of extracellular vesicles. *Biol. Chem.* **2013**, *394*, 1253–1262. [CrossRef]
178. Huang-Doran, I.; Zhang, C.Y.; Vidal-Puig, A. Extracellular Vesicles: Novel Mediators of Cell Communication In Metabolic Disease. *Trends Endocrinol. Metab.* **2017**, *28*, 3–18. [CrossRef]
179. Mitchell, M.D. Placental exosomes in normal and complicated pregnancy. *Am. J. Obstet. Gynecol.* **2015**, *213*, S173–S181. [CrossRef]
180. Adam, S. Review: Fetal-maternal communication via extracellular vesicles Implications for complications of pregnancies. *Placenta* **2017**, *54*, 83–88. [CrossRef]
181. Salomon, C.; Rice, G.E. Role of Exosomes in Placental Homeostasis and Pregnancy Disorders. *Prog. Mol. Biol. Transl. Sci.* **2017**, *145*, 163–179.
182. Nair, S.; Salomon, C. Extracellular vesicles and their immunomodulatory functions in pregnancy. *Semin. Immunopathol.* **2018**, *40*, 425–437. [CrossRef]
183. Sarker, S. Placenta-derived exosomes continuously increase in maternal circulation over the first trimester of pregnancy. *J. Transl. Med.* **2014**, *12*, 204. [CrossRef]
184. Salomon, C.G.D.; Romero, K.S.; Longo, S.; Correa, P.; Illanes, S.E.; Rice, G.E. Placental exosomes as early biomarker of preeclampsia—Potential role of exosomal microRNAs across gestation. *J. Clin. Endocrinol. Metab.* **2017**, *102*, 3182–3194. [CrossRef]
185. Salomon, C. The role of placental exosomes in gestational diabetes mellitus. In *Gestational Diabetes-Causes, Diagnosis and Treatment*; Sobrevia, L., Ed.; IntechOpen: London, UK, 2013.
186. Radu, C.M. Origin and levels of circulating microparticles in normal pregnancy: A longitudinal observation in healthy women. *Scand. J. Clin. Lab. Investig.* **2015**, *75*, 487–495. [CrossRef]
187. Biro, O. Circulating exosomal and Argonaute-bound microRNAs in preeclampsia. *Gene* **2019**, *692*, 138–144. [CrossRef]
188. Truong, G. Oxygen tension regulates the miRNA profile and bioactivity of exosomes released from extravillous trophoblast cells—Liquid biopsies for monitoring complications of pregnancy. *PLoS ONE* **2017**, *12*, e0174514. [CrossRef]
189. Abou-Kheir, W. HTR-8/SVneo cell line contains a mixed population of cells. *Placenta* **2017**, *50*, 1–7. [CrossRef]
190. Tannetta, D.S. Characterisation of syncytiotrophoblast vesicles in normal pregnancy and pre-eclampsia: Expression of Flt-1 and endoglin. *PLoS ONE* **2013**, *8*, e56754. [CrossRef]
191. Germain, S.J. Systemic inflammatory priming in normal pregnancy and preeclampsia: The role of circulating syncytiotrophoblast microparticles. *J. Immunol.* **2007**, *178*, 5949–5956. [CrossRef]
192. Redman, C.W. Review: Does size matter? Placental debris and the pathophysiology of pre-eclampsia. *Placenta* **2012**, *33*, S48–S54. [CrossRef]
193. Tong, M.; Chamley, L.W. Placental Extracellular Vesicles and Feto-Maternal Communication. *Cold Spring Harb. Perspect. Med.* **2015**, *5*, 023028. [CrossRef]
194. Chang, X. Exosomes From Women With Preeclampsia Induced Vascular Dysfunction by Delivering sFlt (Soluble Fms-Like Tyrosine Kinase)-1 and sEng (Soluble Endoglin) to Endothelial Cells. *Hypertension* **2018**, *72*, 1381–1390. [CrossRef]
195. Sammar, M. Reduced placental protein 13 (PP13) in placental derived syncytiotrophoblast extracellular vesicles in preeclampsia A novel tool to study the impaired cargo transmission of the placenta to the maternal organs. *Placenta* **2018**, *66*, 17–25. [CrossRef]
196. Tong, M. Antiphospholipid antibodies increase the levels of mitochondrial DNA in placental extracellular vesicles: Alarmin-g for preeclampsia. *Sci. Rep.* **2017**, *7*, 16556. [CrossRef]
197. Aharon, A. The role of extracellular vesicles in placental vascular complications. *Thromb. Res.* **2015**, *135*, S23–S25. [CrossRef]
198. Miranda, J. Placental exosomes profile in maternal and fetal circulation in intrauterine growth restriction—Liquid biopsies to monitoring fetal growth. *Placenta* **2018**, *64*, 34–43. [CrossRef]

199. Campello, E. Circulating microparticles in umbilical cord blood in normal pregnancy and pregnancy with preeclampsia. *Thromb. Res.* **2015**, *136*, 427–431. [CrossRef]
200. Jia, R. Comparative Proteomic Profile of the Human Umbilical Cord Blood Exosomes between Normal and Preeclampsia Pregnancies with High-Resolution Mass Spectrometry. *Cell Physiol. Biochem.* **2015**, *36*, 2299–2306. [CrossRef]
201. Jadli, A. Combination of copeptin, placental growth factor and total annexin V microparticles for prediction of preeclampsia at 10-14 weeks of gestation. *Placenta* **2017**, *58*, 67–73. [CrossRef]
202. Motta-Mejia, C. Placental Vesicles Carry Active Endothelial Nitric Oxide Synthase and Their Activity is Reduced in Preeclampsia. *Hypertension* **2017**, *70*, 372–381. [CrossRef]
203. Gill, M. Placental Syncytiotrophoblast-Derived Extracellular Vesicles Carry Active NEP (Neprilysin) and Are Increased in Preeclampsia. *Hypertension* **2019**, *73*, 1112–1119. [CrossRef]
204. Kohli, S. Maternal extracellular vesicles and platelets promote preeclampsia via inflammasome activation in trophoblasts. *Blood* **2016**, *128*, 2153–2164. [CrossRef]
205. Motawi, T.M.K. Role of mesenchymal stem cells exosomes derived microRNAs; miR-136, miR-494 and miR-495 in pre-eclampsia diagnosis and evaluation. *Arch. Biochem. Biophys.* **2018**, *659*, 13–21. [CrossRef]
206. Hu, C.C. Pre-eclampsia is associated with altered expression of the renal sodium transporters NKCC2, NCC and ENaC in urinary extracellular vesicles. *PLoS ONE* **2018**, *13*, e0204514. [CrossRef]
207. Moro, L. Placental Microparticles and MicroRNAs in Pregnant Women with Plasmodium falciparum or HIV Infection. *PLoS ONE* **2016**, *11*, e0146361. [CrossRef]
208. Xiong, Z.H. Protective effect of human umbilical cord mesenchymal stem cell exosomes on preserving the morphology and angiogenesis of placenta in rats with preeclampsia. *Biomed. Pharmacother.* **2018**, *105*, 1240–1247. [CrossRef]
209. Zhao, M. Melatonin prevents preeclamptic sera and antiphospholipid antibodies inducing the production of reactive nitrogen species and extrusion of toxic trophoblastic debris from first trimester placentae. *Placenta* **2017**, *58*, 17–24. [CrossRef]
210. Tong, M. Aggregated transthyretin is specifically packaged into placental nano-vesicles in preeclampsia. *Sci. Rep.* **2017**, *7*, 6694. [CrossRef]
211. Gilani, S.I. Urinary Extracellular Vesicles of Podocyte Origin and Renal Injury in Preeclampsia. *J. Am. Soc. Nephrol.* **2017**, *28*, 3363–3372. [CrossRef]
212. O'Brien, M.; Baczyk, D.; Kingdom, J.C. Endothelial Dysfunction in Severe Preeclampsia is Mediated by Soluble Factors, Rather than Extracellular Vesicles. *Sci. Rep.* **2017**, *7*, 5887. [CrossRef]
213. Xu, J. Vitamin D Reduces Oxidative Stress-Induced Procaspase-3/ROCK1 Activation and MP Release by Placental Trophoblasts. *J. Clin. Endocrinol. Metab.* **2017**, *102*, 2100–2110. [CrossRef]
214. Goetzl, E.J. Human plasma platelet-derived exosomes: Effects of aspirin. *Faseb. J.* **2016**, *30*, 2058–2063. [CrossRef]
215. Connor, D.E. Effects of antiplatelet therapy on platelet extracellular vesicle release and procoagulant activity in health and in cardiovascular disease. *Platelets* **2016**, *27*, 805–811. [CrossRef]
216. Chiva-Blanch, G. Microparticle Shedding by Erythrocytes, Monocytes and Vascular Smooth Muscular Cells Is Reduced by Aspirin in Diabetic Patients. *Rev. Esp. Cardiol.* **2016**, *69*, 672–680. [CrossRef]
217. Ambrose, A.R. Comparison of the release of microRNAs and extracellular vesicles from platelets in response to different agonists. *Platelets* **2017**, *29*, 446–454. [CrossRef]
218. Tannetta, D.S. Syncytiotrophoblast Extracellular Vesicles from Pre-Eclampsia Placentas Differentially Affect Platelet Function. *PLoS ONE* **2015**, *10*, e0142538. [CrossRef]
219. Patil, R. Effect of anticoagulant therapy on cell-derived microparticles and pregnancy outcome in women with pregnancy loss. *Br. J. Haematol.* **2015**, *171*, 892–896. [CrossRef]

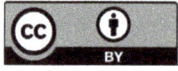

© 2019 by the authors. Licensee MDPI, Basel, Switzerland. This article is an open access article distributed under the terms and conditions of the Creative Commons Attribution (CC BY) license (http://creativecommons.org/licenses/by/4.0/).

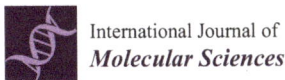

Review

Angiogenesis, Lymphangiogenesis, and the Immune Response in South African Preeclamptic Women Receiving HAART

Thajasvarie Naicker [1,*,†], Wendy N. Phoswa [2,*,†], Onankoy A. Onyangunga [1], Premjith Gathiram [3] and Jagidesa Moodley [3]

1. Optics and Imaging Centre, Doris Duke Medical Research Institute, University of KwaZulu-Natal, Durban 4013, South Africa
2. Discipline of Obstetrics and Gynecology, Nelson R Mandela School of Medicine, University of KwaZulu-Natal, Durban 4013, South Africa
3. Women's Health and HIV Research Group. Department of Obstetrics and Gynecology, School of Clinical Medicine, University of KwaZulu-Natal, Durban 4013, South Africa
* Correspondence: naickera@ukzn.ac.za (T.N.); phoswawendy@gmail.com (W.N.P.)
† These authors contributed equally to this work.

Received: 17 April 2019; Accepted: 22 May 2019; Published: 30 July 2019

Abstract: **Purpose of the review:** This review highlights the role of angiogenesis, lymphangiogenesis, and immune markers in human immunodeficiency virus (HIV)-associated preeclamptic (PE) pregnancies in an attempt to unravel the mysteries underlying the duality of both conditions in South Africa. **Recent findings:** Studies demonstrate that HIV-infected pregnant women develop PE at a lower frequency than uninfected women. In contrast, women receiving highly active anti-retroviral therapy (HAART) are more inclined to develop PE, stemming from an imbalance of angiogenesis, lymphangiogenesis, and immune response. **Summary:** In view of the paradoxical effect of HIV infection on PE development, this study examines angiogenesis, lymphangiogenesis, and immune markers in the highly HIV endemic area of KwaZulu-Natal. We believe that HAART re-constitutes the immune response in PE, thereby predisposing women to PE development. This susceptibility is due to an imbalance in the angiogenic/lymphangiogenic/immune response as compared to normotensive pregnant women. Further large-scale studies are urgently required to investigate the effect of the duration of HAART on PE development.

Keywords: angiogenesis; highly active anti-retroviral therapy; human immunodeficiency virus; lymphangiogenesis; immune response; preeclampsia

1. Problem Identification

Maternal Mortality and Hypertension in South Africa

The adoption of the Millennium Development Goals from 1990–2015 led to a decline in global maternal mortality by 44%; however, South Africa (SA) was unable to reach the target set by the United Nations (Millenium Development Goals, 2015 Report). South Africa has since embraced the Sustainable Development Goals 2016–2030 to reduce its maternal mortality ratio to <70 deaths/100,000 live births [1]. Despite a decline in maternal deaths from human immunodeficiency virus (HIV) infection and obstetric hemorrhage over the period 2008–2016, no change in mortality emanating from hypertensive diseases in pregnancy (HDP) occurred [2]. In fact, deaths from HDP is the commonest direct cause of maternal mortality as reported by the Confidential Report of Saving Mothers in 2017 [2]. Hypertensive diseases in pregnancy account for 18% of all maternal deaths in SA [3]. In developed countries, HDP has a prevalence of 5–10% [4]; however, in developing countries, it occurs more frequently. The incidence of preeclampsia (PE) was 12% amongst all primigravidae who delivered at a large regional hospital in SA [5]. In SA, PE significantly affects both the mother and perinatal morbidity and death. The World Health Organization (WHO) reported that this multisystem pregnancy disorder accounts for 1.6% of maternal deaths in developed countries [6] and 1.8–16.7% in developing countries such as South Africa, Egypt, Tanzania, and Ethiopia [7,8].

2. Human Immunodeficiency Virus Infection in South Africa

HIV infection is a grave public health challenge globally. Sub-Saharan Africa constitutes 56% of the HIV-infected global population [9]. In 2017, women accounted for a disparate 59% of new adult HIV infections (>15 years) [10]. In SA, 13.1% of the total population is HIV-positive, of which 20% involves women in their childbearing age (15–49 years) [11]. Greater than 40% of the global HIV-infected population includes adults residing in the region of KwaZulu-Natal (KZN) [9]. Moreover, the Antenatal HIV and Syphilis Surveillance Report indicates that >37% of antenatal attendees in KZN province are infected [12]. Hence, healthcare professionals providing maternity care are challenged with a double burden of HIV infection and HDP.

The association between HIV infection and PE emanates from the different immune responses [13]. In light of the pervasive nature of both conditions in KZN, this association warrants urgent investigation. Notably, in SA, our group performed extensive research on the effect of angiogenesis and lymphangiogenesis in HIV-infected PE women. Therefore, this review serves to highlight the effect of pregnancy type and HIV status on angiogenesis and lymphangiogenesis using South African cohorts. We also provide compelling evidence of the mechanism(s) that HIV utilizes to exploit the angiogenic system. Furthermore, we provide data based on highly active anti-retroviral treatment (HAART) on reconstituting the immune system and its influence on PE development.

3. Angiogenesis

Angiogenesis is defined as the migration, development, and differentiation of endothelial cells to form new blood vessels [14]. It is initiated by pro-angiogenic vascular endothelial growth factors (VEGFs) and placental growth factors (PlGFs), which increase vessel permeability and promote proteolysis of the extracellular matrix via proteases, resulting in endothelial cell proliferation. Thereafter, endothelial cells migrate and invade the lumen, followed by endothelial maturation [15,16].

In normal pregnancy, the need for increased blood supply to the fetus is met by the physiological transformation of spiral arteries in both the decidua and myometrium. In contrast, as a result of deficient trophoblast invasion, spiral artery remodeling is restricted to the decidua in PE [17] and is often associated with adverse birth outcome.

Angiogenesis is also dysregulated in HIV-1 infected patients [18]. Notably, adverse birth outcome is elevated upon receipt of anti-retroviral therapy (ART) compared to HIV-uninfected women [19,20]. Since SA has the largest anti-retroviral rollout in the world, it is important to recognize any link(s) between HAART usage in pregnancy and the risk for PE development. In a novel study, Powis et al. (2013) assessed angiogenesis in preeclamptic women that initiated HAART during pregnancy [21]. They demonstrated that women who developed PE had an upregulation of anti-angiogenic factors prior to HAART usage. Moreover, a recent report correlated altered angiogenesis with ARV usage in the second and third trimesters as a progenitor of preterm birth, small for gestational age, and stillbirth [22].

3.1. Soluble Fms-Like Tyrosine Kinase 1 (sFlt1), Placental Growth Factor (PlGF), and Soluble Endoglin (Eng)

It is well documented that placental sFlt1 is elevated in PE, resulting in a rise in systemic levels with a concomitant decline in VEGF and PlGF [23]. The anti-angiogenic factor sFlt-1 is a scavenger receptor for VEGF and PlGF, thereby dampening their constructive effects on the maternal endothelium [24]. Moreover, in pregnant rats, the administration of sFlt1 induces the clinical symptoms of PE [25]. Flt-1 and sFlt-1 levels in the placenta are upregulated in PE compared to controls, irrespective of HIV infection [26]. Working in our laboratory, Govender et al. (2013) demonstrated increasing levels of serum sFlt1 and sEng in PE, regardless of HIV infection [27]. sFlt1 and sEng are implicated in the endothelial dysfunction of PE. Moreover the downregulation of serum sFlt1 and sEng within HIV-infected women advocates counterbalance of the immune hyperactivity in PE [27]. sEng weakens the binding of TGF-β1 to its receptors and blocks the activation of the endothelial nitric oxide synthase 3 (eNOS) pathways downstream, thereby inducing hypertension [28]. The recent use of sFlt-1:PlGF ratio for the clinical prediction of severe early-onset PE is encouraging [29].

3.2. Vascular Endothelial Growth Factor (VEGF)

The permeability of blood vessels is enhanced by VEGF, thereby inducing angiogenesis and vasculogenesis [30]. The VEGF family comprises VEGF-A, VEGF-B, VEGF-C, VEGF-D, and PlGF [31]. VEGF receptors include VEGFR-1 (Flt-1) and VEGFR-2 (Flk-1/KDR) [31]. VEGF-A and VEGF-B bind to VEGFR-1 (Flt-1); however, in PE, binding is blocked by the antagonist sFlt-1 or sVEGFR-1, a spliced soluble variant of VEGFR-1 [32]. VEGFR-2 is an antagonist to VEGF and increases arterial pressure [33]. Both VEGF-C and VEGF-D bind to VEGFR-3, thus expediting lymphangiogenesis [34].

3.3. Platelet Endothelial Cell Adhesion Molecule 1 (PECAM-1)

Vascular development is influenced by PECAM-1 through the formation of a complex with VEGFR-2 and VE cadherin [35]. In PE, PECAM-1 induces neutrophil and platelet activation, thereby promoting vascular damage [36]. Thakoordeen et al. (2017) demonstrated a similar level of PECAM-1 between control and preeclamptic pregnancies ($p = 0.07$), while no correlation was found based on HIV infection ($p = 0.68$) or across study groups ($p = 0.24$) [37].

3.4. Angiopoietin (Ang)-2

The angiopoietin family includes Ang-1, Ang-2, Ang-3, and Ang-4 types, which are vital for embryonic angiogenesis. These growth factors are ligands for the vascular endothelial receptor tyrosine kinase (Tie-2), required for vascular activation [38]. Mbhele et al. (2017) demonstrated that, in contrast to PlGF, increased levels of Ang-2 and Eng were noted in PE. The gestational period (early- or late-onset PE) had no effect on Ang-2 expression; yet, it was associated with Eng ($p < 0.0001$) and PlGF ($p = 0.0033$). HIV infection did not affect Ang-2 ($p = 0.4$), Eng ($p = 0.4$), and PlGF ($p = 0.7$) levels [39].

3.5. sTie-2

During development, vascular endothelial cells express the transmembrane tyrosine kinase receptors Tie-1 and Tie-2, which are responsible for vascular maturation and angiogenesis [40]. Angiopoietin-1 via Tie-2 signaling facilitates endothelial development, whilst Ang-2 acts as an Ang-1 antagonist by binding to the Tie-2 receptor [41].

However, whilst vessel growth is dependent on Tie-2 [19], Tie-2 may be proteolytically cleaved to produce sTie-2. This soluble form inhibits Tie-2 signaling by averting angiogenesis [19,20]. Mazibuko et al. (2019) demonstrated that soluble Tie-2 levels were dissimilar between preeclamptic and control pregnancies ($p = 0.0403$). In contrast, HIV status did not affect sTie2 and soluble human epidermal growth factor receptor 2 (sHER2) manifestation [42]. Also, HER2 is a membrane-bound receptor tyrosine kinase that is shed via proteolytic cleavage into body fluids [43]. Mazibuko et al. (2019) reported that sHER2 levels were similar between pregnancy types (control vs. PE; $p = 0.3677$), regardless of HIV status ($p = 0.5249$). These results may be due to the hypoxic pro-oxidative milieu of both PE and HIV infection, as sHER2 interferes with mitogen-activated protein kinase (MAPK) and Phosphatidylinositol-3-kinase/ protein kinase B (P13K/Akt) signaling [42].

3.6. Vascular Endothelial Growth Factor and HIV Tat protein

The accessory protein Tat of HIV-1 interferes with intracellular function by evading host response mechanisms, and may, therefore, contribute to the high inflammatory reaction in HIV-infected PE [44].

The Tat protein is a trans-activator of viral gene expression and is released extracellularly during HIV acute infection [45]. Since Tat has a similar arginine- and lysine-rich sequence to VEGF, it is recognized as a powerful angiogenic factor [46]. Tat imitates VEGF by attaching to and stimulating Flk-1/KDR [47]. Tat promotes endothelial cell adhesion through the binding of its arginine–glycine–aspartic acid region to the $\alpha_v\beta_3$ and $\alpha_5\beta_1$ integrins and VEGFR-2/KDR via its basic domain [46]. Also, a combined Tat/FGF-2 effect is attributed to fibroblast growth factor (FGF-2), which induces the expression of the $\alpha_v\beta_3$ and $\alpha_5\beta_1$ integrins, which aids Tat binding [48].

Additionally, HIV-1 via gp120 binds to heparin sulphate proteoglycans (HSPG) on endothelial cells, amplifying viral infectivity and thereby expediting the release of Tat [49]. Tat induces endothelial cells to migrate, adhere, and grow as a capillary-like network in vitro [50]. HIV Tat was also shown to bind F1k-1/KDR, one of the receptors for VEGF, suggesting an additional mechanism for Tat to exert its angiogenic effect [47].

Defective cell signaling by the Tat protein alters endothelial cell morphology, gene expression, and survival by stimulating the MAPK pathway. The movement from the gap 0 to gap 1 (G0 to G1) phase of naïve T cells enables productive HIV infection [51]. The HIV-1 Tat protein facilitates MAPK activity by promoting a change from the G0 to G1 phase of naïve T cells, thereby stimulating HIV infection [51].

4. Lymphangiogenesis

Lymphatic vessels were first described in the 17th century and consists of a vascular-like network. They play a pivotal role in maintaining tissue fluid homeostasis, transport of proteins, macromolecules, and cells such as leucocytes and activated antigen-presenting cells for immune protection [52]. This vascular-like network consists of a monolayer of blind-ended capillaries transferring "lymph" to the collecting lymphatics. The expansion of new lymphatic vessels from pre-existing ones, called lymphangiogenesis, is controlled mainly by growth factors, i.e., VEGFs such as VEGF-C and its ligand VEGFR-3, VEGF-D [53–55], and other factors, i.e., hypoxia-inducible factor 1-α (HIF-1α), the Tie/angiopoietin system, neuropilin-2, and integrin-α_9 [56–61]. However, until recently, there was a paucity of data on the lymphatic profile during pregnancy and in PE [62–64].

4.1. Lymphatic System in the Placenta

The human placenta is an hemochorial organ and is highly vascularized; yet, there are conflicting reports on the presence of lymphatic vessels in the placenta. However, Gu et al. (2006) [65], Wang et al. (2011) [66], and Liu et al. (2015) [67], as well as our recent observations [68], do not confirm the presence of lymphatic vessels in the placenta. The aforementioned groups instead observed a stromal network immunostained with podoplanin. Lymphangiogenesis was observed at the decidua [68–72] and the uterine wall [64,73].

4.2. Lymphangiogenesis and Preeclampsia

In PE, a dysfunctional fluid clearance manifests as an excessive accumulation of interstitial fluid causing edema [74]. B cells, macrophages, and reticular stromal cells activate the production of VEGF A, C, and D, thereby affecting signaling pathways for the induction of lymphangiogenesis [74]. Increased lymphangiogenesis (pro VEGF-C) is a compensatory response to the heightened exaggerated inflammatory state of PE [75,76]. Indeed, VEGF induces lymphangiogenesis [65]. Nevertheless, Shange et al. (2017) reported no significant difference between VEGF-C and D from PE mothers and control [74]. This upregulation of VEGF-C in PE was observed in early-onset PE; however, one needs to note that patients were on dual ARV therapy [73].

Furthermore, hypoxia-inducible factor-1 (HIF-1) plays an important role in the pathogenesis of PE, and indirectly enhances the molecular regulation of VEGF [66,67,77]. The upregulated *HIF-1* gene plays a critical role in the pathogenesis of PE [58,78–80] and contributes to the lymphangiogenesis in PE.

4.3. Lymphangiogenesis and HIV Infection

At the mucosal level, HIV-1 uses endothelial cell co-receptors CXCR4 and CCR5 before disseminating through lymphatic endothelial channels to the lymph nodes and, thereafter, moving into the general blood circulation. HIV infection plays a crucial role in lymphatic development; nevertheless, its functional integrity is complex and not fully understood. Three HIV-1 proteins, notably the envelope glycoprotein (gp120), transactivator of transcription (Tat), and the matrix protein (p17), may contribute to HIV-associated vascular disorders. HIV-1 gp120 induces apoptosis in endothelial cells. Tat triggers angiogenesis by using the matrix protein p17 [81] to stimulate the endothelin-1/endothelin B receptor axis [82], thereby activating the protein kinase Akt and extracellular signal-regulated kinase (ERK) signaling pathways [66,77,82,83].

The secretory protein (Slit2) and its receptor roundabout protein (Robo4) expressed on endothelial cells also serve to modulate endothelial cell permeability and, hence, have a determinant participation in the pathophysiological mechanism of lymphangiogenesis [84]. Although Slit2/Robo4 interactions are not fully elucidated, a previous study reported an inhibition of VEGF-C and a blockage of VEGFR-3 [85]. Additionally, HIV-1 gp120 leads to hyperpermeability of lymphatic cells in vitro via modulation of fibronectin expression and activation of $\alpha_5\beta_1$ integrins. On the other hand, Slit2 blocks the interaction between $\alpha_5\beta_1$ and Robo4, thus inhibiting lymphatic hyperpermeability [81].

This results in an imbalance of the Akt and ERK signaling pathways, which leads to dysregulation of lymphangiogenesis in PE, since it was shown that, during the pathophysiology of PE, there is decreased P13K/Akt signaling [86].

4.4. Lymphangiogenesis in the Duration of HAART and the Risk of Preeclampsia

By enhancing pro-inflammatory cytokines and chemokines, HIV-1 infection mimics PE, thereby influencing the prevalence of PE among HIV positive women. The HAART intervention improves endothelial function and decreases the inflammatory milieu of PE. However, that is not evident, as the timing and duration of the HAART is not clear in most the studies. Despite long-term use of HAART improving mortality among HIV positive patients, the morbidity (particularly vascular and metabolic in nature) is still a serious concern [87]. Two HIV-1 proteins seem to undermine the beneficial action of HAART in the restoration of endothelial cell (EC) function: HIV-1 Tat and matrix protein p17, which impair the endothelial cells. A recent study on HAART showed that angiogenesis and lymphangiogenesis are downregulated with Nucleoside reverse transcriptase inhibitors (NRTIs) by inducing mitochondrial oxidative stress and subsequently impairing receptor tyrosine kinase (RTK) signaling in EC [88], suggesting that NRTIs might trigger the development of PE.

The prevalence of PE in HIV-infected pregnancies is lower; however, upon HAART administration, the risk of PE development increases [13,89]. The association between lymphangiogenesis in the duration of HAART and the risk of PE development is unclear; hence, more research on lymphangiogenesis at the maternal and fetal interface is vital, particularly in immune transfer and ARV usage.

5. Highly Active Anti-Retroviral Therapy

Protease inhibitors (PI) induce the progression of Kaposi sarcoma [90]. PIs are potent anti-angiogenic factors that block FGF action [91]. PIs deter HIV aspartyl protease and, hence, the production of HIV virions, thus promoting immune restoration. Also, glucose transporter (GLUT)-4, inhibits glucose uptake and affects the cellular proteasome by triggering p53 protein intracellular accumulation, resulting in apoptosis. Finally, the functional impairment of activator protein (AP)-1, specificity protein (SP)-1 or nuclear factor kappa b (NF-κB) transcription factors leads to a decline in MMP and VEGF expression, thereby preventing angiogenesis.

Anti-retroviral drugs regimens are associated with the development of metabolic disorders such as insulin resistance, dyslipidemia, impaired glucose tolerance, and abnormal body fat distribution, which predispose HIV-infected individuals to cardiovascular-related diseases [92]. Anti-retroviral therapy was also shown to lead to endothelial dysfunction [93,94] and decreased nitric oxide, ultimately resulting in induced endothelial oxidative stress [95], which is similarly observed during the pathophysiology of PE [96]. It is, therefore, possible that predisposition to PE may result from endothelial dysfunction and reduced nitric oxide synthase induced by HAART exposure.

Although some studies report on the endothelial HAART-induced endothelial dysfunction, conflicting reports exist. A study done by Torriani et al. (2008) showed improved endothelial function after ARV administration [97]. Additionally, Savvidou et al. (2011) found normal placental perfusion among HIV-infected women, with uncomplicated pregnancies, receiving and not receiving HAART [98]. In contrast, a study done by Sebitloane et al. (2017) evaluating the effect of HAART on HDP showed that, among all women with HIV, a greater risk of mortality due to HDP was reported among those who received HAART compared with those who did not [99].

6. Immune Maladaptation

6.1. Natural Killer Cells in Normal versus Preeclamptic Pregnancies

Natural killer (NK) cells are dysregulated in the presence of preeclampsia and HIV infection. In normal pregnancy, these cells promote placental development by balancing the immune response at the maternal–fetal interface [100]. The function of NK cells is controlled by inhibitory receptors [101] and activating receptors, C-type lectin receptors, and Ig-like receptors (2B4)] [102–104].

During normal pregnancy, the interaction between the maternal NK cells and fetal cells is controlled by NK cell inhibitory receptors, which prevents inadequate trophoblast invasion. However, this action is prevented in PE pregnancies since activating receptors are predominant, leading to shallow trophoblast invasion [105]. Similarly, the function of NK cells during HIV infection is downregulated or similar to NK cells in a healthy pregnancy state [106]. A study conducted by Mela and Goodier showed reduced activation peripheral NK cells of HIV-infected individuals [107].

6.2. Role of HAART on NK Cells and Risk of Preeclampsia Development

Natural killer cells play a role in controlling HIV [108] and are also reported to play a role in pregnancy complications such as miscarriage, implantation failure, and PE development [109–111]. In the duration of HAART, NK cells control HIV by secreting CC chemokines. These chemokines inhibit HIV replication via activation of non-cytolytic mechanisms [112]. Several studies reported on the influence of changes that may occur on NK cells in the duration of HAART exposure, and found conflicting results. A study by Valentin et al. (2002) reported higher frequency of NK cells after HAART initiation [113]. Similar findings were shown by Ballan et al. (2007) and Michaelsson et al. (2008) [114,115]. In contrast, a study done by Fria et al. (2015) examining the HAART effect on T-cell recovery versus NK cells found low NK subset recovery after HAART exposure when compared with T-cell recovery during the early months of therapy [116], suggesting that HIV infection of NK cells is important for viral persistence [113].

NK cells are also implicated in pregnancy complications; it was documented that NK cell activation may lead to inadequate trophoblast invasion and may result in exaggerative immune response, which is commonly associated with PE development [117]. Therefore, the possible mechanism responsible for PE development in HIV-infected women might be due to T-cell activation rather than NK cell subset recovery. More studies are needed to confirm how NK cells are regulated in the duration of HAART in order to understand the pathogenesis of PE in HIV-associated pregnancies.

7. Cytokines in Normal Pregnancy, Preeclampsia, HIV Infection, and in the Duration of HAART

7.1. T Helper Cell 1 and T Helper Cell 2 (Th1 and Th2)

During normal pregnancy, anti-inflammatory (Th2) cytokines are predominant [118], whereas, during the pathogenesis of PE, pro-inflammatory (Th1) cytokines are predominant [119]. However, during the progression of HIV infection, Th2 cytokines are predominant (Figure 1) [120,121].

HIV-infected pregnant women on HAART present a shift toward Th1 immune response [122]. Therefore, HIV-infected pregnant women on HAART have increased risk of developing PE [123].

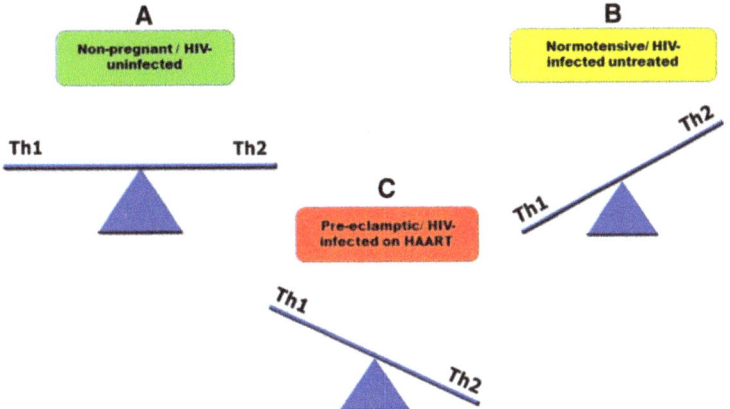

Figure 1. Schematic diagram representing how pro-inflammatory (Th1) and anti-inflammatory (Th2) cytokine are regulated in **A** non-pregnant or HIV-uninfected, **B** normotensive or HIV-infected untreated and **C** pre-eclamptic or HIV-infected on HAART. **A** Shows a balance in the distribution of Th1 and Th2. In **B** there is an imbalance of cytokines with more Th2 release than Th1. This imbalance increases of HIV infection in untreated women. In **C** Th1 levels are higher than Th2. HAART induces Th1 response and leads to pre-eclampsia development [123].

7.2. T Helper Cell 17 (Th17) and T Regulatory Cells (Treg)

Immune cells involved in pregnancy extend from Th1/Th2 into the Th1/Th2/Th17 and regulatory T cells (Treg), introducing Treg as regulators of Th17 lymphocytes and other immune cell types involved in placental development and maintenance [118,124].

Th17 cells are characterized by the secretion of IL-17/IL-17A and are also associated with inducing Th1 cytokine production. An upregulation of Th17 cells is associated with the pathophysiology of autoimmune, chronic inflammatory diseases, allergic disorders, and graft-rejection reactions [125]. Furthermore, it was reported that Th17 cells are upregulated in PE compared to normotensive pregnancies [126,127] and downregulated during the progression of HIV infection [128]. Currently, no studies investigated how IL-17A is regulated in the presence of both PE and HIV infection; more studies are needed in order to have a better understanding of how this cytokine is regulated in the pathophysiology of both conditions, especially in the duration of HAART.

Regulatory T cells are another type of lymphocytes involved in the pathophysiology of PE. In pregnancy, upregulation of these cells is important for maintaining normal pregnancy development [129–131]. Downregulation of Treg cells was reported in PE [132].

In the presence of HIV infection, the frequency of Treg cells is increased, implying their role in the progression of the disease [133–135]. In the duration of HAART, the frequency of Treg cells was shown to be decreased or similar to that of HIV-uninfected individuals [136,137]. Currently, there are no studies that investigated how Treg cells are regulated in the presence of both PE and HIV infection. Therefore, more studies are needed in order to improve management of PE in the presence of HIV infection, and in order to have a better understanding of the pathophysiology of PE in the presence of HIV infection.

8. Conclusions

This paper elaborated on the paradigm shift of HIV's effect on angiogenesis in normotensive and preeclamptic pregnancy. Whilst an imbalance in the angiogenic and lymphangiogenic transference predominates in PE, we highlight the parodist effect of HIV as it utilizes its accessory proteins to exploit VEGF's effect. Furthermore, due to the ubiquitous nature of HIV infection in South Africa, this paper also outlines the effect of HAART on the risk of PE development, albeit not on the duration of the therapy. Current literature is controversial on the effect of HAART on T-cell reconstitution, with regard to NK cell subset recovery and the influence of Th1/Th2/Th17 and Treg cell dysregulation during HIV infection in pregnancy. Since cytokine stimulation is disparate in HIV infection, PE, and during ARV usage, it is important that future research outlines the archetypal effect in pregnancy. Finally, this will improve therapeutic interventions in HIV-associated preeclamptic pregnancies, thus reducing maternal and fetal morbidity and mortality.

Author Contributions: All authors made contributions to the article and approved it for publication.

Funding: This research received no external funding.

Acknowledgments: The authors wish to acknowledge the placental research team at the University of KwaZulu-Natal.

Conflicts of Interest: The authors declare no conflicts of interest.

Abbreviations

Ang-1	Angiopoietin-1
Ang-2	Angiopoietin-2
Ang-3	Angiopoietin-3
Ang-4	Angiopoietin-4
AP-1	Activator protein 1
ARV	Anti-retroviral therapy
CD94	Cluster of differentiation 94
CTLA-4	Cytotoxic T-lymphocyte antigen 4
CXCR1	Chemokine (C–X–C motif) receptor 1
CXCR2	Chemokine (C–X–C motif) receptor 2
ENOS	Endothelial nitric oxide synthase
FGF-2	Fibroblast growth factor
FIK-1	Vascular endothelial growth factor receptor 2 (VEGFR22, kinase domain receptor)
FOXP3	Forkhead box P3
Gp120	Glycoprotein 120
HIF-1	Hypoxic-inducible factor 1
HAART	Highly active anti-retroviral therapy
HDP	Hypertensive disorders of pregnancy
HELLP	Hemolysis, elevated liver enzymes, and low platelets
HIV	Human immuno-deficiency virus
IL-17	Interleukin-17
KDR	Kinase insert domain receptor
KIR2DS	Killer-cell immunoglobulin-like receptor 2DS
KZN	KwaZulu-Natal
LAIR-1	Leukocyte-associated immunoglobulin-like receptor 1
LIR1	Leukocyte immunoglobulin-like receptor 1
MAPKs	Mitogen-activated protein kinases
MMP	Matrix metalloproteases
NF-κB	Nuclear factor kappa B
NKG2	Natural killer cell G2

NKG2C	Natural killer cell G2A
NKG2D	Natural killer cell G2D
NKp30	Natural killer cell precursor 30
NKp44	Natural killer cell precursor 44
NKp46	Natural killer cell precursor 46
PE	Preeclampsia
PECAM-1	Platelet endothelial cell adhesion molecule 1
PLGF	Placental growth factor
SEng	Soluble endoglin
SFlt1	Soluble fms-like tyrosine kinase 1
Slit2/Robo4	Slit/Roundabout (Robo)
Sp-1	Specificity protein 1
Tat	Transactivating regulatory protein
TGF-ß	Transforming growth factor beta
TIE1	Tyrosine protein kinase receptor 1
TIE2	Tyrosine protein kinase receptor 2
Th1	T helper cell type 1
Th2	T helper cell type 2
Th17	T helper type 17
Treg	Regulatory T cells
UNAIDS	United Nations Program on HIV/AIDS
VE cadherin	Vascular endothelial cadherin
VEGF	Vascular endothelial growth factor
VEGFR-1	Vascular endothelial growth factor receptor 1
VEGFR-2	Vascular endothelial growth factor receptor 2
VEGFR-3	Vascular endothelial growth factor receptor 3
WHO	World Health Organization

References

1. World Health Organization. *World Health Statistics 2016: Monitoring Health for the Sdgs Sustainable Development Goals*; World Health Organization: Geneva, Switzerland, 2016.
2. Pretoria: National Department of Health. *Saving Mothers 2014–2016: Seventh Triennial Report on Confidential Enquiries into Maternal Deaths in South Africa: Executive Summary*; National Department of Health: Pretoria, South Africa, 2018.
3. Moodley, J. Maternal deaths due to hypertensive disorders in pregnancy: Saving mothers report 2002–2004. *Cardiovasc. J. Afr.* **2007**, *18*, 358–361. [PubMed]
4. Payne, B.; Hanson, C.; Sharma, S.; Magee, L.; von Dadelszen, P. Epidemiology of the hypertensive disorders of pregnancy. In *The FIGO textbook of pregnancy hypertension*; Magee, L.A., von Dadelszen, P., Stones, W., Mathai, M., Eds.; Global Library of Women's Medicine: London, UK, 2016.
5. Moodley, J.; Onyangunga, O.; Maharaj, N. Hypertensive disorders in primigravid black south african women: A one-year descriptive analysis. *Hypertens. Pregnancy* **2016**, *35*, 529–535. [CrossRef] [PubMed]
6. Khan, K.S.; Wojdyla, D.; Say, L.; Gülmezoglu, A.M.; van Look, P.F. Who analysis of causes of maternal death: A systematic review. *Lancet* **2006**, *367*, 1066–1074. [CrossRef]
7. Osungbade, K.O.; Ige, O.K. Public health perspectives of preeclampsia in developing countries: Implication for health system strengthening. *J. Pregnancy* **2011**, *2011*. [CrossRef] [PubMed]
8. Lakew, Y.; Reda, A.A.; Tamene, H.; Benedict, S.; Deribe, K. Geographical variation and factors influencing modern contraceptive use among married women in ethiopia: Evidence from a national population based survey. *Reprod. Health* **2013**, *10*, 52. [CrossRef] [PubMed]
9. UNAIDS. The Joint United Nations Programme on HIV/AIDS. Available online: https://www.unAIDS.org/en (accessed on 19 December 2018).
10. UNAIDS. Global HIV & AIDS Statistics—2018 Fact Sheet. Available online: https://www.unAIDS.org/en (accessed on 16 April 2019).

11. Human Sciences Research Council. South African National HIV Prevalence Incidence and Behaviour Survey. Human Sciences Research Council: Pretoria, South Africa, 2008.
12. National Department of Health. *National Antenatal Sentinel HIV & Syphilis Survey Report*; National Department of Health: Pretoria, South Africa, 2017.
13. Kalumba, V.M.; Moodley, J.; Naidoo, T.D. Is the prevalence of pre-eclampsia affected by HIV/AIDS? A retrospective case-control study. *Cardiovasc. J. Afr.* **2013**, *24*, 24–27. [CrossRef]
14. Kubis, N.; Levy, B.I. Vasculogenesis and angiogenesis: Molecular and cellular controls. Part 1: Growth factors. *Int. Neuroradiol. J. Perith. Neuroradiol. Surg. Proc. Relat. Neurosci.* **2003**, *9*, 227–237. [CrossRef]
15. Reynolds, L.P.; Killilea, S.; Redmer, D. Angiogenesis in the female reproductive system. *FASEB J.* **1992**, *6*, 886–892. [CrossRef]
16. Risau, W. Mechanisms of angiogenesis. *Nature* **1997**, *386*, 671. [CrossRef]
17. Naicker, T.; Khedun, S.M.; Moodley, J.; Pijnenborg, R. Quantitative analysis of trophoblast invasion in preeclampsia. *Acta Obstet. Gynecol. Scand.* **2003**, *82*, 722–729. [CrossRef]
18. Paydas, S.; Ergin, M.; Seydaoglu, G.; Erdogan, S.; Yavuz, S. Pronostic significance of angiogenic/lymphangiogenic, anti-apoptotic, inflammatory and viral factors in 88 cases with diffuse large b cell lymphoma and review of the literature. *Leuk. Res.* **2009**, *33*, 1627–1635. [CrossRef] [PubMed]
19. Chen, J.Y.; Ribaudo, H.J.; Souda, S.; Parekh, N.; Ogwu, A.; Lockman, S.; Powis, K.; Dryden-Peterson, S.; Creek, T.; Jimbo, W. Highly active antiretroviral therapy and adverse birth outcomes among HIV-infected women in botswana. *J. Infect. Dis.* **2012**, *206*, 1695–1705. [CrossRef] [PubMed]
20. Wimalasundera, R.; Larbalestier, N.; Smith, J.; De Ruiter, A.; Thom, S.M.; Hughes, A.; Poulter, N.; Regan, L.; Taylor, G. Pre-eclampsia, antiretroviral therapy, and immune reconstitution. *Lancet* **2002**, *360*, 1152–1154. [CrossRef]
21. Powis, K.M.; McElrath, T.F.; Hughes, M.D.; Ogwu, A.; Souda, S.; Datwyler, S.A.; von Widenfelt, E.; Moyo, S.; Nádas, M.; Makhema, J. High viral load and elevated angiogenic markers associated with increased risk of preeclampsia among women initiating highly active antiretroviral therapy (haart) in pregnancy in the Mma Bana study, Botswana. *J. Acquir. Immune Defic. Syndr.* **2013**, *62*, 517. [CrossRef] [PubMed]
22. Conroy, A.L.; McDonald, C.R.; Gamble, J.L.; Olwoch, P.; Natureeba, P.; Cohan, D.; Kamya, M.R.; Havlir, D.V.; Dorsey, G.; Kain, K.C. Altered angiogenesis as a common mechanism underlying preterm birth, small for gestational age, and stillbirth in women living with HIV. *Am. J. Obstet. Gynecol.* **2017**, *217*, 684.e1–684.e17. [CrossRef] [PubMed]
23. Nnabuike Chibuoke Ngene, J.M.a.T.N. The performance of pre-delivery serum concentrations of angiogenic factors in predicting postpartum antihypertensive drug therapy following abdominal delivery in severe preeclampsia and normotensive pregnancy. *PLoS ONE* **2019**, *14*, e0215807. [CrossRef]
24. Roberts, J.M.; Rajakumar, A. Preeclampsia and soluble fms-like tyrosine kinase 1. *J. Clin. Endocrinol. Metab.* **2009**, *94*, 2252–2254. [CrossRef]
25. Masuda, Y.; Shimizu, A.; Mori, T.; Ishiwata, T.; Kitamura, H.; Ohashi, R.; Ishizaki, M.; Asano, G.; Sugisaki, Y.; Yamanaka, N. Vascular endothelial growth factor enhances glomerular capillary repair and accelerates resolution of experimentally induced glomerulonephritis. *Am. J. Pathol.* **2001**, *159*, 599–608. [CrossRef]
26. Govender, N.; Moodley, J.; Gathiram, P.; Naicker, T. Soluble fms-like tyrosine kinase-1 in HIV infected pre-eclamptic south african black women. *Placenta* **2014**, *35*, 618–624. [CrossRef]
27. Govender, N.; Naicker, T.; Rajakumar, A.; Moodley, J. Soluble fms-like tyrosine kinase-1 and soluble endoglin in HIV-associated preeclampsia. *Eur. J. Obstet. Gynecol. Reprod. Biol.* **2013**, *170*, 100–105. [CrossRef]
28. Perucci, L.O.; Gomes, K.B.; Freitas, L.G.; Godoi, L.C.; Alpoim, P.N.; Pinheiro, M.B.; Miranda, A.S.; Teixeira, A.L.; Dusse, L.M.; Sousa, L.P. Soluble endoglin, transforming growth factor-beta 1 and soluble tumor necrosis factor alpha receptors in different clinical manifestations of preeclampsia. *PLoS ONE* **2014**, *9*, e97632. [CrossRef]
29. Govender, N.; Moodley, J.; Naicker, T. The use of soluble fms-like tyrosine kinase 1/placental growth factor ratio in the clinical management of pre-eclampsia. *Afr. J. Reprod. Health* **2018**, *22*, 135–143. [PubMed]
30. Bates, D.O. An unexpected tail of vegf and plgf in pre-eclampsia. *Biochem. Soc. Trans.* **2011**, 1576–1582. [CrossRef] [PubMed]
31. Helmo, F.R.; Lopes, A.M.M.; Carneiro, A.; Campos, C.G.; Silva, P.B.; dos Reis Monteiro, M.L.G.; Rocha, L.P.; dos Reis, M.A.; Etchebehere, R.M.; Machado, J.R.; et al. Angiogenic and antiangiogenic factors in preeclampsia. *Pathol. Res. Pract.* **2018**, *214*, 7–14. [CrossRef] [PubMed]

32. Cerdeira, A.S.; Agrawal, S.; Staff, A.C.; Redman, C.W.; Vatish, M. Angiogenic factors: Potential to change clinical practice in pre-eclampsia? *BJOG Int. J. Obstet. Gynaecol.* **2018**, *125*, 1389–1395. [CrossRef] [PubMed]
33. Ngene, N.C.; Moodley, J. Role of angiogenic factors in the pathogenesis and management of pre-eclampsia. *Int. J. Gynaecol. Obstet. Off. Organ Int. Fed. Gynaecol. Obstet.* **2018**, *141*, 5–13. [CrossRef]
34. Shibuya, M. Vascular endothelial growth factor and its receptor system: Physiological functions in angiogenesis and pathological roles in various diseases. *J. Biochem.* **2013**, *153*, 13–19. [CrossRef]
35. Coon, B.G.; Baeyens, N.; Han, J.; Budatha, M.; Ross, T.D.; Fang, J.S.; Yun, S.; Thomas, J.-L.; Schwartz, M.A. Intramembrane binding of ve-cadherin to vegfr2 and vegfr3 assembles the endothelial mechanosensory complex. *J. Cell Biol.* **2015**, *208*, 975–986. [CrossRef]
36. Sahin, S.; Ozakpinar, O.B.; Eroglu, M.; Tetik, S. Platelets in preeclampsia: Function and role in the inflammation. *Clin. Exp. Health Sci.* **2014**, *4*, 111. [CrossRef]
37. Thakoordeen, S.; Moodley, J.; Naicker, T. Serum levels of platelet endothelial cell adhesion molecule-1 (pecam-1) and soluble vascular endothelial growth factor receptor (svegfr)-1 and-2 in HIV associated preeclampsia. *Hypertens. Pregnancy* **2017**, *36*, 168–174. [CrossRef]
38. Findley, C.M.; Cudmore, M.J.; Ahmed, A.; Kontos, C.D. Vegf induces tie2 shedding via a phosphoinositide 3-kinase/akt–dependent pathway to modulate tie2 signaling. *Arterioscler. Thrombo. Vasc. Biol.* **2007**, *27*, 2619–2626. [CrossRef] [PubMed]
39. Mbhele, N.; Moodley, J.; Naicker, T. Role of angiopoietin-2, endoglin, and placental growth factor in HIV-associated preeclampsia. *Hypertens. Pregnancy* **2017**, *36*, 240–246. [CrossRef] [PubMed]
40. Fagiani, E.; Christofori, G. Angiopoietins in angiogenesis. *Cancer Lett.* **2013**, *328*, 18–26. [CrossRef] [PubMed]
41. Findley, C.M.; Mitchell, R.G.; Duscha, B.D.; Annex, B.H.; Kontos, C.D. Plasma levels of soluble tie2 and vascular endothelial growth factor distinguish critical limb ischemia from intermittent claudication in patients with peripheral arterial disease. *J. Am. Coll. Cardiol.* **2008**, *52*, 387–393. [CrossRef] [PubMed]
42. Mazibuko, M.; Moodley, J.; Naicker, T. Dysregulation of circulating stie2 and sher2 in HIV-infected women with preeclampsia. *Hypertens. Pregnancy* **2019**, *38*, 89–95. [CrossRef] [PubMed]
43. Chen, M.K.; Hung, M.C. Proteolytic cleavage, trafficking, and functions of nuclear receptor tyrosine kinases. *FEBS J.* **2015**, *282*, 3693–3721. [CrossRef] [PubMed]
44. Abbas, W.; Herbein, G. T-cell signaling in HIV-1 infection. *Open Virol. J.* **2013**, *7*, 57. [CrossRef] [PubMed]
45. Romani, B.; Engelbrecht, S.; Glashoff, R.H. Functions of tat: The versatile protein of human immunodeficiency virus type 1. *J. Gen. Virol.* **2010**, *91*, 1–12. [CrossRef] [PubMed]
46. Zhou, F.; Xue, M.; Qin, D.; Zhu, X.; Wang, C.; Zhu, J.; Hao, T.; Cheng, L.; Chen, X.; Bai, Z. HIV-1 tat promotes kaposi's sarcoma-associated herpesvirus (kshv) vil-6-induced angiogenesis and tumorigenesis by regulating pi3k/pten/akt/gsk-3β signaling pathway. *PLoS ONE* **2013**, *8*, e53145. [CrossRef] [PubMed]
47. Albini, A.; Soldi, R.; Giunciuclio, D.; Giraudo, E.; Benelli, R.; Primo, L.; Noonan, D.; Salio, M.; Camussi, G.; Rock, W.; et al. The angiogenesis induced by HIV–1 tat protein is mediated by the flk–1/kdr receptor on vascular endothelial cells. *Nat Med.* **1996**, *2*, 1371. [CrossRef] [PubMed]
48. Alghisi, G.C.; Rüegg, C. Vascular integrins in tumor angiogenesis: Mediators and therapeutic targets. *Endothel. Cell Res.* **2006**, *13*, 113–135. [CrossRef] [PubMed]
49. Crublet, E.; Andrieu, J.P.; Vives, R.R.; Lortat-Jacob, H. The HIV-1 envelope glycoprotein gp120 features four heparan sulfate binding domains, including the co-receptor binding site. *J. Biol. Chem.* **2008**, *283*, 15193–15200. [CrossRef] [PubMed]
50. Barillari, G.; Sgadari, C.; Palladino, C.; Gendelman, R.; Caputo, A.; Morris, C.B.; Nair, B.C.; Markham, P.; Nel, A.; Stürzl, M. Inflammatory cytokines synergize with the HIV-1 tat protein to promote angiogenesis and kaposi's sarcoma via induction of basic fibroblast growth factor and the αvβ3 integrin. *J. Immunol.* **1999**, *163*, 1929–1935. [PubMed]
51. Li, C.J.; Ueda, Y.; Shi, B.; Borodyansky, L.; Huang, L.; Li, Y.-Z.; Pardee, A.B. Tat protein induces self-perpetuating permissivity for productive HIV-1 infection. *Proc. Natl. Acad. Sci. USA* **1997**, *94*, 8116–8120. [CrossRef] [PubMed]
52. Detry, B.; Bruyère, F.; Erpicum, C.; Paupert, J.; Lamaye, F.; Maillard, C.; Lenoir, B.; Foidart, J.-M.; Thiry, M.; Noël, A. Digging deeper into lymphatic vessel formation in vitro and in vivo. *BMC Cell Biol.* **2011**, *12*, 29. [CrossRef] [PubMed]
53. Zheng, W.; Aspelund, A.; Alitalo, K. Lymphangiogenic factors, mechanisms, and applications. *J. Clin. Investig.* **2014**, *124*, 878–887. [CrossRef]

54. Norrmén, C.; Tammela, T.; Petrova, T.V.; Alitalo, K. Biological basis of therapeutic lymphangiogenesis. *Circulation* **2011**, *123*, 1335–1351. [CrossRef]
55. Lohela, M.; Bry, M.; Tammela, T.; Alitalo, K. Vegfs and receptors involved in angiogenesis versus lymphangiogenesis. *Curr. Opin. Cell Biol.* **2009**, *21*, 154–165. [CrossRef]
56. Kim, H.; Kataru, R.P.; Koh, G.Y. Inflammation-associated lymphangiogenesis: A double-edged sword? *J. Clin. Investig.* **2014**, *124*, 936–942. [CrossRef]
57. Alitalo, K.; Tammela, T.; Petrova, T.V. Lymphangiogenesis in development and human disease. *Nature* **2005**, *438*, 946. [CrossRef]
58. Zampell, J.C.; Yan, A.; Avraham, T.; Daluvoy, S.; Weitman, E.S.; Mehrara, B.J. Hif-1α coordinates lymphangiogenesis during wound healing and in response to inflammation. *FASEB J.* **2012**, *26*, 1027–1039. [CrossRef] [PubMed]
59. Mitchell, R.N.; Kumar, V.; Abbas, A.K.; Fausto, N. Robbins and cotran pathologic basis of disease. *Saun* **2010**, *2011*, 260–262.
60. Jiang, W.G.; Davies, G.; Martin, T.A.; Parr, C.; Watkins, G.; Mansel, R.E.; Mason, M.D. The potential lymphangiogenic effects of hepatocyte growth factor/scatter factor in vitro and in vivo. *Int. J. Mol. Med.* **2005**, *16*, 723–728. [PubMed]
61. Lohela, M.; Saaristo, A.; Veikkola, T.; Alitalo, K. Lymphangiogenic growth factors, receptors and therapies. *Thromb. Haemost.* **2003**, *90*, 167–184. [CrossRef] [PubMed]
62. Kajiya, K.; Hirakawa, S.; Ma, B.; Drinnenberg, I.; Detmar, M. Hepatocyte growth factor promotes lymphatic vessel formation and function. *EMBO J.* **2005**, *24*, 2885–2895. [CrossRef] [PubMed]
63. Cao, R.; Björndahl, M.A.; Gallego, M.I.; Chen, S.; Religa, P.; Hansen, A.J.; Cao, Y. Hepatocyte growth factor is a lymphangiogenic factor with an indirect mechanism of action. *Blood* **2006**, *107*, 3531–3536. [CrossRef] [PubMed]
64. Naghshvar, F.; Torabizadeh, Z.; Moslemi Zadeh, N.; Mirbaha, H.; Gheshlaghi, P. Investigating the relationship between serum level of s-met (soluble hepatic growth factor receptor) and preeclampsia in the first and second trimesters of pregnancy. *ISRN Obstet. Gynecol.* **2013**, *2013*, 925062. [CrossRef]
65. Gu, B.; Alexander, J.S.; Gu, Y.; Zhang, Y.; Lewis, D.F.; Wang, Y. Expression of lymphatic vascular endothelial hyaluronan receptor-1 (lyve-1) in the human placenta. *Lymphat. Res. Biol.* **2006**, *4*, 11–17. [CrossRef]
66. Wang, Y.; Sun, J.; Gu, Y.; Zhao, S.; Groome, L.J.; Alexander, J.S. D2-40/podoplanin expression in the human placenta. *Placenta* **2011**, *32*, 27–32. [CrossRef]
67. Liu, H.; Li, Y.; Zhang, J.; Rao, M.; Liang, H.; Liu, G. The defect of both angiogenesis and lymphangiogenesis is involved in preeclampsia. *Placenta* **2015**, *36*, 279–286. [CrossRef]
68. Cele, S.; Odun-Ayo, F.; Onyangunga, O.; Moodley, J.; Naicker, T. Analysis of hepatocyte growth factor immunostaining in the placenta of HIV-infected normotensive versus preeclamptic pregnant women. *Eur. J. Obstet. Gynecol. Reprod. Biol.* **2018**, *227*, 60–66. [CrossRef] [PubMed]
69. Platonova, N.; Miquel, G.; Regenfuss, B.; Taouji, S.; Cursiefen, C.; Chevet, E.; Bikfalvi, A. Evidence for the interaction of fibroblast growth factor-2 with the lymphatic endothelial cell marker lyve-1. *Blood* **2013**, *121*, 1229–1237. [CrossRef] [PubMed]
70. Brown, H.; Russell, D. Blood and lymphatic vasculature in the ovary: Development, function and disease. *Hum. Reprod. Update* **2013**, *20*, 29–39. [CrossRef] [PubMed]
71. Jerman, L.F.; Hey-Cunningham, A.J. The role of the lymphatic system in endometriosis: A comprehensive review of the literature. *Biol. Reprod.* **2015**, *92*, 1–10. [CrossRef] [PubMed]
72. Red-Horse, K. Lymphatic vessel dynamics in the uterine wall. *Placenta* **2008**, *29*, 55–59. [CrossRef] [PubMed]
73. Cao, R.; Ji, H.; Feng, N.; Zhang, Y.; Yang, X.; Andersson, P.; Sun, Y.; Tritsaris, K.; Hansen, A.J.; Dissing, S. Collaborative interplay between fgf-2 and vegf-c promotes lymphangiogenesis and metastasis. *Proc. Natl. Acad. Sci. USA* **2012**, *109*, 15894–15899. [CrossRef] [PubMed]
74. Shange, G.P.; Moodley, J.; Naicker, T. Effect of vascular endothelial growth factors a, c, and d in HIV-associated pre-eclampsia. *Hypertens. Pregnancy* **2017**, *36*, 196–203. [CrossRef]
75. Volchek, M.; Girling, J.E.; Lash, G.E.; Cann, L.; Kumar, B.; Robson, S.C.; Bulmer, J.N.; Rogers, P.A. Lymphatics in the human endometrium disappear during decidualization. *Hum. Reprod.* **2010**, *25*, 2455–2464. [CrossRef]
76. Lely, A.T.; Salahuddin, S.; Holwerda, K.M.; Karumanchi, S.A.; Rana, S. Circulating lymphangiogenic factors in preeclampsia. *Hypertens. Pregnancy* **2013**, *32*, 42–49. [CrossRef]

77. Onyangunga, O.A.; Moodley, J.; Merhar, V.; Ofusori, D.A.; Naicker, T. Lymphatic vascular endothelial hyaluronan receptor-1 immunoexpression in placenta of HIV infected pre-eclamptic women. *J. Reprod. Immunol.* **2016**, *117*, 81–88. [CrossRef]
78. Spradley, F.T.; Palei, A.C.; Anderson, C.D.; Granger, J.P. Melanocortin-4 receptor deficiency attenuates placental ischemia-induced hypertension in pregnant rats. *Hypertension* **2019**, *73*, 162–170. [CrossRef] [PubMed]
79. Morfoisse, F.; Renaud, E.; Hantelys, F.; Prats, A.-C.; Garmy-Susini, B. Role of hypoxia and vascular endothelial growth factors in lymphangiogenesis. *Mol. Cell. Oncol.* **2014**, *1*, e29907. [CrossRef] [PubMed]
80. Tal, R. The role of hypoxia and hypoxia-inducible factor-1alpha in preeclampsia pathogenesis. *Biol. Reprod.* **2012**, *87*, 131–138. [CrossRef] [PubMed]
81. Zhang, X.; Yu, J.; Kuzontkoski, P.M.; Zhu, W.; Li, D.Y.; Groopman, J.E. Slit2/robo4 signaling modulates HIV-1 gp120-induced lymphatic hyperpermeability. *PLoS Path.* **2012**, *8*, e1002461. [CrossRef]
82. Caccuri, F.; Rueckert, C.; Giagulli, C.; Schulze, K.; Basta, D.; Zicari, S.; Marsico, S.; Cervi, E.; Fiorentini, S.; Slevin, M. HIV-1 matrix protein p17 promotes lymphangiogenesis and activates the endothelin-1/endothelin b receptor axis. *Arterioscl. Thromb. Vasc. Biol.* **2014**, *34*, 846–856. [CrossRef] [PubMed]
83. Basta, D.; Latinovic, O.; Lafferty, M.K.; Sun, L.; Bryant, J.; Lu, W.; Caccuri, F.; Caruso, A.; Gallo, R.; Garzino-Demo, A. Angiogenic, lymphangiogenic and adipogenic effects of HIV-1 matrix protein p17. *Path. Dis.* **2015**, *73*, ftv062. [CrossRef]
84. Park, K.W.; Morrison, C.M.; Sorensen, L.K.; Jones, C.A.; Rao, Y.; Chien, C.-B.; Wu, J.Y.; Urness, L.D.; Li, D.Y. Robo4 is a vascular-specific receptor that inhibits endothelial migration. *Dev. Biol.* **2003**, *261*, 251–267. [CrossRef]
85. Yu, J.; Zhang, X.; Kuzontkoski, P.M.; Jiang, S.; Zhu, W.; Li, D.Y.; Groopman, J.E. Slit2n and robo4 regulate lymphangiogenesis through the vegf-c/vegfr-3 pathway. *Cell Commun. Sign.* **2014**, *12*, 25. [CrossRef]
86. Khaliq, O.P.; Murugesan, S.; Moodley, J.; Mackraj, I. Differential expression of mirnas are associated with the insulin signaling pathway in preeclampsia and gestational hypertension. *Clin. Exp. Hypertens.* **2018**, *40*, 744–751. [CrossRef]
87. Marincowitz, C. The Effects of HIV-1-Proteins and Antiretroviral Therapy on Aortic Endothelial Cells (Aecs)—A Mechanistic In Vitro Approach. Master's Thesis, Stellenbosch University, Stellenbosch, South Africa, 2019.
88. Song, L.; Ding, S.; Ge, Z.; Zhu, X.; Qiu, C.; Wang, Y.; Lai, E.; Yang, W.; Sun, Y.; Chow, S.A. Nucleoside/nucleotide reverse transcriptase inhibitors attenuate angiogenesis and lymphangiogenesis by impairing receptor tyrosine kinases signalling in endothelial cells. *Br. J. Pharm.* **2018**, *175*, 1241–1259. [CrossRef]
89. Sansone, M.; Sarno, L.; Saccone, G.; Berghella, V.; Maruotti, G.M.; Migliucci, A.; Capone, A.; Martinelli, P. Risk of preeclampsia in human immunodeficiency virus–infected pregnant women. *Obstet. Gynecol.* **2016**, *127*, 1027–1032. [CrossRef] [PubMed]
90. Krischer, J.; Rutschmann, O.; Hirschel, B.; Vollenweider-Roten, S.; Saurat, J.-H.; Pechère, M. Regression of kaposi's sarcoma during therapy with HIV-1 protease inhibitors: A prospective pilot study. *J. Am. Acad. Dermatol.* **1998**, *38*, 594–598. [CrossRef]
91. Sgadari, C.; Barillari, G.; Toschi, E.; Carlei, D.; Bacigalupo, I.; Baccarini, S.; Palladino, C.; Leone, P.; Bugarini, R.; Malavasi, L. HIV protease inhibitors are potent anti-angiogenic molecules and promote regression of kaposi sarcoma. *Nat. Med.* **2002**, *8*, 225. [CrossRef] [PubMed]
92. Filardi, P.P.; Paolillo, S.; Marciano, C.; Iorio, A.; Losco, T.; Marsico, F.; Scala, O.; Ruggiero, D.; Ferraro, S.; Chiariello, M. Cardiovascular effects of antiretroviral drugs: Clinical review. *Cardiovasc. Haematol. Disord. Drug Targets.* **2008**, *8*, 238–244. [CrossRef]
93. Fiala, M.; Murphy, T.; MacDougall, J.; Yang, W.; Luque, A.; Iruela-Arispe, L.; Cashman, J.; Buga, G.; Byrns, R.E.; Barbaro, G. Haart drugs induce mitochondrial damage and intercellular gaps and gp 120 causes apoptosis. *Cardiovasc. Toxicol.* **2004**, *4*, 327–337. [CrossRef] [PubMed]
94. Zhong, D.-s.; Lu, X.-h.; Conklin, B.S.; Lin, P.H.; Lumsden, A.B.; Yao, Q.; Chen, C. HIV protease inhibitor ritonavir induces cytotoxicity of human endothelial cells. *Arterioscler. Thromb. Vasc. Biol.* **2002**, *22*, 1560–1566. [CrossRef]
95. Chai, H.; Yang, H.; Yan, S.; Li, M.; Lin, P.H.; Lumsden, A.B.; Yao, Q.; Chen, C. Effects of 5 HIV protease inhibitors on vasomotor function and superoxide anion production in porcine coronary arteries. *J. Acquir. Immune Defic. Syndr.* **2005**, *40*, 12–19. [CrossRef]

96. Aouache, R.; Biquard, L.; Vaiman, D.; Miralles, F. Oxidative stress in preeclampsia and placental diseases. *Int. J. Mol. Sci.* **2018**, *19*, 1496. [CrossRef]
97. Torriani, F.J.; Komarow, L.; Parker, R.A.; Cotter, B.R.; Currier, J.S.; Dubé, M.P.; Fichtenbaum, C.J.; Gerschenson, M.; Mitchell, C.K.; Murphy, R.L. Endothelial function in human immunodeficiency virus-infected antiretroviral-naive subjects before and after starting potent antiretroviral therapy: The actg (AIDS clinical trials group) study 5152's. *J. Am. Coll. Cardiol.* **2008**, *52*, 569–576. [CrossRef]
98. Savvidou, M.; Samuel, M.; Akolekar, R.; Poulton, M.; Nicolaides, K. First trimester maternal uterine artery doppler examination in HIV—positive women. *HIV Med.* **2011**, *12*, 632–636. [CrossRef]
99. Sebitloane, H.M.; Moodley, J.; Sartorius, B. Associations between HIV, highly active anti-retroviral therapy, and hypertensive disorders of pregnancy among maternal deaths in south africa 2011–2013. *Int. J. Gynecol. Obstet.* **2017**, *136*, 195–199. [CrossRef] [PubMed]
100. Dosiou, C.; Giudice, L.C. Natural killer cells in pregnancy and recurrent pregnancy loss: Endocrine and immunologic perspectives. *Endocr. Rev.* **2005**, *26*, 44–62. [CrossRef] [PubMed]
101. King, A.; Allan, D.S.; Bowen, M.; Powis, S.J.; Joseph, S.; Verma, S.; Hiby, S.E.; McMichael, A.J.; Loke, Y.W.; Braud, V.M. HLA-E is expressed on trophoblast and interacts with CD94/NKG2 receptors on decidual nk cells. *Eur. J. Immunol.* **2000**, *30*, 1623–1631. [CrossRef]
102. Wu, J.; Lanier, L.L. Natural killer cells and cancer. *Adv. Cancer Res.* **2003**, *90*, 127–156. [PubMed]
103. Cerwenka, A.; Lanier, L.L. Natural killer cells, viruses and cancer. *Nat. Rev. Immunol.* **2001**, *1*, 41. [CrossRef] [PubMed]
104. Mandal, A.; Viswanathan, C. Natural killer cells: In health and disease. *Hematol. Oncol. Stem Cell Ther.* **2015**, *8*, 47–55. [CrossRef]
105. Wallace, A.E.; Fraser, R.; Cartwright, J.E. Extravillous trophoblast and decidual natural killer cells: A remodelling partnership. *Hum. Reprod. Update* **2012**, *18*, 458–471. [CrossRef]
106. Smith, C.; Jalbert, E.; de Almeida, V.; Canniff, J.; Lenz, L.L.; Mussi-Pinhata, M.M.; Cohen, R.A.; Yu, Q.; Amaral, F.R.; Pinto, J.; et al. Altered natural killer cell function in HIV-exposed uninfected infants. *Front. Immun.* **2017**, *8*, 470. [CrossRef]
107. Mela, C.M.; Goodier, M.R. The contribution of cytomegalovirus to changes in nk cell receptor expression in HIV-1–infected individuals. *J. Infect. Dis.* **2007**, *195*, 158–159. [CrossRef]
108. Alter, G.; Altfeld, M. Nk cells in HIV-1 infection: Evidence for their role in the control of HIV-1 infection. *J. Int. Med.* **2009**, *265*, 29–42. [CrossRef]
109. Sharma, S. Natural killer cells and regulatory t cells in early pregnancy loss. *Int. J. Dev. Biol.* **2014**, *58*, 219–229. [CrossRef] [PubMed]
110. Tang, A.-W.; Alfirevic, Z.; Quenby, S. Natural killer cells and pregnancy outcomes in women with recurrent miscarriage and infertility: A systematic review. *Hum. Reprod.* **2011**, *26*, 1971–1980. [CrossRef] [PubMed]
111. Hashemi, V.; Dolati, S.; Hosseini, A.; Gharibi, T.; Danaii, S.; Yousefi, M. Natural killer t cells in preeclampsia: An updated review. *Biomed. Pharmacother.* **2017**, *95*, 412–418. [CrossRef] [PubMed]
112. Kottilil, S. Natural killer cells in HIV-1 infection: Role of nk cell-mediated non-cytolytic mechanisms in pathogenesis of HIV-1 infection. *Indian J. Exp. Biol.* **2003**, *41*, 1219–1225. [PubMed]
113. Valentin, A.; Rosati, M.; Patenaude, D.J.; Hatzakis, A.; Kostrikis, L.G.; Lazanas, M.; Wyvill, K.M.; Yarchoan, R.; Pavlakis, G.N. Persistent HIV-1 infection of natural killer cells in patients receiving highly active antiretroviral therapy. *Proc. Natl. Acad. Sci. USA* **2002**, *99*, 7015–7020. [CrossRef] [PubMed]
114. Michaëlsson, J.; Long, B.R.; Loo, C.P.; Lanier, L.L.; Spotts, G.; Hecht, F.M.; Nixon, D.F. Immune reconstitution of cd56dim nk cells in individuals with primary HIV-1 infection treated with interleukin-2. *J. Infect. Dis.* **2008**, *197*, 117–125. [CrossRef] [PubMed]
115. Ballan, W.M.; Vu, B.-A.N.; Long, B.R.; Loo, C.P.; Michaëlsson, J.; Barbour, J.D.; Lanier, L.L.; Wiznia, A.A.; Abadi, J.; Fennelly, G.J.; et al. Natural killer cells in perinatally HIV-1-infected children exhibit less degranulation compared to HIV-1-exposed uninfected children and their expression of KIR2DL3, NKG2C, and NKP46 correlates with disease severity. *J. Immun.* **2007**, *179*, 3362–3370. [CrossRef]
116. Frias, M.; Rivero-Juarez, A.; Gordon, A.; Camacho, A.; Cantisan, S.; Cuenca-Lopez, F.; Torre-Cisneros, J.; Peña, J.; Rivero, A. Persistence of pathological distribution of nk cells in HIV-infected patients with prolonged use of haart and a sustained immune response. *PLoS ONE* **2015**, *10*, e0121019. [CrossRef]

117. Bachmayer, N.; Sohlberg, E.; Sundström, Y.; Hamad, R.R.; Berg, L.; Bremme, K.; Sverremark-Ekström, E. Women with pre-eclampsia have an altered NKG2A and NKG2C receptor expression on peripheral blood natural killer cells. *Am. J. Reprod. Immunol.* **2009**, *62*, 147–157. [CrossRef]
118. Laresgoiti-Servitje, E.; Gómez-López, N.; Olson, D.M. An immunological insight into the origins of pre-eclampsia. *Hum. Reprod. Update* **2010**, *16*, 510–524. [CrossRef]
119. Hu, W.; Wang, H.; Wang, Z.; Huang, H.; Dong, M. Elevated serum levels of interleukin-15 and interleukin-16 in preeclampsia. *J. Reprod. Immunol.* **2007**, *73*, 166–171. [CrossRef] [PubMed]
120. Fiore, S.; Newell, M.-L.; Trabattoni, D.; Thorne, C.; Gray, L.; Savasi, V.; Tibaldi, C.; Ferrazzi, E.; Clerici, M. Antiretroviral therapy-associated modulation of th1 and th2 immune responses in HIV-infected pregnant women. *J. Reprod. Immunol.* **2006**, *70*, 143–150. [CrossRef]
121. Phoswa, W.N.; Naicker, T.; Ramsuran, V.; Moodley, J. Pre-eclampsia: the role of highly active antiretroviral therapy and immune markers. *Inflamm. Res.* **2019**, *68*, 47–57. [CrossRef]
122. Maharaj, N.R.; Phulukdaree, A.; Nagiah, S.; Ramkaran, P.; Tiloke, C.; Chuturgoon, A.A. Pro-inflammatory cytokine levels in HIV infected and uninfected pregnant women with and without preeclampsia. *PLoS ONE* **2017**, *12*, e0170063. [CrossRef] [PubMed]
123. Machado, E.S.; Krauss, M.R.; Megazzini, K.; Coutinho, C.M.; Kreitchmann, R.; Melo, V.H.; Pilotto, J.H.; Ceriotto, M.; Hofer, C.B.; Siberry, G.K. Hypertension, preeclampsia and eclampsia among HIV-infected pregnant women from latin america and caribbean countries. *J. Infect.* **2014**, *68*, 572–580. [CrossRef] [PubMed]
124. Saito, S.; Nakashima, A.; Shima, T.; Ito, M. Th1/th2/th17 and regulatory *t*-cell paradigm in pregnancy. *Am. J. Reprod. Immunol.* **2010**, *63*, 601–610. [CrossRef] [PubMed]
125. Tesmer, L.A.; Lundy, S.K.; Sarkar, S.; Fox, D.A. Th17 cells in human disease. *Immunol. Rev.* **2008**, *223*, 87–113. [CrossRef] [PubMed]
126. Darmochwal-Kolarz, D.; Kludka-Sternik, M.; Tabarkiewicz, J.; Kolarz, B.; Rolinski, J.; Leszczynska-Gorzelak, B.; Oleszczuk, J. The predominance of th17 lymphocytes and decreased number and function of treg cells in preeclampsia. *J. Reprod. Immunol.* **2012**, *93*, 75–81. [CrossRef]
127. Al-Nafea, H.M.; Hamdy, N.M.; Aref, N.M. Evaluation of interleukin 17 level as a prognostic marker in active antiviral treated human immunodeficiency virus in saudi patients. *Am. J. Biochem.* **2017**, *7*, 13–22.
128. Campillo-Gimenez, L.; Cumont, M.-C.; Fay, M.; Kared, H.; Monceaux, V.; Diop, O.; Müller-Trutwin, M.; Hurtrel, B.; Lévy, Y.; Zaunders, J. AIDS progression is associated with the emergence of il-17–producing cells early after simian immunodeficiency virus infection. *J. Immunol.* **2010**, *184*, 984–992. [CrossRef]
129. Terness, P.; Kallikourdis, M.; Betz, A.G.; Rabinovich, G.A.; Saito, S.; Clark, D.A. Tolerance signaling molecules and pregnancy: Ido, galectins, and the renaissance of regulatory t cells. *Am. J. Reprod. Immunol.* **2007**, *58*, 238–254. [CrossRef] [PubMed]
130. Saito, S.; Shima, T.; Nakashima, A.; Shiozaki, A.; Ito, M.; Sasaki, Y. What is the role of regulatory t cells in the success of implantation and early pregnancy? *J. Assist. Reprod. Genet.* **2007**, *24*, 379–386. [CrossRef] [PubMed]
131. Saito, S.; Shiozaki, A.; Sasaki, Y.; Nakashima, A.; Shima, T.; Ito, M. Seminars in immunopathology. In *Regulatory t Cells and Regulatory Natural Killer (nk) Cells Play Important Roles in Feto-Maternal Tolerance*; Arck, P.C., Elkon, K.B., Hasler, P., Miyazaki, T., Eds.; Springer: Berlin, Germany, 2007; pp. 115–122.
132. Sasaki, Y.; Darmochwal-Kolarz, D.; Suzuki, D.; Sakai, M.; Ito, M.; Shima, T.; Shiozaki, A.; Rolinski, J.; Saito, S. Proportion of peripheral blood and decidual cd4+ cd25bright regulatory t cells in pre-eclampsia. *Clin. Exp. Immunol.* **2007**, *149*, 139–145. [CrossRef] [PubMed]
133. Andersson, J.; Boasso, A.; Nilsson, J.; Zhang, R.; Shire, N.J.; Lindback, S.; Shearer, G.M.; Chougnet, C.A. Cutting edge: The prevalence of regulatory t cells in lymphoid tissue is correlated with viral load in HIV-infected patients. *J. Immunol.* **2005**, *174*, 3143–3147. [CrossRef] [PubMed]
134. Suchard, M.S.; Mayne, E.; Green, V.A.; Shalekoff, S.; Donninger, S.L.; Stevens, W.S.; Gray, C.M.; Tiemessen, C.T. Foxp3 expression is upregulated in cd4+ t cells in progressive HIV-1 infection and is a marker of disease severity. *PLoS ONE* **2010**, *5*, e11762. [CrossRef] [PubMed]
135. Eggena, M.P.; Barugahare, B.; Jones, N.; Okello, M.; Mutalya, S.; Kityo, C.; Mugyenyi, P.; Cao, H. Depletion of regulatory t cells in HIV infection is associated with immune activation. *J. Immunol.* **2005**, *174*, 4407–4414. [CrossRef] [PubMed]

136. Pozo-Balado, M.M.; Martínez-Bonet, M.; Rosado, I.; Ruiz-Mateos, E.; Méndez-Lagares, G.; Rodríguez-Méndez, M.M.; Vidal, F.; Muñoz-Fernández, M.A.; Pacheco, Y.M.; Leal, M. Maraviroc reduces the regulatory t-cell frequency in antiretroviral-naive HIV-infected subjects. *J. Infect. Dis.* **2014**, *210*, 890–898. [CrossRef]
137. Montes, M.; Sanchez, C.; Lewis, D.E.; Graviss, E.A.; Seas, C.; Gotuzzo, E.; White, A.C., Jr. Normalization of foxp3+ regulatory t cells in response to effective antiretroviral therapy. *J. Inf. Dis.* **2010**, *203*, 496–499. [CrossRef]

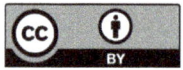

© 2019 by the authors. Licensee MDPI, Basel, Switzerland. This article is an open access article distributed under the terms and conditions of the Creative Commons Attribution (CC BY) license (http://creativecommons.org/licenses/by/4.0/).

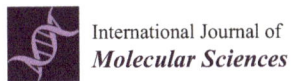

Article

Hydroxychloroquine Mitigates the Production of 8-Isoprostane and Improves Vascular Dysfunction: Implications for Treating Preeclampsia

Rahana Abd Rahman [1,2,3,*], Padma Murthi [2,4,*,†], Harmeet Singh [2], Seshini Gurungsinghe [1], Bryan Leaw [2], Joanne C. Mockler [1], Rebecca Lim [1,2] and Euan M. Wallace [1,2,*]

1. Department of Obstetrics and Gynaecology, School of Clinical Sciences, Monash University, Monash Medical Centre, Clayton, Victoria 3168, Australia; seshini.gurusinghe@monash.edu (S.G.); joanne.mockler@monash.edu (J.C.M.); rebecca.lim@hudson.org.au (R.L.)
2. The Ritchie Centre, Hudson Institute of Medical Research, Clayton, Victoria 3168, Australia; harmeet73@gmail.com (H.S.); bryan.leaw@hudson.org.au (B.L.)
3. Department of Obstetrics and Gynaecology, Faculty of Medicine, National University of Malaysia, Kuala Lumpur 56000, Malaysia
4. Department of Obstetrics and Gynaecology, University of Melbourne, Parkville, Victoria 3052, Australia
* Correspondence: drrahana@ppukm.ukm.edu.my (R.A.R.); padma.murthi@monash.edu (P.M.); euan.wallace@monash.edu (E.M.W.)
† Current address: Cardiovascular Research Program, Monash Biomedicine Discovery Institute and Department of Pharmacology, Monash University, Clayton, Victoria, Australia.

Received: 19 March 2020; Accepted: 31 March 2020; Published: 3 April 2020

Abstract: In preeclampsia, widespread maternal endothelial dysfunction is often secondary to excessive generation of placental-derived anti-angiogenic factors, including soluble fms-like tyrosine kinase-1 (sFlt-1) and soluble endoglin (sEng), along with proinflammatory cytokines such as tumour necrosis factor-α (TNF-α) and activin A, understanding of which offers potential opportunities for the development of novel therapies. The antimalarial hydroxychloroquine is an anti-inflammatory drug improving endothelial homeostasis in lupus. It has not been explored as to whether it can improve placental and endothelial function in preeclampsia. In this in vitro study, term placental explants were used to assess the effects of hydroxychloroquine on placental production of sFlt-1, sEng, TNF-α, activin A, and 8-isoprostane after exposure to hypoxic injury or oxidative stress. Similarly, human umbilical vein endothelial cells (HUVECs) were used to assess the effects of hydroxychloroquine on in vitro markers of endothelial dysfunction. Hydroxychloroquine had no effect on the release of sFlt-1, sEng, TNF-α, activin A, or 8-isoprostane from placental explants exposed to hypoxic injury or oxidative stress. However, hydroxychloroquine mitigated TNF-α-induced HUVEC production of 8-isoprostane and Nicotinanamide adenine dinucleotide phosphate (NADPH) oxidase expression. Hydroxychloroquine also mitigated TNF-α and preeclamptic serum-induced HUVEC monolayer permeability and rescued the loss of zona occludens protein zona occludens 1 (ZO-1). Although hydroxychloroquine had no apparent effects on trophoblast function, it may be a useful endothelial protectant in women presenting with preeclampsia.

Keywords: hydroxychloroquine; preeclampsia; sFlt-1; sEng; TNF-α; endothelial dysfunction

1. Introduction

Preeclampsia complicates 3%–5% of all pregnancies and remains one of the leading causes of maternal and perinatal morbidity and mortality [1]. In particular, pregnancies complicated by early onset preeclampsia (prior to 34 weeks gestation) are associated with a 20-fold increase in maternal death [2] and considerably increased rates of maternal and perinatal morbidities [3]. As such, the management of early onset preeclampsia continues to pose significant challenges to obstetricians attempting to balance maternal risks with fetal benefits of prolonging pregnancy.

Although not fully understood, the pathophysiology of preeclampsia is generally agreed to originate with poor placentation [4]. Inadequate trophoblast invasion and failure of maternal spiral arterial remodeling leads to impaired placental development, including exposure to chronic progressive ischaemia–reperfusion injury characterized by evidence of excessive oxidative stress. In turn, this induces excessive placental release of anti-angiogenic factors such as soluble fms-like tyrosine kinase-1 (sFlt-1) and soluble endoglin (sEng), coupled with inflammatory cytokines including tumour necrosis factor-α (TNF-α) and activin A [5–8]. These various factors target the maternal vasculature and contribute significantly to the widespread maternal vascular dysfunction, which is often associated with oxidative injury [9–12]. Dysfunctional cells of the vasculature are characterized by increased endothelial cell permeability, altered distribution of endothelial junctional proteins, and reduced endothelium-dependent relaxation [13,14].

Antimalarials, such as hydroxychloroquine, were first formally used as a treatment for cutaneous lupus in 1894. Following the observation in the 1940s that they had improved rheumatoid arthritis, they became a popular therapy in rheumatic diseases [15]. However, research has only recently unraveled some of the mechanisms of hydroxychloroquine's therapeutic effect, as observed by Wallace et al. 2012 [16]. Hydroxychloroquine is classified as C under the U.S. Food and Drug Administration pregnancy category because it crosses the placenta but has not been reported to cause any teratogenic effects to the fetus [17,18]. It has both anti-inflammatory and immunomodulatory properties [19–21], and is widely used in autoimmune disorders such as systemic lupus erythematosus (SLE), rheumatoid arthritis (RA), and Sjogren's syndrome. The exact mechanisms by which hydroxychloroquine improves the activity of these disorders are still not fully understood. However, in women with SLE, it has been shown to decrease circulating levels of pro-inflammatory cytokines IL-6, IL-8, and TNF-α [22], as well as IL-17 and IL-22, which are cytokines produced by helper T cells [23]. Recently, in a female mouse model of SLE, it was reported that hydroxychloroquine decreased endothelial oxidative stress by reducing Nicotinamide adenine dinucleotide phosphate (NADPH) oxidase activity, which led to improved endothelial function, lower blood pressure, and a reduction in proteinuria [24].

In preeclampsia, NADPH oxidase-dependent oxidative stress is one of the pathways underlying the maternal endothelial dysfunction [12]. Accordingly, we hypothesize that hydroxychloroquine may confer beneficial effects in women diagnosed with preeclampsia by reducing placental production of potentially deleterious mediators, thus improving the overall maternal endothelial homeostasis.

2. Results

2.1. Effects of Hydroxychloroquine on Placental Secretion

Hypoxia significantly increased the secretion of sFlt-1 (Figure 1a, $p = 0.02$), sEng (Figure 1b, $p = 0.02$), and TNF-α (Figure 1c, $p = 0.02$) from explant cultures after 24 h incubation. In the presence of X-XO (xanthine/xanthine oxidase system), explants cultured for 48 h significantly increased secretions of 8-isoprostane (Figure 2a, $p = 0.03$) and activin A (Figure 2b, $p = 0.01$) compared to controls. Co-incubation with 1 µg/mL hydroxychloroquine did not alter either the hypoxia-induced secretion of sFlt-1 (Figure 1a), sEng (Figure 1b), or TNF-α (Figure 1c), or the X-XO-induced increase in 8-isoprostane (Figure 2a) and activin A (Figure 2b).

2.2. Effect of Hydroxychloroquine on HUVEC Viability

Previously we have demonstrated that, compared to untreated controls, there was no effect of hydroxychloroquine on human umbilical vein endothelial cell (HUVEC) viability across a dose range of 0.1, 1, and 10 µg/mL over 120 h in culture [25]. However, treatment of cells with

100 µg/mL hydroxychloroquine significantly reduced cell viability at 24 h ($p < 0.001$) [25]. Dosing of hydroxychloroquine for all subsequent experiments were based on these results.

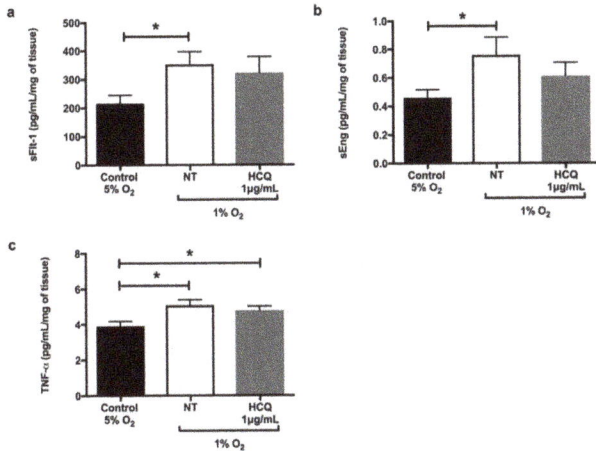

Figure 1. Release of (**a**) soluble fms-like tyrosine kinase-1 (sFlt-1), (**b**) soluble endoglin (sEng), and (**c**) tumour necrosis factor-α (TNF-α) by placental explants of human term normal pregnancy placentae after 24 h incubation at 5% oxygen concentration (normoxia) versus 1% oxygen (hypoxia). The explants were incubated in the hypoxic environment in the absence or presence of 1 µg/mL hydroxychloroquine. Data are mean ± standard error of the mean (SEM) from 10 independent biological replicates. * denotes $p < 0.05$. NT: non treated, HCQ: hydroxychloroquine.

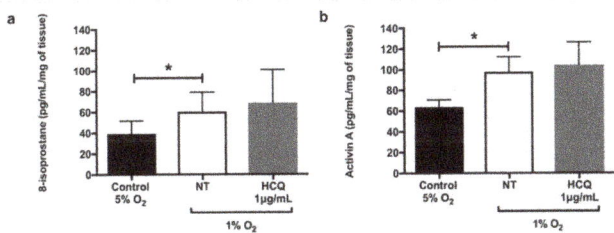

Figure 2. Release of (**a**) 8-isoprostane and (**b**) activin A by placental explants of human term normal pregnancy placentae after 48 h incubation at 20% oxygen concentration with 5% CO_2. The explants were incubated in media containing xanthine (2.3 mM) + xanthine oxidase (15 mU/mL) in the absence or presence of 1 µg/mL hydroxychloroquine. Data are mean ± SEM from 10 independent biological replicates. * denotes $p < 0.05$. X/XO: xanthine/xanthine oxidase, HCQ: hydroxychloroquine.

2.3. Effects of Hydroxychloroquine on Endothelial Function In Vitro

HUVECs were treated in the absence or presence of (i) TNF-α (100 ng/mL), (ii) sera from normal pregnancies (20%), or (iii) sera from preeclamptic women (20%) in the presence or absence of hydroxychloroquine (1 µg/mL) to assess endothelial dysfunction (Figure 3). Compared to controls, incubation of HUVECs with TNF-α (Figure 3a,c) or sera from preeclamptic women (Figure 3b,d) significantly increased both NADPH oxidase 2 (NOX2) mRNA expression ($p < 0.001$ and $p = 0.01$, respectively) and 8-isoprostane secretion ($p = 0.02$ and $p = 0.04$, respectively). Co-treatment of HUVECs with TNF-α and hydroxychloroquine significantly reduced NOX2 mRNA expression (Figure 3a, $p = 0.03$) and secretion of 8-isoprostane (Figure 3c, $p = 0.04$). Co-treatment of HUVECs with serum from preeclamptic women and hydroxychloroquine did not significantly alter the expression of NOX2 mRNA or 8-isoprostane. However, 100 µM apocynin, a NOX inhibitor, significantly reduced the NOX2 mRNA expression and 8-isoprostane release induced by serum from preeclamptic women (Figure 3b,d, respectively, $p < 0.01$ for both).

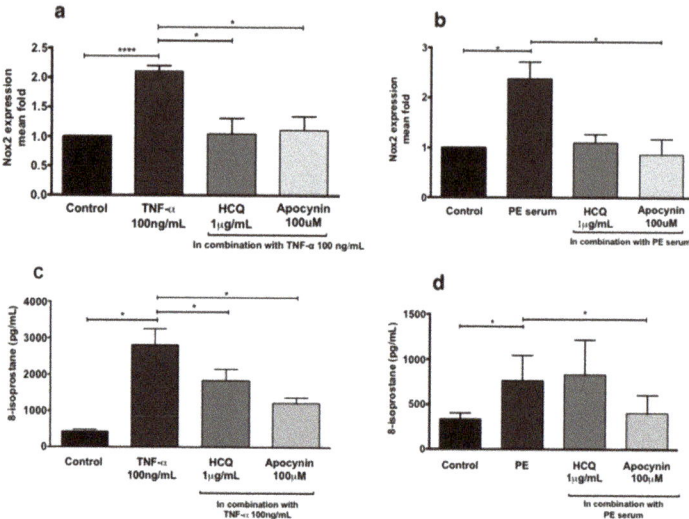

Figure 3. NADPH oxidase 2 (NOX2) RNA expression of human umbilical vein endothelial cells (HUVECs) treated with 100 ng/mL TNF-α (**a**) and 20% preeclampsia (PE) sera (**b**). Release of 8-isoprostane by HUVECs treated with 100 ng/mL recombinant TNF-α (**c**) and 20% preeclampsia sera (**d**). Data are mean ± SEM from eight independent biological replicates. * denotes $p < 0.05$; ****$p < 0.001$.

Compared to controls, incubation of HUVECs with TNF-α (Figure 4a) or 20% sera from preeclamptic women (Figure 4b) increased immunoreactivity for NOX2 protein. Once again, co-treatment of HUVECs with TNF-α and either apocynin or hydroxychloroquine reduced immunoreactive NOX2 protein expression (Figure 4a). Similarly, co-treatment of HUVECs with sera from preeclamptic women and either apocynin or hydroxychloroquine also showed reduced immunoreactive NOX2 protein expression (Figure 4b).

Figure 4. Western blot representative for NOX2 protein expression of HUVECs untreated (cont) or treated with 100 ng/mL TNF-α (**a**) or 20% preeclampsia (PE) sera (**b**) with or without apocynin (apo, 100 µM) or hydroxychloroquine (HCQ, 1 µg/mL). β-actin was used as a loading control.

2.4. Effect of Hydroxychloroquine on Vascular Permeability

Both TNF-α (Figure 5a) and sera from preeclamptic women (Figure 5b) significantly increased HUVEC monolayer permeability compared to controls ($p = 0.02$ and $p = 0.005$, respectively). These effects were mitigated by co-treatment with hydroxychloroquine ($p = 0.04$ and $p = 0.007$, respectively). Hydroxychloroquine prevented the significant loss of zonula occludens 1 (ZO-1) induced by both TNF-α (Figure 5c, $p = 0.003$) and sera from preeclamptic women (Figure 5d, $p = 0.02$).

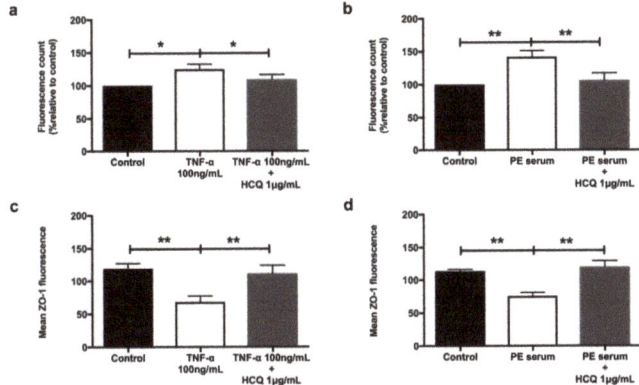

Figure 5. HUVECs' permeability when treated with 100 ng/mL recombinant TNF-α (**a**) and 20% preeclampsia sera (**b**) ($n = 9$). Mean zonula occludens 1 (ZO-1) fluorescence when treated with 100 ng/mL recombinant TNF-α (**c**) and 20% preeclampsia sera (**d**) ($n = 6$). Data are means ± SEM from nine and six independent biological replicates, respectively. * denotes $p < 0.05$, and ** denotes $p < 0.005$.

2.5. Effect of Hydroxychloroquine on Zonula Occludens 1 (ZO-1) Immunohistochemistry

Figure 6 contains representative images of ZO-1 immunostaining. There was normal ZO-1 immunostaining in untreated or HUVECs treated with sera from normal pregnancies (Figure 6A,D), with the loss of immunostaining in cells treated with either TNF-α (Figure 6B) or preeclampsia sera (Figure 6E). Hydroxychloroquine rescued the loss of ZO-1 induced by both TNF-α (Figure 6C) and preeclampsia sera (Figure 6F).

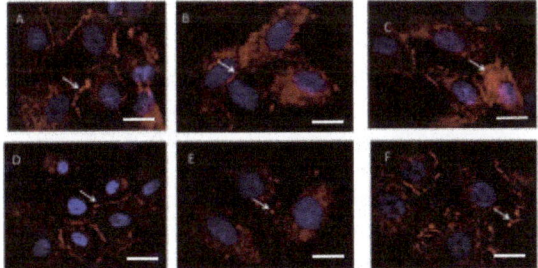

Figure 6. Immunofluorescent staining of ZO-1 on HUVECs treated with 100 ng/mL recombinant TNF-α or 20% preeclampsia sera for 16–22 h. Representative images from one of six experiments are shown. (**A**) Control untreated HUVECs, (**B**) TNF-α 100 ng/mL, (**C**) TNF-α 100 ng/mL with hydroxychloroquine 1 μg/mL, (**D**) control HUVECs treated with 20% normal pregnancy sera, (**E**) 20% preeclampsia sera, and (**F**) preeclampsia sera with hydroxychloroquine 1 μg/mL. Arrows show the ZO-1 staining on the endothelial cell border.

3. Discussion

We undertook the study to explore the potential of hydroxychloroquine as a novel targeted therapy addressing key pathophysiological pathways in preeclampsia. We demonstrated that this antimalarial drug affords no apparent protection against hypoxia or oxidative stress in placental explants but that it does have endothelial protective properties. These observations suggest that hydroxychloroquine is a potential therapy for women with established preeclampsia but is unlikely to be useful as a preventative treatment.

We hypothesized that hydroxychloroquine would protect placental tissue from hypoxia-induced injury ex vivo. Specifically, we sought to show that hydroxychloroquine could mitigate the effects of hypoxia and hyperoxia on the placental release of the anti-angiogenic factors sFlt-1 and sEng, as well as on the release of the pro-inflammatory cytokines, TNF-α, and activin A. However, we found this not to be the case. Hydroxychloroquine had no effect on modulating hypoxia-induced placental injury. These findings support those of others who tested hydroxychloroquine in a trophoblast-derived cell line exposed to antiphospholipid antibodies as a model of antiphospholipid syndrome [26]. They found that although hydroxychloroquine was able to mitigate trophoblast secretion of IL-6, it had no effect on sEng release [26]. Collectively, this suggests that in an established diagnosis of preeclampsia, the use of hydroxychloroquine may not confer any beneficial effects.

The maternal symptoms of preeclampsia are largely due to widespread maternal endothelial dysfunction [27,28]. Lupus shares this feature as the key mechanism underlying hypertension, renal dysfunction, and other organ injury [29]. Indeed, the endothelial dysfunction in both preeclampsia and lupus have also been shown to be due, at least in part, to excessive oxidative stress secondary to NOX activation [12,30,31]. Recently, in murine models of lupus, hydroxychloroquine was shown to reverse endothelial dysfunction via the downregulation of NOX, and subsequently, oxidative stress [24,32]. Here, we showed that hydroxychloroquine may have similar effects in an in vitro model of preeclampsia-like endothelial dysfunction. Specifically, hydroxychloroquine was able to prevent the TNF-α induction of NOX2 and subsequent oxidative stress in HUVECs but, importantly, was not able to block similar effects induced by sera from preeclamptic women. Interestingly, apocynin, a NOX inhibitor, was able to prevent the effects of both TNF-α and sera from preeclamptic women on NOX2. This confirms the pro-oxidative effects of the sera of preeclamptic women are mediated via NOX2 [12]. Müller-Calleja et al. demonstrated the inhibition of reactive oxygen species (ROS) generated by endosomal NOX in human monocytic cells [33]. However, the concentration used was much higher (10 µM) but still within therapeutic range as compared to ours (3.6 µM). It is apparent that the concentration of hydroxychloroquine differs in various cell types in in vitro experiments. Although several isoforms of NOX family members including NOX1, NOX2 (also called gp91phox), NOX3, NOX 4, and NOX 5 have been reported to date, in endothelial cells, NOX1, NOX2, and NOX4 isoforms are reported to be involved in the inflammatory response and cytokine expression, triggered by angiotensin II treatment, through different mitogen activated protein kinases (MAPK) pathway activation (phosphorylated form of p38 MAPK, extracellular signal regulated kinases, ERK-1/2 and stress-activated protein kinases and c-jun N-terminal kinase, SAPK/JNK) [34].

We have shown before that follistatin, an activin binding protein, can block the endothelial effects of sera from preeclamptic women [12,35]. Compared to women with a normal pregnancy, maternal circulating levels of activin are increased approximately 10-fold in women with preeclampsia [36]. We have not yet explored whether hydroxychloroquine can block activin-mediated effects. However, the current study suggests that sera from preeclamptic women contains factors capable of inducing NOX, which cannot be mitigated by hydroxychloroquine.

Intriguingly, hydroxychloroquine was able to mitigate the effects of both TNF-α and sera from preeclamptic women on the loss of endothelial ZO-1 and integrity. Endothelial ZO-1 is a protein present in endothelial cell–cell junction known to regulate cellular permeability [37]. Any changes in ZO-1 protein, such as induced by a response to inflammatory cytokines, will alter the endothelial cell permeability. The loss of ZO-1 induced by TNF-α is known to be mediated via the activation of NOX [38,39]. Hydroxychloroquine was able to prevent the loss of ZO-1 and the subsequently increased endothelial permeability induced by both TNF-α and sera from preeclamptic women, suggesting these effects may be mediated through a TNF-α-dependent upregulation of NOX. Further evaluation is required to verify this theory, perhaps using TNF-α receptor antagonists co-incubated with the sera of preeclamptic women.

Circulating levels of TNF-α increase in normal pregnant women and are further raised in preeclamptic women [40–42]. These levels are much lower than the concentrations tested in the present study (15 pg/mL vs. 100 ng/mL, respectively). Although in the in vitro model of acute exposure of cells to single high dose may not be a good representation of the in vivo situation, previous studies have reported that 100 ng/mL of TNF-α in cultured HUVEC enhanced endothelial cell activation, similar to that observed in preeclampsia [43].

The effect of hydroxychloroquine on other pathogenic pathways of preeclampsia have not been explored in this study. For example, it is now thought that a key mechanism of action of antimalarial drugs is the antagonism of toll-like receptor (TLR) signaling and subsequent downstream activation of pro-inflammatory cytokines [16,44]. In preeclampsia, placental expression of TLR3, TLR7, and TLR8 are upregulated [45,46]. The treatment of pregnant rodents with TLR agonists induces a preeclampsia-like phenotype, providing further evidence of other mechanistic pathways that hydroxychloroquine treatment could also target.

In addition to the effects of antimalarial agents on TLRs, these drugs have other benefits, such as inhibition of phospholipase A2 (PLA2) enzyme. PLA2 has been implicated in the pathogenesis of preeclampsia and is found to be elevated in both decidual tissue and the sera of preeclamptic women [47,48]. Similarly, in patients with active SLE, there is a 4.6-fold increase in the mean activity of PLA2 [49]. Lipid peroxidation occurs because of oxidative stress induced by the elevated levels of reactive oxygen species. This leads to membrane phospholipid degradation and hence release of arachidonic acid [50]. Zabul et al. have described the potential role of arachidonic acid hydroperoxide underlying the molecular mechanism of oxidative stress in preeclampsia [51]. Arachidonic acid stimulates release of superoxide from neutrophils and macrophages [52]. Antimalarial drugs have been shown to inhibit PLA2 activity and therefore reduce the generation of superoxide, which will be beneficial for improving endothelial dysfunction in preeclamptic patients [50,53].

4. Materials and Methods

4.1. Blood and Tissue Collection

Preeclampsia is defined as elevation of blood pressure of 140/90 mmHg or more, and proteinuria of more than 0.3 g in a 24 h urine collection or random urine dipstick test of more than 2+ according to the Society of Obstetric Medicine of Australia and New Zealand guidelines [54]. All blood and placental tissues were collected from pregnant women, as detailed below. Written and informed consent was obtained from all individual participants included in the study with the approval of the Monash Health Human Research Ethics Committee (HREC no. 13357B, dated 6 August 2015). Venous blood was collected from women with a singleton healthy pregnancy and from women with established preeclampsia at 24 to 34 weeks of gestation. Women who had received intravenous magnesium sulphate, or had pre-existing or secondary hypertension, diabetes, or a multiple pregnancy, were excluded. None of the women with preeclampsia were in labor at the time of blood sampling. The control (healthy) women were matched for gestation (≤34 weeks). Sera were separated and pooled into two groups: healthy term pregnancy serum and preeclampsia serum. For all in vitro experiments, 20% pooled sera from preeclampsia pregnancies were used for treatment of endothelial cells and were compared with that of the normotensive sera treated cells. There were significant differences in the systolic and diastolic blood pressure and proteinuria between normotensive and preeclamptic patients ($p = 0.007$), as previously presented [25].

4.2. Placental Explant Cultures Ex Vivo

Placental villous explants ($n = 10$) were collected from term uncomplicated pregnancies at elective caesarean section within 20 min of delivery of the placenta. Briefly, placental villous tissue was excised by removing maternal decidua. Villous explants (approximately 50–70 mg wet weight) were then thoroughly washed with cold Hank's balanced salt solution (HBSS, 1:10, Life Technologies/Thermo Fisher Scientific, Waltham, MA, USA) and placed in 24-well plates in M199 supplemented with 1% antibiotics/antimycotics (penicillin G, streptomycin sulphate, and amphotericin B) and 1% of

4.3. Placental Hypoxia

Placental hypoxia was modeled by incubating placental explants in 1% oxygen with 5% CO_2 at 37°C in the presence or absence of 1µg/mL hydroxychloroquine (Sigma-Aldrich, St. Louis, Missouri, USA). Controls were incubated in 5% oxygen. The conditioned media were collected after 24 h and stored at -80°C for sFlt-1, sEng, TNF-α, and activin A assay.

4.4. Placental Oxidative Stress

The explants were treated with 2.3 mM xanthine (X) and 0.015 U/mL xanthine oxidase (XO) (Sigma-Aldrich) to induce oxidative stress [8,55]. Explants were incubated in X/XO in the presence or absence of 1 µg/mL hydroxychloroquine for 48 h at 37 °C in 20% oxygen, 5% CO_2. Untreated cultures served as controls. Conditioned media were collected and stored at -80 °C in the presence of 0.005% butylated hydroxytoluene (BHT) (Sigma-Aldrich, St. Louis, Missouri, USA) to prevent autoxidation for activin A and 8-isoprostane assay measurements. Elevated levels of 8-isoprostane are a marker for lipid peroxidation caused by oxidative stress [56] and, in addition, high levels of activin A have been implicated in the pathway of placental oxidative stress [12].

4.5. Measurement of sFlt-1, sEng, TNF-α, and Activin A with ELISA

Levels of sFlt-1, sEng, TNF-α, and activin A were measured in placental explant ($n = 10$) conditioned media using Quantikine immunoassay ELISAs (R&D systems, Minneapolis, Minnesota, USA) according to the manufacturer's protocol. All samples were assayed in duplicate. Briefly, for the measurement of sFlt-1, sEng, TNF-α, and activin A, the conditioned media was diluted (1:40, 1:10, 1:5, and 1:30, respectively) with assay diluent. Results were normalized per milligram weight of tissue.

4.6. Human Umbilical vein Endothelial Cell (HUVEC) Isolation

Umbilical cords were also obtained from healthy women with term singleton pregnancies ($n = 8$) undergoing elective caesarean. HUVECs were isolated and cultured, as previously described, with minor modifications [8,57]. Briefly, the umbilical cord was severed from the placenta within an hour of collection. All areas with clamp marks were removed and the umbilical vein was cannulated and tied with thread. After removal of blood, the umbilical veins were infused with type II collagenase (0.5 mg/mL, Sigma-Aldrich) and incubated for 10 min at 37°C to isolate the endothelial cells. They were maintained in M199 complete media containing 20% heat-inactivated fetal calf serum, 1% antibiotics/antimycotics (penicillin G, streptomycin sulphate, and amphotericin B), and 1% L-glutamine with endothelial and fibroblast growth factor (10 ng/mL each). Only cells at passage 2 to 4 were used for experiments.

4.7. HUVEC Viability Assay

We first determined the effect of different concentrations of hydroxychloroquine on HUVEC viability. Cells were plated at 2×10^4 cells per well in 96-well plates ($n = 8$, Corning) and grown to confluence in 100 µL culture media with hydroxychloroquine added at different concentrations (0.1, 1, 10, 100 µg/mL) and further incubated for 24 h. Viability was assessed by adding 20 µL MTS (3-(4,5-dimethylthiazol-2-yl)-2,5-diphenyltetrazolium bromide) reagent (Promega, Madison, WI, USA) to each well. After 1 h at 37 °C, the absorbance at 490 nm was read using a plate reader (SpectraMax i3, Molecular Devices, San Jose, CA 95134 USA).

4.8. Oxidative Stress as Assessed by 8-Isoprostane

Cells were grown to confluence in 96-well plates (2×10^4 cells per well) for 24 h in M199 complete media. Cells were treated with media (control), 100 ng/mL TNF-α (Life Technologies/Thermo Fisher Scientific, Waltham, MA, USA), 20% normal pregnancy sera, or 20% preeclampsia sera, in the presence or absence of hydroxychloroquine (0, 0.1, 1, and 10 μg/mL) for a further 24 h. Conditioned media were then stored at -80°C in the presence of 0.005% butylated hydroxytoluene (BHT) as described above. Total 8-isoprostane was measured using a commercial enzyme immunoassay (Cayman Chemical, Ann Arbor, MI, USA) according to the manufacturer's instructions. Samples were assayed in duplicate after diluting 1:5 with assay diluent. On the basis of the results from this experiment, in all subsequent experiments 1 μg/mL hydroxychloroquine was used. The cells were treated with either 100 ng/mL of recombinant TNF-α or 20% preeclampsia sera in combination with either 1 μg/mL hydroxychloroquine or 100 μM apocynin (NADPH oxidase inhibitor) (Sigma-Aldrich) for 24 h.

4.9. Measurement of NADPH Oxidase (NOX2) mRNA Expression

Cells were grown to confluence in 6-well plates (1×10^5 cells per well) for 48–72 h in M199 complete media. Cells were treated with 100 ng/mL recombinant TNF-α or 20% preeclampsia serum combined with either 100 μM apocynin or 1 μg/mL hydroxychloroquine for 6 and 12 h, respectively. The treatment groups were compared with untreated HUVECs or cells treated with 20% sera from normotensive pregnant women. Total cellular RNA was isolated with Ambion (Life Technologies/Thermo Fisher Scientific, Waltham, MA, USA) according to the manufacturer's protocols. The cDNA was prepared with 1 μg of cellular mRNA and reverse-transcribed using SuperScript III first strand synthesis system (Life Technologies). Quantitative PCR was performed on Rotorgene (Qiagen, Hilden, Germany) in a reaction mixture (20 μL) containing Sensimix SYBR Green PCR master mix (Bioline Meridian Biosciences, Heidelberg, Germany). The reactions were performed with the following conditions: 95 °C for 10 min then 40 cycles of 95°C for 20 s, 60 °C for 30 s, and 72 °C for 30 s. NOX2 was amplified using primers 5'-TGG CAC CCT TTT ACA CTG-3' and 5'-CCA CTA ACA TCA CCA CCT CA-3'. The housekeeping gene 18S was amplified using primers 5'-GTC TGT GAT GCC CTT AGA TGT C-3' and 5'-AAG CTT ATG ACC CGC ACT TAC-3'. Relative gene expression was determined using the delta delta – cycle threshold (CT) method.

4.10. Measurement of NOX2 Protein Expression

HUVECs were grown to confluence and treated with either 100 ng/mL recombinant TNF-α or 20% preeclampsia serum combined with 100 μM apocynin or 1 μg/mL hydroxychloroquine for 6 and 12 h, respectively. HUVECs were assessed for total NOX2 protein. Protein extracts of nucleic and cytoplasmic fractions were obtained using the nuclear and cytoplasmic reagents (Life Technologies/Thermo Fisher Scientific, Waltham, MA, USA) according to manufacturer's instructions. Protein quantification was performed using the Pierce Bicinchoninic acid (BCA) kit (Life Technologies/Thermo Fisher Scientific, Waltham, MA, USA)). For Western blots, 40μg protein was loaded for each sample. Membranes were then blocked with 5% (*w/v*) skim milk in phosphate-buffered saline with 0.1% (*v/v*) Tween-20 for 1 h prior to probing with antibodies. Membranes were stripped in a mild stripping buffer (1.5% *w/v* glycine, 0.1% *w/v* sodium dodecyl sulfate, 1% *v/v* Tween-20 in distilled water) for 5 min between antibodies. The primary antibodies and concentrations used were Nox2 at 0.025 ng/mL (anti-NOX2/gp91phox antibody (ab80508, Abcam, Cambridge, United Kingdom) and the control β-actin at 0.01 ng/mL (IMG-5142A, Imgenex). Antibodies were diluted in blocking buffer and incubated overnight at 4 °C. Chemiluminiscence detection was performed using Clarity Western Electrochemiluminescence (ECL) blotting Substrates (Bio-Rad, Hercules, CA, USA).

4.11. Endothelial Permeability Assay

An endothelial permeability assay was performed as previously described with minor modifications [58]. Briefly, culture inserts (0.4 µm pore size, 6.5 mm diameter; Corning) were coated with 0.2% gelatin (Sigma-Aldrich) for 30 min at room temperature. HUVECs (50,000 cells per well) were plated on the inserts and cultured to form a tight monolayer with 100 µL M199 complete media in the upper chamber and 600 µL in the lower chamber at 37 °C, 5% CO_2 for 72 h. Inserts were then transferred to a fresh plate and cell monolayers were treated in fresh media containing 100 ng/mL recombinant TNF-α alone or with 1 µg/mL hydroxychloroquine for 16–22 h. Treatment groups were compared with untreated HUVECs. The conditioned media were collected and 100 µL fresh media containing fluorescein isothiocyanate (FITC)-conjugated dextran (MW 40000, final concentration 1 mg/mL, Sigma-Aldrich) was added to the upper chamber. The plate was incubated while protected from light for 60 min. The media from the lower chamber were diluted (1:20) in HBSS for measurement of fluorescence at 485/535 nm using a plate reader (SpectraMax i3, Molecular Devices). Results (fluorescence units) were expressed as percent changes relative to control.

Assessment of cell permeability when treated with 20% sera from healthy or preeclamptic women was performed using in vitro permeability assay kit from Millipore (Merck Millipore) in the absence or presence of 1 µg/mL hydroxychloroquine for 16–22 h. The treatment groups were compared with HUVECs treated with serum from women who had normal pregnancies (NP). Briefly, the transwells, which were coated with collagen, were rehydrated with 250 µL endothelial growth media (EGM, Lonza) and left at room temperature for 15 min. Subsequently, 200 µL of the media was removed and replaced with an equal volume of cell stock (1×10^5). Then, 500 µL of media was added to the receiver plate and incubated for 72 h to form a tight monolayer. Following this, fresh media was replaced in the receiver plate. The cells were treated accordingly and further incubated for 16–22 h. Media in the upper chamber was replaced with fresh media (150 µL) containing fluorescein isothiocyanate (FITC)-conjugated dextran, and the plate was incubated for 30 min and protected from light. The media from the lower chamber was diluted (1:20) with HBSS for measurement of fluorescence at 485/535 nm using a plate reader (SpectraMax i3, Molecular Devices). Results (fluorescence units) were expressed as percent changes relative to control.

4.12. Zonula Occludens (ZO-1) Immunohistochemistry for the Assessment of Endothelial Integrity

HUVECs were grown on 14 mm glass coverslips (4×10^4 cells/well) placed in 24 well plates. Cells were treated with 100 ng/mL recombinant TNF-α or 20% sera from preeclamptic women in the presence or absence of 1 µg/mL hydroxychloroquine for 16–22 h prior to fixing with 4% paraformaldehyde (Sigma-Aldrich) for 30 min at room temperature. The treatment groups were compared with untreated HUVECs or cells treated with 20% normal pregnancy sera. Cells were blocked with 0.5% bovine serum albumin (BSA, Sigma-Aldrich) for 30 min, incubated first with rabbit anti-ZO-1 (1:50, Zymed) overnight at 4°C, then with donkey anti-rabbit Alexa Fluor 568 (1:100, Invitrogen) for 1 h in the dark. Cell nuclei were stained with 2 µm 4′,6-diamidino-2-phenyindole dilactate (DAPI, Sigma Aldrich) for 10 min and mounted with fluorescent mounting media (DakoCytomation). Staining was examined with an Olympus BX60 fluorescent microscope and images were taken using an Olympus DP70 camera and Olympus CellSens software (Olympus). The primary antibody was replaced with an isotype-matched control antibody in the negative controls. The mean intensity of the staining was assessed using ImageJ software (version 2.0.0-rc-43/1.50i, http://imagej.net/Fiji/Downloads, Bethesda, MD).

5. Conclusions

Hydroxychloroquine has a significant protective impact on endothelial function acting via the suppression of NOX-induced oxidative stress; it is unable to mitigate all of the effects of preeclamptic sera-induced injury in vitro or to mitigate ex vivo placental injury. Further evaluation is warranted to determine other molecular pathways by which hydroxychloroquine may prevent endothelial dysfunction in preeclampsia. The results of this study strongly suggest that hydroxychloroquine seems likely to be clinically effective as adjuvant therapy in women diagnosed with preeclampsia.

Author Contributions: All authors have read and agree to the published version of the manuscript. Conceptualization, R.A.R., P.M., and E.M.W.; methodology, R.A.R. and P.M.; software, B.L.; validation, H.S. and P.M.; formal analysis, R.A.R., H.M., and P.M.; investigation, R.L.; data curation, S.G.; writing and editing—original draft preparation, R.A.R.; writing—review and editing, P.M. and E.M.W.; visualization, H.M.; supervision, P.M. and E.M.W.; project administration, E.M.W.; funding acquisition, E.M.W.

Funding: R.A.R. was supported by The Ministry of Higher Education of Malaysia.

Acknowledgments: We would like to acknowledge all mothers who donated their placenta and the staff at Monash Medical Centre, Clayton, Australia, for their assistance with collecting these tissue samples. Monash Health is supported by the Victorian Government's Operational Infrastructure Support Program.

Conflicts of Interest: The authors declare no conflict of interest.

References

1. Sibai, B.; Dekker, G.; Kupfermine, M. Pre-eclampsia. *Lancet* **2005**, *365*, 785–799. [CrossRef]
2. Mackay, A.; Berg, C.; Atrash, H. Pregnancy-related mortality from preeclampsia and eclampsia. *Obstet. Gynecol.* **2001**, *97*, 533–538. [PubMed]
3. Kucukgoz Gulec, U.; Ozgunen, F.T.; Buyukkurt, S.; Guzel, A.B.; Urunsak, I.F.; Demir, S.C.; Evruke, I.C. Comparison of clinical and laboratory findings in early- and late-onset preeclampsia. *J. Matern. Fetal Neonatal Med.* **2013**, *26*, 1228–1233. [CrossRef] [PubMed]
4. Lisonkova, S.; Sabr, Y.; Mayer, C.; Young, C.; Skoll, A.; Joseph, K.S. Maternal morbidity associated with early-onset and late-onset preeclampsia. *Obstet. Gynecol.* **2014**, *124*, 771–781. [CrossRef] [PubMed]
5. Redman, C.W. Preeclampsia: A multi-stress disorder. *Rev. Med. Interne* **2011**, *32*, S41–S44. [CrossRef]
6. Nagamatsu, T.; Fujii, T.; Kusumi, M.; Zou, L.; Yamashita, T.; Osuga, Y.; Momoeda, M.; Kozuma, S.; Taketani, Y. Cytotrophoblasts up-regulate soluble fms-like tyrosine kinase-1 expression under reduced oxygen: An implication for the placental vascular development and the pathophysiology of preeclampsia. *Endocrinology* **2004**, *145*, 4838–4845. [CrossRef]
7. Gilbert, J.S.; Gilbert, S.A.; Arany, M.; Granger, J.P. Hypertension produced by placental ischemia in pregnant rats is associated with increased soluble endoglin expression. *Hypertension* **2009**, *53*, 399–403. [CrossRef]
8. Jain, A.; Schneider, H.; Aliyev, E.; Soydemir, F.; Baumann, M.; Surbek, D.; Hediger, M.; Brownbill, P.; Albrecht, C. Hypoxic treatment of human dual placental perfusion induces a preeclampsia-like inflammatory response. *Lab Investig.* **2014**, *94*, 873–880. [CrossRef]
9. Mandang, S.; Manuelpillai, U.; Wallace, E.M. Oxidative stress increases placental and endothelial cell activin A secretion. *J. Endocrinol.* **2007**, *192*, 485–493. [CrossRef]
10. Tam Tam, K.B.; Lamarca, B.; Arany, M.; Cockrell, K.; Fournier, L.; Murphy, S.; Martin, J.N., Jr.; Granger, J.P. Role of reactive oxygen species during hypertension in response to chronic antiangiogenic factor (sFlt-1) excess in pregnant rats. *Am. J. Hypertens.* **2011**, *24*, 110–113. [CrossRef]
11. Onda, K.; Tong, S.; Nakahara, A.; Kondo, M.; Monchusho, H.; Hirano, T.; Kaitu'u-Lino, T.; Beard, S.; Binder, N.; Tuohey, L.; et al. Sofalcone upregulates the nuclear factor (erythroid-derived 2)-like 2/heme oxygenase-1 pathway, reduces soluble fms-like tyrosine kinase-1, and quenches endothelial dysfunction: Potential therapeutic for preeclampsia. *Hypertension* **2015**, *65*, 855–862. [CrossRef] [PubMed]
12. Brownfoot, F.C.; Tong, S.; Hannan, N.J.; Hastie, R.; Cannon, P.; Tuohey, L.; Kaitu'u-Lino, T.J. YC-1 reduces placental sFlt-1 and soluble endoglin production and decreases endothelial dysfunction: A possible therapeutic for preeclampsia. *Mol. Cell. Endocrinol.* **2015**, *413*, 202–208. [CrossRef] [PubMed]
13. Lim, R.; Acharya, R.; Delpachitra, P.; Hobson, S.; Sobey, C.G.; Drummond, G.R.; Wallace, E.M. Activin and NADPH-oxidase in preeclampsia: Insights from in vitro and murine studies. *Am. J. Obstet. Gynecol.* **2015**, *212*, e1–e12. [CrossRef] [PubMed]
14. Myers, J.; Mires, G.; Macleod, M.; Baker, P. In preeclampsia, the circulating factors capable of altering in vitro endothelial function precede clinical disease. *Hypertension* **2005**, *45*, 258–263. [CrossRef] [PubMed]

15. Wang, Y.; Gu, Y.; Zhang, Y.; Lewis, D.F. Evidence of endothelial dysfunction in preeclampsia: Decreased endothelial nitric oxide synthase expression is associated with increased cell permeability in endothelial cells from preeclampsia. *Am. J. Obstet. Gynecol.* **2004**, *190*, 817–824. [CrossRef]
16. Wallace, D.J. The history of antimalarials. *Lupus* **1996**, *5*, S2–S3. [CrossRef]
17. Wallace, D.J.; Gudsoorkar, V.S.; Weisman, M.H.; Venuturupalli, S.R. New insights into mechanisms of therapeutic effects of antimalarial agents in SLE. *Nat. Rev. Rheumatol.* **2012**, *8*, 522–533. [CrossRef]
18. US Food and Drug Administration Pregnancy Category. Available online: http://www.accessdata.fda.gov/scripts/cdrh/cfdocs/cfCFR/CFRSearch.cfm?fr=201.57 (accessed on 6 August 2015).
19. Costedoat-Chalumeau, N.; Amoura, Z.; Duhaut, P.; Huong, D.L.; Sebbough, D.; Wechsler, B.; Vauthier, D.; Denjoy, I.; Lupoglazoff, J.M.; Piette, J.C. Safety of hydroxychloroquine in pregnant patients with connective tissue diseases: A study of one hundred thirty-three cases compared with a control group. *Arthritis Rheum.* **2003**, *48*, 3207–3211. [CrossRef]
20. Miyachi, Y.; Yoshioka, A.; Imamura, S.; Niwa, Y. Antioxidant action of antimalarials. *Ann. Rheum. Dis.* **1986**, *45*, 244–248. [CrossRef]
21. Zhu, X.; Ertel, W.; Ayala, A.; Morrison, M.; Perrin, M.; Chaudry, I. Chloroquine inhibits macrophage tumour necrosis factor-α mRNA transcription. *Immunology* **1993**, *80*, 122–126.
22. Karres, I.; Kremer, J.; Dietl, I.; Steckholzer, U.; Jochum, M.; Ertel, W. Chloroquine inhibits proinflammatory cytokine release into human whole blood. *Am. J. Physiol.* **1998**, *43*, R1058–R1064. [CrossRef] [PubMed]
23. Willis, R.; Seif, A.M.; McGwin, G., Jr.; Martinez-Martinez, L.A.; Gonzalez, E.B.; Dang, N.; Papalardo, E.; Liu, J.; Vila, L.M.; Reveille, J.D.; et al. Effect of hydroxychloroquine treatment on pro-inflammatory cytokines and disease activity in SLE patients: Data from LUMINA (LXXV), a multiethnic US cohort. *Lupus* **2012**, *21*, 830–835. [CrossRef] [PubMed]
24. Silva, J.C.; Mariz, H.A.; Rocha Jr, L.F.; Oliveira, P.S.; Dantas, A.T.; Duarte, A.L.; Pitta, I.R.; Galdino, S.L.; Pitta, M.G. Hydroxychloroquine decreases Th17-related cytokines in systemic lupus erythematosus and rheumatoid arthritis patients. *Clinics* **2013**, *68*, 766–771. [CrossRef]
25. Gomez-Guzman, M.; Jimenez, R.; Romero, M.; Sanchez, M.; Zarzuelo, M.J.; Gomez-Morales, M.; O'Valle, F.; Lopez-Farre, A.J.; Algieri, F.; Galvez, J.; et al. Chronic hydroxychloroquine improves endothelial dysfunction and protects kidney in a mouse model of systemic lupus erythematosus. *Hypertension* **2014**, *64*, 330–337. [CrossRef]
26. Rahman, R.; Murthi, P.; Singh, H.; Gurusinghe, S.; Mockler, J.C.; Lim, R.; Wallace, E.M. The effects of hydroxychloroquine on endothelial dysfunction. *Pregnancy Hypertens. Int. J. Women's Cardiovasc. Health* **2016**, *6*, 259–262. [CrossRef]
27. Albert, C.R.; Schlesinger, W.J.; Viall, C.A.; Mulla, M.J.; Brosens, J.J.; Chamley, L.W.; Abrahams, V.M. Effect of hydroxychloroquine on antiphospholipid antibody-induced changes in first trimester trophoblast function. *Am. J. Reprod. Immunol.* **2014**, *71*, 154–164. [CrossRef]
28. Roberts, J.; Taylor, R.; Musci, T.; Rodgers, G.; Hubel, C.; McLaughlin, M. Preeclampsia-an endothelial disorder. *Am. J. Obstet. Gynecol.* **1989**, *161*, 1200–1204. [CrossRef]
29. LaMarca, B. Endothelial dysfunction; an important mediator in the pathophysiology of hypertension during preeclampsia. *Minerva Ginecol.* **2012**, *64*, 309–320.
30. Bilodeau, J.F.; Qin Wei, S.; Larose, J.; Greffard, K.; Moisan, V.; Audibert, F.; Fraser, W.D.; Julien, P. Plasma F2-isoprostane class VI isomers at 12-18 weeks of pregnancy are associated with later occurrence of preeclampsia. *Free Radic. Biol. Med.* **2015**, *85*, 282–287. [CrossRef]
31. George, E.M.; Hosick, P.A.; Stec, D.E.; Granger, J.P. Heme oxygenase inhibition increases blood pressure in pregnant rats. *Am. J. Hypertens.* **2013**, *26*, 924–930. [CrossRef]
32. Miesel, R.; Hartung, R.; Kroeger, H. Priming Of NADPH oxidase by tumor necrosis factor-α in patients with inflammatory and autoimmune rheumatic diseases. *Inflammation* **1996**, *20*, 427–438. [CrossRef] [PubMed]
33. Virdis, A.; Tani, C.; Duranti, E.; Vagnani, S.; Carli, L.; Kuhl, A.A.; Solini, A.; Baldini, C.; Talarico, R.; Bombardieri, S.; et al. Early treatment with hydroxychloroquine prevents the development of endothelial dysfunction in a murine model of systemic lupus erythematosus. *Arthritis Res. Ther.* **2015**, *17*, 277. [CrossRef] [PubMed]
34. Muller-Calleja, N.; Manukyan, D.; Canisius, A.; Strand, D.; Lackner, K.J. Hydroxychloroquine inhibits proinflammatory signalling pathways by targeting endosomal NADPH oxidase. *Ann. Rheum. Dis.* **2017**, *76*, 891–897. [CrossRef]

35. Dan, I.; Watanabe, M.N.; Kusumi, A. The Ste20 group kinases as regulators of MAP kinase cascades. *Trends Cell Biol.* **2001**, *11*, 220–230. [CrossRef]
36. Hobson, S.R.; Acharya, R.; Lim, R.; Chan, S.T.; Mockler, J.; Wallace, E.M. Role of activin A in the pathogenesis of endothelial cell dysfunction in preeclampsia. *Pregnancy Hypertens.* **2016**, *6*, 130–133. [CrossRef] [PubMed]
37. Muttukrishna, S.; Knight, P.G.; Groome, N.P.; Redman, C.W.G.; Ledger, W.L. Activin A and inhibin A as possible endocrine markers for pre-eclampsia. *Lancet* **1997**, *349*, 1285–1288. [CrossRef]
38. Kakei, Y.; Akashi, M.; Shigeta, T.; Hasegawa, T.; Komori, T. Alteration of cell-cell junctions in cultured human lymphatic endothelial cells with inflammatory cytokine stimulation. *Lymphat. Res. Biol.* **2014**, *12*, 136–143. [CrossRef]
39. Aveleira, C.; Lin, C.; Abcouwer, S.; Ambrosio, A.; Antonetti, D. TNF-α signals through PKC/NFkB to alter the tight junction complex and increase retinal endothelial cell permeability. *Diabetes* **2010**, *59*, 2872–2882. [CrossRef]
40. Abdullah, Z.; Bayraktutan, U. NADPH oxidase mediates TNF-α-evoked in vitro brain barrier dysfunction: Roles of apoptosis and time. *Mol. Cell. Neurosci.* **2014**, *61*, 72–84. [CrossRef]
41. Vince, S.G.; Starkey, M.P.; Austgulen, R.; Kowiatkowski, D.; Redman, C.W.G. Interleukin-6, turnour necrosis factor and soluble tumour necrosis factor receptors in women with pre-eclampsia. *Br. J. Obstet. Gynaecol.* **1995**, *102*, 20–25. [CrossRef]
42. Conrad, K.P.; Miles, T.M.; Benyo, D.F. Circulating levels of immunoreactive cytokines in women with preeclampsia. *Am. J. Reprod. Immunol.* **1998**, *40*, 102–111. [CrossRef] [PubMed]
43. Teran, E.; Escudero, C.; Moya, W.; Flores, M.; Vallance, P.; Lopez-Jaramillo, P. Elevated C-reactive protein and pro-inflammatory cytokines in Andean women with pre-eclampsia. *Int. J. Gynecol. Obstet.* **2001**, *75*, 243–249. [CrossRef]
44. Tannetta, D.S.; Muttukrishna, S.; Groome, N.P.; Redman, C.W.; Sargent, I.L. Endothelial cells and peripheral blood mononuclear cells are a potential source of extraplacental activin a in preeclampsia. *J. Clin. Endocrinol. Metab.* **2003**, *88*, 5995–6001. [CrossRef] [PubMed]
45. Kuznik, A.; Bencina, M.; Svajger, U.; Jeras, M.; Rozman, B.; Jerala, R. Mechanism of endosomal TLR inhibition by antimalarial drugs and imidazoquinolines. *J. Immunol.* **2011**, *186*, 4794–4804. [CrossRef]
46. Chatterjee, P.; Weaver, L.E.; Doersch, K.M.; Kopriva, S.E.; Chiasson, V.L.; Allen, S.J.; Narayanan, A.M.; Young, K.J.; Jones, K.A.; Kuehl, T.J.; et al. Placental Toll-like receptor 3 and Toll-like receptor 7/8 activation contributes to preeclampsia in humans and mice. *PLoS ONE* **2012**, *7*, e41884. [CrossRef]
47. Tinsley, J.H.; Chiasson, V.L.; Mahajan, A.; Young, K.J.; Mitchell, B.M. Toll-like receptor 3 activation during pregnancy elicits preeclampsia-like symptoms in rats. *Am. J. Hypertens.* **2009**, *22*, 1314–1319. [CrossRef]
48. Pulkkinen, M.; Kivikoski, A.; Nevalainen, T. Group 1 and group II phospholipase A2 in serum during normal and pathological pregnancy. *Gynecol. Obstet. Investig.* **1993**, *36*, 96–101. [CrossRef]
49. Staff, A.; Ranheim, T.; Halvorsen, B. Augmented PLA2 activity in pre-eclamptic decidual tissue—A key player in the pathophysiology of 'acute atherosis' in pre-eclampsia? *Placenta* **2003**, *24*, 965–973. [CrossRef]
50. Pruzanski, W.; Goulding, N.; Flower, R.; Gladman, D.; Urowitz, M.; Goodman, P.; Scott, K.; Vadas, P. Circulating group II phospholipase A2 activity and antilipocortin antibodies in systemic lupus erythematosus. Correlative study with disease activity. *J. Rheumatol.* **1994**, *21*, 252–257.
51. Au, A.; Chan, P.; Fishman, R. Stimulation of phospholipase A2 activity by oxygen-derived free radicals in isolated brain capillaries. *J. Cell. Biochem.* **1985**, *27*, 449–453. [CrossRef]
52. Zabul, P.; Wozniak, M.; Slominski, A.T.; Preis, K.; Gorska, M.; Korozan, M.; Wieruszewski, J.; Zmijewski, M.A.; Zabul, E.; Tuckey, R.; et al. A proposed molecular mechanism of high-dose vitamin D3 supplementation in prevention and treatment of preeclampsia. *Int. J. Mol. Sci.* **2015**, *16*, 13043–13064. [CrossRef] [PubMed]
53. Maridonneau-Parini, I.; Tauber, A. Activation of NADPH-oxidase by arachidonic acid involves phospholipase A2 in intact human neutrophils but not in the cell-free system. *Biochem. Biophys. Res. Commun.* **1986**, *138*, 1099–1105. [CrossRef]
54. Henderson, L.; Chappell, J.; Jones, O. Superoxide generation is inhibited by phospholipase A2 inhibitors. *Biochem. J.* **1989**, *264*, 249–255. [CrossRef] [PubMed]
55. Lowe, S.; Bowyer, L.; Lust, K.; McMahon, L.; Morton, M.; North, R.; Paech, M.; Said, J. Guidelines for the management of hypertensive disorders of pregnancy 2014. *Aust. N. Z. J. Obstet. Gynaecol.* **2014**, *49*, 242–246. [CrossRef]

56. Murata, M.; Fukushima, K.; Seki, H.; Takeda, S.; Wake, N. Oxidative stress produced by xanthine oxidase induces apoptosis in human extravillous trophoblast cells. *J. Reprod. Dev.* **2013**, *59*, 7–13. [CrossRef]
57. Montuschi, P.; Barnes, P.J.; Roberts, L.J., 2nd. Isoprostanes: Markers and mediators of oxidative stress. *FASEB J.* **2004**, *18*, 1791–1800. [CrossRef]
58. Jaffe, E.A.; Nachman, R.L.; Becker, C.G.; Minick, C.R. Culture of human endothelial cells derived from umbilical veins. Identification by morphologic and immunologic criteria. *J. Clin. Investig.* **1973**, *52*, 2745–2756. [CrossRef]

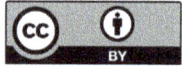

© 2020 by the authors. Licensee MDPI, Basel, Switzerland. This article is an open access article distributed under the terms and conditions of the Creative Commons Attribution (CC BY) license (http://creativecommons.org/licenses/by/4.0/).

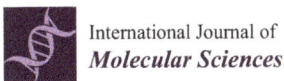

Article

Speckle Tracking Echocardiography: New Ways of Translational Approaches in Preeclampsia to Detect Cardiovascular Dysfunction

Kristin Kräker [1,2,3,4,5], Till Schütte [3,4,5,6], Jamie O'Driscoll [7,8,9], Anna Birukov [5,10], Olga Patey [7,8,11], Florian Herse [1,2,3,4], Dominik N. Müller [1,2,3,4,5], Basky Thilaganathan [7,8], Nadine Haase [1,2,3,4,5] and Ralf Dechend [1,3,4,5,12],*

1. Experimental and Clinical Research Center, a joint cooperation between the Max – Delbrück—Center for Molecular Medicine and the Charité—Universitätsmedizin Berlin, 13125 Berlin, Germany; kristin.kraeker@charite.de
2. Max – Delbrück—Center for Molecular Medicine in the Helmholtz Association, 13125 Berlin, Germany
3. Charité—Universitätsmedizin Berlin, corporate member of Freie Universität Berlin, Humboldt—Universität zu Berlin, and Berlin Institute of Health, 10117 Berlin, Germany
4. Berlin Institute of Health (BIH), 10178 Berlin, Germany
5. DZHK (German Centre for Cardiovascular Research), partner site Berlin, 10785 Berlin, Germany
6. Institute of Pharmacology, Charité—Universitätsmedizin Berlin, corporate member of Freie Universität Berlin, Humboldt—Universität zu Berlin, and Berlin Institute of Health, 10115 Berlin, Germany
7. Molecular & Clinical Sciences Research Institute, St George's University of London, London SW17 0RE, UK
8. Fetal Medicine Unit, St. George's University Hospitals NHS Foundation Trust, London SW17 0QT, UK
9. Canterbury Christ Church University, School of Human and Life Sciences, Kent CT1 1QU, UK
10. Department of Molecular Epidemiology, German Institute of Human Nutrition Potsdam-Rehbrücke, 14558 Nuthetal, Germany
11. Brompton Centre for Fetal Cardiology, Royal Brompton and Harefield Hospitals NHS Foundation Trust, London SW3 6NP, UK
12. HELIOS-Klinikum, 13125 Berlin, Germany
* Correspondence: ralf.dechend@charite.de; Tel.: +49-30-450540303

Received: 2 December 2019; Accepted: 3 February 2020; Published: 10 February 2020

Abstract: Several studies have shown that women with a preeclamptic pregnancy exhibit an increased risk of cardiovascular disease. However, the underlying molecular mechanisms are unknown. Animal models are essential to investigate the causes of this increased risk and have the ability to assess possible preventive and therapeutic interventions. Using the latest technologies such as speckle tracking echocardiography (STE), it is feasible to map subclinical changes in cardiac diastolic and systolic function as well as structural changes of the maternal heart. The aim of this work is to compare cardiovascular changes in an established transgenic rat model with preeclampsia-like pregnancies with findings from human preeclamptic pregnancies by STE. The same algorithms were used to evaluate and compare the changes in echoes of human and rodents. Parameters of functionality such as global longitudinal strain (animal −23.54 ± 1.82% vs. −13.79 ± 0.57%, human −20.60 ± 0.47% vs. −15.45 ± 1.55%) as well as indications of morphological changes such as relative wall thickness (animal 0.20 ± 0.01 vs. 0.25 ± 0.01, human 0.34 ± 0.01 vs. 0.40 ± 0.02) are significantly altered in both species after preeclamptic pregnancies. Thus, the described rat model simulates the human situation quite well and is a valuable tool for future investigations regarding cardiovascular changes. STE is a unique technique that can be applied in animal models and humans with a high potential to uncover cardiovascular maladaptation and subtle pathologies.

Keywords: preeclampsia; pregnancy; speckle tracking echocardiography; cardiovascular dysfunction; animal models of human disease

1. Introduction

A pathological pregnancy, including preterm birth, gestational diabetes mellitus, and preeclampsia (PE), is the first gender-specific risk factor for cardiovascular disease (CVD) later in life [1]. PE, with its typical symptoms including the onset of hypertension and signs of end-organ damage, has a fourfold increase regarding the risk for long-term CVD [2]. In the last years, cardiovascular changes during a preeclamptic pregnancy and especially persistent alterations in maternal cardiac structure and function moved into the focus of scientific research [3]. It has been demonstrated that former preeclamptic women show relaxation abnormalities, diastolic dysfunction, left ventricular (LV) hypertrophy [4–6], and abnormal response to volume expansion and exercise [7–9]. In most of the studies, symptoms are rather mild and sometimes even asymptomatic. It remains unclear whether the increased risk for future CVD is related to PE or predisposing and preexisting factors [10], and thus PE represents a window to compromised future cardiovascular health. The mechanism for pathological functional and structural remodeling in the maternal heart after a pathological pregnancy is also not fully understood.

For this reason, representative animal models are of increasing importance. A well-established rodent model for PE is the rat model, whose female is transgenic for human angiotensinogen and is mated with a transgenic male for human renin. Both animals are phenotypically inconspicuous until mating. Interestingly, dams develop typical symptoms of PE such as high blood pressure and albuminuria in the last trimester of pregnancy [11,12]. In addition, placenta-induced pathology with intrauterine growth retardation [12,13], elevated sFlt-1 levels [14], and existing AT1 autoantibodies [15] are presented in this animal model. Although PE is not caused by a monocausal pathology, this model reflects appropriately the human aspects of the disease. The use of rodent models such as this will help us to understand the mechanisms of disease-related alterations in cardiac function and structure that influence maternal long-term health after a pathological pregnancy. Furthermore, potential novel preventive and therapeutic strategies can be evaluated. Nevertheless, the gap between animal models and the human disease is wide, and translational research strategies are warranted to narrow the bridge.

In this study, we tested the hypothesis of whether the transgenic rat model is suitable for the investigation of the cardiovascular burden after PE. Recently, we showed that the preeclamptic rat suffers from hypertrophy and diastolic dysfunction [16]. Next, we compared this animal model with the systolic and the diastolic functions of the human maternal heart after a preeclamptic pregnancy. Speckle tracking echocardiography (STE), a state-of-the-art technique considered as the gold standard for early detection of cardiac dysfunction, is the current key tool for the non-invasive measurement of changes in cardiac function and structure. In this ultrasound imaging technique, the movement of heart tissue is analyzed using the naturally occurring speckle pattern in the heart muscle or in the blood. This mixture of interference patterns and natural acoustic reflections makes it possible to document the movement of the heart muscle by defining vectors and speed. These reflections are also known as speckles, which have a unique pattern for each region of the myocardium and make it possible to follow the region from one image to the next. Strain is defined as the percentage change in the dimension of an object compared to the original shape. Similarly, strain rate can be defined as the speed at which the deformation occurs. When applied to the LV, the deformation is defined by the three strains: longitudinal, circumferential, and radial. There is a systolic longitudinal and circumferential shortening and a radial thickening. Therefore, longitudinal and circumferential parameters have negative values, whereas radial parameters have positive values.

Formerly preeclamptic women were examined by STE 50 weeks after delivery and compared with age-matched controls. Transgenic rats were subjected to echocardiography and the same post processing algorithms four weeks after a preeclamptic pregnancy, which corresponds to two years in the human situation [17].

2. Results

Speckle tracking echocardiography (STE) was performed four weeks postpartum in formerly pregnant rats with PE-specific symptoms such as high blood pressure and albuminuria. In comparison, the same method was performed in formerly preeclamptic women 50 weeks after delivery (Figure 1). Both former preeclamptic species (PE) were compared with matched controls after healthy pregnancy (control).

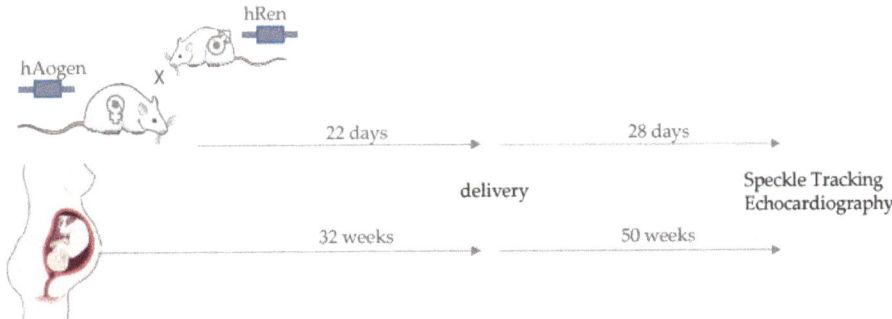

Figure 1. Formerly preeclamptic women and rats from a transgenic animal model were characterized postpartum regarding cardiac alterations in function and structure. Early onset preeclamptic women showed a lower gestational age than controls but were matched on scanning time after delivery.

2.1. Speckle Tracking Echocardiography in the Transgenic Animal Model Simulates the Human Situation

The most important readout in STE is the global strain data. It describes the degree of deformation of the myocardium in different directions. The most sensitive parameter, the global longitudinal strain (GLS), was reduced after PE in both the animal model (control −23.5 ± 1.8% vs. PE −13.8 ± 0.6%) and the human (control −20.6 ± 0.5% vs. PE −15.5 ± 1.6%) postpartum situation (Figure 2A), and it was the same regarding the global longitudinal strain rate (Figure 2B). The global radial strain (Figure 2C) and the corresponding strain rate (Figure 2D) showed only a decreased tendency in the animal post-PE model and were unchanged in the human situation. The global circumferential strain (Figure 2E) and the corresponding strain rate (Figure 2F) were reduced in the animal model but showed no changes after human preeclamptic pregnancy. Moreover, former PE animals demonstrated a clear reduction of the ejection fraction (EF) with control 66.3 ± 2.3% vs. PE 55.5 ± 1.3%. The human data confirm the trend (Figure 2G). The stroke volume (Figure 2H) as well as the cardiac output (Figure 2I) and the end diastolic volume (Figure 2J) were not altered postpartum in any of the species. The end systolic volume only showed a slight increase in the animal model but not in the human postpartum situation (Figure 2K). In addition, echocardiography provided the first initial evidence of morphological changes. The posterior wall was clearly thickened in the animal post-PE model; in the human situation, it showed a borderline p-value of 0.06 (Figure 2L). If the relative wall thickness was considered, both species showed a postpartum increase (Figure 2M) with control 0.20 ± 0.01 vs. PE 0.25 ± 0.01 in the animal model and control 0.34 ± 0.01 vs. PE 0.40 ± 0.02 in the human postpartum situation. Interestingly, formerly preeclamptic animals showed an increase in LV masses (control 983.5 ± 19.0 mg vs. PE 1138.0 ± 40.6 mg); however, formerly preeclamptic women did not (Figure 2N). The LV diameter in the end diastole was not significantly changed in either species (Figure 2O). The heart rate was significantly increased in the animal model after preeclamptic pregnancy (control 306.6 ± 6.8 bpm vs. PE 356.2 ± 11.0 bpm). With a p-value of 0.08, this trend was also evident in the human situation (Figure 2P).

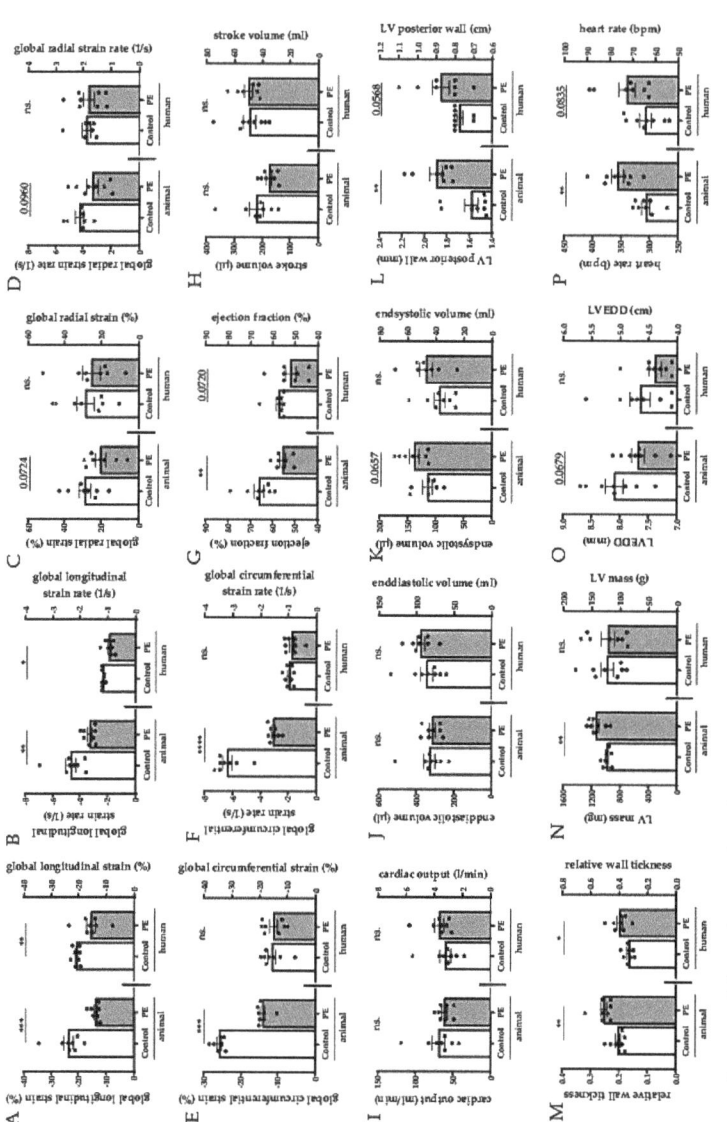

Figure 2. The transgenic rat model simulates cardiac alterations of a human preeclamptic pregnancy. Global longitudinal strain (**A**) and global longitudinal strain rate (**B**) were decreased after preeclampsia (PE). Global radial strain (**C**) and the corresponding strain rate (**D**) were not altered after PE. Global circumferential strain (**E**) and global circumferential strain rate (**F**) were reduced in the post-PE animals but not in the human cohort. Ejection fraction was reduced in animals and showed the same trend in the human PE data (**G**). Stroke volume (**H**), cardiac output (**I**), end-diastolic (**J**), and end-systolic volume (**K**) were not altered in either species after PE. Left ventricle (LV) posterior wall (**L**) and relative wall thickness (**M**) were increased due to PE in both species. LV mass (**N**) was only increased in the post-PE animals. LV end-diastolic diameter (**O**) was unaltered. Heart rate was higher in PE animals and showed increasing trends in humans (**P**). Mean values ± SEM, unpaired students t-test, ns. Non-significant, * $p < 0.05$, ** $p < 0.01$, *** $p < 0.001$, **** $p < 0.0001$.

Figure 3 summarizes the described measurements in relative changes after a preeclamptic pregnancy compared to the healthy controls by a spider's web plot. Here, the examined parameters are noted in the corners. The controls were normalized to the reference value 1.0, which is shown as a grey line. Changes in the animal post-PE model are reflected by the red line, and the purple line refers to the changes in the human post-PE situation compared to healthy controls. Concludingly, similar deviations after pathological pregnancy in both species can be observed. Several functional parameters, such as EF, were reduced, and parameters representing structural remodeling, such as relative wall thickness, were increased in both species compared to controls.

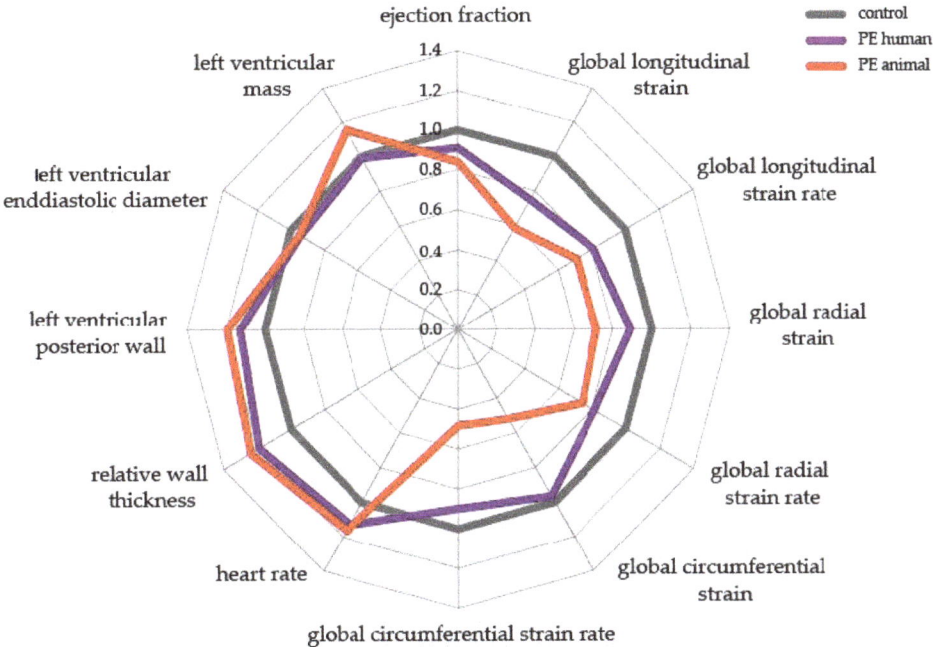

Figure 3. Relative values of post-preeclamptic changes in the animal model and in the human situation. Controls of each species were normalized to one. Grey line = controls, purple line = PE human, red line = PE animal; PE preeclampsia.

2.2. Intraobserver Variability Shows an Excellent Correlation within One Observer

Analyses of the intraobserver variability in the animal data showed an excellent correlation between two repeated evaluations of EF, $r = 0.97$, $p < 0.0001$ (Figure 4A), and GLS, $r = 0.98$, $p < 0.0001$ (Figure 4B) within one observer. The very strong agreement between repeated evaluations was substantiated in the corresponding Bland–Altman plots, which showed only a marginal bias mean difference (95% CI for limits of agreement): 0.75 (4.50 to −3.00) for EF (Figure 4C) and −0.50 (1.30 to −2.31) for GLS (Figure 4D). In the human data analyses, there was likewise an excellent intraobserver correlation regarding measurements of EF, $r = 0.94$, $p < 0.0001$ (Figure 4E), and GLS, $r = 0.98$, $p < 0.0001$ (Figure 4F). Only a minor bias was seen in the corresponding Bland–Altman plots: 0.44 (4.48 to −3.61) for repeated evaluation of human EF (Figure 4G) and −0.11 (1.36 to −1.58) for human GLS (Figure 4H). The intraclass correlation coefficients (ICCs) for reliability of the evaluations were excellent both in animal and in human analyses (95% CI): 0.96 (0.89 to 0.99) for animal EF, 0.97 (0.92 to 0.99) for animal GLS, 0.93 (0.83 to 0.98) for human EF, 0.98 (0.95 to 0.99) for human GLS evaluations.

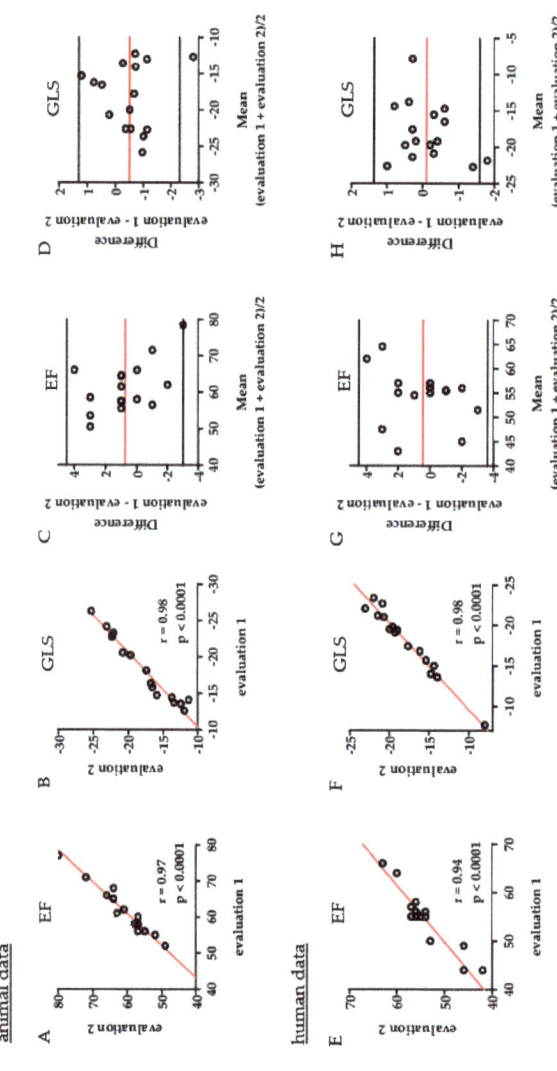

Figure 4. Intraobserver comparison. In analyses of animal data, there was an excellent correlation between the two repeated evaluations of ejection fraction, r = 0.97, $p < 0.0001$ (**A**), and global longitudinal strain, r = 0.98, $p < 0.0001$ (**B**) within one observer. The excellent agreement between the two evaluations was substantiated in the corresponding Bland–Altman plots, which showed only a marginal bias, mean difference (95% CI for limits of agreement) 0.75 (4.50 to −3.00) for ejection fraction (**C**) and −0.50 (1.30 to −2.31) for global longitudinal strain (**D**). In human data analyses, there was likewise an excellent intraobserver correlation regarding measurements of ejection fraction, r = 0.94, $p < 0.0001$ (**E**), and global longitudinal strain, r = 0.98, $p < 0.0001$ (**F**). Only minor bias was seen in the corresponding Bland–Altman plots: 0.44 (4.48 to −3.61) for repeated evaluation of human ejection fraction (**G**) and −0.11 (1.36 to −1.58) for global longitudinal strain (**H**). EF = ejection fraction, GLS = global longitudinal strain.

2.3. Interobserver Comparison Displays Strong Correlation between Two Different Observers

The interobserver variability comparison showed moderate to strong correlation between the assessments of the two observers for animal EF (Figure 5A) and GLS (Figure 5B) with a moderate bias, as shown in the Bland–Altman plots, mean difference (95% CI for limits of agreement) of 1.56 (−4.96 to 8.09) for animal EF (Figure 5C) and −1.01 (−9.30 to 7.28) for animal GLS (Figure 5D). A moderate to strong correlation was also shown between the assessments of the two observers for human EF (Figure 5E) and GLS (Figure 5F) with a moderate bias, as shown in the Bland–Altman plots, mean difference of −4.50 (−12.27 to 3.27) for human EF (Figure 5G) and −1.08 (−5.79 to 3.64) for human GLS (Figure 5H). The repeatability of the interobserver assessments fluctuated between good ICC (95% CI) for interobserver animal EF assessments: 0.89 (0.69 to 0.96) and 0.63 (−0.04 to 0.88) for human EF, 0.68 (0.31 to 0.88) for animal GLS, and 0.73 (0.39 to 0.90) for human GLS interobserver assessments.

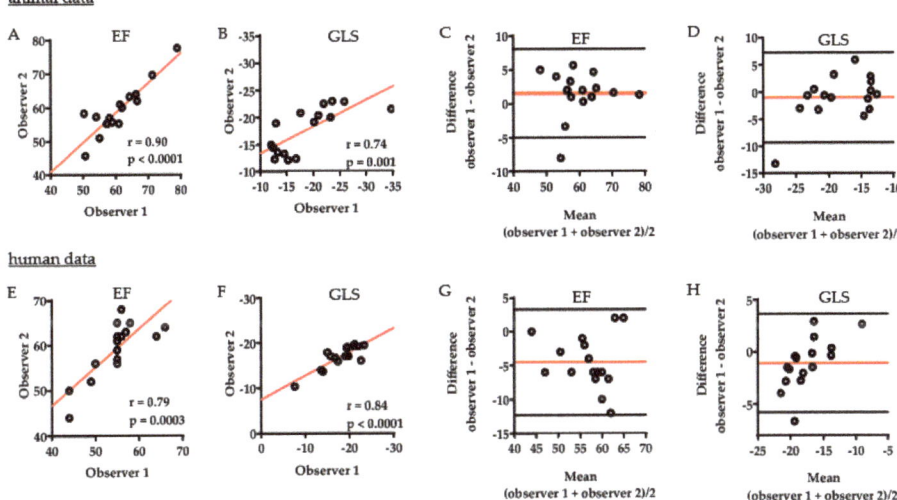

Figure 5. Interobserver comparison. In analysis by two experts, variability comparison showed moderate to strong correlation between the assessments for animal EF (**A**) and GLS (**B**) with a moderate bias, as shown in the Bland–Altman plots, mean difference (95% CI for limits of agreement) of 1.56 (−4.96 to 8.09) for animal EF (**C**) and −1.01 (−9.30 to 7.28) for animal GLS (**D**). A moderate to strong correlation was also shown between the assessments of the two observers for human EF (**E**) and GLS (**F**) with a moderate bias, as shown in the Bland–Altman plots, mean difference of −4.50 (−12.27 to 3.27) for human EF (**G**) and −1.08 (−5.79 to 3.64) for human GLS (**H**).

3. Discussion

The aim of this study was to compare cardiac alterations in a transgenic rat model for PE with the human post-PE situation. In order to describe cardiovascular changes after pregnancy in both species, STE was performed by blinded observers. The reported data reflect equivalent changes in the transgenic rat model and the human situation. Functional parameters such as EF and GLS were reduced in both species post-PE. We observed an increase in relative wall thickness and an increase in the posterior wall thickness of the LV as signs of structural remodeling. Melchiorre et al. were among the first who described permanent cardiovascular changes concerning relaxation abnormalities, diastolic dysfunction, and alterations according to LV geometry during and after PE in humans [4,18,19]. They evaluated LV dysfunction and geometry according to the European Association and American Society of Echocardiography guidelines, not mentioning the individual parameters that were altered. The novelty of our study is based on the very sensitive method of measuring myocardial function using STE. Former preeclamptic women often suffer from asymptomatic cardiac abnormalities with prevalence of asymptomatic heart failure stage B including concentric remodeling and mildly impaired EF [6]. STE offers more sensitive parameters by describing the deformation of the myocardium and is even able to distinguish between individually contracting muscle layers of the heart. Previous publications demonstrated the extensive ability of STE to differentiate between physiological and pathological hypertrophic changes of the heart [20]. With the unique possibility of targeted myocardial specification, STE is being used more frequently in animal models [21–23]. The GLS, as the most sensitive parameter, was induced much earlier than EF [24] and showed a reduction of cardiac functionality post-PE in both species of our translational comparison. To our knowledge, this is the only animal model investigating cardiovascular changes postpartum by STE. An important open and unacknowledged question is whether the changes seen in humans are reversible [25] or permanent after delivery [26], and, if this is going to be an irreversible remodeling, whether replacement fibrosis is also present. We observed perivascular and interstitial fibrosis in the transgenic animal model [16], suggesting that a persisting structural remodeling post-PE and thus permanent cardiovascular abnormalities after preeclamptic pregnancy might be present after human preeclamptic pregnancy. Cardiovascular magnetic resonance (CMR) displays a high potential in the detection of myocardial fibrosis. One of our latest publications about CMR in formerly preeclamptic women describes the structural remodeling postpartum and underlines the burden of increased cardiovascular risk in later life. In this four year postpartum study, diffuse injury of the myocardium was assessed by parametric mapping, focal injury by late gadolinium enhancement imaging, and cardiac function was evaluated by cine imaging and tissue tracking (strain). The post-preeclamptic group showed increased left-atrial end-diastolic volume stroke volume with a slight increase in left ventricular hypertrophy. We could not detect differences in focal or diffuse myocardial tissue composition between the groups. Follow up studies are needed to identify the critical window when morphologic tissue differentiation, such as progression to myocardial fibrosis or inflammation, occurs in post-preeclamptic patients. Beside replacement fibrosis, another indication for permanent alterations in the maternal heart is the concentric remodeling. LV posterior wall and the extrapolated relative wall thickness increased in this study in both post-PE species. Intriguingly, the LV mass only increased significantly in the animal model. However, already published human studies show a permanent hypertrophy of the maternal heart [4,18,27].

The importance of PE as a risk factor in the development of chronic heart disease has been reinforced, and the future cardiovascular health of formerly preeclamptic women is getting more and more attention. Since 2011, the American Heart Association concludes that a pathological pregnancy is an important novel risk factor for later CVD [1]. While California was the only state in the USA to reduce maternal mortality due to hemorrhage using disease-specific toolkits and evidence-based protocol [28], death rates from maternal CVD are rising in the rest of the country. That demonstrates the urgent need for a cardiovascular follow-up after preeclamptic pregnancy and a preventive strategy worldwide. New guidelines from the European Society of Cardiology for the management of CVD during pregnancy [29] recommend lifestyle modifications and annual visits to a primary care physician to check blood pressure and metabolic factors. A sufficient strategy for cardiovascular prevention and postpartum treatment is still missing. To investigate the disease related remodeling process of the maternal heart, animal models are essential. The transgenic rat model mimics a preeclamptic pregnancy in several important aspects [11–15] and shows characteristic features of cardiac dysfunction after a preeclamptic pregnancy, as shown in this study.

In conclusion, our data indicate that the transgenic rat model and the use of STE depicts the cardiovascular abnormalities in the human situation well. That provides the basis investigating the causes of structural changes and functional disorders and gives the opportunity to test promising interventions. To underpin the methodical safety, we used one single observer for STE analysis in both species and demonstrated excellent intraobserver comparison. Interobserver agreements differed between EF and GLS and underlined the important aspect of fixed observers within a study.

However, it should be mentioned that preeclampsia is not a monocausal disease, and there is no model that completely reflects the heterogeneous clinical picture of this disorder. Another limitation is the postpartum observation time point of four weeks in the animal model. Further studies with longer postpartum periods corresponding to 10–20 human years will be necessary in the future to be able to make further statements about the cardiovascular risk after a preeclamptic pregnancy.

4. Materials and Methods

4.1. Animal Cohort

A transgenic rat model was used for simulation of a preeclamptic pregnancy. Female Sprague-Dawley rats harboring the human angiotensinogen gene [TGR(hAogen)L1623] were mated with male rats transgenic for the human renin gene [TGR(hRen)L10J] and developed the disease related phenotype during the last trimester of pregnancy. Age- and body weight-matched wild-type Sprague-Dawley rats constituted the control group. Both groups were housed in a temperature-controlled environment of 22 ± 2 °C, 12:12-hour light/dark cycle, and a humidity of 55 ± 15%. The animals had access to water and food (Sniff V1324-300) ad libitum. Rats were sacrificed 28 days postpartum by decapitation with prior isoflurane anesthesia or due to predefined stopping. The study was approved by local authorities (G0273/16; State Office of Health and Social Affairs Berlin).

4.2. Animal Echocardiography

Transthoracic echocardiography in both groups (control $n = 8$, PE $n = 8$) was performed postpartum in anesthetized animals (1.5% isoflurane via an oxygen mask). Temperature, ECG, and respiration were monitored. By a heated platform, rectal temperature was maintained at 37 ± 2 °C. Abdominal hair was removed by depilatory cream. Pre-warmed gel was used as an ultrasound-coupling medium. For imaging, a Vevo3100 high-resolution imaging system (Fujifilm, VisualSonics Inc., Toronto, ON, Canada) mounted with a 21 MHz transducer (MS250) was used. All images were acquired and stored for offline analysis. Analysis was done by two blinded observers using VisualSonics VevoStrain software (Version 2.2.0, Toronto, ON, Canada). In parasternal long and short axis view, B-Mode cine loops were used to assess speckle tracking analysis. Images were checked for quality with regard to absence of artifacts and differentiation of wall borders. The endocardium of the left ventricle was traced manually in end-diastole. The epicardium was automatically traced by the software, checked and manually adjusted if necessary, for maximum tracking accuracy. Global strain values were obtained from the average of the six segments of the left ventricle. M-mode was obtained to measure cardiac wall and chamber dimensions. Relative wall thickness was calculated by the formula (2*PWd)/LVEDD. Analysis was performed on three consecutive cardiac cycles; mean values from three measurements were calculated.

4.3. Human Cohort

This prospective case-control study was carried out at St. George's University Hospitals NHS Foundation Trust in London over a 12-month period from April 2016 until March 2017. The local institutional review committee approved the study (ID 12/LO/0810; NRES Committee London—Stanmore; date: 30-06-2012), and all participants provided written informed consent. Women with singleton pregnancy were recruited as cases. There were no cases of primigravida. Only women without any cardiovascular co-morbidity and before starting any antihypertensive medication were asked to take part in the study. Preeclampsia was defined according to the guidelines of the International Society for the Study of Hypertension in Pregnancy (ISSHP) [30,31]. Normotensive healthy term pregnant women without any co-morbidity were recruited as controls. Blood pressure was measured manually from the brachial artery according to the guidelines of the National High Blood Pressure

Education Program Working Group on High Blood Pressure in Pregnancy [32]. Maternal data of the human cohort are given in Table 1.

Table 1. Maternal data of human cohort. Cases and controls are matched in age, body mass index (BMI), and scan time after delivery. Preeclamptic women show lower gestational age of delivery. Data given as mean ± SEM.

	Control ($n = 8$)	Preeclamptic ($n = 8$)	p-Value
Age (years)	36.3 ± 1.71	35.0 ± 1.45	0.5860
Weight (kg)	70.9 ± 5.2	77.8 ± 7.3	0.4569
Height (m)	1.7 ± 0.0	1.6 ± 0.0	0.2014
BMI (kg/m^2)	25.1 ± 1.58	28.8 ± 2.17	0.1870
Gestational age of delivery (weeks)	40.4 ± 0.60	31.5 ± 1.49	<0.0001
Scan after delivery (weeks)	45.5 ± 5.45	49.8 ± 3.34	0.5169

4.4. Human Echocardiography

Echocardiographic examination and analysis were performed by a single operator (BSB) using a GE Vivid Q ultrasound machine equipped with a 3.5 MHz transducer (GE Healthcare, Boston, MA, USA). Images were acquired at rest in the left lateral decubitus position from standard parasternal and apical views. Digital loops of 3 cardiac cycles with associated electrocardiogram information were stored on the hard disk of the ultrasound machine and transferred to a GE EchoPac workstation (GE Healthcare, Boston, MA, USA) for offline analysis. Analysis was performed according to existing guidelines [33]. Interventricular septum thickness, left ventricular posterior wall thickness, and left ventricular systolic and diastolic diameter were measured in the parasternal long axis view. Left atrial volume (LAV) and left ventricular volume in diastole (LVEDV) were calculated from apical views. Left ventricular mass was calculated using the Devereux formula $0.8(1.04[([LVEDD + IVSd + PWd]^3 - LVEDD^3)]) + 0.6v$, where LVEDD is left ventricular end diastolic diameter, IVSd is thickness of the intraventricular septum in diastole, and PWd is posterior wall thickness in diastole. Relative wall thickness was calculated with the formula $(2*PWd)/LVEDD$. For speckle tracking echocardiography, the myocardium was traced manually, and the EchoPac software then suggested an area of interest by delimiting the endocardium and the epicardium. The operator readjusted this area before the software calculated deformation. LV endocardial and epicardial global strain as well as LV longitudinal, LV early, and LV late diastolic strain rates were calculated from apical views. Negative values indicate fiber shortening, and positive values indicate fiber lengthening. If >1 segment was rejected, subjects were excluded from statistical analysis.

4.5. Statistics

Statistical analyses were performed by using SPSS version 25 (IBM, Armonk, NY, USA) and Prism 7.0 software (GraphPad Software Inc., San Diego, CA, USA). ROUT method was performed for outlier identification with an average false discovery rate less than 1%. After testing for normal distribution group differences were analyzed by 2-tailed unpaired t-test or by Mann–Whitney U test. All data are presented as means ± SEM. To describe the quality and the sensitivity of the STE measurements in both species, intra- and interobserver comparisons were presented for EF and GLS. Intra- and interobserver variability was assessed on all animals and all study participants by the repeated evaluation of the EF and GLS. Pearson correlation, Bland–Altman plots, and intraclass correlation were performed to assess the agreement and the reliability within and between the observers. For interobserver comparison, two experts evaluated parameters of EF and GLS independently in a blinded manner concerning the animal model as well as in the human participants. For intraobserver comparison, one observer repeatedly evaluated EF and GLS in a blinded fashion. Bland–Altman plots were reported including the mean difference (bias) with corresponding 95% limits of agreement between the evaluations of the two observers (interobserver agreement) or the repeated evaluations of one observer (intraobserver agreement). For the calculation of the intraclass correlation coefficient, a two-way random-effect model based on single measurements and absolute agreement assessed the interobserver repeatability, and a two-way mixed-effect model based on single measurements assessed the intraobserver repeatability for one observer. Mean estimators with 95% confidence intervals (CI) were reported for each ICC. Interpretation of ICC and Pearson correlation coefficients was elaborated as the following: <0.50 = poor; between 0.50 and 0.75 = moderate; between 0.75 and 0.90 = strong; >0.90 = excellent. A two-sided $p < 0.05$ was considered statistically significant.

5. Conclusions

The use of STE has shown that the transgenic animal model reflects the changes after preeclamptic pregnancy in a human situation. By applying the state-of-the-art technique STE, especially marginal changes can be detected due to its sensitivity. This will be of paramount importance for future studies on the cause of early cardiac remodeling and the evaluation of potential interventions.

Author Contributions: Conceptualization, K.K. and R.D.; Methodology, K.K. and J.O.; Validation, T.S. and O.P.; Formal Analysis, K.K. and A.B.; Investigation, K.K. and J.O.; Data Curation, K.K.; Writing—Original Draft Preparation, K.K.; Writing—Review & Editing, K.K., T.S., J.O., A.B., O.P., F.H., D.N.M., B.T., N.H. and R.D.; Visualization, K.K.; Supervision, R.D.; Project Administration, K.K.; Funding Acquisition, R.D. and B.T. All authors have read and agreed to the published version of the manuscript.

Funding: K.K. was funded through a translational Ph.D. project grant by Berlin Institute of Health. B.T. was supported by the European Union's Horizon 2020 research and innovation program under the Marie Skłodowska-Curie grant agreement No. 765274 – iPlacenta. The Deutsche Forschungsgemeinschaft supported F.H. (HE 6249/5-1).

Acknowledgments: We thank Jutta Meisel, Astrid Schiche and Arnd Heuser for their excellent technical assistance. Images in Figure 1 were taken from https://smart.servier.com (Les Laboratoires Servier, Suresnes, France).

Conflicts of Interest: The authors declare no conflict of interest.

Abbreviations

CVD	Cardiovascular disease
EF	Ejection fraction
GLS	Global longitudinal strain
hAogen	Human angiotensinogen
hRen	Human renin
ICC	Intraclass correlation coefficient
IVSd	Intraventricular septum diastole
LV	Left ventricle
LVEDD	Left ventricle end diastolic diameter
ns	Non-significant
PE	Preeclampsia
PWd	Posterior wall diastole
SEM	Standard error mean
sFlt-1	Soluble fms-like tyrosine kinase I
STE	Speckle Tracking Echocardiography

References

1. Mosca, L.; Benjamin, E.J.; Berra, K.; Bezanson, J.L.; Dolor, R.J.; Lloyd-Jones, D.M.; Newby, L.K.; Pina, I.L.; Roger, V.L.; Shaw, L.J.; et al. Effectiveness-based guidelines for the prevention of cardiovascular disease in women–2011 update: A guideline from the american heart association. *Circulation* **2011**, *123*, 1243–1262. [CrossRef]
2. Bellamy, L.; Casas, J.P.; Hingorani, A.D.; Williams, D.J. Pre-eclampsia and risk of cardiovascular disease and cancer in later life: Systematic review and meta-analysis. *BMJ* **2007**, *335*, 974. [CrossRef]
3. Melchiorre, K.; Sharma, R.; Thilaganathan, B. Cardiovascular implications in preeclampsia: An overview. *Circulation* **2014**, *130*, 703–714. [CrossRef]

4. Melchiorre, K.; Sutherland, G.R.; Liberati, M.; Thilaganathan, B. Preeclampsia is associated with persistent postpartum cardiovascular impairment. *Hypertension* **2011**, *58*, 709–715. [CrossRef]
5. Strobl, I.; Windbichler, G.; Strasak, A.; Weiskopf-Schwendinger, V.; Schweigmann, U.; Ramoni, A.; Scheier, M. Left ventricular function many years after recovery from pre-eclampsia. *BJOG* **2011**, *118*, 76–83. [CrossRef]
6. Ghossein-Doha, C.; van Neer, J.; Wissink, B.; Breetveld, N.M.; de Windt, L.J.; van Dijk, A.P.; van der Vlugt, M.J.; Janssen, M.C.; Heidema, W.M.; Scholten, R.R.; et al. Pre-eclampsia: An important risk factor for asymptomatic heart failure. *Ultrasound. Obstet. Gynecol.* **2017**, *49*, 143–149. [CrossRef]
7. Lampinen, K.H.; Ronnback, M.; Kaaja, R.J.; Groop, P.H. Impaired vascular dilatation in women with a history of pre-eclampsia. *J. Hypertens* **2006**, *24*, 751–756. [CrossRef]
8. Krabbendam, I.; Maas, M.L.; Thijssen, D.H.; Oyen, W.J.; Lotgering, F.K.; Hopman, M.T.; Spaanderman, M.E. Exercise-induced changes in venous vascular function in nonpregnant formerly preeclamptic women. *Reprod. Sci.* **2009**, *16*, 414–420. [CrossRef]
9. Spaan, J.J.; Ekhart, T.; Spaanderman, M.E.; Peeters, L.L. Remote hemodynamics and renal function in formerly preeclamptic women. *Obstet. Gynecol.* **2009**, *113*, 853–859. [CrossRef]
10. Foo, F.L.; Mahendru, A.A.; Masini, G.; Fraser, A.; Cacciatore, S.; MacIntyre, D.A.; McEniery, C.M.; Wilkinson, I.B.; Bennett, P.R.; Lees, C.C. Association Between Prepregnancy Cardiovascular Function and Subsequent Preeclampsia or Fetal Growth Restriction. *Hypertension* **2018**, *72*, 442–450. [CrossRef]
11. Bohlender, J.; Ganten, D.; Luft, F.C. Rats transgenic for human renin and human angiotensinogen as a model for gestational hypertension. *J. Am. Soc. Nephrol.* **2000**, *11*, 2056–2061.
12. Hering, L.; Herse, F.; Geusens, N.; Verlohren, S.; Wenzel, K.; Staff, A.C.; Brosnihan, K.B.; Huppertz, B.; Luft, F.C.; Muller, D.N.; et al. Effects of circulating and local uteroplacental angiotensin II in rat pregnancy. *Hypertension* **2010**, *56*, 311–318. [CrossRef]
13. Geusens, N.; Verlohren, S.; Luyten, C.; Taube, M.; Hering, L.; Vercruysse, L.; Hanssens, M.; Dudenhausen, J.W.; Dechend, R.; Pijnenborg, R. Endovascular trophoblast invasion, spiral artery remodelling and uteroplacental haemodynamics in a transgenic rat model of pre-eclampsia. *Placenta* **2008**, *29*, 614–623. [CrossRef]
14. Andersen, L.B.; Golic, M.; Przybyl, L.; Sorensen, G.L.; Jorgensen, J.S.; Fruekilde, P.; von Versen-Hoynck, F.; Herse, F.; Hojskov, C.S.; Dechend, R.; et al. Vitamin D depletion does not affect key aspects of the preeclamptic phenotype in a transgenic rodent model for preeclampsia. *J. Am. Soc. Hypertens.* **2016**, *10*, 597–607. [CrossRef]
15. Dechend, R.; Gratze, P.; Wallukat, G.; Shagdarsuren, E.; Plehm, R.; Brasen, J.H.; Fiebeler, A.; Schneider, W.; Caluwaerts, S.; Vercruysse, L.; et al. Agonistic autoantibodies to the AT1 receptor in a transgenic rat model of preeclampsia. *Hypertension* **2005**, *45*, 742–746. [CrossRef]
16. Kraker, K.; O'Driscoll, J.M.; Schutte, T.; Herse, F.; Patey, O.; Golic, M.; Geisberger, S.; Verlohren, S.; Birukov, A.; Heuser, A.; et al. Statins Reverse Postpartum Cardiovascular Dysfunction in a Rat Model of Preeclampsia. *Hypertension* **2020**, *75*, 202–210. [CrossRef]
17. Sengupta, P. The Laboratory Rat: Relating Its Age With Human's. *Int. J. Prev. Med.* **2013**, *4*, 624–630.
18. Melchiorre, K.; Sutherland, G.R.; Baltabaeva, A.; Liberati, M.; Thilaganathan, B. Maternal cardiac dysfunction and remodeling in women with preeclampsia at term. *Hypertension* **2011**, *57*, 85–93. [CrossRef]
19. Melchiorre, K.; Sutherland, G.R.; Watt-Coote, I.; Liberati, M.; Thilaganathan, B. Severe myocardial impairment and chamber dysfunction in preterm preeclampsia. *Hypertens. Pregnancy* **2012**, *31*, 454–471. [CrossRef]
20. An, X.; Wang, J.; Li, H.; Lu, Z.; Bai, Y.; Xiao, H.; Zhang, Y.; Song, Y. Speckle Tracking Based Strain Analysis Is Sensitive for Early Detection of Pathological Cardiac Hypertrophy. *PLoS ONE* **2016**, *11*, e0149155. [CrossRef]
21. Bauer, M.; Cheng, S.; Jain, M.; Ngoy, S.; Theodoropoulos, C.; Trujillo, A.; Lin, F.C.; Liao, R. Echocardiographic speckle-tracking based strain imaging for rapid cardiovascular phenotyping in mice. *Circ. Res.* **2011**, *108*, 908–916. [CrossRef]
22. Peng, Y.; Popovic, Z.B.; Sopko, N.; Drinko, J.; Zhang, Z.; Thomas, J.D.; Penn, M.S. Speckle tracking echocardiography in the assessment of mouse models of cardiac dysfunction. *Am. J. Physiol. Heart. Circ. Physiol.* **2009**, *297*, H811–H820. [CrossRef]
23. De Lucia, C.; Wallner, M.; Eaton, D.M.; Zhao, H.; Houser, S.R.; Koch, W.J. Echocardiographic Strain Analysis for the Early Detection of Left Ventricular Systolic/Diastolic Dysfunction and Dyssynchrony in a Mouse Model of Physiological Aging. *J. Gerontol. A Biol. Sci. Med. Sci.* **2019**, *74*, 455–461. [CrossRef]
24. Imbalzano, E.; Zito, C.; Carerj, S.; Oreto, G.; Mandraffino, G.; Cusma-Piccione, M.; Di Bella, G.; Saitta, C.; Saitta, A. Left ventricular function in hypertension: New insight by speckle tracking echocardiography. *Echocardiography* **2011**, *28*, 649–657. [CrossRef]

25. Cong, J.; Fan, T.; Yang, X.; Squires, J.W.; Cheng, G.; Zhang, L.; Zhang, Z. Structural and functional changes in maternal left ventricle during pregnancy: A three-dimensional speckle-tracking echocardiography study. *Cardiovasc. Ultrasound.* **2015**, *13*, 6. [CrossRef]
26. Orabona, R.; Vizzardi, E.; Sciatti, E.; Bonadei, I.; Valcamonico, A.; Metra, M.; Frusca, T. Insights into cardiac alterations after pre-eclampsia: An echocardiographic study. *Ultrasound. Obstet. Gynecol.* **2017**, *49*, 124–133. [CrossRef]
27. Orabona, R.; Sciatti, E.; Vizzardi, E.; Prefumo, F.; Bonadei, I.; Valcamonico, A.; Metra, M.; Lorusso, R.; Ghossein-Doha, C.; Spaanderman, M.E.A.; et al. Inappropriate left ventricular mass after preeclampsia: Another piece of the puzzle Inappropriate LVM and PE. *Hypertens Res.* **2019**, *42*, 522–529. [CrossRef]
28. Main, E.K.; Cape, V.; Abreo, A.; Vasher, J.; Woods, A.; Carpenter, A.; Gould, J.B. Reduction of severe maternal morbidity from hemorrhage using a state perinatal quality collaborative. *Am. J. Obstet. Gynecol.* **2017**, *216*, 298.e1–298.e11. [CrossRef]
29. Regitz-Zagrosek, V.; Roos-Hesselink, J.W.; Bauersachs, J.; Blomstrom-Lundqvist, C.; Cifkova, R.; De Bonis, M.; Iung, B.; Johnson, M.R.; Kintscher, U.; Kranke, P.; et al. 2018 ESC Guidelines for the management of cardiovascular diseases during pregnancy. *Eur. Heart J.* **2018**, *39*, 3165–3241. [CrossRef]
30. Tranquilli, A.L.; Brown, M.A.; Zeeman, G.G.; Dekker, G.; Sibai, B.M. The definition of severe and early-onset preeclampsia. Statements from the International Society for the Study of Hypertension in Pregnancy (ISSHP). *Pregnancy Hypertens.* **2013**, *3*, 44–47. [CrossRef]
31. Tranquilli, A.L.; Dekker, G.; Magee, L.; Roberts, J.; Sibai, B.M.; Steyn, W.; Zeeman, G.G.; Brown, M.A. The classification, diagnosis and management of the hypertensive disorders of pregnancy: A revised statement from the ISSHP. *Pregnancy Hypertens.* **2014**, *4*, 97–104. [CrossRef]
32. National High Blood Pressure Education Program Working Group on High Blood Pressure in Pregnancy. Report of the National High Blood Pressure Education Program Working Group on High Blood Pressure in Pregnancy. *Am. J. Obstet. Gynecol.* **2000**, *183*, S1–S22. [CrossRef]
33. Nagueh, S.F.; Smiseth, O.A.; Appleton, C.P.; Byrd, B.F., 3rd; Dokainish, H.; Edvardsen, T.; Flachskampf, F.A.; Gillebert, T.C.; Klein, A.L.; Lancellotti, P.; et al. Recommendations for the Evaluation of Left Ventricular Diastolic Function by Echocardiography: An Update from the American Society of Echocardiography and the European Association of Cardiovascular Imaging. *Eur. Heart J. Cardiovasc. Imaging* **2016**, *17*, 1321–1360. [CrossRef]

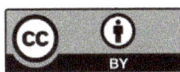

© 2020 by the authors. Licensee MDPI, Basel, Switzerland. This article is an open access article distributed under the terms and conditions of the Creative Commons Attribution (CC BY) license (http://creativecommons.org/licenses/by/4.0/).

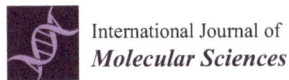

Article

The Effects of Early-Onset Pre-Eclampsia on Placental Creatine Metabolism in the Third Trimester

Stacey J. Ellery [1,*], Padma Murthi [1,2], Paul A. Della Gatta [3], Anthony K. May [3], Miranda L. Davies-Tuck [1], Greg M. Kowalski [3], Damien L. Callahan [4], Clinton R. Bruce [3], Euan M. Wallace [1], David W. Walker [5], Hayley Dickinson [1] and Rod J. Snow [3]

1. The Ritchie Centre, Hudson Institute of Medical Research, and Department of Obstetrics & Gynaecology, Monash University, Clayton 3168 Australia; padma.murthi@monash.edu (P.M.); miranda.davies@hudson.org.au (M.L.D.-T.); euan.wallace@monash.edu (E.M.W.); TheScienceOfPregnancy@gmail.com (H.D.)
2. Department of Pharmacology, Monash University, and Department of Obstetrics and Gynaecology, University of Melbourne, Parkville, Melbourne 3010, Australia
3. Institute for Physical Activity and Nutrition, School of Exercise and Nutrition Sciences, Deakin University, Geelong 3216, Australia; paul.dellagatta@deakin.edu.au (P.A.D.G.); a.may@deakin.edu.au (A.K.M.); greg.kowalski@deakin.edu.au (G.M.K.); clinton.bruce@deakin.edu.au (C.R.B.); rod.snow@deakin.edu.au (R.J.S.)
4. Centre for Cellular and Molecular Biology, School of Life and Environmental Science, Deakin University, Burwood, Melbourne 3125, Australia; damien.callahan@deakin.edu.au
5. School of Health & Biomedical Sciences, RMIT University, Melbourne 3082, Australia; david.walker@rmit.edu.au
* Correspondence: stacey.ellery@hudson.org.au

Received: 10 December 2019; Accepted: 24 January 2020; Published: 26 January 2020

Abstract: Creatine is a metabolite important for cellular energy homeostasis as it provides spatio-temporal adenosine triphosphate (ATP) buffering for cells with fluctuating energy demands. Here, we examined whether placental creatine metabolism was altered in cases of early-onset pre-eclampsia (PE), a condition known to cause placental metabolic dysfunction. We studied third trimester human placentae collected between 27–40 weeks' gestation from women with early-onset PE ($n = 20$) and gestation-matched normotensive control pregnancies ($n = 20$). Placental total creatine and creatine precursor guanidinoacetate (GAA) content were measured. mRNA expression of the creatine synthesizing enzymes arginine:glycine aminotransferase (*GATM*) and guanidinoacetate methyltransferase (*GAMT*), the creatine transporter (*SLC6A8*), and the creatine kinases (mitochondrial *CKMT1A* & cytosolic *BBCK*) was assessed. Placental protein levels of arginine:glycine aminotransferase (AGAT), GAMT, CKMT1A and BBCK were also determined. Key findings; total creatine content of PE placentae was 38% higher than controls ($p < 0.01$). mRNA expression of *GATM* ($p < 0.001$), *GAMT* ($p < 0.001$), *SLC6A8* ($p = 0.021$) and *BBCK* ($p < 0.001$) was also elevated in PE placentae. No differences in GAA content, nor protein levels of AGAT, GAMT, BBCK or CKMT1A were observed between cohorts. Advancing gestation and birth weight were associated with a down-regulation in placental *GATM* mRNA expression, and a reduction in GAA content, in control placentae. These relationships were absent in PE cases. Our results suggest PE placentae may have an ongoing reliance on the creatine kinase circuit for maintenance of cellular energetics with increased total creatine content and transcriptional changes to creatine synthesizing enzymes and the creatine transporter. Understanding the functional consequences of these changes warrants further investigation.

Keywords: placental bioenergetics 1; phosphocreatine 2; metabolism 3; obstetrics 4

1. Introduction

Pre-eclampsia (PE) is a pregnancy-specific hypertensive disorder that affects about 5% of all pregnancies and is responsible for more than 50,000 maternal deaths each year worldwide [1–4]. It is hypothesized that the pathophysiology of early-onset pre-eclampsia (<34 weeks' gestation) has its origins in the placental and uterine vasculature, where inadequate vascular remodeling leads to repeated ischemic-reperfusion (I/R) events within placental tissue [5]. This chronic impaired placental perfusion is thought to promote the production and release of inflammatory and anti-angiogenic factors that are known to be elevated in the maternal circulation of PE cases [6]. These factors damage the maternal vasculature inducing wide-spread endothelial dysfunction, hypertension and, in severe cases, organ injury and maternal death [7].

Impaired oxygen delivery to the placenta also destabilizes placental metabolism and bioenergetics, which in turn limits ATP-dependent processes and promotes the production of reactive oxygen species, often leading to functional insufficiencies in the placenta that can negatively impact the developing fetus. Indeed, the risk of fetal growth restriction and preterm birth, either spontaneous or through iatrogenic delivery, is increased with PE [2,8].

A recent wide-spectrum metabolomic analysis identified increased creatine and creatinine in cord plasma in PE pregnancies [9] indicating that, among other metabolic changes, fetal and potentially placental creatine homeostasis is altered in PE. Creatine—N-(aminoiminomethyl)N-methyl glycine—is a nitrogenous amino acid derivative obtained from our diet and endogenously synthesized by some tissues, including the placenta [10]. Through a reversible phosphorylation/dephosphorylation reaction catalyzed by mitochondrial (CKMT1A) and cytosolic (BBCK) creatine kinases, creatine stabilizes cellular bioenergetics through both spatial and temporal maintenance of adenosine diphosphate and triphosphate (ADP/ATP) ratios [11].

Our understanding of the importance of creatine provision to the developing placenta and fetus in healthy pregnancies has expanded in recent years [12–16]. We have previously demonstrated that the term human placenta expresses both enzymes (arginine:glycine aminotransferase [AGAT] and guanidinoacetate methyltransferase [GAMT]) required to synthesize creatine *de novo*, and can produce both creatine and the creatine precursor guanidinoacetate (GAA) ex vivo, thus bypassing a complete reliance on dietary creatine or endogenous synthesis by the maternal kidney and liver for its creatine supply [10]. Our further investigations into creatine metabolism in cases of third trimester placental insufficiency and fetal growth restriction in the absence of PE suggest that the compromised placenta adapts by increasing tissue creatine concentrations, which may reflect a heightened reliance on the creatine kinase circuit to stabilize placental bioenergetics under chronic hypoxic conditions [17]. Whether placental metabolic changes associated with PE induce changes in placental creatine metabolism, and potentially creatine transfer to the fetus, is unknown.

This study examined whether early-onset PE altered placental creatine metabolism. Specifically, we assessed placental creatine and GAA content, the expression of the enzymes required for creatine synthesis, creatine intracellular uptake and utilization via the creatine kinase circuit. We hypothesized that PE would have effects on placental creatine homeostasis that would include pathways involved in its synthesis and transport. Our findings are discussed in relation to a possible placental response to minimize PE-induced injury, which could have the dual benefit of reducing the maternal syndrome of PE and improving fetal wellbeing.

2. Results

2.1. Population Characteristics

Table 1 summarizes the maternal characteristics and pregnancy outcomes for the normotensive control and early-onset PE cohorts. Women with PE were hypertensive (162.3 ± 11.8/102.9 ± 5.9 mmHg) with confirmed proteinuria. These women were younger than controls ($p < 0.01$) and more likely to be nulliparous ($p < 0.01$). There was no significant difference in gestational age between control and PE cohorts. However, infants born from pregnancies complicated by PE had lower birth ($p < 0.05$) and placenta ($p < 0.05$) weights compared to controls.

Table 1. Population Characteristics.

Characteristics	Control ($n = 20$)	PE ($n = 20$)	p Value
Maternal Age (years)	33.5 (5.0) [1]	28.9 (4.4) [1]	<0.01
Nulliparous	6.0 (30.0) [2]	15.0 (75.0) [2]	<0.01
Gestation (weeks)	34.2 (4.1) [1]	32.7 (4.0) [1]	NS
Systolic Blood Pressure (mmHg)	<140	162.3 (11.8) [1]	-
Diastolic Blood Pressure (mmHg)	<90	102.9 (5.9) [1]	-
Mode of Delivery			
Vaginal Delivery	5.0 (25.0) [2]	5.0 (25.0) [2]	NS
C-Section not in Labor	14.0 (70.0) [2]	5.0 (25.0) [2]	<0.01
C-Section in Labor	1.0 (5.0) [2]	10.0 (50.0) [2]	<0.01
Birth Weight (g)	3140 (2762–3620) [3]	1443 (1155–3520) [3]	<0.05
Placental Weight (g)	463.5 (402–830) [3]	380.0 (323–600) [3]	<0.05
Baby Sex (male)	10 (50.0) [2]	14 (70.0) [2]	NS

[1] Mean (standard deviation); [2] Number (%) total number; [3] Median (interquartile range); NS: not significant.

2.2. Placental Creatine and GAA Content

Total creatine content of PE placentae was significantly higher (+38%) than controls (Figure 1A; $p < 0.01$). Placental content of GAA (creatine precursor) was not significantly different between PE and control cohorts (Figure 1B). Baby sex had no effect on placental creatine or GAA content in either control or PE pregnancies.

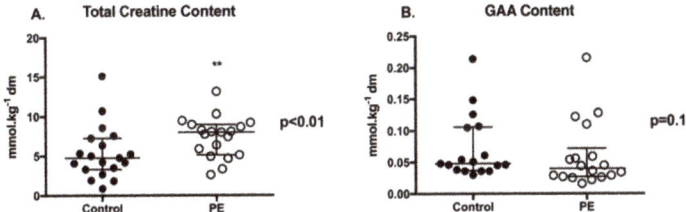

Figure 1. Placental Creatine and Creatine Precursor Guanidinoacetate (GAA) Content. Total creatine (**A**) and GAA (**B**) content of $n = 19$ healthy control (closed circle) and $n = 19$ PE (open circle) placentae. Two sample t-tests were used for statistical comparison. Data are present means ± SD. ** $p < 0.01$.

2.3. Creatine Synthesis and Transport Genes and Proteins

GATM and *GAMT* mRNA expression were up-regulated 2-fold in PE placentae compared to controls (Figure 2A $p < 0.001$ and Figure 2B $p < 0.001$, respectively). We also observed a two-fold increase in mRNA expression for the creatine transporter (*SLC6A8*) and a 4-fold increase in cytosolic *BBCK* mRNA expression in PE placentae compared to controls (Figure 2C $p = 0.021$ and Figure 2D $p < 0.001$, respectively). Conversely, mitochondrial creatine kinase (*CKMT1A*) mRNA expression was significantly decreased in PE placentae (Figure 2E $p < 0.01$). Despite changes in mRNA expression of the creatine synthesizing enzymes and creatine kinases, there were no significant differences in protein abundance of AGAT, GAMT, BBCK or CKMT1A between the PE and control placentae (Figure 3, blots available in Supplementary Information as Figures S1–S4). Baby sex had no impact on placental gene and protein expression in either control or PE pregnancies.

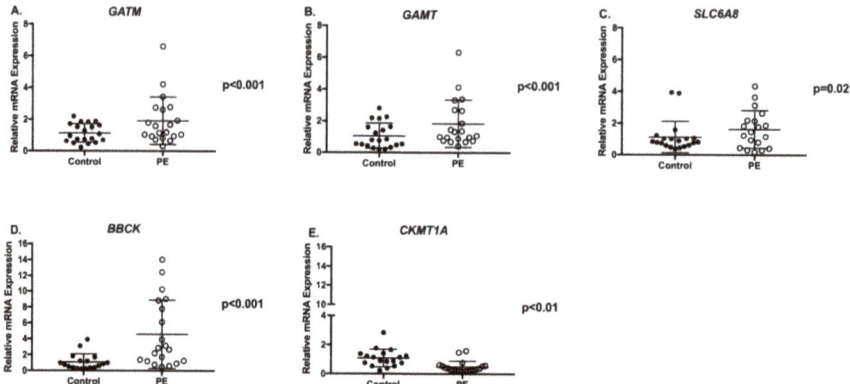

Figure 2. Placental Gene Expression of the Creatine Synthesizing Enzymes, the Creatine Transporter and Kinases. Creatine synthesizing enzymes *GATM* gene that codes for AGAT (**A**) and *GAMT* (**B**), the creatine transporter *SLC6A8* (**C**), cytosolic creatine kinase *BBCK* (**D**) and mitochondrial creatine kinase *CKMT1A* (**E**). $n = 20$ normotensive control (closed circle) and $n = 20$ PE (open circle). Data are presented relative to the control cohort. Values are mean ± SD. Wilcoxon Rank Sum was used for statistical comparison. Significance was set at $p \leq 0.025$, following a Benjamini-Hochberg adjustment for false-positives.

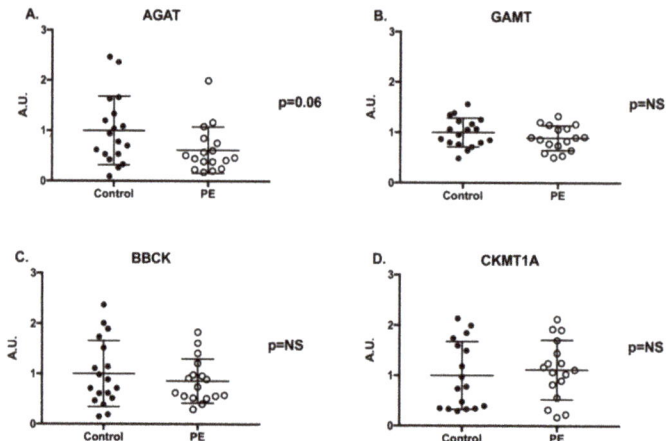

Figure 3. Placental Protein Expression of the Creatine Synthesizing Enzymes and Kinases. Creatine synthesis enzymes AGAT (**A**) and GAMT (**B**), cytosolic creatine kinase BBCK (**C**) and mitochondrial creatine kinase CKMT1A (**D**). $n = 19$ normotensive control (closed circle) and $n = 19$ PE (open circle). Data were normalized to total protein and a control sample run across blots. Data are expressed in arbitrary units (A.U.) relative to the control cohort. Wilcoxon Rank Sum was used for statistical comparison. Significance was set at $p \leq 0.025$, following a Benjamini-Hochberg adjustment for false-positives. NS: not significant.

2.4. Correlations between Creatine Metabolism and Pregnancy Outcomes

We explored associations between placental metabolite content, gene and protein expression, and then these laboratory measures with maternal characteristics (age, parity, mode of delivery) and pregnancy outcomes (baby sex, gestational age, birth weight and placental weight). There was a significant decrease in placental *GATM* mRNA expression with advancing gestational age (Figure 4A, $r = -0.681$; $p < 0.001$) and birth weight (Figure 4B, $r = -0.610$; $p < 0.001$) in controls. These gene associations were absent in the PE cohort (Figure 4C,D). Similar correlations were observed with placental GAA, with tissue content declining with advancing gestational age (Figure 4E, $r = -0.720$; $p < 0.002$) and birth weight (Figure 4F, $r = -0.687$; $p < 0.003$) in normotensive controls. These associations were again absent in the PE cohort (Figure 4G,H). Placental creatine content was not significantly associated with any other maternal characteristics or pregnancy outcomes. Nor were mRNA expression patterns of *GAMT, SLC6A8, BBCK, CKMT1A* or AGAT, GAMT, BBCK or CKMT1A protein abundance.

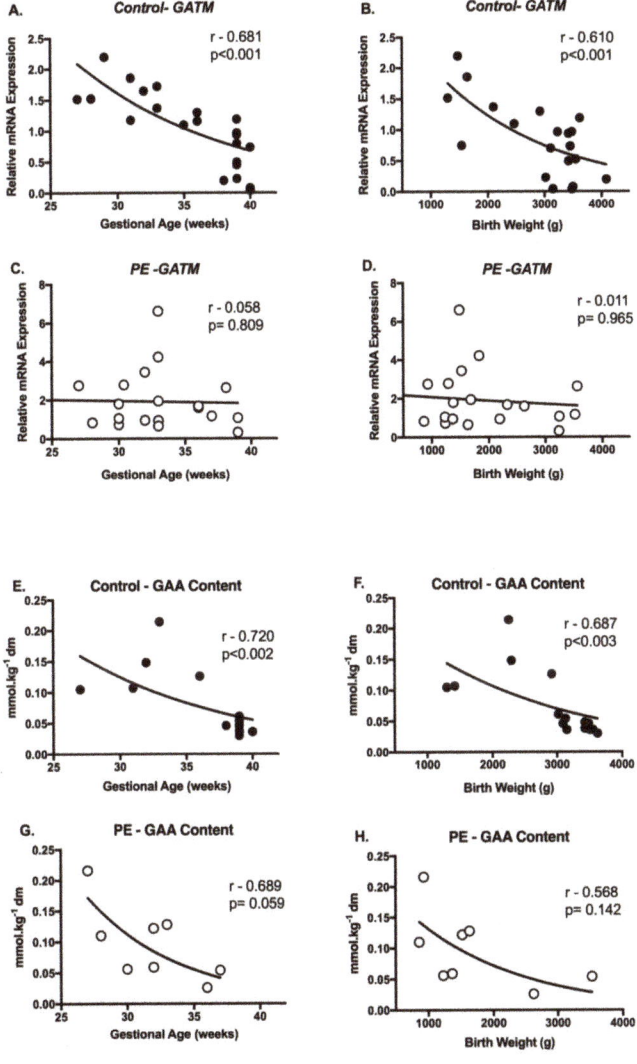

Figure 4. Associations (r) between placental *GATM* mRNA and gestational age (**A**) and birth weight (**B**) in the control cohort; placental *GATM* mRNA and gestational age (**C**) and birth weight (**D**) in the PE cohort; placental GAA content and gestational age (**E**) and birth weight (**F**) in the control cohort and GAA content and gestational age (**G**) and birth weight (**H**) in the PE cohort. *r* values were generated using Spearman's correlation coefficient. Normotensive placenta data are represented by closed circles and PE placentae open circles. Significance was set at $p \leq 0.004$, following a Benjamini-Hochberg adjustment for false-positives.

3. Discussion

In addition to widespread endothelial dysfunction, alterations to maternal, placental and fetal metabolism are hallmarks of PE [18]. In this study, we explored third trimester placental creatine metabolism in early-onset PE and gestation-matched normotensive pregnancies. Our findings confirm the recent metabolomic reports of altered creatine homeostasis with PE [9]; moreover, we identified significant changes in expression of genes associated with the synthesis and transport of creatine within the placenta. Our main finding was that total creatine content of the third trimester PE placentae was significantly higher than controls. Similar adaptations have recently been described in placental insufficiency leading to fetal growth restriction (FGR) in the absence of PE [17] and in pregnancies that occurred at high altitude [19]. To the best of our knowledge, these studies are the first to describe increased creatine content in human tissue exposed to perturbations in oxygen delivery, in vivo.

There are three potential mechanisms for changes in placental creatine content between normotensive and PE placentae. These include changes to creatine to creatinine degradation rates, increased endogenous synthesis and/or increased cellular uptake of creatine from the circulation. It is unlikely that changes to the rate of creatine degradation to creatinine would have led to differences in placental creatine content between cohorts, as this is a spontaneous, non-enzymatically driven process that occurs at a near constant rate of ~1.7% of total body creatine content per day [20]. This leaves changes to endogenous placental creatine synthesis and/or rates of cellular up-take as potential mechanisms for increasing placental creatine content with PE. As cellular metabolism is in a constant state of flux, it is difficult to ascertain exactly which of these processes (de novo synthesis or cellular up-take, or both) resulted in the increased total creatine content of the PE placenta in this retrospective study. However, we make the following observations.

PE up-regulated placental gene expression of the creatine synthesizing enzymes *GATM* and *GAMT*. Modulation of *de novo* creatine synthesis is usually discussed in the context of AGAT (i.e., *GATM* mRNA expression and/or AGAT activity) as this is thought to be the rate-limiting step of creatine biosynthesis [21]. Mediators of AGAT expression and activity include thyroid hormone, growth hormone, and circulating levels of arginine, citrulline and creatine [22,23]. The influence of arginine, citrulline and creatine on the rate of endogenous creatine synthesis has mainly been described as a down-regulation of *GATM* and AGAT when these metabolites are in excess, which is the opposite to what has been observed in the PE placentae [22]. On the contrary, adequate concentrations of thyroid and growth hormone are required to maintain AGAT activity, with studies in thyroidectomy or hypophysectomy rats observing decreased AGAT renal activity [24]. Whether increases in thyroid or growth hormone above basal levels can increase AGAT activity is unknown. There is the potential that increased placental growth factor production by the PE placenta may be influencing these transcriptional pathways, and maintaining the placental *GATM* mRNA expression with advancing gestational age and birth weight observed in the current study, a finding that was absent in normotensive controls [25].

Despite increases in gene expression of both *GATM* and *GAMT* and the increased total creatine content, there were no detectable changes in AGAT or GAMT protein levels, indicating a mismatch in transcription and abundance of the enzymatic machinery of creatine synthesis in the PE placentae. It may be that placental endoplasmic reticulum stress reported with PE may hinder increased production of AGAT and GAMT enzymes [26]. There is also the potential of an increased rate of *de novo* creatine synthesis by increased activity of the AGAT and GAMT enzymes in the absence of changes to overall protein abundance. As no change in placental GAA content was observed between cohorts, we would contend that any changes in AGAT and GAMT activity would have been in equilibrium. We cannot rule out how histomorphological differences between control and PE placentae may have influenced measured AGAT and GAMT expression, as our assessments were conducted on tissue homogenates. An increase in terminal villi density, but an overall decline to villous surface area are characteristic of placental PE histology [27]. AGAT is expressed in stromal and endothelial cells of the fetal capillaries and GAMT in the syncytiotrophoblast of the fetal villi [10], so it is plausible that levels of AGAT and GAMT could be altered by changes to cell populations. However, one would anticipate that the known histological changes within the PE placenta would lead to a down-regulation in expression, not the increases in mRNA expression and no change in protein levels observed in the current cohort.

The alternate route of increasing placental creatine content is by increased transport of creatine into the placental cells via the creatine transporter [28]. This could simply be the result of increased maternal circulating creatine levels with PE. While no studies have characterized changes in maternal creatine levels in PE cases, increased creatine in cord plasma has been reported [9]. The retrospective nature of the current study and lack of maternal blood sampling inhibited our ability to explore this hypothesis further. Assessment of maternal circulating concentrations of creatine should be a focus of future prospective cohort studies. The current study did find a 2-fold increase mRNA expression of the creatine transporter *SLC6A8* in PE placentae compared to controls. A potential mechanistic pathway for increased creatine transporter expression and activity in the placenta is via AMP-activated protein kinase (AMPK), a key regulator of cellular energy metabolism that has been implicated in the pathophysiology of PE [29]. In cardiomyocytes, activation of AMPK pathways has been shown to up-regulate creatine transporter expression and activity, ultimately increasing cellular creatine up-take [30]. This effect is thought to be indirect, as the creatine transporter does not contain substrate sites for AMPK mediated phosphorylation. Potential intermediates are co-activator peroxisome activated receptor γ coactivator-1 alpha (PGC-1α) and estrogen-related receptor α (ERRα), both known to be regulated by AMPK and induce the expression of genes involved in cellular bioenergetics, including mitogenesis [31]. Studies in skeletal muscle cells (L6 myotubes) have described direct interactions between PGC-1α/ERRα, increased creatine transporter mRNA expression and cellular creatine up-take [32]. As there have been mixed reports of increases and decreases to placental mitochondrial content and PGC-1α expression with PE [33,34], further exploration of this mechanistic pathway is required before conclusions about AMPK's role in driving changes to creatine transport and cellular up-take in PE placentae can be drawn. In vitro techniques should be employed for these analyses to control for changes in placental metabolism associated with tissue collection and processing times.

It is probable that placental mitochondrial dysfunction [8], and thus changes in AMPK expression, are also influencing how the PE placenta is utilizing the available creatine for ATP homeostasis. AMPK is a known regulator of the expression of the cytosolic isoform of creatine kinase *BBCK* (responsible for the hydrolysis of phosphocreatine and phosphorylation of ADP to form ATP) [35]. This finding is consistent with the increased *BBCK* mRNA expression observed in PE placentae in the current study. Activation of the HIF-2α hypoxia response element, which has been shown to be up-regulated in PE, may also contribute to changes in *BBCK* mRNA expression, as activation of HIF-2α enhances BBCK expression in apical intestinal epithelial cells with inflammatory bowel disease [36]. Again, there was no detectable difference in protein abundance in the current study. Thus, further interrogation of these mechanisms is required to elucidate the interactions between metabolic regulatory pathways and creatine metabolism in the PE placenta. Known variations in mitochondrial function and thus capacity to generate ATP between pre-term and term PE placentae should be considered within this context [37].

Interestingly, the mechanism (de novo synthesis and/or cellular uptake) for increasing placental creatine levels may be different between the PE and FGR pathologies. Placentae of growth restricted infants had lowered GAA levels and reduced mRNA expression of *GATM* and *GAMT*, compared to the PE placentae that showed no change in GAA content and an up-regulation in *GATM* and *GAMT* [17]. It is generally accepted that the level of placental insult is higher in PE than in FGR, producing a more substantial burden of placental pro-inflammatory and anti-angiogenic factors and their interactions on maternal endothelium in multiple-organ systems [38]. As maternal kidney injury is a primary manifestation of the PE syndrome, changes to maternal systemic creatine synthesis, mainly GAA production by AGAT activity in the renal proximal tubules, may alter maternal creatine homeostasis, placing a more significant burden on the placenta to maintain adequate creatine levels for placental and fetal requirements.

Increased de novo creatine synthesis, either by the placenta or maternal production by the kidney and liver could have further implications for the pathogenesis of PE. The methylation of GAA by GAMT produces creatine and S-Adenosylhomocysteine, contributing to around 40% of total homocysteine production under basal conditions [39]. Elevated maternal homocysteine levels have been identified in several PE cohort studies. As homocysteine can cause endothelial dysfunction, it is thought that hyperhomocysteinemia could contribute to maternal vascular dysfunction with PE [40,41]. Considering that a consequence of increased *de novo* creatine synthesis in response to PE could be the over-production of homocysteine, understanding these pathways may have implications for the management of the maternal PE syndrome beyond placental bioenergetics.

There were several limitations to this study. Villous tissue was dissected from a central placental cotyledon only, and not randomly sampled from several sites across the placenta, as is now the recommendation for molecular studies [42]. The retrospective nature of this study also meant that some maternal demographic information that may have been relevant (i.e., ethnicity) was not available. Finally, the lack of an appropriate antibody inhibited our ability to quantify creatine transporter protein concentrations, via western blot [28].

4. Materials and Methods

4.1. Human Research Ethics, Sample Collection and Storage

Archived placental villous samples, from 20 normotensive controls and 20 women with early-onset PE, were collected at the Royal Women's Hospital Melbourne, Australia for research purposes, and explicitly accessed for this study. The Society of Obstetric Medicine of Australia and New Zealand (SOMANZ) research definition of PE was used to select the PE cohort [43]. Gestation-matched controls were selected from normotensive term pregnancies, idiopathic preterm deliveries or preterm elective deliveries for indications not associated with placental function. All controls were absent of placental pathology and delivered babies with birth weights appropriate for gestational age [44]. The collection and archiving of all samples had the approval of the relevant institutional human research ethics committees in 2000 and 2001 (HREC# 01/46, 00/27). Each woman gave written informed consent for tissue collection and the recording of de-identified demographic information and pregnancy outcomes. Where available, information on maternal age, parity, gestational age, mode of delivery, baby sex, birth weight and placental weight were extracted from electronic records. Sample processing was within 20 min of placental delivery. Villous tissue was dissected from a central placental cotyledon. The decidua was removed before tissues were divided into pieces, snap-frozen in liquid nitrogen and stored at −80 °C for future analysis [45].

4.2. Sample Processing

4.2.1. Creatine and GAA Analysis

Snap frozen placental tissues of sufficient weight ($n = 19$ control and $n = 19$ PE) were freeze dried overnight at −80 °C. Powdered samples were then weighed (3–4 mg) and extracted on ice using 0.5 M perchloric acid/1mM Ethylenediaminetetraacetic acid (EDTA) before being neutralized with 2.1 M potassium hydrogen carbonate as previously described [17]. Total creatine content (creatine + phosphocreatine) was measured using fluorometric assays [46]. GAA was measured by liquid chromatography tandem mass spectrometry (LC-MS/MS) through a slight modification of the method of Tran et al. (2014) [47]. Briefly, 10 µL of unlabeled standard, placental tissue lysate or lysis solution (extraction blank) were deproteinized with 200 µL of methanol containing 2.5 µM $2,2$-d_2-GAA (Sigma, Rowville, Victoria, Australia deuterium labelled internal standard. Samples were vortexed for 20 min before centrifugation at 15,000 rpm for 5 min, followed by the transfer of 180 µL of the supernatant into 250 µL glass inserts. Samples were then dried in a speed vacuum prior to being derivatized (butylated) by the addition of 100 µL of 3 M butanol-hydrochloric acid and incubation at 60 °C for

30 min. After derivatization, samples were dried under speed vacuum and the residue re-suspended in 100 µL of methanol: water (1:1 v/v). The LC-MS/MS system comprised a vacuum degasser, binary pumps, column oven and a temperature-controlled autosampler (Shimadzu, Nexera® UPLC, Rowville, Victoria, Australia) interfaced with a triple quadrupole mass spectrometer (Shimadzu, LC-MS-8040) with positive electrospray ionization and operated in multiple reaction monitoring (MRM) mode. The MRM transitions for the [M+H$^+$]$^+$ butylated derivatives were: GAA 174.1 m/z–101.1 m/z, d$_2$-GAA 176.1 m/z–103.1 m/z, the collision energy (−15 V) and quad bias voltages were optimized using standards. The LC column was a 2.1 mm × 100 mm, 1.8 µm C18 Zorbax Elipse plus (Agilent, Mulgrave, Victoria, Australia) maintained at 30 °C. The sample and standard injection volume was 5 µL. Samples were eluted with a binary mobile gradient at 0.4 mL/min (mobile phase A water 0.1% formic acid, mobile phase B acetonitrile 0.1% formic acid) with the following program: initial composition was 5% B followed by a linear increase to 50% B over 5 min. The column was then washed at 100% B for 2 min then re-equilibrated at 5% B for 3 min. Total run time was 11 min. GAA eluted at 2.6 min. Peak areas were determined using Lab Solutions Post-run Browser software (Shimadzu). The GAA concentration in the tissue lysate was calculated via linear regression of a serially diluted external (unlabeled) standard series using the isotope dilution technique, after which the concentration was adjusted to the total lysate volume, dilution factor and then normalized to tissue dry mass.

4.2.2. Gene Expression Analysis

Total RNA was extracted from placental tissues ($n = 20$ control and $n = 20$ PE) using RNeasy Kits (Qiagen, Glen Forrest, Australia) and reverse transcribed to form cDNA with SuperScript III Reverse Transcriptase (Invitrogen, ThermoFisher Scientific, Scoresby, Australia), according to manufacturer's protocol. mRNA expression of the creatine synthesizing enzymes (*GATM*-the gene that expresses AGAT & *GAMT*), the creatine transporter (*SLC6A8*) and creatine kinase isoforms (*BBCK* & *CKMT1A*) was determined using Fluidigm Biomark HD system with TaqMan chemistry. TaqMan probe sequences are detailed in Table 2. *RN18S* was used as the housekeeping gene, after conserved expression between the cohorts was validated. Data from qPCR was analyzed according to the $^{\Delta\Delta}C_T$ method [48] and results are expressed relative to the control cohort.

Table 2. TaqMan probe Sequences.

	Gene of Interest	TaqMan Probes
Creatine Synthesis	GATM	Hs00933793_m1
	GAMT	Hs00355745_g1
Creatine Transport	SLC6A8	Hs00940515_m1
Creatine Kinases	BBCK	Hs00176484_m1
	CKMT1A	Hs00179727_m1
Housekeeping	RN18S1	Hs03003631_g1

4.2.3. Protein Analysis

The abundance of AGAT, GAMT, BBCK and CKMT1A in placental protein extracts ($n = 19$ control and $n = 19$ PE) was measured by western immunoblotting, as previously described [17]. Briefly, 40 µg protein/sample was separated on 4%–15% Criterion™ TGX Stain-Free™ precast gels in 10× Tris/Glycine/SDS buffer solution (Bio-Rad, Gladesville, Australia) (for sample arrangement see Supplementary Information Tables S1 and S2). Two micrograms of human liver protein extract (Santa Cruz Biotechnologies sc-363766, Dallas, TX, USA) were included on gels for AGAT and GAMT assessment, as a positive control. Gels for creatine kinase B type and creatine kinase u-type mitochondrial assessment included 2 µg of human brain protein extract (Santa Cruz Biotechnologies sc-364375, Dallas, TX, USA) as the positive control. Proteins samples were transferred for 30 min onto Immobilin-FL PVDF membranes (Millipore, Billerica, MA, USA) and membranes scanned to quantify the total protein transferred using a Bio-Rad Gel Doc™ XR+ (Bio-Rad Laboratories, Hercules, CA, USA). Membranes were then blocked for 1 h with 5% skim milk powder/10% Tris-buffered saline with 0.1% Tween 20 (TBST) at room temperature. After blocking, membranes were incubated overnight at 4 °C with primary antibodies for AGAT (1:100; Atlas Antibodies HPA026077, Bromma, Sweden); GAMT (1:1000; Monash Antibody Technologies Facility, Melbourne, Australia); Creatine kinase B type (1:5000; Abcam BBCK ab92452, Cambridge, UK) or creatine kinase u-type mitochondrial (1:1000; Atlas CKMT1A HPA043491) in 5% skim milk powder/TBST.

Membranes were incubated for 1 h with fluorescent secondary antibodies (Anti-Mouse IgG (H+L) Daylight™ 680 Conjugate or Anti-Rabbit IgG (H+L) Daylight™ 800 Conjugate; Cell Signalling Technologies®, Danvers, MA, USA). Membranes were exposed on an Odyssey® Infrared Imaging System (LI-COR Biosciences, Lincoln, NE, USA) and individual protein band optical densities were determined using Image Studio Lite software (V5.2.5; LI-COR Biosciences, Lincoln, Nebraska, USA). Optical densities for each sample were quantified and then normalized to the total protein transferred onto the blot for that sample [49]. To account for any inter-blot variability, results were then normalized further using the optical density generated by an internal control (healthy term human placenta sample) run on each blot. Data is expressed relative to the control cohort.

4.3. Statistical Analysis

All data were assessed for normality using the Shapiro-Wilk test. Population characteristics (maternal age, parity, gestational age, mode of delivery, baby sex, birth weight and placenta weight) were tabulated. Data are presented as mean ± SD if normally distributed or median and interquartile range (IQR) if non-parametric. Potential confounders, including maternal age, mode of delivery, birth weight and placental weight were assessed with univariate analysis for each of the outcome variables prior to group comparisons being completed. None of these factors were independently associated with changes in outcomes measures. Statistical differences in placental creatine and GAA content, mRNA and protein expression between groups were established with either t-tests or Wilcoxon rank-sum, as appropriate. Baby sex was considered as a covariate for each of these analyses. Correlations between creatine and GAA content, mRNA and protein expression data, with maternal characteristics and birth outcomes were determined using the Spearman rank correlation coefficient. $p \leq 0.025$ was considered statistically significant for direct comparisons and $p \leq 0.004$ for correlations after a Benjamini-Hochberg adjustment for false-positives due to multiple comparisons. All analyses were undertaken using SPSS® (Version 23, IBM Corporation, 2015, Armonk, NY, USA).

5. Conclusions

Placentae from pregnancies affected by early-onset PE have increased total creatine content compared to normotensive controls. Although the current study did not identify changes to protein abundance, the metabolic stress of PE induced gene expression increases in creatine synthesizing enzymes and cytosolic creatine kinase. These initial observations suggest that the PE placenta may adapt to perturbations in oxygen delivery and reduced ATP production at the site of the mitochondria by heightening its reliance on the creatine kinase circuit to stabilize bioenergetics. These processes should be further explored in the context of mitochondrial and endoplasmic reticulum stress, particularly AMPK activation, which has been shown in other tissues to up-regulate creatine metabolism in response to metabolic stress.

Supplementary Materials: Supplementary Materials can be found at http://www.mdpi.com/1422-0067/21/3/806/s1.

Author Contributions: All authors have read and agreed to the published version of the manuscript. Conceptualization, S.J.E. and R.J.S.; methodology, M.L.D.-T., G.M.K., D.L.C., C.R.B.; validation, formal analysis, S.J.E., A.K.M. and P.A.D.G.; investigation, S.J.E.; resources, P.M.; writing—original draft preparation, S.J.E.; writing—review and editing, P.M., P.A.D.G., A.K.M., M.L.D.-T., G.M.K., D.L.C., C.R.B., E.M.W., D.W.W., H.D., R.J.S.; supervision, E.M.W., D.W.W.; project administration, H.D.; funding acquisition, S.J.E., H.D., R.J.S., D.W.W.

Funding: S.J.E. and M.L.D.-T. were NHMRC Early Career Fellows and H.D., an NHMRC Career Development Fellow during the completion of this study. G.M.K. (DE180100859) and C.R.B. (FT160100017) were supported by Australian Research Council Fellowships. A grant from the NHMRC to H.D., D.W.W. and R.J.S. and the Victorian Government Infrastructure Support Fund to the Hudson Institute of Medical Research supported this work.

Acknowledgments: The authors would like to acknowledge the efforts of all research support staff involved in the consenting and collecting of biological samples at the Royal Women's Hospital Melbourne, as well as the MHTP Medical Genomics Facility for providing sequencing services.

Conflicts of Interest: The authors declare no conflict of interest.

Abbreviations

PE	Pre-eclampsia
GAA	Guanidinoacetate
GATM	Gene—arginine:glycine aminotransferase
AGAT	Protein—arginine:glycine aminotransferase
SLC6A8	Gene—creatine transporter
GAMT	Guanidinoacetate methyltransferas
BBCK	Cytosolic creatine kinase
CKMT1A	Mitochondrial creatine kinase
ADP	Adenosine Diphosphate
ATP	Adenosine Triphosphate
I/R	Ischemic-reperfusion
FGR	Fetal Growth Restriction
mRNA	Messenger Ribonucleic Acid
AMPK	AMP-activated protein kinase
PGC-1α	Peroxisome activated receptor γ coactivator-1 alpha
ERRα	Estrogen-related receptor α
HIF-2α	Hypoxia-inducible factor 2 α

References

1. Ananth, C.V.; Keyes, K.M.; Wapner, R.J. Pre-eclampsia rates in the United States, 1980–2010: Age-period-cohort analysis. *BMJ* **2013**, *347*, f6564. [CrossRef] [PubMed]
2. Mol, B.W.; Roberts, C.T.; Thangaratinam, S.; Magee, L.A.; De Groot, C.J.; Hofmeyr, G.J. Pre-eclampsia. *Lancet* **2016**, *387*, 999–1011. [CrossRef]
3. Abalos, E.; Cuesta, C.; Grosso, A.L.; Chou, D.; Say, L. Global and regional estimates of preeclampsia and eclampsia: A systematic review. *Eur. J. Obstet. Gynecol. Reprod. Biol.* **2013**, *170*, 1–7. [CrossRef] [PubMed]
4. Ghulmiyyah, L.; Sibai, B. Maternal mortality from preeclampsia/eclampsia. *Semin. Perinatol.* **2012**, *36*, 56–59. [CrossRef] [PubMed]
5. Cartwright, J.E.; Fraser, R.; Leslie, K.; Wallace, A.E.; James, J.L. Remodelling at the maternal-fetal interface: Relevance to human pregnancy disorders. *Reproduction* **2010**, *140*, 803. [CrossRef] [PubMed]
6. Karumanchi, S.A. Angiogenic factors in preeclampsia: From diagnosis to therapy. *Hypertension* **2016**, *67*, 1072–1079. [CrossRef] [PubMed]
7. Redman, C.W.; Sacks, G.P.; Sargent, I.L. Preeclampsia: An excessive maternal inflammatory response to pregnancy. *Am. J. Obstet. Gynecol.* **1999**, *180*, 499–506. [CrossRef]
8. Holland, O.; Nitert, M.D.; Gallo, L.A.; Vejzovic, M.; Fisher, J.J.; Perkins, A.V. Placental mitochondrial function and structure in gestational disorders. *Placenta* **2017**, *54*, 2–9. [CrossRef]
9. Jääskeläinen, T.; Kärkkäinen, O.; Jokkala, J.; Litonius, K.; Heinonen, S.; Auriola, S.; Lehtonen, M.; Hanhineva, K.; Laivuori, H. A non-targeted LC-MS profiling reveals elevated levels of carnitine precursors and trimethylated compounds in the cord plasma of pre-eclamptic infants. *Sci. Rep.* **2018**, *8*, 14616. [CrossRef]
10. Ellery, S.J.; Della Gatta, P.A.; Bruce, C.R.; Kowalski, G.M.; Davies-Tuck, M.; Mockler, J.C.; Murthi, P.; Walker, D.W.; Snow, R.J.; Dickinson, H. Creatine biosynthesis and transport by the term human placenta. *Placenta* **2017**, *52*, 86–93. [CrossRef]
11. Wallimann, T.; Tokarska-Schlattner, M.; Schlattner, U. The creatine kinase system and pleiotropic effects of creatine. *Amino Acids* **2011**, *40*, 1271–1296. [CrossRef] [PubMed]

12. Braissant, O.; Henry, H.; Villard, A.-M.; Speer, O.; Wallimann, T.; Bachmann, C. Creatine synthesis and transport during rat embryogenesis: Spatiotemporal expression of AGAT, GAMT and CT1. *BMC Dev. Biol.* **2005**, *5*, 9. [CrossRef] [PubMed]
13. Thomure, M. Regulation of creatine kinase isoenzymes in human placenta during early, mid-, and late gestation. *J. Soc. Gynecol. Investig.* **1996**, *3*, 322–327. [CrossRef]
14. Dickinson, H.; Davies-Tuck, M.; Ellery, S.; Grieger, J.; Wallace, E.; Snow, R.; Walker, D.; Clifton, V. Maternal creatine in pregnancy: A retrospective cohort study. *Bjog: Int. J. Obstet. Gynaecol.* **2016**, *123*, 1830–1838. [CrossRef] [PubMed]
15. Heazell, A.E.; Bernatavicius, G.; Warrander, L.; Brown, M.C.; Dunn, W.B. A metabolomic approach identifies differences in maternal serum in third trimester pregnancies that end in poor perinatal outcome. *Reprod. Sci.* **2012**, *19*, 863–875. [CrossRef] [PubMed]
16. Evangelou, I.E.; Du Plessis, A.J.; Vezina, G.; Noeske, R.; Limperopoulos, C. Elucidating metabolic maturation in the healthy fetal brain using 1H-MR spectroscopy. *Am. J. Neuroradiol.* **2016**, *37*, 360–366. [CrossRef] [PubMed]
17. Ellery, S.J.; Murthi, P.; Davies-Tuck, M.L.; Gatta, P.D.; May, A.K.; Kowalski, G.M.; Callahan, D.L.; Bruce, C.R.; Alers, N.O.; Miller, S.L. Placental Creatine Metabolism in Cases of Placental Insufficiency and Reduced Fetal Growth. *Mol. Hum. Reprod.* **2019**, *25*, 495–505. [CrossRef] [PubMed]
18. Burton, G.J.; Redman, C.W.; Roberts, J.M.; Moffett, A. Pre-eclampsia: Pathophysiology and clinical implications. *BMJ* **2019**, *366*, l2381. [CrossRef]
19. Tissot van Patot, M.C.; Murray, A.J.; Beckey, V.; Cindrova-Davies, T.; Johns, J.; Zwerdlinger, L.; Jauniaux, E.; Burton, G.J.; Serkova, N.J. Human placental metabolic adaptation to chronic hypoxia, high altitude: Hypoxic preconditioning. *Am. J. Physiol. Regul. Integr. Comp. Physiol.* **2009**, *298*, R166–R172. [CrossRef]
20. Brosnan, J.; Brosnan, M. Creatine: Endogenous metabolite, dietary, and therapeutic supplement. *Annu. Rev. Nutr.* **2007**, *27*, 241–261. [CrossRef]
21. Wyss, M.; Kaddurah-Daouk, R. Creatine and creatinine metabolism. *Physiol. Rev.* **2000**, *80*, 1107–1213. [CrossRef] [PubMed]
22. Edison, E.E.; Brosnan, M.E.; Meyer, C.; Brosnan, J.T. Creatine synthesis: Production of guanidinoacetate by the rat and human kidney in vivo. *Am. J. Physiol. Ren. Physiol.* **2007**, *293*, F1799–F1804. [CrossRef] [PubMed]
23. McGuire, D.M.; Tormanen, C.; Segal, I.; Van Pilsum, J. The effect of growth hormone and thyroxine on the amount of L-arginine: Glycine amidinotransferase in kidneys of hypophysectomized rats. Purification and some properties of rat kidney transamidinase. *J. Biol. Chem.* **1980**, *255*, 1152–1159. [PubMed]
24. Guthmiller, P.; Van Pilsum, J.; Boen, J.R.; McGuire, D.M. Cloning and sequencing of rat kidney L-arginine: Glycine amidinotransferase. Studies on the mechanism of regulation by growth hormone and creatine. *J. Biol. Chem.* **1994**, *269*, 17556. [PubMed]
25. Mittal, P.; Espinoza, J.; Hassan, S.; Kusanovic, J.P.; Edwin, S.S.; Nien, J.K.; Gotsch, F.; Than, N.G.; Erez, O.; Mazaki-Tovi, S. Placental growth hormone is increased in the maternal and fetal serum of patients with preeclampsia. *J. Matern. Fetal Neonatal Med.* **2007**, *20*, 651–659. [CrossRef] [PubMed]
26. Yung, H.-w.; Calabrese, S.; Hynx, D.; Hemmings, B.A.; Cetin, I.; Charnock-Jones, D.S.; Burton, G.J. Evidence of placental translation inhibition and endoplasmic reticulum stress in the etiology of human intrauterine growth restriction. *Am. J. Pathol.* **2008**, *173*, 451–462. [CrossRef]
27. Sankar, K.D.; Bhanu, P.S.; Ramalingam, K.; Kiran, S.; Ramakrishna, B. Histomorphological and morphometrical changes of placental terminal villi of normotensive and preeclamptic mothers. *Anat. Cell Biol.* **2013**, *46*, 285–290. [CrossRef]
28. Snow, R.J.; Murphy, R.M. Creatine and the creatine transporter: A review. *Mol. Cell. Biochem.* **2001**, *224*, 169–181. [CrossRef]
29. Yang, X.; Xu, P.; Zhang, F.; Zhang, L.; Zheng, Y.; Hu, M.; Wang, L.; Han, T.-l.; Peng, C.; Wang, L. AMPK Hyper-Activation Alters Fatty Acids Metabolism and Impairs Invasiveness of Trophoblasts in Preeclampsia. *Cell. Physiol. Biochem.* **2018**, *49*, 578–594. [CrossRef]

30. Darrabie, M.D.; Arciniegas, A.J.L.; Mishra, R.; Bowles, D.E.; Jacobs, D.O.; Santacruz, L. AMPK and substrate availability regulate creatine transport in cultured cardiomyocytes. *Am. J. Physiol. Endocrinol. Metab.* **2011**, *300*, E870–E876. [CrossRef]
31. Huss, J.M.; Torra, I.P.; Staels, B.; Giguere, V.; Kelly, D.P. Estrogen-related receptor α directs peroxisome proliferator-activated receptor α signaling in the transcriptional control of energy metabolism in cardiac and skeletal muscle. *Mol. Cell. Biol.* **2004**, *24*, 9079–9091. [CrossRef] [PubMed]
32. Brown, E.L.; Snow, R.J.; Wright, C.R.; Cho, Y.; Wallace, M.A.; Kralli, A.; Russell, A.P. PGC-1α and PGC-1β increase CrT expression and creatine uptake in myotubes via ERRα. *Biochim. Biophys. Acta* **2014**, *1843*, 2937–2943. [CrossRef] [PubMed]
33. Vishnyakova, P.A.; Volodina, M.A.; Tarasova, N.V.; Marey, M.V.; Tsvirkun, D.V.; Vavina, O.V.; Khodzhaeva, Z.S.; Kan, N.E.; Menon, R.; Vysokikh, M.Y. Mitochondrial role in adaptive response to stress conditions in preeclampsia. *Sci. Rep.* **2016**, *6*, 32410. [CrossRef] [PubMed]
34. He, L.; Wang, Z.; Sun, Y. Reduced amount of cytochrome c oxidase subunit I messenger RNA in placentas from pregnancies complicated by preeclampsia. *Acta Obstet. Et Gynecol. Scand.* **2004**, *83*, 144–148. [CrossRef]
35. Schlattner, U.; Klaus, A.; Rios, S.R.; Guzun, R.; Kay, L.; Tokarska-Schlattner, M. Cellular compartmentation of energy metabolism: Creatine kinase microcompartments and recruitment of B-type creatine kinase to specific subcellular sites. *Amino Acids* **2016**, *48*, 1751–1774. [CrossRef]
36. Glover, L.E.; Bowers, B.E.; Saeedi, B.; Ehrentraut, S.F.; Campbell, E.L.; Bayless, A.J.; Dobrinskikh, E.; Kendrick, A.A.; Kelly, C.J.; Burgess, A. Control of creatine metabolism by HIF is an endogenous mechanism of barrier regulation in colitis. *Proc. Natl. Acad. Sci. USA* **2013**, *110*, 19820–19825. [CrossRef]
37. Holland, O.J.; Cuffe, J.S.; Nitert, M.D.; Callaway, L.; Cheung, K.A.K.; Radenkovic, F.; Perkins, A.V. Placental mitochondrial adaptations in preeclampsia associated with progression to term delivery. *Cell Death Dis.* **2018**, *9*, 1150. [CrossRef]
38. Burton, G.J.; Jauniaux, E. Pathophysiology of placental-derived fetal growth restriction. *Am. J. Obstet. Gynecol.* **2018**, *218*, S745–S761. [CrossRef]
39. Stead, L.M.; Au, K.P.; Jacobs, R.L.; Brosnan, M.E.; Brosnan, J.T. Methylation demand and homocysteine metabolism: Effects of dietary provision of creatine and guanidinoacetate. *Am. J. Physiol. Endocrinol. Metab.* **2001**, *281*, E1095–E1100. [CrossRef]
40. Lai, W.K.C.; Kan, M.Y. Homocysteine-induced endothelial dysfunction. *Ann. Nutr. Metab.* **2015**, *67*, 1–12. [CrossRef]
41. Powers, R.W.; Evans, R.W.; Majors, A.K.; Ojimba, J.I.; Ness, R.B.; Crombleholme, W.R.; Roberts, J.M. Plasma homocysteine concentration is increased in preeclampsia and is associated with evidence of endothelial activation. *Am. J. Obstet. Gynecol.* **1998**, *179*, 1605–1611. [CrossRef]
42. Pidoux, G.; Gerbaud, P.; Laurendeau, I.; Guibourdenche, J.; Bertin, G.; Vidaud, M.; Evain-Brion, D.; Frendo, J.-L. Large variability of trophoblast gene expression within and between human normal term placentae. *Placenta* **2004**, *25*, 469–473. [CrossRef] [PubMed]
43. Lowe, S.; Brown, M.; Dekker, G.; Gatt, S.; McLintock, C.; McMahon, L. *Guidelines for the Management of Hypertensive Disorders of Pregnancy*; SOMANZ: Sydney, Australia, 2008; pp. 12–23.
44. Murthi, P.; Said, J.; Doherty, V.; Donath, S.; Nowell, C.; Brennecke, S.; Kalionis, B. Homeobox gene DLX4 expression is increased in idiopathic human fetal growth restriction. *Mhr: Basic Sci. Reprod. Med.* **2006**, *12*, 763–769. [CrossRef] [PubMed]
45. Chui, A.; Murthi, P.; Brennecke, S.; Ignjatovic, V.; Monagle, P.; Said, J.M. The expression of placental proteoglycans in pre-eclampsia. *Gynecol. Obstet. Investig.* **2012**, *73*, 277–284. [CrossRef]
46. Harris, R.C.; Soderlund, K.; Hultman, E. Elevation of creatine in resting and exercised muscle of normal subjects by creatine supplementation. *Clin. Sci* **1992**, *83*, 367–374. [CrossRef]
47. Tran, C.; Yazdanpanah, M.; Kyriakopoulou, L.; Levandovskiy, V.; Zahid, H.; Naufer, A.; Isbrandt, D.; Schulze, A. Stable isotope dilution microquantification of creatine metabolites in plasma, whole blood and dried blood spots for pharmacological studies in mouse models of creatine deficiency. *Clin. Chim. Acta* **2014**, *436*, 160–168. [CrossRef]

48. Vandesompele, J.; De Preter, K.; Pattyn, F.; Poppe, B.; Van Roy, N.; De Paepe, A.; Speleman, F. Accurate normalization of real-time quantitative RT-PCR data by geometric averaging of multiple internal control genes. *GenomeBiologycom* **2002**, *3*, 31–34.
49. Eaton, S.L.; Roche, S.L.; Hurtado, M.L.; Oldknow, K.J.; Farquharson, C.; Gillingwater, T.H.; Wishart, T.M. Total protein analysis as a reliable loading control for quantitative fluorescent Western blotting. *PLoS ONE* **2013**, *8*, e72457. [CrossRef]

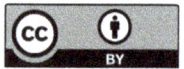

© 2020 by the authors. Licensee MDPI, Basel, Switzerland. This article is an open access article distributed under the terms and conditions of the Creative Commons Attribution (CC BY) license (http://creativecommons.org/licenses/by/4.0/).

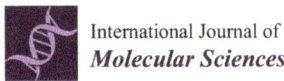

Communication

Expression of Retinoid Acid Receptor-Responsive Genes in Rodent Models of Placental Pathology

Alexander Mocker [1], Marius Schmidt [1], Hanna Huebner [2], Rainer Wachtveitl [3], Nada Cordasic [3], Carlos Menendez-Castro [1], Andrea Hartner [1] and Fabian B. Fahlbusch [1,*]

1. Department of Pediatrics and Adolescent Medicine, Friedrich-Alexander University Erlangen-Nuremberg, 91054 Erlangen, Germany; alexmocker@t-online.de (A.M.); mschmidtdav@gmail.com (M.S.); Carlos.Menendez-Castro@uk-erlangen.de (C.M.-C.); andrea.hartner@uk-erlangen.de (A.H.)
2. Department of Gynaecology and Obstetrics/Comprehensive Cancer Center Erlangen-EMN, Friedrich-Alexander University Erlangen-Nuremberg, 91054 Erlangen, Germany; hanna.huebner@uk-erlangen.de
3. Department of Nephrology and Hypertension, Friedrich-Alexander University Erlangen-Nuremberg, 91054 Erlangen, Germany; Rainer.Wachtveitl@uk-erlangen.de (R.W.); Nada.Cordasic@uk-erlangen.de (N.C.)
* Correspondence: fabian.fahlbusch@uk-erlangen.de; Tel.: +49-9131-853-3118; Fax: +49-9131-853-3714

Received: 24 October 2019; Accepted: 27 December 2019; Published: 29 December 2019

Abstract: In humans, retinoic acid receptor responders (RARRES) have been shown to be altered in third trimester placentas complicated by the pathologies preeclampsia (PE) and PE with intrauterine growth restriction (IUGR). Currently, little is known about the role of placental Rarres in rodents. Therefore, we examined the localization and expression of Rarres1 and 2 in placentas obtained from a Wistar rat model of isocaloric maternal protein restriction (E18.5, IUGR-like features) and from an eNOS-knockout mouse model (E15 and E18.5, PE-like features). In both rodent models, Rarres1 and 2 were mainly localized in the placental spongiotrophoblast and giant cells. Their placental expression, as well as the expression of the Rarres2 receptor chemokine-like receptor 1 (*CmklR1*), was largely unaltered at the examined gestational ages in both animal models. Our results have shown that RARRES1 and 2 may have different expression and roles in human and rodent placentas, thereby underlining immanent limitations of comparative interspecies placentology. Further functional studies are required to elucidate the potential involvement of these proteins in early placentogenesis.

Keywords: RARRES; chemerin; placenta; IUGR; PE; eNOS-knockout; CmklR1; IL-11; low protein diet; pregnancy

---

1. Introduction

Our previous human studies indicated a dysregulation of the tumor suppressor genes retinoic acid receptor responsive proteins (retinoic acid receptor responders, RARRES) 1 and 2 in the third trimester placentas complicated by preeclampsia (PE) and PE conjoined with intrauterine growth restriction (IUGR) [1,2]. We observed an induction of RARRES1 expression in primary villous cytotrophoblasts isolated from PE and PE/IUGR placentas with a concomitant increase in RARRES1 syncytial staining. RARRES2 mRNA expression, on the contrary, seemed reduced, yet unaltered at the protein level in third trimester villous placental samples [1]. These results are controversial, as others have found increased RARRES2 protein expression in samples from total placentas in pregnancies complicated by PE [3]. Furthermore, we had previously determined that RARRES1 and 2 were located in distinct functional placental compartments [1]. RARRES1 (also known as Tazarotene-induced gene 1 (TIG1), Latexin-like (LXNL), or Phorbol Ester-induced gene 1 (PERG-1) [4]) was located in human villous and extravillous trophoblast cells (EVT) [1], while RARRES2 (also known as chemerin, HP10433, and TIG2 [5]) was specifically expressed in human placental EVTs [1]. In contrast, Garces et al. described an additional placental RARRES2 expression in cytotrophoblasts and Hofbauer cells [6].

RARRES1 stimulates the expression of antioxidant enzymes, inhibits angiogenesis, and stimulates autophagy via mTOR [7]. In line with its proposed tumor suppressor function [8–10], RARRES1, along with RARRES2, was reduced in choriocarcinoma [2] and its expression was also significantly reduced in certain choriocarcinoma cell lines (i.e., Jeg-3 and BeWo) [1].

While RARRES1 is located intracellularly [10,11], RARRES2 is a secreted adipocytokine that requires activation of its pro-form by proteolytic cleavage to exert its functions via chemokine-like receptor 1 (CMKLR1, ChemR23) [12,13]. Wang et al. [3] were able to show that RARRES2 exerts anti-inflammatory functions by inducing endothelial nitric oxide synthase (eNOS) expression in human umbilical vein endothelial cells (HUVECs) and by significantly decreasing TNF-α-induced nuclear factor (NF)-kappa B, and vascular cell adhesion molecule (VCAM)-1 production [3]. RARRES2 further modulates chemotaxis and activation of dendritic cells and macrophages via CMKLR1 [14,15], which is expressed in various leukocyte populations [16].

Pregnancy represents a state of constant metabolic adaptation and increased inflammation. In this respect, IUGR and PE represent two extreme gestational disturbances [17–19]. In PE the production of placental inflammatory cytokines [18,19] is increased. It is known that adipocytokine and interleukin signaling interact [20–22]. Recently IL-11, a member of the IL-6 family also known as adipogenesis inhibitory factor (AGIF) [23], has been found by others to be upregulated in PE and leads to inflammation and preeclampsia-like features in mice [24]. Treatment of mice with IL-11 negatively affects placentation, including trophoblast invasion and spiral artery remodeling, a key process in the pathogenesis of human PE [24,25]. IL-11 further increases systolic maternal blood pressure and leads to PE-like proteinuria in dams [24,25]. Mice with an eNOS-deficiency (eNOS$^{-/-}$ [26–29]) display PE-like features (e.g., vascular placental impairment [19,27,30] and an increased inflammatory state [31–34]).

To confirm this, we tested placental IL-11 expression in these mice. Moreover, we analyzed Rarres expression in second and third trimester placenta of eNOS$^{-/-}$ mice, because Garces et al. detected a maximum of placental Rarres2 expression at this gestational age in rodents [6].

To expand our findings from third trimester human placenta [1], we investigated Rarres1, Rarres2, and Cmklr1 expression in third trimester rodent placenta. Moreover, we analyzed the influence of maternal protein restriction in rats (IUGR-like features [35,36]) on placental Rarres1 and 2 expression. We additionally compared placentas in the context of fetal sex, given the differences in Rarres2 expression that were already described by Watts et al. [37] for male and female fetuses.

2. Results

2.1. Auxology

Animal data are displayed in Table 1. Maternal protein restriction led to a significant decrease in fetal weight ($p = 0.03$) and a significant increase in placental/fetal ratio ($p = 0.03$) at E18.5 in rats. This had no significant influence on placental weight ($p = 0.11$). In our eNOS$^{-/-}$ mice, fetal and placental weights were examined at E15 and E18.5. The animals showed a significant decrease of fetal weight at both time points compared to wildtype controls ($p < 0.001$). Mouse placental weights were significantly decreased at E18.5 ($p = 0.006$), with a similar trend at E15 ($p = 0.08$). The placental-to-fetal weight ratio was unaffected by eNOS deficiency (Table 1).

Table 1. Animal auxology. NP: normal protein diet; LP: low protein diet.

Rat [†]	E18.5 NP	E18.5 LP	p Value			
fetal weight (fw)	1.38 ± 0.09	0.86 ± 0.05	**0.03** *			
placental weight (pw)	0.34 ± 0.04	0.30 ± 0.01	0.11 *			
pw/fw ratio	0.25 ± 0.02	0.35 ± 0.02	**0.03** *			
Mouse [‡]	**E15 C57BL/6**	**E15 eNOS$^{-/-}$**	**p Value**	**E18.5 C57BL/6**	**E18.5 eNOS$^{-/-}$**	**p Value**
fetal weight (fw)	0.34 ± 0.07	0.28 ± 0.03	0.08 *	1.19 ± 0.15	0.97 ± 0.08	**0.006** *
placental weight (pw)	0.10 ± 0.01	0.08 ± 0.01	**<0.001** *	0.09 ± 0.01	0.07 ± 0.01	**<0.001** *
pw/fw ratio	0.31 ± 0.06	0.29 ± 0.06	0.58 *	0.08 ± 0.02	0.07 ± 0.01	0.63 *

* Mann-Whitney U-Test. [†] For rats, each group consisted of n = 4 dams each with n = 6 NP/LP pups/damn, respectively. [‡] For mice, groups consisted of n = 6 eNOS$^{-/-}$ vs. n = 5 C57BL/6 dams at both time points with n = 2 pups/dam. Legend: bold values denote statistical significance.

2.2. Localization of Rarres1 and 2

Representative images of Rarres1 and 2 immunohistochemical (IHC) stains are given in Figure 1A,D and Figure 2A,D, respectively. Both proteins shared similar localization in functional placental compartments. In contrast to Rarres1 (cytoplasmic stain, Figure 1), Rarres2 (Figure 2) additionally showed nuclear staining. IHC did not reveal species differences between rat (Figures 1A and 2A) and mouse (Figures 1D and 2D) placentas regarding Rarres1 and 2 localization. Positive staining was mostly present in the cytoplasm of trophoblast giant cells (GC) and spongiotrophoblasts (ST) of rat (Figure 1A) and mouse (Figure 1D) placentas at E18.5. In mice, we did not note differences in Rarres1 and 2 staining in comparison to E15 (data not shown). We additionally found positive staining for both proteins in the yolk sac, decidual stroma, and the umbilical cord lining membrane (data not shown). Glycogen cells and the labyrinth zone (LZ) stained negative for Rarres1 and 2.

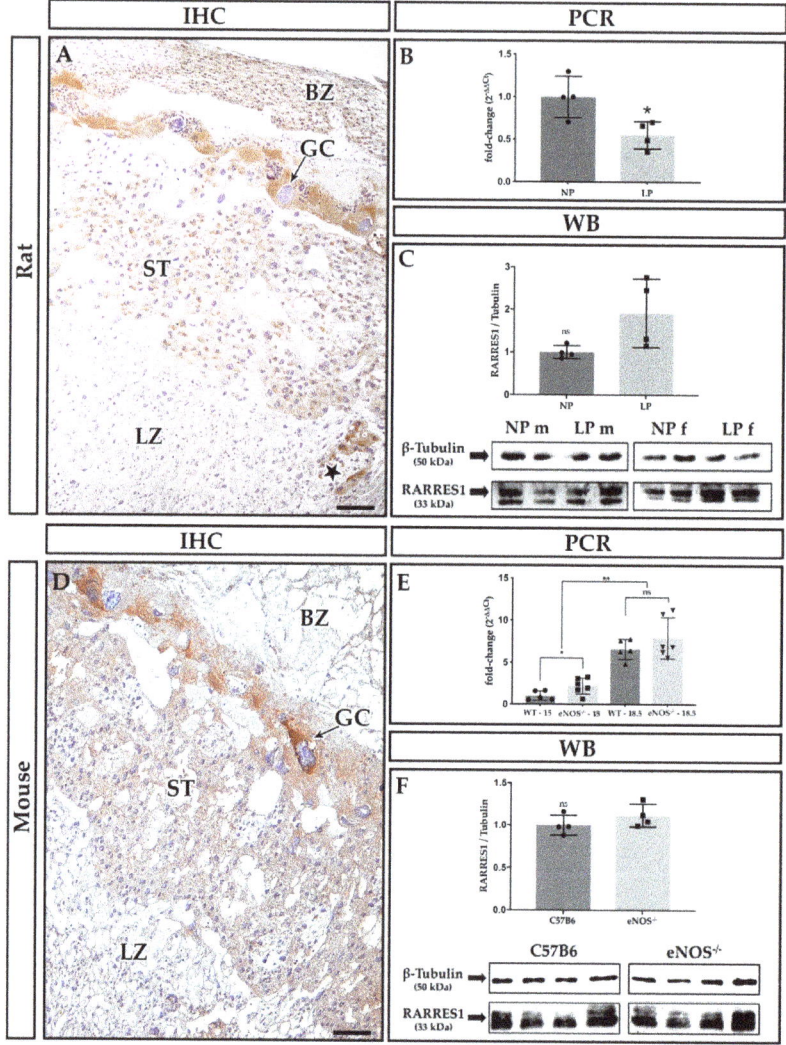

Figure 1. Rarres1 expression in rat and mouse placenta. (**A–C**) Rat placenta, (**D–F**) mouse placenta. (**A,D**) Immunohistochemical (IHC) stains of methyl Carnoy-fixed placental paraffin sections. Abbreviations: GC = giant cell, BZ = basal zone, ST = spongiotrophoblast, LZ = labyrinth zone, star = glycogen cells. The bar equals 100 μm. (**B**) Maternal protein restriction rat model: placental *Rarres1* mRNA expression on E18.5 (*p = 0.03, Mann-Whitney U-Test, n = 4 NP/LP dams with 6 pups each). E) eNOS$^{-/-}$ mouse model: placental *Rarres1* mRNA expression on E15 and E18.5 (* p = 0.03, ** p = 0.008 for C57BL/6 and p = 0.002 for eNOS$^{-/-}$, ns: p = 0.66, Mann-Whitney U-Test, WT: n = 5 dams, eNOS$^{-/-}$: n = 6 dams with 2 pups each). C + F) Analysis of Rarres1 protein expression versus β-Tubulin housekeeper by Western blotting (WB, Rat: ns: p = 0.057, Mann-Whitney U-Test, n = 4 NP/LP dams with n = 2 pups each, E18.5; Mouse: ns: p = 0.20, Mann-Whitney U-Test, n = 4 C57B6 and eNOS$^{-/-}$ dams per group with n = 1 pup each, E18.5). Abbreviations: LP = low protein diet, NP = normal protein diet in the rat IUGR model with m = male fetus, f = female fetus; C57B6 = C57BL/6 wild type (WT) control strain, eNOS$^{-/-}$ = preeclampsia (PE)/intrauterine growth restriction (IUGR) model eNOS knockout mouse, ns = not significant. RARRES = retinoic acid receptor responders.

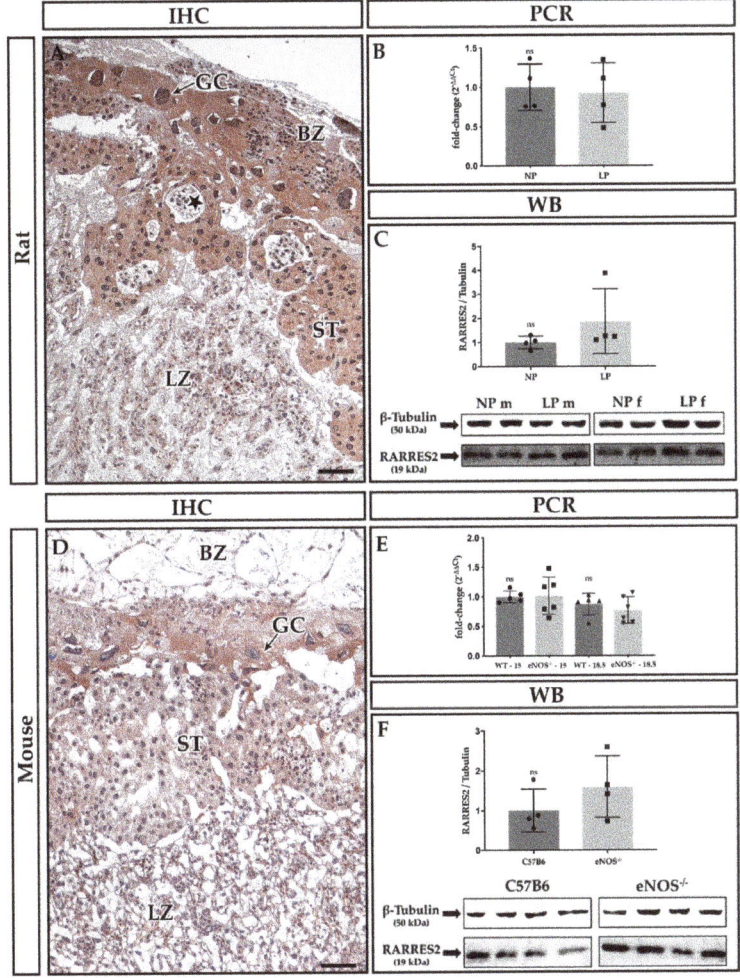

Figure 2. Rarres2 expression in rat and mouse placenta. (**A–C**) Rat placenta, (**D–F**) mouse placenta. (**A,D**) Immunohistochemical (IHC) stains of methyl Carnoy-fixed placental paraffin sections. Abbreviations: GC = giant cell, BZ = basal zone, ST = spongiotrophoblast, LZ = labyrinth zone, star = glycogen cells. The bar equals 100 µm. (**B**) Maternal protein restriction rat model: placental *Rarres2* mRNA expression on E18.5 (ns: $p = 0.89$, Mann-Whitney U-Test, $n = 4$ NP/LP dams with 6 pups each). E) eNOS$^{-/-}$ mouse model: placental *Rarres2* mRNA expression on E15 and E18.5 (E15: ns: $p = 0.31$, E19: ns: $p = 0.66$, Mann-Whitney U-test, WT: $n = 5$ dams, eNOS$^{-/-}$: $n = 6$ dams with 2 pups each). C + F) Analysis of Rarres1 protein expression versus β-Tubulin housekeeper by Western blotting (WB, Rat: ns: $p = 0.10$, Mann-Whitney U-Test, $n = 4$ NP/LP dams with $n = 2$ pups each, E18.5; Mouse: ns: $p = 0.49$, Mann-Whitney U-Test, $n = 4$ C57B6 and eNOS$^{-/-}$ dams per group with $n = 1$ pup each, E18.5). Abbreviations: LP = low protein diet, NP = normal protein diet in the rat IUGR model with m = male fetus, f = female fetus; C57B6 = C57BL/6 wild type (WT) control strain, eNOS$^{-/-}$ = PE/IUGR model eNOS knockout mouse, ns = not significant.

2.3. Expression Analyses of Rarres1/2, CmklR1 Receptor, and IL-11

We detected a small but significant decrease of placental *Rarres1* mRNA expression in our maternal protein restriction rat model at E18.5 ($p = 0.03$, Figure 1B). Sex did not show any significant influence on the expression of *Rarres1*, *2* and *CmklR1* mRNA expression levels (Table 2). In contrast to the rat, we could determine significant differences in *Rarres1* mRNA expression between eNOS$^{-/-}$ mice and C57BL/6 wildtype controls at E15 ($p = 0.03$) but not on E18.5 ($p = 0.66$) (Figure 1E). However, a 3.6-fold (eNOS$^{-/-}$) and 6.5-fold (C57BL/6) temporal increase of placental *Rarres1* mRNA expression was detected from E15 to E18.5 ($p = 0.008$ for C57BL6 mice and $p = 0.002$ for eNOS$^{-/-}$ mice, Figure 1E). Western blot analysis did not reveal significant differences in placental Rarres1 protein expression E18.5 in both animal models (rat: $p = 0.057$, mouse: $p = 0.20$, Figure 1C,F).

Placental *Rarres2* mRNA (Figure 2B,E) and protein expression (Figure 2C,F) was neither affected by maternal protein restriction in the rat (PCR: $p = 0.89$, WB: $p = 0.10$, Figure 2B,C), nor eNOS$^{-/-}$ in the mice (PCR: E15: $p = 0.31$, E19: $p = 0.66$, WB: $p = 0.49$, Figure 2E,F). Also, the expression of *Rarres2* remained unchanged from E15 to E18.5 in the mouse ($p = 0.31$ for C57BL6 mice and $p = 0.13$ for eNOS$^{-/-}$ mice, Figure 2E).

Placental *CmklR1* expression was unchanged by maternal protein restriction in the rat and eNOS$^{-/-}$ in the mouse. Gestational age seemed to have no significant influence on *CmklR1* expression in the mouse (Table 3). However, a significant increase of placental interleukin 11 (*IL-11*) mRNA expression at E15 (2.3-fold, $p = 0.004$, Figure 3) was observed in eNOS$^{-/-}$ mice compared to controls. No such change in *IL-11* expression was noted at E18.5 ($p = 0.99$).

Table 2. Sex differences in mRNA expression (fold-change).

Rat	NP m	NP f	*p* Value	LP m	LP f	*p* Value
Rarres1	1.00 ± 0.36	0.97 ± 0.17	0.89 *	0.48 ± 0.26	0.58 ± 0.19	0.69 *
Rarres2	1.00 ± 0.30	1.30 ± 0.41	0.49 *	0.90 ± 0.75	1.52 ± 0.42	0.23 *
CmklR1	1.00 ± 0.44	0.89 ± 0.60	0.99 *	1.10 ± 0.51	0.95 ± 0.29	0.99 *

* Mann-Whitney U-Test; For Rarres1 and 2, groups consisted of n = 4 NP/LP dams with n = 3 female/male pups, respectively. For CmklR1, groups consisted n = 3 NP/LP dams with n = 2 female/male pups, respectively. Abbreviations: LP = low protein diet, NP = normal protein diet in the rat IUGR model; m = male fetus, f = female fetus.

Table 3. Placental *CmklR1* mRNA expression (fold-change).

Rat †	E18.5 NP	E18.5 LP	*p* Value			
	1.00 ± 0.53	1.08 ± 0.32	0.99 *			
Mouse ‡	E15 C57BL/6	E15 eNOS$^{-/-}$	*p* Value	E18.5 C57BL/6	E18.5 eNOS$^{-/-}$	*p* Value
	1.00 ± 0.43	0.9 ± 0.42	0.93 *	0.51 ± 0.1	0.41 ± 0.18	0.18 *

* Mann-Whitney U-Test. † For rats, groups consisted of n = 3 dams per group (NP/LP) with n = 5 pups each; ‡ For mice, groups consisted of n = 6 eNOS$^{-/-}$ vs. n = 5 C57BL/6 dams at both time-points with n = 2 pups/dam. Abbreviations: LP = low protein diet, NP = normal protein diet in the rat IUGR model; C57BL/6 = Wild type (WT) control, eNOS$^{-/-}$ = PE/IUGR model knockout mouse.

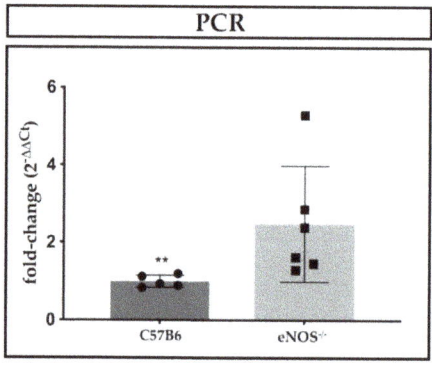

Figure 3. Placental *IL-11* mRNA expression in eNOS$^{-/-}$ mice on E15. (** $p = 0.004$, Mann-Whitney U-test, WT: n = 5 dams, eNOS$^{-/-}$: n = 6 dams with 2 pups each) Abbreviations: C57B6 = C57BL/6 wild type (WT) control strain, eNOS$^{-/-}$ = PE/IUGR model knockout mouse.

3. Discussion

Summarizing our findings, we demonstrate a sufficient induction of intrauterine growth restriction in both rodent models, as determined by fetal weight reduction, when compared to the respective controls. Rarres1 and 2 were pre-dominantly located in the spongiotrophoblast and giant cells of both rat and mouse placenta. In the rat, no consistent regulation of Rarres1/2 was detected under maternal protein restriction. Similarly, we did not find changes in *Rarres1* and 2 mRNA or protein expressions in eNOS$^{-/-}$ mice. In the mouse, we observed a temporal increase in placental *Rarres1* mRNA expression from E15 to E18.5 independent of their genotype. Moreover, we found an IL-11 induction at E15 in the eNOS$^{-/-}$ mice, suggestive of increased placental inflammation, a common feature of human PE [24].

3.1. Expression of Rarres1 in Rodent Placenta

Based on its localization in the human placenta, we have previously hypothesized that RARRES1, as a tumor-suppressor gene, might slow down invasion and migration of EVTs in terminal placentas and that it might regulate proliferation, syncytialization, and apoptosis of villous trophoblasts [1,2]. Thus, an increased RARRES1 expression in human PE might represent a state of reduced trophoblast proliferation and syncytialization with increased apoptosis [1,38,39].

In our current study, we determined that rodent Rarres1 was predominantly located in the placental junctional zone (giant cells and the spongiotrophoblast) with only minor expression in the labyrinth layer (resembling the human syncytiotrophoblast). Based on this observation, it could be assumed that Rarres1 plays a minor role in rodent placental syncytial physiology at the examined gestational stages. Other than a common hemochorial nature, murine placental anatomy shares limited features with the human placenta [40,41]. Nevertheless, the rodent placenta junctional zone (JZ) shares similarities with the human extravillous compartment [42–45], as it is positioned between the labyrinth and the maternal decidua [46]. From ~E12.5 onwards, trophoblast cells of the JZ invade into the decidua, where they become associated with maternal blood spaces. As a counterpart to the human placental syncytium, the JZ also constitutes the main placental endocrine compartment affecting both maternal and fetal physiology [46]. We have previously demonstrated that the placental distribution pattern of RARRES1 changes throughout human gestation [1]. Since we were able to detect temporal changes in the gestational expression of Rarres1 in mice, an involvement of Rarres1 in placental development and growth seems feasible, potentially regulating invasiveness of JZ trophoblast.

In contrast to our previous results from human PE placentas, *Rarres1* expression was not induced in placentas of eNOS$^{-/-}$ mice. In fact, late gestational expression of placental *Rarres1* was rather reduced by dietary-induced IUGR in the rat. However, our *Rarres1* mRNA data were not supported by Western blot analysis, potentially owing to alterations in translation rate/protein degradation or transcription/mRNA stability (reviewed by [47]).

Our findings argue for a species-specific role of RARRES1 in the human syncytium and its involvement in PE [48,49]. While in the murine placenta temporal changes of placental *Rarres1* expression were noted, gestational changes in Rarres1 expression in the rat were not studied. No differences in Rarres1 expression were detected in placentas of male or female fetuses.

3.2. Expression of Rarres2 in Rodent Placenta

We found that our Wistar rats expressed Rarres2 in the same placental compartments as Rarres1 (see above). The pronounced localization of Rarres2 in rat trophospongium supports our previous findings in human placenta [1], where RARRES2 was specifically expressed in extravillous trophoblasts (see above).

The expression and regulation of Rarres2 during rat pregnancy has been previously studied by Garces et al. [6] in Sprague Dawley rats at multiple gestational timepoints. In contrast to our findings, Garces et al. [6] found relevant Rarres2 staining in the labyrinthine trophoblast, besides the trophospongium in rats, which might have been due to the difference in employed rat species (Wistar vs. Sprague Dawley). Similarly, they found syncytial RARRES2 expression besides its extravillous localization in the human placenta, which was not supported by our previous studies [1]. This difference requires further investigation. It might be due to divergent IHC techniques (fixation: methyl Carnoy's solution (our study) versus paraformaldehyde [6], rabbit antibody vs. recombinant full length human RARRES2 (our study) versus goat antibody vs. N-terminal human RARRES2 [6]). The placental *Rarres2* expression increased until E16 in rats and then decreased until term, while rat maternal serum levels (ELISA) steadily decreased over the course of pregnancy in their animals [6]. This finding is in contrast to analyses of the same research group in humans, where RARRES2 levels were shown to rise significantly over the course of pregnancy [50]. This might argue for species-specific differences in the regulation of gestational Rarres2 expression and/or different functions of Rarres2 in murine and human placenta. The expression of *Rarres2* in rat mesenteric adipose tissue remained mainly constant, despite a singular increase at E19 [6]. IUGR (30% of total ad libitum maternal diet) resulted in a ~50% reduction of placental *Rarres2* expression in Sprague Dawley rats. The gestational expression pattern of *Rarres2* (i.e., maximum of placental expression around E16), however, remained unchanged [6]. Rarres2 expression in rodents was higher at the end of the second trimester, than at the end of the third trimester. This is in line with our findings of a more prominent Rarres2 expression in mouse placenta at gestational E15 compared to gestational day E18.5.

In contrast to Garces et al. [6], we did not observe a reduction of *Rarres2* in our isocaloric rat model of maternal protein restriction. This might be due to the divergent use of maternal diets (i.e., isocaloric protein restriction vs. total caloric reduction). We have just recently shown that our diet does not resemble a stress-model, unlike other models of total intake restriction [36]. Furthermore, models with total calorie restriction [51,52] seem more prone to develop insulin resistance after IUGR. Thus, the observed placental reduction of rat *Rarres2* expression under the condition of profound maternal food restriction [6] might underscore its proposed role as placental adipocytokine [6,53], with putative involvement in the development of maternal insulin resistance [54,55] and in feto-maternal metabolic homeostasis during pregnancy [56]. However, this hypothesis and the association of markers of insulin sensitivity with circulating RARRES2 is controversially discussed [50,57]. Unfortunately, there was no description of the influence of IUGR on *Rarres2* levels in rat maternal adipose tissue or serum by Garces et al. [6].

In vitro findings of Wang et al. [3] indicated that RARRES2 induces NO production in HUVECs. Our PE mouse model did not show local induction of *Rarres2* despite the knockout of eNOS, which suggests a lack of local negative feedback. At this point, systemic feedback-signaling cannot be ruled out, as circulating Rarres2 remained undetermined in our study.

3.3. Expression of CmklR1 in Rodent Placenta

Our finding of stable placental *CmklR1* expression levels in our Wistar rats resembled the gestational findings of Sanchez-Rebordelo et al. in Sprague Dawley rats [58]. Similarly, we could not detect significant differences or gestational changes of *CmklR1*-expression in our eNOS$^{-/-}$ mice. This finding is of interest, as CMKLR1 activation has been shown to induce vasoconstriction of peripheral vessels [59] and a reduced uterine blood flow is characteristic in eNOS$^{-/-}$ mice [60]. Thus, CmklR1 might play a minor role in the dysregulation of vascular tone in these mice. However, as knockout of CmklR1 seems to induce higher abortion rates in mice [61], different mechanisms of action need to be taken into consideration.

3.4. IL-11 as a Novel Regulatory Cytokine in eNOS$^{-/-}$ Mice

The level of IUGR in our rats, as determined by fetal weight, was comparable to our previous experience with this model [36,62]. Additionally, the observed level of fetal and placental weight reduction in eNOS$^{-/-}$ mice (18% and 22%, respectively; E18.5) was similar to findings from the literature (11% and 10%, respectively; E17 [28]), when compared to C57BL/6 control mice.

Interestingly, we found an induction of placental *IL-11* in our eNOS$^{-/-}$ mice at midgestation, which has not been shown previously. As IL-11 has been demonstrated to contribute to the development of inflammation in PE and placental vascular changes in mice [24,25], our finding might indicate respective changes in our rodent placentas, which are found in a similar manner in human PE.

4. Materials and Methods

4.1. Animals and Diets

This study was carried out following the recommendations of the National Institute of Health (NIH) *Guide for the Care and Use of Laboratory Animals* and the Directive 2010/63/EU. All procedures and protocols were governmentally approved by the corresponding board (Regierung von Mittelfranken, AZ #54-2531.31-31/09 (10 November 2010) and AZ #55.2-2532-2-820 (17 January 2019)). Surgical procedures were performed under isoflurane anesthesia and all efforts were made to minimize suffering.

4.1.1. Alimentary Rat Model with IUGR-Like Features

Animal procedures and the dietary regimen were carried out as previously described by us in detail [36]. Wistar rats were ordered from Charles River (Sulzfeld, Germany). Weighing 240–260 g, rats were mated, and the beginning of gestation was determined via assessment of vaginal plug expulsion. Subsequently, dams were randomly assigned into two groups consisting of six animals each and received semi-purified diets (Altromin Spezialfutter GmbH & Co. KG, Lage, Germany) of either low protein diet (LP group, 25 g/d of Altromin C1003, 8% protein) or an isocaloric diet of normal protein content (NP group, 25 g/d of Altromin C1000, 17% protein) from day 1 of gestation. This results in reduced birth weight and increased placental-to-fetal weight ratio, indicating preserved placental efficiency [63]. Rat placentas were obtained at E18.5. Animal characteristics are displayed in Table 1. Sex verification was carried out via sex-determining region Y (Sry) gene PCR, as previously described by us in detail [36].

4.1.2. Mouse Model with PE/IUGR-Like Features

The eNOS-knockout (eNOS$^{-/-}$) mice came from Jackson Laboratories (Bar Harbor, Maine, USA). The recommended wild-type (WT) C57BL/6 mice were ordered from Charles River (Sulzfeld, Germany). A homozygous breeding strategy was followed. Both strains were kept over ten generations in our animal facility before being utilized in experiments. Mice were housed at 22 ± 2 °C and a 12 h light/dark cycle in our animal facilities. Animals had unlimited access to standard chow (SSNIFF V1534, ssniff Spezialdiäten GmbH, Soest, Germany) and tap water. The animal model of eNOS$^{-/-}$ mice was previously described in detail by others [28,64,65]. The placental dysfunction in eNOS$^{-/-}$ mice [26,64,65] is caused with an impaired systemic vascularization of the dam [29]: eNOS deficiency significantly reduces the essential maternal cardiovascular adaptive capacity via reduction of circulating nitric oxide [28]. Thus, maintenance of constant uterine and feto-placental blood flow and of low feto-placental vascular resistance via modulation of smooth muscle myogenic tone is disabled [19,27,30]. Moreover, eNOS deficiency seems to be associated with an increased inflammatory state [31–34]. We chose eNOS$^{-/-}$ mice over various other rodent models of PE (reviewed by [18]) as placentas of this model lack gross anatomic alterations [28] similar to our low protein rat model [66]. Each group of mice was mated, and the presence of a copulation plug was denoted as day 0.5 of pregnancy. Mouse placentas were obtained from these mice at day E15 and E18.5. Animal characteristics are displayed in Table 1. Based on our finding that sex seemed to have no influence on *Rarres1/2* expression in the rat placenta, we did not include it as a variable in the mouse model analysis. The placental *eNOS* mRNA expression was well detectable in control mice but was below the detection limit in eNOS$^{-/-}$ mice (data not shown).

All rodent placentas were fixed in methyl Carnoy's solution (Roth, Karlsruhe, Germany) for embedding in paraffin or were snap frozen and stored at −80 °C for messenger RNA (mRNA) preparation and protein extraction.

4.2. RNA Extraction, RT-PCR, and Real-Time Quantitative PCR

Gene expression analysis has previously been described by us in detail [36]. PCR was performed in $n = 5$ pups (mean) per litter from 4 NP/LP dams, respectively. In our mouse model, $n = 2$ pups per litter from $n = 6$ eNOS$^{-/-}$ dams and $n = 5$ C57BL/6 wild type controls, respectively, were examined at two different time points (E15; E18.5). Snap-frozen placental tissues were minced using a Mikro-Dismembrator (Sartorius Stedim Biotech GmbH, Göttingen, Germany). RNA purification of our rat placentas was achieved with peqGold TriFast reagent (Peqlab, Erlangen, Germany), and RNA pretreatment with DNase I (Sigma-Aldrich, Darmstadt, Germany) was used. For mouse samples, the frozen tissue was homogenized by grinding with a T10 basic ULTRA TURRAX disperser (IKA, Staufen im Breisgau, Germany), and total RNA was extracted using the RNeasy Mini Kit with DNase treatment (Qiagen, Hilden, Germany) according to the manufacturer's instructions. RNA concentration was determined by NanoDrop spectrophotometry (Peqlab, Erlangen, Germany) and adjusted to 100 ng/mL for all rodent placenta samples. Complementary DNA (cDNA) synthesis was conducted using TaqMan Reverse Transcription (Applied Biosystems, Waltham, MA, USA) in a Biometra Trio thermal cycler (Analytik Jena, Jena, Germany). Quantification of *Rarres1*, *Rarres2*, *CmlkR1*, and *IL11* mRNA expression was achieved by qRT PCR analysis using the Fast SYBR Green Master Mix and Sequence Detector StepOnePlus (Applied Biosystems, Waltham, MA, USA) with *r18s* RNA as a reference gene. Measurements were performed in duplicate. Primers were designed using Primer Express software (version 3.0.1, Applied Biosystems, Waltham, MA, USA) or Primer-BLAST (NCBI, NIH). Primers were ordered from Eurofins (Eurofins Genomics Germany GmbH, Ebersberg, Germany) and sequences are listed in Table 4.

Table 4. Primer sequences.

Rat	Forward	Reverse
Rarres1	5′-AGGTGGACCTGGTGTTTAGCA-3′	5′-AACACCCTCGCAGAACATTTG-3′
Rarres2	5′-AAATGGGAGGAAGCGGAAAT-3′	5′-CCATCCGGCCTAGAACTTTACC-3′
CmlkR1	5′-AAGAGATGGAGTACGAGGGTTACAA-3′	5′-GATGTAGTCCGAGCCGTCAGA-3′
r18s	5′-TTGATTAAGTCCCTGCCCTTTGT-3′	5′-CGATCCGAGGGCCTCACTA-3′
Mouse		
Rarres1	5′-AGCGGCTGAAAACGGATGA-3′	5′-CCAAGTGAATACGGCAGGGA-3′
Rarres2	5′-CACTGCCCAATTCTGAAGCAA-3′	5′-CGCCAGCCTGTGCTATCTTAA-3′
Cmlkr1	5′- CAACGGTGAACAGTGAAAGGTC-3′	5′- TTGTAAGCGTCGTACTCCATCTCT-3′
eNos	5′-CACCAGGAAGAAGACCTTTAAGGA-3′	5′-CACCGTGCCCATGAGTGA-3′
IL-11	5′-GCTCCCCTCGAGTCTCTTCA-3′	5′-TGTCTCTCATCTGTGCAGCTAGTTG-3′
r18s	5′-TTGATTAAGTCCCTGCCCTTTGT-3′	5′-CGATCCGAGGGCCTCACTA-3′

4.3. Western Blot Analysis

For protein expression analysis, placental tissue of rat NP/LP (4 dams with 2 pups/dam) and mouse E18.5 eNOS$^{-/-}$ versus C57BL/6 control (8 dams with 1 pup each) was homogenized by mincing in 20 mL RIPA buffer, consisting of 50 mM Tris (pH 7.2), 10 mM EDTA, 150 mM NaCl, 0.1% SDS, 1.0% Triton X-100, 1.0% sodium deoxycholate, 20 μL/mL proteinase inhibitor (Complete proteinase inhibitor, Santa Cruz Biotechnology Inc., Dallas, TX, USA), and 2 mM Na3VO4. Buffer amount was adjusted to sample weight. The protein concentration was determined by the kit (Pierce, Rockford, IL, USA). Rat samples containing 30 μg/44 μl and mouse samples containing 30 μg/40 μL of protein were boiled at 95 °C for 8 min and separated on a 10% denaturing SDS-PAGE gel (for Rarres1 measurements of rat samples, 12% gel was used). Semi-dry electro-blotting was performed using Hartenstein GB33 PVDF membranes (Bio-Rad Laboratories, Hercules, USA), which were then blocked with Rotiblock (Roth,

Karlsruhe, Germany) for 60 min. The membrane was incubated overnight at 4 °C with a polyclonal rabbit anti-rat antibody to Rarres1 (Biorbyt, Cambridge, UK) at a concentration of 1:250, or polyclonal rabbit anti-rat antibody to Rarres2 (Thermo Fisher, Waltham, MA, USA) at a concentration of 1:500 (rat)/1:1000 (mouse). Subsequently, the membrane was incubated for 60 min at room temperature with a secondary donkey anti-rabbit antibody (GE Healthcare, Amersham, UK) in the concentration 1:10,000 (for Rarres1 rat–blots 5% milk powder was added). As a reference, a monoclonal mouse anti-vinculin antibody at a concentration of 1:2000 and a monoclonal mouse anti-β-Tubulin antibody at a concentration of 1:10,000 (both from Sigma Aldrich, St. Louis, MO, USA) followed by a secondary sheep anti-mouse antibody (GE Healthcare, Amersham, UK) were used. As both reference genes resulted in similar results, only β-Tubulin blots were displayed. Immunoreactivity was visualized using the fluorescent ECL Plus Western Blotting Substrate according to the manufacturer's instructions (Thermo Fisher Scientific, Waltham, MA, USA) and quantified with a luminescent imager (LAS-1000, Fujifilm, Berlin, Germany) and AIDA Image Analysis software (version 2.1, Elysia-raytest GmbH, Straubenhardt Germany).

Coomassie Brilliant Blue staining served as the loading control.

4.4. Immunohistochemistry

For immunohistochemical (IHC) analysis, tissues were fixed in methyl Carnoy's solution and embedded in paraffin, as previously described [67]. Each group consisted of 6 placentas (3 sections of the central region, each) from 2 dams. Two-micrometer paraffin sections were prepared with a HM340E microtome (Thermo Fisher Scientific, Waltham, MA, USA). After de-paraffinization and rehydration with intermittent Tris-buffered saline (TBS) washing, tissue sections were unmasked by cooking in target retrieval solution (TRS, Dako Agilent, Santa Clara, CA, USA) for 10 min. Endogenous peroxidase activity was blocked with 3% H_2O_2 for 20 min at room temperature. Sections were then incubated in fetal calf serum (FCS) at 37 °C for 30 min and coated with the primary antibody (Rarres1: MyBioSource, San Diego, CA, USA, 1:50; Rarres2: Thermo Fisher, Waltham, MA, USA 1:100). After incubation at 4 °C overnight, sections were washed in TBS and layered with the secondary antibody (dilution 1:500; biotin-conjugated, goat anti-rabbit immunoglobulin G; Vector Laboratories, Burlingame, CA, USA) at room temperature for 30 min. Subsequently, sections were incubated with avidin-biotinylated horseradish peroxidase complex (Vectastain PK-6100; Vector Laboratories) at RT for 30 min and with a DAB (diaminobenzidine tetrahydrochloride) kit (SK-4100; Vector Laboratories, both supplied by Linaris, Dossenheim, Germany) for 15 min and counterstained with hematoxylin (Merck, Darmstadt, Germany). After embedding in Entellan (Merck, Darmstadt, Germany), imaging was performed with a DMC 6200 camera mounted on a Leica DMR microscope (Type 020-525.731) using LASX 3.4.2.18368 image software (all from Leica Microsystems, Wetzlar, Germany). Representative photomicrographs for antibody specificity testing are shown in supplementary Figure S1.

4.5. Statistical Analysis

Results were expressed as mean ± standard deviation (SD) unless stated otherwise. Statistical analyses were performed using GraphPad Prism software (version 7.0, GraphPad Software, San Diego, CA, USA). We checked for outliers by using the PRISM "robust regression and outlier removal" (ROUT) method (Q = 1%, equivalent to a false discovery rate of 1%), as described by Motulsky and Brown [68] and Hughes and Hekimi [69]. Excluded data points ($n = 0$ in rats; $n = 1$ for mouse PCR of *Rarres1*, *CmklR1*, and *IL-11*, respectively) were not included in the calculation of the mean per litter. Subsequently, the means per litter were subjected to further statistical analysis. Before performing groupwise comparisons, outliers were removed [36] and a non-parametric Mann–Whitney U-test was executed. A p value <0.05 was considered statistically significant. Data processing and imaging was performed with Microsoft Office 2016 (Microsoft, Redmond, WA, USA) and Adobe Photoshop CS6 (Adobe Systems, San José, CA, USA).

5. Limitations

In our study, rodent placental tissue was analyzed in toto. Thus, compartment specific changes might have been masked. We did not analyze circulating Rarres2 levels in maternal or fetal serum. Thus, at this point, our conclusions regarding Rarres1/2 are limited to the placental level only. In line with this limitation, no other local sources of Rarres1/2 (e.g., adipose tissue) were evaluated in our study and only certain gestational time-points were examined. Thus, temporal changes in placental expression profiles remain elusive. The choice to analyze mid-/late-gestational placental tissue was based on our previous findings in human third trimester placentas and trophoblasts [1,2]. Consequently, a potential involvement of Rarres1/2 in placentation and early gestation of our animal models remains to be determined. Furthermore, the use of eNOS$^{-/-}$ as a model for IUGR or preeclampsia has been controversially discussed [70,71]. This model is characterized by impaired endothelial function with uterine artery dysfunction and a lack of blood vessel expansion, as well as a placental transport phenotype [26]. Therefore, eNOS$^{-/-}$ might only represent certain early subtypes of human PE and/or IUGR, which on the other hand may not be relevant to rodents themselves.

6. Conclusions

To our knowledge, we were the first to examine Rarres1 localization in the rodent placenta. Also, Rarres1 and 2 expressions have not been studied in the above rodent models.

Rarres1/2 findings in both animal models did not resemble placental alterations of RARRES1/2 observed by us in human PE or PE/IUGR. These results might indicate species-specific differences in placental regulation and compartmentation. The fact that others observed reduced placental Rarres2 expression following more profound maternal food restriction suggests metabolic functions of the peptide beyond its potential tumor-suppressor role that need further investigation. Furthermore, the clarification of a potential feto-maternal crosstalk via adipocytokine Rarres2 and its possible role in the regulation of immunologic and inflammatory processes at the placental interface requires further functional studies. Moreover, the role of IL-11 in the placental pathophysiology of eNOS$^{-/-}$ mice remains to be determined.

Supplementary Materials: The following are available online at http://www.mdpi.com/1422-0067/21/1/242/s1, Figure S1: Specificity testing of the antibody to RARRES1, Figure S2: Specificity testing of the antibody to RARRES2.

Author Contributions: Conceptualization, Validation and Project Administration by F.B.F. and A.H.; Methodology and Visualization by M.S., R.W., H.H., and N.C.; Investigation, Data Acquisition and Analysis, Software and Preparation of Original Draft by A.M.; Reviewing and Editing by C.M.-C.; Supervision and Resources by A.H. Revision by F.B.F., A.H., and A.M. All authors have read and agreed to the published version of the manuscript.

Funding: This research was funded by Deutsche Forschungsgemeinschaft and Friedrich-Alexander-University Erlangen-Nürnberg (FAU) within the funding program Open Access Publishing.

Acknowledgments: Data acquisition was performed by Alexander F. C. Mocker in fulfillment of the requirements for obtaining the degree "med." at the Friedrich-Alexander University of Erlangen-Nürnberg, Department of Pediatrics and Adolescent Medicine, Germany. We thank M. Kupraszewicz-Hutzler for supervising the immunohistochemistry.

Conflicts of Interest: The authors declare no conflict of interest. Funding by DFG had no role in the design of the study; in the collection, analyses, or interpretation of data; in the writing of the manuscript, or in the decision to publish the results.

References

1. Huebner, H.; Hartner, A.; Rascher, W.; Strick, R.R.; Kehl, S.; Heindl, F.; Wachter, D.L.; Beckmann Md, M.W.; Fahlbusch, F.B.; Ruebner, M. Expression and Regulation of Retinoic Acid Receptor Responders in the Human Placenta. *Reprod. Sci.* **2018**, *25*, 1357–1370. [CrossRef] [PubMed]
2. Huebner, H.; Strick, R.; Wachter, D.L.; Kehl, S.; Strissel, P.L.; Schneider-Stock, R.; Hartner, A.; Rascher, W.; Horn, L.C.; Beckmann, M.W.; et al. Hypermethylation and loss of retinoic acid receptor responder 1 expression in human choriocarcinoma. *J. Exp. Clin. Cancer Res.* **2017**, *36*, 165. [CrossRef] [PubMed]

3. Wang, L.; Yang, T.; Ding, Y.; Zhong, Y.; Yu, L.; Peng, M. Chemerin Plays a Protective Role by Regulating Human Umbilical Vein Endothelial Cell-Induced Nitric Oxide Signaling in Preeclampsia. *Endocrine* **2015**, *48*, 299–308. [CrossRef] [PubMed]
4. Nagpal, S.; Patel, S.; Asano, A.T.; Johnson, A.T.; Duvic, M.; Chandraratna, R.A. Tazarotene-Induced Gene 1 (TIG1), a Novel Retinoic Acid Receptor-Responsive Gene in Skin. *J. Investig. Dermatol.* **1996**, *106*, 269–274. [CrossRef] [PubMed]
5. Nagpal, S.; Patel, S.; Jacobe, H.; Disepio, D.; Ghosn, C.; Malhotra, M.; Teng, M.; Duvic, M.; Chandraratna, R.A. Tazarotene-induced gene 2 (TIG2), a novel retinoid-responsive gene in skin. *J. Investig. Dermatol.* **1997**, *109*, 91–95. [CrossRef]
6. Garces, M.; Sánchez, E.; Acosta, B.; Angel, E.; Ruiz, A.; Rubio-Romero, J.; Diéguez, C.; Nogueiras, R.; Caminos, J. Expression and regulation of chemerin during rat pregnancy. *Placenta* **2012**, *33*, 373–378. [CrossRef]
7. Roy, A.; Ramalinga, M.; Kim, O.J.; Chijioke, J.; Lynch, S.; Byers, S.; Kumar, D. Multiple roles of RARRES1 in prostate cancer: Autophagy induction and angiogenesis inhibition. *PLoS ONE* **2017**, *12*, 0180344. [CrossRef]
8. Wang, X.; Saso, H.; Iwamoto, T.; Xia, W.; Gong, Y.; Pusztai, L.; Woodward, W.A.; Reuben, J.M.; Warner, S.L.; Bearss, D.J.; et al. TIG1 Promotes the Development and Progression of Inflammatory Breast Cancer through Activation of Axl Kinase. *Cancer Res.* **2013**, *73*, 6516–6525. [CrossRef]
9. Liu-Chittenden, Y.; Jain, M.; Gaskins, K.; Wang, S.; Merino, M.J.; Kotian, S.; Kumar Gara, S.; Davis, S.; Zhang, L.; Kebebew, E. Rarres2 Functions as a Tumor Suppressor by Promoting Beta-Catenin Phosphorylation/Degradation and Inhibiting P38 Phosphorylation in Adrenocortical Carcinoma. *Oncogene* **2017**, *36*, 3541–3552. [CrossRef]
10. Oldridge, E.E.; Walker, H.F.; Stower, M.J.; Simms, M.S.; Mann, V.M.; Collins, A.T.; Pellacani, D.; Maitland, N.J. Retinoic acid represses invasion and stem cell phenotype by induction of the metastasis suppressors RARRES1 and LXN. *Oncogenesis* **2013**, *2*, e45. [CrossRef]
11. Sahab, Z.J.; Hall, M.D.; Me Sung, Y.; Dakshanamurthy, S.; Ji, Y.; Kumar, D.; Byers, S.W. Tumor Suppressor Rarres1 Interacts with Cytoplasmic Carboxypeptidase Agbl2 to Regulate the Alpha-Tubulin Tyrosination Cycle. *Cancer Res.* **2011**, *71*, 1219–1228. [CrossRef] [PubMed]
12. Meder, W.; Wendland, M.; Busmann, A.; Kutzleb, C.; Spodsberg, N.; John, H.; Richter, R.; Schleuder, D.; Meyer, M.; Forssmann, W. Characterization of human circulating TIG2 as a ligand for the orphan receptor ChemR23. *FEBS Lett.* **2003**, *555*, 495–499. [CrossRef]
13. Zabel, B.A.; Silverio, A.M.; Butcher, E.C. Chemokine-like receptor 1 expression and chemerin-directed chemotaxis distinguish plasmacytoid from myeloid dendritic cells in human blood. *J. Immunol.* **2005**, *174*, 244–251. [CrossRef] [PubMed]
14. Lehrke, M.; Becker, A.; Greif, M.; Stark, R.; Laubender, R.P.; Von Ziegler, F.; Lebherz, C.; Tittus, J.; Reiser, M.; Becker, C.; et al. Chemerin is associated with markers of inflammation and components of the metabolic syndrome but does not predict coronary atherosclerosis. *Eur. J. Endocrinol.* **2009**, *161*, 339–344. [CrossRef]
15. Wittamer, V.; Franssen, J.D.; Vulcano, M.; Mirjolet, J.F.; Le Poul, E.; Migeotte, I.; Brezillon, S.; Tyldesley, R.; Blanpain, C.; Detheux, M.; et al. Specific Recruitment of Antigen-Presenting Cells by Chemerin, a Novel Processed Ligand from Human Inflammatory Fluids. *J. Exp. Med.* **2003**, *198*, 977–985. [CrossRef]
16. Bondue, B.; Wittamer, V.; Parmentier, M. Chemerin and its receptors in leukocyte trafficking, inflammation and metabolism. *Cytokine Growth Factor Rev.* **2011**, *22*, 331–338. [CrossRef]
17. Redman, C.; Sargent, I. Pre-eclampsia, the Placenta and the Maternal Systemic Inflammatory Response—A Review. *Placenta* **2003**, *24* (Suppl. A), S21–S27. [CrossRef]
18. Podjarny, E.; Losonczy, G.; Baylis, C. Animal Models of Preeclampsia. *Semin. Nephrol.* **2004**, *24*, 596–606. [CrossRef]
19. Sladek, S.M.; Magness, R.R.; Conrad, K.P. Nitric Oxide and Pregnancy. *Am. J. Physiol.* **1997**, *272*, R441–R463. [CrossRef]
20. Depoortere, I.; Thijs, T.; Keith, J.; Peeters, T.L. Treatment with interleukin-11 affects plasma leptin levels in inflamed and non-inflamed rabbits. *Regul. Pept.* **2004**, *122*, 149–156. [CrossRef]
21. Makrilakis, K.; Fragiadaki, K.; Smith, J.; Sfikakis, P.P.; Kitas, G.D. Interrelated Reduction of Chemerin and Plasminogen Activator Inhibitor-1 Serum Levels in Rheumatoid Arthritis after Interleukin-6 Receptor Blockade. *Clin. Rheumatol.* **2015**, *34*, 419–427. [CrossRef] [PubMed]

22. Fatima, S.S.; Alam, F.; Chaudhry, B.; Khan, T.A. Elevated Levels of Chemerin, Leptin, and Interleukin-18 in Gestational Diabetes Mellitus. *J. Matern. Fetal Neonatal Med.* **2017**, *30*, 1023–1028. [CrossRef] [PubMed]
23. Kawashima, I.; Ohsumi, J.; Mita-Honjo, K.; Shimoda-Takano, K.; Ishikawa, H.; Sakakibara, S.; Miyadai, K.; Takiguchi, Y. Molecular cloning of cDNA encoding adipogenesis inhibitory factor and identity with interleukin-11. *FEBS Lett.* **1991**, *283*, 199–202. [CrossRef]
24. Winship, A.; Dimitriadis, E. Interleukin 11 is upregulated in preeclampsia and leads to inflammation and preeclampsia features in mice. *J. Reprod. Immunol.* **2018**, *125*, 32–38. [CrossRef]
25. Winship, A.L.; Koga, K.; Menkhorst, E.; Van Sinderen, M.; Rainczuk, K.; Nagai, M.; Cuman, C.; Yap, J.; Zhang, J.-G.; Simmons, D.; et al. Interleukin-11 alters placentation and causes preeclampsia features in mice. *Proc. Natl. Acad. Sci.USA* **2015**, *112*, 15928–15933. [CrossRef]
26. Kusinski, L.C.; Stanley, J.L.; Dilworth, M.R.; Hirt, C.J.; Andersson, I.J.; Renshall, L.J.; Baker, B.C.; Baker, P.N.; Sibley, C.P.; Wareing, M.; et al. eNOS knockout mouse as a model of fetal growth restriction with an impaired uterine artery function and placental transport phenotype. *Am. J. Physiol. Integr. Comp. Physiol.* **2012**, *303*, R86–R93. [CrossRef]
27. Anumba, D.O.C.; Robson, S.C.; Boys, R.J.; Ford, G.A. Nitric oxide activity in the peripheral vasculature during normotensive and preeclamptic pregnancy. *Am. J. Physiol. Content* **1999**, *277*, H848–H854. [CrossRef]
28. Hefler, L.A.; Reyes, C.A.; O'Brien, W.E.; Gregg, A.R. Perinatal development of endothelial nitric oxide synthase-deficient mice. *Boil. Reprod.* **2001**, *64*, 666–673. [CrossRef]
29. Hefler, L.A.; Tempfer, C.B.; Moreno, R.M.; O'Brien, W.E.; Gregg, A.R. Endothelial-derived nitric oxide and angiotensinogen: Blood pressure and metabolism during mouse pregnancy. *Am. J. Physiol. Integr. Comp. Physiol.* **2001**, *280*, R174–R182. [CrossRef]
30. Veerareddy, S.; Cooke, C.-L.M.; Baker, P.N.; Davidge, S.T. Vascular adaptations to pregnancy in mice: Effects on myogenic tone. *Am. J. Physiol. Circ. Physiol.* **2002**, *283*, H2226–H2233. [CrossRef]
31. Flaherty, M.P.; Brown, M.; Grupp, I.L.; El Schultz, J.; Murphree, S.S.; Jones, W.K. eNOS Deficient Mice Develop Progressive Cardiac Hypertrophy with Altered Cytokine and Calcium Handling Protein Expression. *Cardiovasc. Toxicol.* **2007**, *7*, 165–177. [CrossRef] [PubMed]
32. Bucci, M.; Gratton, J.-P.; Rudic, R.D.; Acevedo, L.; Roviezzo, F.; Cirino, G.; Sessa, W.C. In vivo delivery of the caveolin-1 scaffolding domain inhibits nitric oxide synthesis and reduces inflammation. *Nat. Med.* **2000**, *6*, 1362–1367. [CrossRef] [PubMed]
33. Bucci, M.; Roviezzo, F.; Posadas, I.; Yu, J.; Parente, L.; Sessa, W.C.; Ignarro, L.J.; Cirino, G. Endothelial nitric oxide synthase activation is critical for vascular leakage during acute inflammation in vivo. *Proc. Natl. Acad. Sci. USA* **2005**, *102*, 904–908. [CrossRef] [PubMed]
34. Han, L.; Zhang, M.; Liang, X.; Jia, X.; Jia, J.; Zhao, M.; Fan, Y. Interleukin-33 Promotes Inflammation-Induced Lymphangiogenesis via St2/Traf6-Mediated Akt/Enos/No Signalling Pathway. *Sci. Rep.* **2017**, *7*, 10602. [CrossRef]
35. Beinder, L.; Faehrmann, N.; Wachtveitl, R.; Winterfeld, I.; Hartner, A.; Menendez-Castro, C.; Rauh, M.; Ruebner, M.; Huebner, H.; Noegel, S.C.; et al. Detection of Expressional Changes Induced by Intrauterine Growth Restriction in the Developing Rat Mammary Gland via Exploratory Pathways Analysis. *PLoS ONE* **2014**, *9*, e100504. [CrossRef]
36. Schmidt, M.; Rauh, M.; Schmid, M.C.; Huebner, H.; Ruebner, M.; Wachtveitl, R.; Cordasic, N.; Rascher, W.; Menendez-Castro, C.; Hartner, A.; et al. Influence of Low Protein Diet-Induced Fetal Growth Restriction on the Neuroplacental Corticosterone Axis in the Rat. *Front. Endocrinol.* **2019**, *10*, 124. [CrossRef]
37. Watts, S.W.; Darios, E.S.; Mullick, A.E.; Garver, H.; Saunders, T.L.; Hughes, E.D.; Filipiak, W.E.; Zeidler, M.G.; McMullen, N.; Sinal, C.J.; et al. The Chemerin Knockout Rat Reveals Chemerin Dependence in Female, but Not Male, Experimental Hypertension. *FASEB J.* **2018**, fj201800479. [CrossRef]
38. Langbein, M.; Strick, R.; Strissel, P.L.; Vogt, N.; Parsch, H.; Beckmann, M.W.; Schild, R.L. Impaired Cytotrophoblast Cell-Cell Fusion Is Associated with Reduced Syncytin and Increased Apoptosis in Patients with Placental Dysfunction. *Mol. Reprod. Dev.* **2008**, *75*, 175–183. [CrossRef]
39. Burton, G.J.; Jones, C.J. Syncytial Knots, Sprouts, Apoptosis, and Trophoblast Deportation from the Human Placenta. *Taiwan. J. Obstet. Gynecol.* **2009**, *48*, 28–37. [CrossRef]
40. Dilworth, M.; Sibley, C. Review: Transport across the placenta of mice and women. *Placenta* **2013**, *34*, S34–S39. [CrossRef]

41. Silva, J.F.; Serakides, R. Intrauterine trophoblast migration: A comparative view of humans and rodents. *Cell Adhes. Migr.* **2016**, *10*, 88–110. [CrossRef] [PubMed]
42. Hemberger, M.; Cross, J.C. Genes governing placental development. *Trends Endocrinol. Metab.* **2001**, *12*, 162–168. [CrossRef]
43. Cross, J.; Baczyk, D.; Dobric, N.; Hemberger, M.; Hughes, M.; Simmons, D.; Yamamoto, H.; Kingdom, J. Genes, Development and Evolution of the Placenta. *Placenta* **2003**, *24*, 123–130. [CrossRef] [PubMed]
44. Georgiades, P.; Ferguson-Smith, A.; Burton, G. Comparative Developmental Anatomy of the Murine and Human Definitive Placentae. *Placenta* **2002**, *23*, 3–19. [CrossRef] [PubMed]
45. Simmons, D.G.; Cross, J.C. Determinants of trophoblast lineage and cell subtype specification in the mouse placenta. *Dev. Boil.* **2005**, *284*, 12–24. [CrossRef]
46. Woods, L.; Perez-Garcia, V.; Hemberger, M. Regulation of Placental Development and Its Impact on Fetal Growth—New Insights from Mouse Models. *Front. Endocrinol.* **2018**, *9*, 570. [CrossRef]
47. Abreu, R.D.S.; Penalva, L.O.; Marcotte, E.M.; Vogel, C. Global signatures of protein and mRNA expression levels. *Mol. BioSyst.* **2009**, *5*, 1512–1526.
48. Ruebner, M.; Strissel, P.L.; Langbein, M.; Fahlbusch, F.; Wachter, D.L.; Faschingbauer, F.; Beckmann, M.W.; Strick, R. Impaired cell fusion and differentiation in placentae from patients with intrauterine growth restriction correlate with reduced levels of HERV envelope genes. *J. Mol. Med.* **2010**, *88*, 1143–1156. [CrossRef]
49. Ruebner, M.; Strissel, P.L.; Ekici, A.B.; Stiegler, E.; Dammer, U.; Goecke, T.W.; Faschingbauer, F.; Fahlbusch, F.B.; Beckmann, M.W.; Strick, R. Reduced Syncytin-1 Expression Levels in Placental Syndromes Correlates with Epigenetic Hypermethylation of the ERVW-1 Promoter Region. *PLoS ONE* **2013**, *8*, 56145. [CrossRef]
50. Garces, M.F.; Sanchez, E.; Ruíz-Parra, A.I.; Rubio-Romero, J.A.; Angel-Müller, E.; Suarez, M.A.; Bohórquez, L.F.; Bravo, S.B.; Nogueiras, R.; Diéguez, C.; et al. Serum chemerin levels during normal human pregnancy. *Peptides* **2013**, *42*, 138–143. [CrossRef]
51. Snoeck, A.; Hoet, J.J.; Remacle, C.; Reusens, B. Effect of a Low Protein Diet during Pregnancy on the Fetal Rat Endocrine Pancreas. *Biol. Neonate* **1990**, *57*, 107–118. [CrossRef] [PubMed]
52. Blondeau, B.; Lesage, J.; Czernichow, P.; Dupouy, J.P.; Bréant, B. Glucocorticoids impair fetal beta-cell development in rats. *Am. J. Physiol. Metab.* **2001**, *281*, 592–599.
53. Mühlhäusler, B.S. Programming of the Appetite-Regulating Neural Network: A Link Between Maternal Overnutrition and the Programming of Obesity? *J. Neuroendocr.* **2007**, *19*, 67–72. [CrossRef] [PubMed]
54. Valsamakis, G.; Kumar, S.; Creatsas, G.; Mastorakos, G. The effects of adipose tissue and adipocytokines in human pregnancy. *Ann. N. Y. Acad. Sci.* **2010**, *1205*, 76–81. [CrossRef] [PubMed]
55. Ritterath, C.; Rad, N.T.; Siegmund, T.; Heinze, T.; Siebert, G.; Buhling, K.J. Adiponectin During Pregnancy: Correlation with Fat Metabolism, but Not with Carbohydrate Metabolism. *Arch. Gynecol. Obstet.* **2010**, *281*, 91–96. [CrossRef]
56. Briana, D.D.; Malamitsi-Puchner, A. The role of adipocytokines in fetal growth. *Ann. N. Y. Acad. Sci.* **2010**, *1205*, 82–87. [CrossRef]
57. Barker, G.; Lim, R.; Rice, G.E.; Lappas, M. Increased chemerin concentrations in fetuses of obese mothers and correlation with maternal insulin sensitivity. *J. Matern. Neonatal Med.* **2012**, *25*, 2274–2280. [CrossRef]
58. Sanchez-Rebordelo, E.; Cunarro, J.; Perez-Sieira, S.; Seoane, L.M.; Diéguez, C.; Nogueiras, R.; Tovar, S. Regulation of Chemerin and CMKLR1 Expression by Nutritional Status, Postnatal Development, and Gender. *Int. J. Mol. Sci.* **2018**, *19*, 2905. [CrossRef]
59. Kennedy, A.J.; Yang, P.; Read, C.; Kuc, R.E.; Yang, L.; Taylor, E.J.; Taylor, C.W.; Maguire, J.J.; Davenport, A.P. Chemerin Elicits Potent Constrictor Actions Via Chemokine-Like Receptor 1 (Cmklr1), Not G-Protein-Coupled Receptor 1 (Gpr1), in Human and Rat Vasculature. *J. Am. Heart Assoc.* **2016**, *5*. [CrossRef]
60. Kulandavelu, S.; Whiteley, K.J.; Qu, D.; Mu, J.; Bainbridge, S.A.; Adamson, S.L. Endothelial Nitric Oxide Synthase Deficiency Reduces Uterine Blood Flow, Spiral Artery Elongation, and Placental Oxygenation in Pregnant Mice. *Hypertension* **2012**, *60*, 231–238. [CrossRef]
61. Yang, X.; Yao, J.; Wei, Q.; Ye, J.; Yin, X.; Quan, X.; Lan, Y.; Xing, H. Role of chemerin/CMKLR1 in the maintenance of early pregnancy. *Front. Med.* **2018**, *12*, 525–532. [CrossRef] [PubMed]
62. Menendez-Castro, C.; Fahlbusch, F.; Cordasic, N.; Amann, K.; Münzel, K.; Plank, C.; Wachtveitl, R.; Rascher, W.; Hilgers, K.F.; Hartner, A. Early and Late Postnatal Myocardial and Vascular Changes in a Protein Restriction Rat Model of Intrauterine Growth Restriction. *PLoS ONE* **2011**, *6*, e20369. [CrossRef] [PubMed]

63. Hayward, C.E.; Lean, S.; Sibley, C.P.; Jones, R.L.; Wareing, M.; Greenwood, S.L.; Dilworth, M.R. Placental Adaptation: What Can We Learn from Birthweight: Placental Weight Ratio? *Front. Physiol.* **2016**, *7*, 405. [CrossRef] [PubMed]
64. Van Der Heijden, O.W.; Essers, Y.P.; Fazzi, G.; Peeters, L.L.; De Mey, J.G.R.; Van Eys, G.J. Uterine Artery Remodeling and Reproductive Performance Are Impaired in Endothelial Nitric Oxide Synthase-Deficient Mice1. *Boil. Reprod.* **2005**, *72*, 1161–1168. [CrossRef] [PubMed]
65. Pallares, P.; Gonzalez-Bulnes, A. The effect of embryo and maternal genotypes on prolificacy, intrauterine growth retardation and postnatal development of Nos3-knockout mice. *Reprod. Boil.* **2010**, *10*, 241–248. [CrossRef]
66. Herdl, S.; Huebner, H.; Volkert, G.; Marek, I.; Menendez-Castro, C.; Noegel, S.C.; Ruebner, M.; Rascher, W.; Hartner, A.; Fahlbusch, F.B. Integrin Alpha8 Is Abundant in Human, Rat, and Mouse Trophoblasts. *Reprod. Sci.* **2017**, *24*, 1426–1437. [CrossRef] [PubMed]
67. Menendez-Castro, C.; Nitz, D.; Cordasic, N.; Jordan, J.; Bäuerle, T.; Fahlbusch, F.B.; Rascher, W.; Hilgers, K.F.; Hartner, A. Neonatal nephron loss during active nephrogenesis—Detrimental impact with long-term renal consequences. *Sci. Rep.* **2018**, *8*, 4542. [CrossRef]
68. Motulsky, H.J.; E Brown, R. Detecting outliers when fitting data with nonlinear regression—A new method based on robust nonlinear regression and the false discovery rate. *BMC Bioinform.* **2006**, *7*, 123. [CrossRef]
69. Hughes, B.G.; Hekimi, S. Different Mechanisms of Longevity in Long-Lived Mouse andCaenorhabditis elegansMutants Revealed by Statistical Analysis of Mortality Rates. *Genetics* **2016**, *204*, 905–920. [CrossRef]
70. Pallares, P.; Gonzalez-Bulnes, A. Intrauterine Growth Retardation in Endothelial Nitric Oxide Synthase-Deficient Mice Is Established from Early Stages of Pregnancy. *Boil. Reprod.* **2008**, *78*, 1002–1006. [CrossRef]
71. Shesely, E.G.; Gilbert, C.; Granderson, G.; Carretero, C.; Carretero, O.A.; Beierwaltes, W.H. Nitric oxide synthase gene knockout mice do not become hypertensive during pregnancy. *Am. J. Obstet. Gynecol.* **2001**, *185*, 1198–1203. [CrossRef] [PubMed]

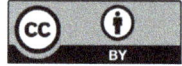

© 2019 by the authors. Licensee MDPI, Basel, Switzerland. This article is an open access article distributed under the terms and conditions of the Creative Commons Attribution (CC BY) license (http://creativecommons.org/licenses/by/4.0/).

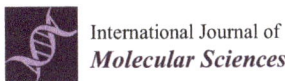

Article

Involvement of Receptor for Advanced Glycation Endproducts in Hypertensive Disorders of Pregnancy

Juria Akasaka [1], Katsuhiko Naruse [1], Toshiyuki Sado [1], Tomoko Uchiyama [2], Mai Makino [2], Akiyo Yamauchi [2], Hiroyo Ota [2], Sumiyo Sakuramoto-Tsuchida [2], Asako Itaya-Hironaka [2], Shin Takasawa [2,*] and Hiroshi Kobayashi [1]

[1] Department of Obstetrics and Gynecology, Nara Medical University, 840 Shijo-cho, Kashihara, Nara 634-8522, Japan; juria@naramed-u.ac.jp (J.A.); naruse@naramed-u.ac.jp (K.N.); tsado@naramed-u.ac.jp (T.S.); hirokoba@nmu-gw.naramed-u.ac.jp (H.K.)
[2] Department of Biochemistry, Nara Medical University, 840 Shijo-cho, Kashihara, Nara 634-8521, Japan; uchiyama0403@naramed-u.ac.jp (T.U.); m.makino@naramed-u.ac.jp (M.M.); yamauchi@naramed-u.ac.jp (A.Y.); hiroyon@naramed-u.ac.jp (H.O.); ssumiyo@naramed-u.ac.jp (S.S.-T.); iasako@naramed-u.ac.jp (A.I.-H.)
* Correspondence: shintksw@naramed-u.ac.jp; Tel.: +81-744-22-3051 (ext. 2227); Fax: +81-744-24-9525

Received: 29 August 2019; Accepted: 28 October 2019; Published: 1 November 2019

Abstract: Preeclampsia/hypertensive disorders of pregnancy (PE/HDP) is a serious and potentially life-threatening disease. Recently, PE/HDP has been considered to cause adipose tissue inflammation, but the detailed mechanism remains unknown. We exposed human primary cultured adipocytes with serum from PE/HDP and healthy controls for 24 h, and analyzed mRNA expression of several adipokines, cytokines, and ligands of the receptor for advanced glycation endproducts (RAGE). We found that the mRNA levels of interleukin-6 (*IL-6*), C-C motif chemokine ligand 2 (*CCL2*), high mobility group box 1 (*HMGB1*), and *RAGE* were significantly increased by the addition of PE/HDP serum. Among RAGE ligands, advanced glycation endproducts (AGE) and HMGB1 increased mRNA levels of *IL-6* and *CCL2* in SW872 human adipocytes and mouse 3T3-L1 cells. The introduction of small interfering RNA for *RAGE* (siRAGE) into SW872 cells abolished the AGE- and HMGB1-induced up-regulation of IL-6 and CCL2. In addition, lipopolysaccharide (LPS), a ligand of RAGE, increased the expression of IL-6 and CCL2 and siRAGE attenuated the LPS-induced expression of IL-6 and CCL2. These results strongly suggest that the elevated AGE, HMGB1, and LPS in pregnant women up-regulate the expression of IL-6 and CCL2 via the RAGE system, leading to systemic inflammation such as PE/HDP.

Keywords: hypertensive disorders of pregnancy; RAGE; AGE; adipocyte; IL-6; CCL2; LPS

1. Introduction

Preeclampsia/hypertensive disorders of pregnancy (PE/HDP) is a serious and potentially life-threatening disease appearing as a complication in about 2–12% of all pregnancies and associated with significant perinatal and maternal mortality [1,2]. It is estimated that more than 60,000 women worldwide die of the disease each year; it is one of the main causes of maternal mortality [3]. There is considerable evidence that maternal obesity, increased insulin resistance, inflammation, and aberrant fatty acid metabolism are involved in the pathogenesis of PE/HDP [4,5]. Inflammatory reactions have recently been attracting attention as the pathophysiological characteristics of PE/HDP, including vascular endothelial dysfunction and placental abnormalities [6–14]. Shallow trophoblast invasion and inadequate artery remodeling in pregnancy may cause placental hypoperfusion, hypoxia, or ischemia, which play an important role in the pathogenesis of PE/HDP [15]. The link between adiposity, inflammation, and insulin resistance has been increasingly acknowledged since Spiegelman and his colleagues demonstrated the relationship [16]. White adipose tissue secretes pro-inflammatory cytokines which contribute significantly to the chronic inflammatory state and metabolic complications of obesity [17]. It is plausible that similar disturbances in adipocyte function might contribute to the development of the clinical syndrome of PE/HDP, a state of inflammation and insulin resistance.

Adipose tissue, complex tissue composed of preadipocytes, adipocytes, and stromal vascular cells, is one of the representative organs to contribute to worsening insulin resistance through inflammation and subsequent dysfunction. Visceral adiposity correlates with metabolic risk factor [18] and adverse metabolic outcomes in pregnancy including gestational diabetes mellitus and PE/HDP [19–21]. Adipokines are cytokines expressed in and secreted from adipocytes in response to the systemic nutritional status, and some of them induce macrophage infiltration and inflammatory cytokine secretion [22,23]. In the present study, we analyzed expression of adipokines including inflammatory cytokines in adipocytes and found the involvement of receptor for advanced glycation endproducts (RAGE) in expression of interleukin-6 (IL-6) and C-C motif chemokine ligand 2 (CCL2) in adipocytes.

2. Results

2.1. PE/HDP Patient Sera Up-Regulated Gene Expression of IL-6, CCL2, High Mobility Group Box (HMGB)1, S100 Ca^{2+}-Binding Protein B (S100B), and Receptor for Advanced Glycation Endproducts (RAGE) in Primary Cultured Human Adipocytes

Obesity increases PE/HDP risk. Maternal obesity, increased insulin resistance, and inflammation are involved in the pathogenesis of PE/HDP [24,25]. Furthermore, PE/HDP risk has been reported to increase 2–4-fold among women with diabetes [26]. We therefore hypothesized that the PE/HDP patient sera contain some of these factors that induce insulin resistance and/or inflammation. We incubated primary cultured human adipocytes with sera from disease-free pregnant women (control) or those from PE/HDP (patients) for 24 h, and the gene expression of *IL-6*, *CCL2*, *tumor necrosis factor α (TNFα)*, *leptin (LEP)*, *adiponectin (ADIP)*, *resistin (RETN)*, *HMGB1*, *S100B*, and *RAGE* in the adipocytes was measured via real-time reverse transcriptase-polymerase chain reaction (RT-PCR). As shown in Figure 1, mRNA levels of *IL-6*, *CCL2*, *HMGB1*, *S100B*, and *RAGE*, but not *TNFα*, *LEP*, *ADIP*, and *RETN* ($P = 0.4496$, $P = 0.1157$, $P = 0.0875$, and $P = 0.2912$, respectively) were significantly increased by the addition of PE/HDP patient sera compared to those cells incubated with control sera.

2.2. Up-Regulation of IL-6 and CCL2 by HMGB1 and Advanced Glycation Endproducts (AGE) in Adipocytes

It is well-known that HMGB1 and S100B are typical ligands for RAGE. RAGE expression was reported in adipocytes and SW872 cells [27,28], and furthermore immunofluorescent staining of RAGE in 3T3-L1 adipocytes was shown [27]. RAGE expression was up-regulated by ligands for RAGE [29], we tested whether ligands for RAGE up-regulate gene expression of inflammatory mediators, such as *IL-6* and *CCL2*, in human SW872 adipocytes. We added HMGB1, AGE, and S100B in SW872 culture medium, incubated for 24 h, and the expression of *IL-6* and *CCL2* was analyzed via real-time RT-PCR. As shown in Figure 2, mRNAs of *IL-6* and *CCL2* were significantly up-regulated by the addition of HMGB1 and AGE. In contrast, S100B, another noted ligand for RAGE, failed to up-regulate mRNA for IL-6 or CCL2.

In order to see whether the up-regulation of mRNAs for *IL-6* and *Ccl2* occurred only in SW872 or other adipocytes, we cultured mouse 3T3-L1 preadipocytes, differentiated them into differentiated adipocytes, and tested whether ligands for RAGE up-regulate gene expression of *IL-6* and *Ccl2* in mouse 3T3-L1 undifferentiated preadipocytes and differentiated adipocytes. As shown in Figure 3, the mRNA levels of *IL-6* were significantly up-regulated by AGE and HMGB1 but not by S100B ($P = 0.6414$) in differentiated 3T3-L1 adipocytes, but unchanged by any of the RAGE ligands (AGE, HMGB1, or S100B) in undifferentiated preadipocytes ($P = 0.8037$ [No addition vs. AGE], $P = 0.4793$ [No addition vs. HMGB1], and $P = 0.3138$ [No addition vs. S100B]). In contrast, the mRNA levels of *Ccl2* remained unchanged in response to AGE, HMGB1, or S100B in 3T3-L1 differentiated adipocytes

(P = 0.1892 [No addition vs. AGE], P = 0.2885 [No addition vs. HMGB1], and P = 0.4024 [No addition vs. S100B]), but significantly up-regulated in the undifferentiated preadipocytes by the addition of AGE but not by HMGB1 and S100B (P = 0.1241 [No addition vs. HMGB1] and P = 0.4305 [No addition vs. S100B]) (Figure 3). Previous studies reported that S100B up-regulated TNFα in adipocytes [30,31]. In contrast, S100B induced neither *IL-6* nor *CCL2* in adipocytes in this study, suggesting that SW872 and 3T3-L1 cells may insensitive to S100B.

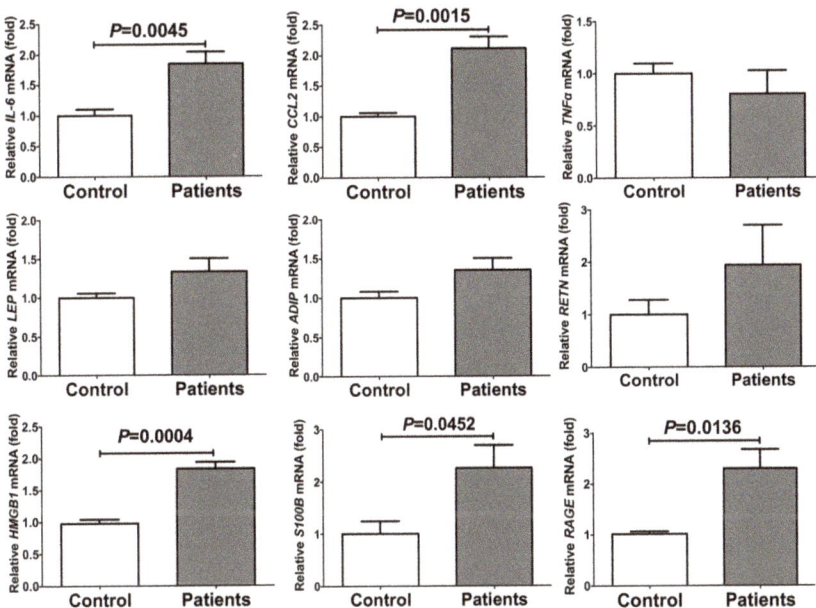

Figure 1. The mRNA levels of *IL-6*, *CCL2*, *TNFα*, *LEP*, *ADIP*, *RETN*, *HMGB1*, *S100B*, and *RAGE* in primary cultured human adipocytes treated with sera from disease-free control (Control) or preeclampsia/hypertensive disorders of pregnancy (PE/HDP) patients (Patients) for 24 h. The levels of the mRNAs were measured via real-time reverse transcriptase-polymerase chain reaction (RT-PCR) using *β-actin* as an endogenous control. Data are expressed as mean ± SE for each group (n = 4). The statistical analyses were performed using Student's *t*-test.

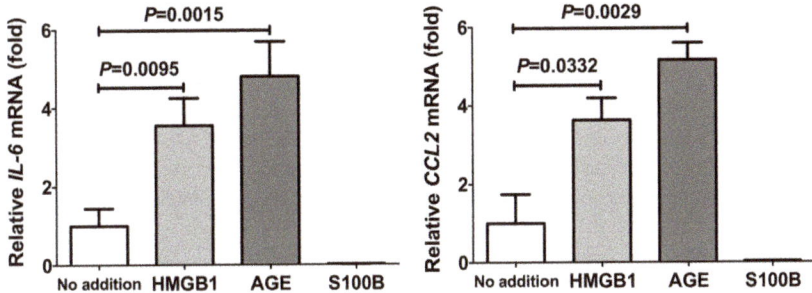

Figure 2. The mRNA levels of *IL-6* and *CCL2* in SW872 human adipocytes treated with 1 μg/mL HMGB1, 150 μg/mL advanced glycation endproducts (AGE), or 100 ng/mL S100B for 24 h. The levels of the mRNAs were measured via real-time RT-PCR using *β-actin* as an endogenous control. Data are expressed as mean ± SE for each group (n = 4). The statistical analyses were performed using Student's *t*-test vs. No addition.

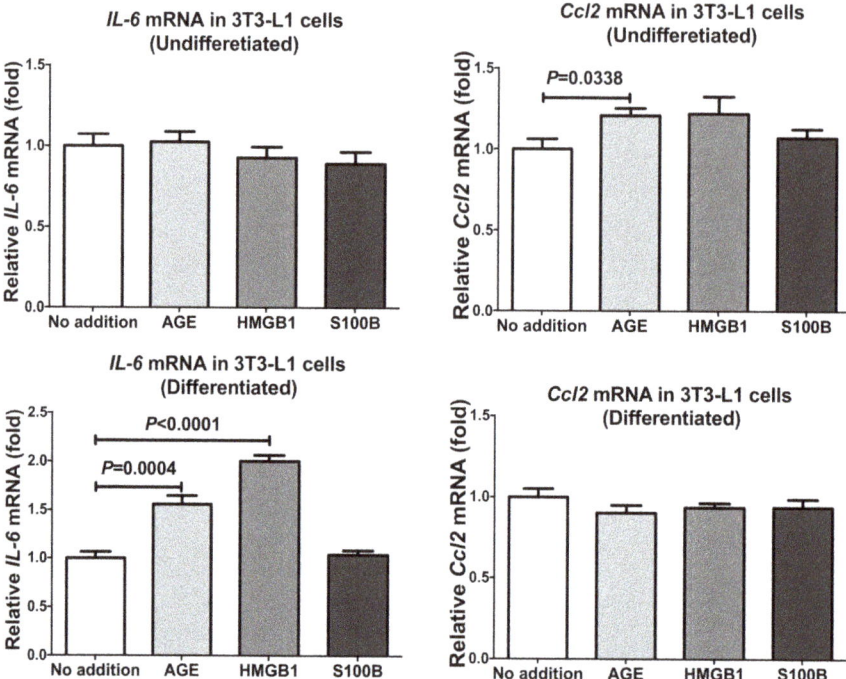

Figure 3. The mRNA levels of *IL-6* and *Ccl2* in 3T3-L1 mouse cells (undifferentiated preadipocytes and differentiated adipocytes) treated with 300 μg/mL AGE, 1 μg/mL HMGB1, or 100 ng/mL S100B for 24 h. The levels of the mRNAs were measured via real-time RT-PCR using *rat insulinoma gene (Rig)/ribosomal protein S15 (RpS15)* as an endogenous control. Data are expressed as mean ± SE for each group ($n = 4$). The statistical analyses were performed using Student's *t*-test vs. No addition.

2.3. Down-Regulation of RAGE Attenuated the Increases of IL-6 and CCL2 in Adipocytes Treated with Small Interfering RNA (siRNA) for RAGE

In order to see the mechanism of HMGB1- and AGE-induced gene expression of *IL-6* and *CCL2*, *RAGE* gene was knocked down by RNA interference. The expression of *IL-6* and *CCL2* was significantly increased by the addition of HMGB1 and AGE even in the presence of scrambled RNA. In contrast, introduction of small interfering RNA (siRNA) for RAGE (*siRAGE*) clearly inhibited the HMGB1- and AGE-induced increases of mRNAs for *IL-6* and *CCL2* in SW872 human adipocytes (Figure 4; $P = 0.2638$ [No addition vs. HMGB1 in *IL-6*], $P = 0.0744$ [No addition vs. AGE in *IL-6*], $P = 0.2559$ [No addition vs. HMGB1 in *CCL2*], and $P = 0.5541$ [No addition vs. AGE in *CCL2*]).

We also measured the concentrations of IL-6 and CCL2 in the RAGE-knocked-down SW872 cell culture medium via enzyme-linked immunosorbent assay (ELISA). The concentrations of IL-6 and CCL2 were significantly increased in response to HMGB1 and AGE in scrambled RNA-introduced cell culture medium. In contrast, the introduction of siRAGE significantly attenuated the HMGB1- and AGE-induced increases of IL-6 and CCL2 in the medium (Figure 5).

2.4. Up-Regulation of IL-6 and CCL2 by Lipopolysaccharide (LPS) in Adipocytes

Recent reports indicated that PE/HDP is also induced by lipopolysaccharide (LPS) [32] and that RAGE mediates LPS signaling and acts as an LPS receptor [33–38]. Thus, we tested whether LPS up-regulate gene expression of *IL-6* and *CCL2* in human SW872 adipocytes. We added 10 ng/mL LPS in SW872 culture medium, incubated for 24 h, and the expression of *IL-6* and *CCL2* was analyzed via real-time RT-PCR. As shown in Figure 6, mRNAs of *IL-6* and *CCL2* were significantly up-regulated by the addition of LPS.

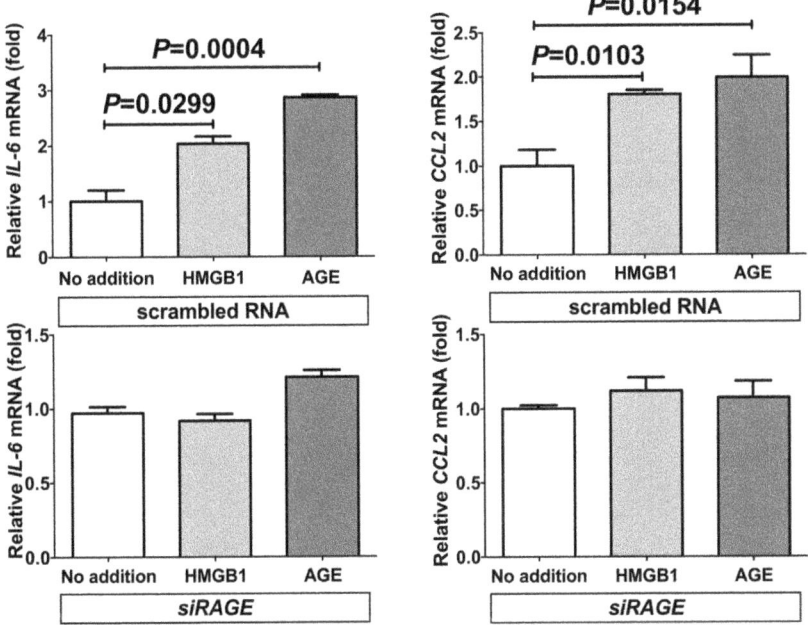

Figure 4. Effects of siRNA against *RAGE* on HMGB1- and AGE-induced gene expression of *IL-6* and *CCL2*. SiRNA for *RAGE* was transfected into SW872 cells and the cells were incubated with HMGB1 or AGE for 24 h. The levels of *IL-6* and *CCL2* mRNA were measured via real-time RT-PCR using β-*actin* as an endogenous control. Data are expressed as mean ± SE for each group (n = 4). The statistical analyses were performed using Student's *t*-test vs. No addition.

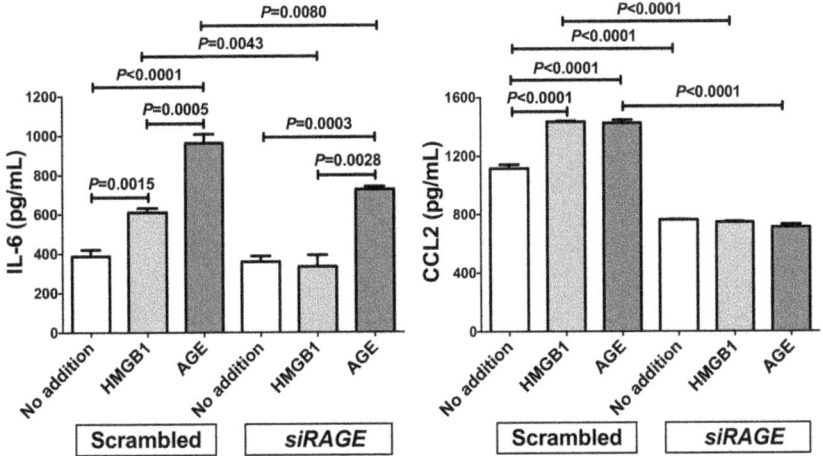

Figure 5. Effect of siRNA against RAGE on the HMGB1- and AGE-induced expression of IL-6 and CCL2. SiRNA for RAGE was transfected into SW872 cells and the cells were incubated with HMGB1 or AGE for 24 h. The levels of IL-6 and CCL2 in the cell culture medium were measured via ELISA. Data are expressed as mean ± SE for each group (n = 4). The statistical analyses were performed using Student's *t*-test vs. No addition.

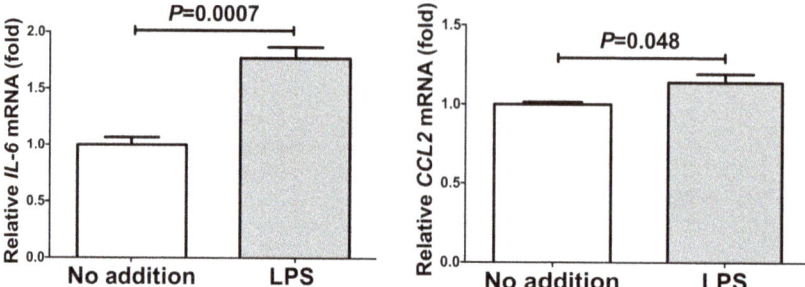

Figure 6. The mRNA levels of IL-6 and CCL2 in SW872 human adipocytes treated with 10 ng/mL lipopolysaccharide (LPS) for 24 h. The levels of the mRNAs were measured via real-time RT-PCR using β-actin as an endogenous control. Data are expressed as mean ± SE for each group ($n = 4$). The statistical analyses were performed using Student's t-test.

We next measured IL-6 and CCL2 in the LPS-stimulated SW872 cell culture medium and found that the levels of IL-6 and CCL2 in the LPS-stimulated SW872 culture medium were also elevated significantly (Figure 7).

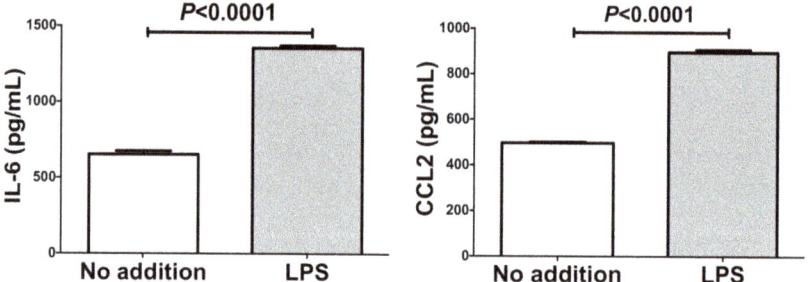

Figure 7. The levels of IL-6 and CCL2 in culture medium of SW872 human adipocytes treated with 10 ng/mL LPS for 24 h. The levels of IL-6 and CCL2 in the cell culture medium were measured via ELISA. Data are expressed as mean ± SE for each group (n = 4). The statistical analyses were performed using Student's t-test.

2.5. Down-Regulation of RAGE Attenuated the LPS-Induced IL-6 and CCL2 Increases in Adipocytes

In order to confirm whether the mechanism of LPS-induced *IL-6* and *CCL2* up-regulation is also mediated by RAGE, *RAGE* gene was knocked down by RNA interference. The expression of *IL-6* and *CCL2* was significantly increased by the addition of LPS even in the presence of scrambled RNA. In contrast, introduction of *siRAGE* clearly inhibited the LPS-induced increases of mRNAs for *IL-6* and *CCL2* in SW872 human adipocytes (Figure 8).

We also measured the concentrations of IL-6 and CCL2 in the RAGE-knocked-down SW872 cell culture medium via ELISA. The concentrations of IL-6 and CCL2 were significantly increased in response to the addition of LPS in scrambled RNA-introduced cell culture medium. In contrast, the introduction of siRAGE significantly attenuated the LPS-induced increases of IL-6 and CCL2 in the medium (Figure 9).

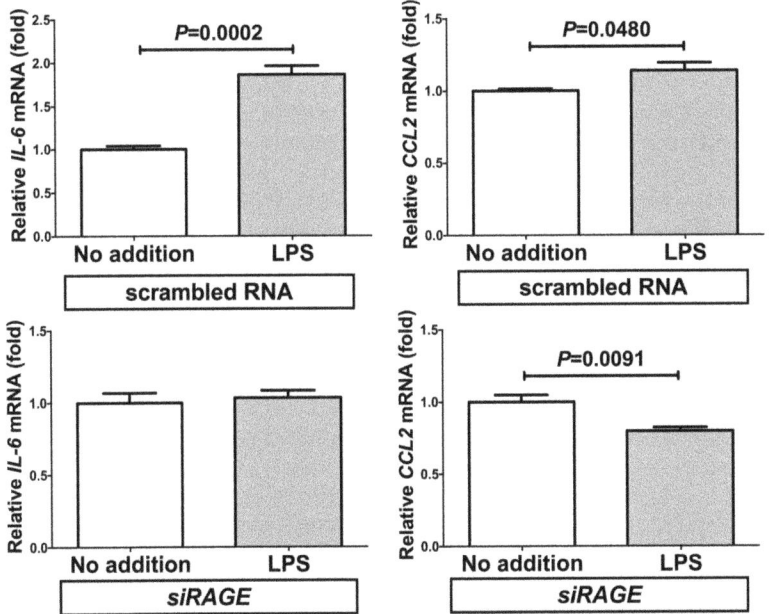

Figure 8. Effects of siRNA against *RAGE* on the LPS-induced gene expression of *IL-6* and *CCL2*. SiRNA for *RAGE* was transfected into SW872 cells and the cells were incubated with 10 ng/mL LPS for 24 h. The levels of *IL-6* and *CCL2* mRNA were measured via real-time RT-PCR using *β-actin* as an endogenous control. Data are expressed as mean ± SE for each group (*n* = 4). The statistical analyses were performed using Student's *t*-test.

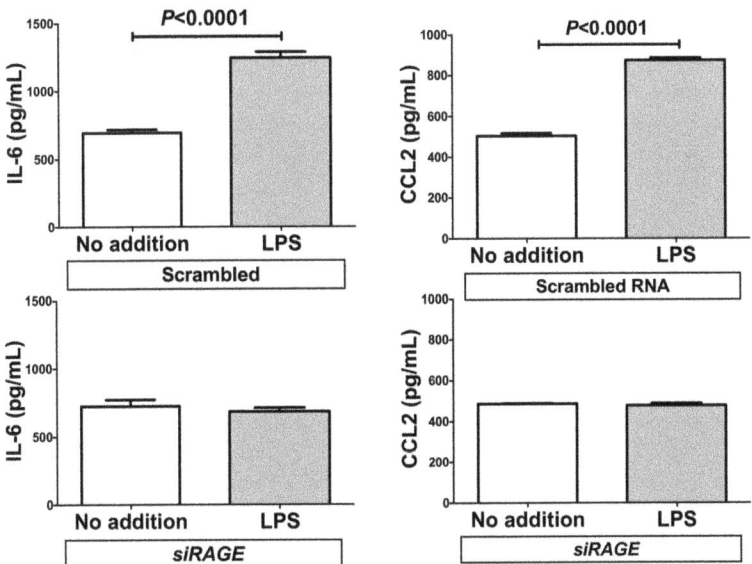

Figure 9. Effect of siRNA against RAGE on the LPS-induced expression of IL-6 and CCL2. SiRNA for RAGE was transfected into SW872 cells and the cells were incubated with LPS for 24 h. The levels of IL-6 and CCL2 in the cell culture medium were measured via ELISA. Data are expressed as mean ± SE for each group (*n* = 4). The statistical analyses were performed using Student's *t*-test.

3. Discussion

Previous studies indicated that body mass index (BMI), anemia, lower education, maternal age, primiparity, multiple pregnancy, PE/HDP in previous pregnancy, gestational diabetes mellitus, preexisting hypertension, preexisting type 2 diabetes mellitus, preexisting urinary tract infection, and a family history of hypertension, type 2 diabetes mellitus, or PE/HDP are potential risk factors for PE/HDP [39,40]. Of the risk factors, obesity is a major risk factor and is associated with an increased risk for obstetrical complications such as gestational diabetes mellitus, PE/HDP, pre-term delivery, and Cesarean section [41–45], and increased neonatal morbidity and mortality [42,46,47]. Maternal obesity has been associated with low-grade metabolic inflammation due to increased release of adipokines, which are believed to contribute to maternal glucose intolerance and insulin resistance and cardiovascular and neuroendocrine modulation associated with increased maternal BMI [48]. Increased cytokine and decreased adiponectin release from adipose tissue have been linked to the meta-inflammatory state of obesity [49,50].

In this study, we measured the mRNA levels for adipokines (*LEP*, *ADIP*, and *RETN*) in human primary adipocytes and found that they were not up-regulated in response to the addition of sera from PE/HDP patients. We also measured mRNA levels of *TNFα*, *IL-6*, and *CCL2*, which have been reported to play important roles in pathogenesis or development of PE/HDP, and found that the expression of *IL-6* and *CCL2* was elevated in response to the addition of PE/HDP sera. In addition, the mRNA levels of RAGE system members (*HMGB1*, *S100B*, and *RAGE*) were significantly elevated by the addition of PE/HDP patient sera, suggesting possible involvement of the RAGE system in the up-regulation of *IL-6* and *CCL2* in adipocytes. In order to verify this possibility, we tested whether RAGE ligands up-regulate expression of *IL-6* and *CCL2* using human SW872 adipocytes and mouse 3T3-L1 cells and found that AGE and HMGB1 but not S100B significantly up-regulated gene expression of *IL-6* and *CCL2* in SW872 cells. In contrast to SW872 cells, AGE and HMGB1 up-regulated the gene expression of *IL-6* in differentiated 3T3-L1 cells but not in undifferentiated cells, and the addition of AGE, but neither HMGB1 nor S100B, up-regulated *Ccl2* expression in undifferentiated 3T3-L1 cells but any of them up-regulated *Ccl2* in differentiated cells. These results indicate that RAGE ligands, especially AGE and HMGB1, stimulate adipocytes to induce gene expression of *IL-6* and *CCL2*.

IL-6 is a key player in tissue inflammation and insulin resistance, and was observed in higher serum concentrations in PE/HDP patients [51]. CCL2, also referred as monocyte chemoattractant protein-1, is a key regulator of monocyte infiltration of adipose tissue, and it plays a central role in the development and maintenance of chronic adipose tissue inflammation and insulin resistance [23,52,53]. Therefore, IL-6 and CCL2 could be key players produced from adipocytes to induce tissue damages in PE/HDP patients.

Exposure of the amino acid residues of proteins to reducing sugars, such as glucose, results in non-enzymatic glycation, which forms reversible Schiff bases and subsequently Amadori compounds. A series of further complex molecular rearrangements including dehydration, condensation, and crosslinking, yield irreversible and heterogeneous derivatives termed AGE. AGEs are chemically heterogeneous groups of compounds. Apart from endogenously formed AGEs, exogenous AGEs from foods are absorbed in the gastrointestinal tract and reportedly constitute ~10% of total AGE in the body. In animal studies, the restriction of dietary AGE intake significantly improved insulin sensitivity and extended lifespan.

HMGB1 is a nuclear protein that stabilizes nucleosome formation and facilitates transcription. HMGB1 is a strong inflammatory trigger from necrotic cells as a result of passive leakage, and can be actively secreted by activated monocytes, macrophages, dendritic cells, natural killer cells, and endothelial cells, though there is no canonical signal sequence in the HMGB1 protein. It is well-known that the levels of AGE in serum such as hemoglobin A1c (HbA1c) are increased in diabetes (hyperglycemia) patients and that diabetes is a typical risk factor for PE/HDP. Elevated HMGB1 was observed in pregnant women with other pro-inflammatory conditions as obesity and pre-term labor. It is well established that labor is associated with a pro-inflammatory systemic response. Extracellular

HMGB1 exerts its cytokine-like activity by binding to RAGE receptor. In fact, the serum HMGB1 levels were significantly increased in the PE/HDP patients (329.2 ± 93.18 ng/mL) than those in control patients (35.45 ± 25.11 ng/mL) ($P = 0.0473$). In the management of pregnant women, monitoring of blood glucose and HbA1c are very common but HMGB1 levels in serum are rarely monitored. Although the numbers of PE/HDP patients in our study were relatively small, the increased tendency of serum HMGB1 in PE/HDP patients suggests that the serum HMGB1 measuring could be a new marker for screening of PE/HDP risk.

As AGE and HMGB1 are ligands for RAGE, it is quite possible that AGE- and HMGB1-induced up-regulation of *IL-6* and *CCL2* is mediated via RAGE. In fact, the introduction of *siRAGE* abolished the AGE- and HMGB1-mediated increases of gene expression of *IL-6* and *CCL2* in adipocytes (Figures 4 and 5), indicating involvement of AGE and/or HMGB1/RAGE system in the up-regulation of IL-6 and CCL2 in adipocytes. Among major RAGE ligands, we tested S100B, in addition to AGE and HMGB1, but S100B failed to increase gene expression of *IL-6* and *CCL2*. As most but not all the ligands for RAGE up-regulate (pro)inflammatory mediators, such as IL-6 and CCL2, some other RAGE ligands such as macrophage-1 antigen/cluster of differentiation molecule 11b [54], amyloid β peptide [55], β-sheet fibrils [56], advanced oxidation protein products [57], complement C3a [58], LPS [33], and phosphatidylserine on the surface of apoptotic cells [59] might increase the expression of IL-6 and CCL2, leading to PE/HDP in pregnant women. In fact, recent reports showed that PE/HDP was also induced by LPS [32], and that RAGE mediated LPS signaling and acted as an LPS receptor [33–38]. Thus, we tested whether LPS up-regulate gene expression of IL-6 and CCL2 in human SW872 adipocytes, and found that LPS significantly up-regulated the expression of IL-6 and CCL2 in SW872 cells via RAGE (Figures 6–9).

Some soluble products of RAGE such as soluble RAGE (sRAGE) and endogenous secretory RAGE (esRAGE) are generated from *RAGE* gene and modulate the RAGE signaling [60,61]. It was previously reported that the levels of sRAGE were reduced in PE/HDP patient serum and that serum esRAGE and the esRAGE/sRAGE ratio were elevated in PE/HDP patient serum [62]. It was also reported that pregnancy induced a significant increase in RAGE protein levels in both myometrium and omental vasculature and that blood vessels from women with preeclampsia had intense staining for RAGE in both vessel beds [63]. In the present study, we showed the up-regulation of RAGE in adipocytes by PE/HDP sera (Figure 1) but did not see sRAGE and esRAGE. Reduction of sRAGE and elevation of esRAGE/sRAGE ratio could be a potential marker for screening of PE/HDP risk.

Nuclear factor κ-light-chain-enhncer of activated B cells (NF-κB) is a key transcription factor for the expression of IL-6 and CCL2 [64,65]. RAGE ligands usually activate NF-κB [66]. The RAGE-NF-κB-IL-6/CCL2 pathway might function in adipocytes stimulated by RAGE ligands (AGE, HMGB1, and LPS), resulting in the development of inflammation that may lead to PE/HDP in pregnant women.

4. Materials and Methods

4.1. Patient Samples

The study was approved by the Local Ethics Committee at Nara Medical University (Kashihara, Japan; approval number 873, 24 July 2014), and all participants provided written informed consent. We included PE/HDP patients with a pregnancy and disease-free pregnant women with pregnancy were the control (Table 1). The participants' BMI values before pregnancy were less than 25 kg/m^2 with gestational age-matched normal pregnant women at 27 weeks' gestation or later. All subjects were Eastern Asian origin, and none of the subjects were taking any medication or showed evidence of any metabolic diseases or other complications besides PE/HDP. PE/HDP was defined as new onset and diagnosed based on two consecutive measurements of diastolic and systolic blood pressure, diastolic blood pressure greater than or equal to 90 mmHg, or systolic blood pressure was greater than or equal to 140 mmHg, with urine protein over 300 mg/day, occurring diagnosed after 20 weeks of gestation [67]. All subjects (4 patients and 4 controls) provided serum samples for analysis and did not have gestational diabetes mellitus, thyroid malfunction, or other complications. All venous blood samples were obtained after an overnight fast at routine medical examination. The sera were separated immediately and stored at −80 °C for 3 years at the longest and 6 months at the shortest. HMGB1 concentrations of the sera were measured using Human HMGB1 ELISA kit (Arigo Biolaboratories Corp., Hsinchu, Taiwan).

Table 1. Clinical characteristics of patients/controls involved in the study.

Patients/Controls	Age (Years)	BMI	Gestational Age at Blood Sampling (Week)	Parity
PE/HDP #1	33	23.2	30	0
PE/HDP #2	27	21.9	29	1
PE/HDP #3	28	21.3	28	0
PE/HDP #4	29	23.4	27	0
Control #1	30	22.4	28	0
Control #2	29	24.6	28	0
Control #3	26	23.8	27	0
Control #4	33	22.4	28	2

4.2. Cell Culture and Treatment

Human primary visceral preadipocytes were purchased from ZenBio, Inc. (Research Triangle Park, NC, USA). The cells were differentiated to adipocytes according to the supplier's protocol, and their differentiation to mature adipocyte was confirmed by Oil Red O staining. The primary adipocytes were incubated with 10% individual PE/HDP patient serum (#1~#4) and control serum (#1~#4) for 24 h. Human SW872 adipocytes were purchased from American Type Culture Collection (ATCC, Manassas, VA), and cultured at 37 °C with 5% CO_2 in DMEM medium (Wako Pure Chemical Industries, Ltd., Osaka, Japan) supplemented with 10% fetal calf serum (FCS), 100 units/mL penicillin G (Wako) and 100 µg/mL streptomycin (Wako) as described [68]. Mouse 3T3-L1 preadipocytes were purchased from Japanese Collection of Research Bioresources (JCRB) Cell Bank (Ibaraki, Japan), and cell culture and differentiation of 3T3-L1 preadipocytes were performed as described by Ntambi et al. [69,70]. Briefly, confluent 3T3-L1 pre-adipocytes monolayers were incubated for 72 h in DMEM medium containing 10% FCS, 0.5 mM methylisobutylxanthine (IBMX; Wako), 1 µM dexamethasone (Wako), and 10 µg/mL insulin (Wako). After 72 h the cells were washed free of IBMX and dexamethasone and maintained in DMEM medium containing 10% FCS and 10 µg/mL insulin for 72 h. Adipocyte morphology was monitored by the appearance of cytoplasmic triacylglycerol droplets, which is closely correlated with the acquisition of the adipocyte phenotype. For the stimulation experiments, SW872 and 3T3-L1 cells (undifferentiated preadipocytes and differentiated adipocytes) were treated with 150 µg/mL (for SW872) or 300 µg/mL (for 3T3-L1) AGE-bovine serum albumin (BSA) (Calbiochem®, Merck KGaA, Darmstadt, Germany), 1 µg/mL HMGB1 (Bio-Techne, Minneapolis, MN) or 100 ng/mL S100B (Medical & Biological Laboratories Co., Ltd., Nagoya, Japan). SW872 cells were also treated with 10 ng/mL *E. coli* LPS (Wako) for 24 h as described [33].

4.3. Real-Time Reverse Transcriptase-Polymerase Chain Reaction (RT-PCR)

Total RNA was isolated using a RNeasy Protect Cell Mini Kit (Qiagen, Hilden, Germany) from primary cultured human visceral adipocytes, SW872, and 3T3-L1 adipocytes/preadipocytes, and cDNA was synthesized from total RNA as template using a High Capacity cDNA Reverse Transcription kit (Applied Biosystems, Foster City, CA) as described [68,70–82]. Real-time polymerase chain reaction (PCR) was performed using SYBR® Fast qPCR kit (KAPA Biosystems, Boston, MA) and a Thermal Cycler Dice Real Time System (Takara Bio Inc., Kusatsu, Japan). All the PCR primers were synthesized by Nihon Gene Research Laboratories, Inc. (NGRL; Sendai, Japan), and the primer sequences for each primer set are described in Table 2. PCR was performed with an initial step of 3 min at 95 °C followed by 40 cycles of 3 s at 95 °C and 20 s at 60 °C for human *β-actin*, mouse *rat insulinoma gene*

(Rig)/ribosomal protein S15 (RpS15), mouse *IL-6*, human and mouse *CCL2*, human *LEP*, human *ADIP*, human *RETN*, human *S100B*, human *HMGB1*, and human *RAGE*, and with an initial step of 3 min at 95 °C followed by 40 cycles of 3 s at 95 °C and 20 s at 62 °C for human *IL-6* and human *TNFα*. The mRNA expression levels were normalized to the mRNA level of *Rig/RpS15* in mouse samples or *β-actin* in human samples [68,70–85].

Table 2. Primers used for real-time reverse transcriptase-polymerase chain reaction (RT-PCR).

Target mRNA	Primer Sequence (Position)
Human *IL-6* (NM_000600)	5′-GGTACATCCTCGACGGCATC-3′ (289–308)
	5′-GCCTCTTTGCTGCTTTCACAC-3′ (347–367)
Human *CCL2* (NM_002982)	5′-GTCTCTGCCGCCCTTCTGT-3′ (80–98)
	5′-TTGCATCTGGCTGAGCGAG-3′ (137–155)
Human *TNFα* (NM_000594)	5′-CTTCTCCTTCCTGATCGTGG-3′ (280–299)
	5′-TCTCAGCTCCACGCCATT-3′ (518–535)
Human *LEP* (NM_000230)	5′-GGCTTTGGCCCTATCTTTTC-3′ (89–108)
	5′-GGATAAGGTCAGGATGGGGT-3′ (257–276)
Human *ADIP* (NM_001177800)	5′-CATGACCAGGAAACCACGACT-3′ (181–201)
	5′-TGAATGCTGAGCGGTAT-3′ (465–481)
Human *RETN* (NM_020415)	5′-TCCTCCTCCTCCCTGTCCTGG-3′ (63–83)
	5′-CAGTGACATGTGGTCTGGGCG-3′ (298–318)
Human *S100B* (NM_006272)	5′-AGGGAGGGAGACAAGCACAA-3′ (172–191)
	5′-ACTCGTGGCAGGCAGTAGTA-3′ (293–312)
Human *HMGB1* (NM_001313893)	5′-ATATGGCAAAAGCGGACAAG-3′ (1126–1145)
	5′-AGGCCAGGATGTTCTCCTTT-3′ (1281–1300)
Human *RAGE* (NM_001136)	5′-TGGAACCGTAACCCTGACCT-3′ (856–875)
	5′-CGATGATGCTGATGCTGACA-3′ (1045–1064)
Human *β-actin* (NM_001101)	5′-GCGAGAAGATGACCCAGA-3′ (420–437)
	5′-CAGAGGCGTACAGGGATA-3′ (492–509)
Mouse *IL-6* (NM_031168)	5′-GTATGAACAACGATGATGCACTTG-3′ (305–328)
	5′-ATGGTACTCCAGAAGACCAGAGGA-3′ (418–441)
Mouse *Ccl2* (NM_011333)	5′-CCACTCACCTGCTGCTACTCAT-3′ (176–197)
	5′-TGGTGATCCTCTTGTAGCTCTCC-3′ (229–251)
Mouse *Rig/RpS15* (NM_009091)	5′-ACGGCAAGACCTTCAACCAG-3′ (323–342)
	5′-ATGGAGAACTCGCCCAGGTAG-3′ (372–392)

4.4. Measurement of IL-6 and CCL2 Concentrations in Culture Medium via ELISA

Cells were stimulated with HMGB1 (1 µg/mL), AGE (150 and 300 µg/mL), S100B (100 ng/mL), and LPS (10 ng/mL) for 24 h, culture medium was collected, and the concentrations of IL-6 and CCL2 were measured by using a Human IL-6 ELISA kit (RayBiotech, Norcross, GA, USA) for IL-6 and a Quantikine® ELISA Human CCL2/MCP-1 Immunoassay kit (R&D Systems, Inc., Minneapolis, MN, USA) for CCL2, according to the instructions of suppliers.

4.5. RNA Interference (RNAi)

Small interfering RNA (siRNA) directed against human *RAGE* was synthesized by NGRL. The sense sequence of siRNA for human *RAGE* was 5′-AUCUACAAUUUCUGGCUUCtt-3′ (corresponding to 466-484 of NM_001136) as described [76,78]. The Silencer® Select human scrambled siRNA was purchased from Ambion® (Waltham, MA, USA) and used as a control. Transfection of siRNAs to SW872 cells was carried out using Lipofectamine® RNAiMAX Reagent (Life Technologies, Waltham, MA, USA) as described [68,72,74–80]. Cells were transfected with 5 pmol siRNA per 24-well culture dish (4.0×10^5 cells/mL in 24-well plates).

4.6. Data Analysis

Results are expressed as mean ± SE. The data obtained were checked against Shapiro-Wilk normality test, which found that all the *P* values were larger than 0.05, and the statistical significance was determined by Student's *t*-test using GraphPad Prism ver. 6.0 for Mac OSX software (GraphPad Software, La Jolla, CA, USA).

Author Contributions: J.A., K.N., T.S., S.T., and H.K. contributed to the study design. J.A., T.U., M.M., A.Y., H.O., S.S.-T., A.I.-H., and S.T. contributed to data collection. J.A., S.T., and H.K. contributed to data analysis. J.A., S.T., and H.K. contributed to data interpretation. J.A., S.T., and H.K. contributed to manuscript preparation. All the authors contributed to revising and approval of manuscript content.

Funding: This research was funded by JSPS KAKEN Grants JP15K10682 and JP19K09829.

Acknowledgments: This work was supported in part by Grants-in-Aid for Scientific Research from the Ministry of Education, Culture, Sports, Science and Technology (JSPS: 23659161), Japan, JSPS KAKEN Grants JP15K10682 and JP19K09829, and the Japan Science and Technology Agency (JST: 18●06255) and is partial fulfillment by Juria Akasaka of the degree of Doctor of Medical Science at Nara Medical University.

Conflicts of Interest: The authors declare no conflict of interest.

Abbreviations

ADIP	Adiponectin
AGE	Advanced glycation endproduct(s)
BMI	Body mass index
CCL2	C-C motif chemokine ligand 2
ELISA	Enzyme-linked immunosorbent assay
esRAGE	Endogenous secretory RAGE
FCS	Fetal calf serum
HbA1c	Hemoglobin A1c
HMGB1	High mobility group box 1
IBMX	Methylisobutylxanthine
IL-6	Interleukin-6
LEP	Leptin
LPS	Lipopolysaccharide
NF-κB	Nuclear factor κ-light-chain-enhancer of activated B cells
PCR	Polymerase chain reaction
PE/HDP	Preeclampsia/hypertensive disorders of pregnancy
RAGE	Receptor for advanced glycation endproduct(s)
RETN	Resistin
Rig/RpS15	Rat insulinoma gene/Ribosomal protein S15
RT-PCR	Reverse transcriptase-PCR
S100B	S100 Ca^{2+}-binding protein B
siRNA	Small interfering RNA
sRAGE	Soluble RAGE
TNFα	Tumor necrosis factor α

References

1. Walker, J.J. Pre-eclampsia. *Lancet* **2000**, *356*, 1260–1265. [CrossRef]
2. Kintiraki, E.; Papakatsika, S.; Kotronis, G.; Goulis, D.G.; Kotsis, V. Pregnancy-induced hypertension. *Hormones* **2015**, *14*, 211–223. [CrossRef] [PubMed]
3. Goldenberg, R.L.; Culhane, J.F.; Iams, J.D.; Romero, R. Epidemiology and causes of preterm birth. *Lancet* **2008**, *371*, 75–84. [CrossRef]
4. Freeman, D.J.; McManus, F.; Brown, E.A.; Cherry, L.; Norrie, J.; Ramsay, J.E.; Clark, P.; Walker, I.D.; Sattar, N.; Greer, I.A. Short- and long-term changes in plasma inflammatory markers associated with preeclampsia. *Hypertension* **2004**, *44*, 708–714. [CrossRef] [PubMed]
5. Von Versen-Hoeynck, F.M.; Powers, R.W. Maternal-fetal metabolism in normal pregnancy and preeclampsia. *Front. Biosci.* **2007**, *12*, 2457–2470. [CrossRef] [PubMed]
6. Boeldt, D.S.; Bird, I.M. Vascular adaptation in pregnancy and endothelial dysfunction in preeclamsia. *J. Endocrinol.* **2017**, *232*, R27–R44. [CrossRef]

7. Possomato-Vieira, J.S.; Khalil, R.A. Mechanisms of endothelial dysfunction in hypertensive pregnancy and preeclampsia. *Adv. Pharmacol.* **2016**, *77*, 361–431.
8. Brennan, L.J.; Morton, J.S.; Davidge, S.T. Vascular dysfunction in preeclampsia. *Microcirculation* **2014**, *21*, 4–14. [CrossRef]
9. Yang, X.; Guo, L.; Li, H.; Chen, X.; Tong, X. Analysis of the original causes of placental oxidative stress in normal pregnancy and preeclampsia: a hypothesis. *J. Matem. Fetal Neonatal Med.* **2012**, *25*, 884–888. [CrossRef]
10. Fisher, S.J. Why is placentation abnormal in preeclampsia? *Am. J. Obstet. Gynecol.* **2015**, *213*, S115–S122. [CrossRef]
11. Saito, S.; Nakashima, A. A review of the mechanism for poor placentation in early-onset preeclampsia: the role of autophagy in trophoblast invasion vascular remodeling. *J. Reprod. Immunol.* **2014**, *101*, 80–88. [CrossRef] [PubMed]
12. Harmon, A.C.; Cornelius, D.C.; Amaral, L.M.; Faulkner, J.L.; Cunningham, W.W., Jr.; Wallace, K.; LaMarca, B. The role of inflammation in the pathology of preeclampsia. *Clin. Sci.* **2016**, *130*, 409–419. [CrossRef] [PubMed]
13. Kalagiri, R.R.; Carder, T.; Choudhury, S.; Vora, N.; Ballard, A.R.; Govande, V.; Drever, N.; Beeram, M.R.; Uddin, M.N. Inflammation in complicated pregnancy and its outcome. *Am. J. Perinatol.* **2016**, *33*, 1337–1356. [CrossRef] [PubMed]
14. Shamshirsaz, A.A.; Paidas, M.; Krikun, G. Preeclamsia, hypoxia, thrombosis, and inflammation. *J. Pregnancy* **2012**, *2012*, 374047. [CrossRef]
15. Kim, Y.J. Pathogenesis and promising non-invasive markers for preeclampsia. *Obstet. Gynecol. Sci.* **2013**, *56*, 2–7. [CrossRef]
16. Hotamisligil, G.S.; Shargill, N.S.; Spiegelman, B.M. Adipose expression of tumor necrosis factor-α: Direct role in obesity-linked insulin resistance. *Science* **1993**, *259*, 87–91. [CrossRef]
17. Shah, A.; Mehta, N.; Reilly, M.P. Adipose inflammation, insulin resistance, and cardiovascular disease. *JPEN J. Parenter. Enteral Nutr.* **2008**, *32*, 638–644. [CrossRef]
18. Bartha, J.L.; Marín-Segura, P.; González-González, N.L.; Wagner, F.; Aguilar-Diosdado, M.; Hervias-Vivancos, B. Ultrasound evaluation of visceral fat and metabolic risk factors during early pregnancy. *Obesity* **2007**, *15*, 2233–2239. [CrossRef]
19. Taebi, M.; Sadat, Z.; Saberi, F.; Kalahroudi, M.A. Early pregnancy waist-to-hip ratio and risk P preeclampsia: a prospective cohort study. *Hypertens. Res.* **2015**, *38*, 80–83. [CrossRef]
20. De Souza, L.R.; Kogan, E.; Berger, H.; Alves, J.G.; Lebovic, G.; Retnakaran, R.; Maguire, J.L.; Ray, J.G. Abdominal adiposity and insulin resistance in early pregnancy. *J. Obstet. Gynaecol. Can.* **2014**, *36*, 969–975. [CrossRef]
21. Zhang, S.; Folsom, A.R.; Flack, J.M.; Liu, K. Body fat distribution before pregnancy and gestational diabetes: findings from coronary artery risk development in young adults (CARDIA) study. *BMJ* **1995**, *311*, 1139–1140. [CrossRef] [PubMed]
22. Rabe, K.; Lehrke, M.; Parhofer, K.G.; Broedl, U.C. Adipokines and insulin resistance. *Mol. Med.* **2008**, *14*, 741–751. [CrossRef] [PubMed]
23. Maurizi, G.; Babini, L.; Della Guardia, L. Potential role of microRNAs in the regulation of adipocytes liposecretion and adipose tissue physiology. *J. Cell. Physiol.* **2018**, *233*, 9077–9086. [CrossRef] [PubMed]
24. Barden, A. Pre-eclampsia: contribution of maternal constitutional factors and the consequences for cardiovascular health. *Clin. Exp. Pharmacol. Physiol.* **2006**, *33*, 826–830. [CrossRef] [PubMed]
25. Lopez-Jaramillo, P.; Barajas, J.; Rueda-Quijano, S.M.; Lopez-Lopez, C.; Felix, C. Obesity and preeclampsia: Common pathophysiological mechanisms. *Front. Physiol.* **2018**, *9*, 1838. [CrossRef] [PubMed]
26. Weissgerber, T.L.; Mudd, L.M. Preeclampsia and diabetes. *Curr. Diab. Rep.* **2015**, *15*, 9. [CrossRef]
27. Chen, C.-Y.; Abell, A.M.; Moon, Y.S.; Kim, K.-H. An advanced glycation end product (AGE)-receptor for AGEs (RAGE) axis restores adipogenic potential of senescent preadipocytes through modulation of p53 protein function. *J. Biol. Chem.* **2012**, *287*, 44498–44507. [CrossRef]
28. Nativel, R.; Marimoutou, M.; Thon-Hon, V.G.; Guanasekaran, M.K.; Andries, J.; Stanislas, G.; Da Silva, C.R.; Césari, M.; Iwema, T.; Gasque, P.; et al. Soluble HMGB1 is a novel adipokine stimulating IL-6 secretion through RAGE receptor in SW872 preadipocyte cell line: Contribution to chronic inflammation in fat tissue. *PLoS ONE* **2013**, *8*, e76039. [CrossRef]

29. Tanaka, N.; Yonekura, H.; Yamagishi, S.; Fujimori, H.; Yamamoto, Y.; Yamamoto, H. The receptor for advanced glycation end products is induced by the glycation products themselves and tumor necrosis factor-α through nuclear factor-κB, and by 17β-estradiol through Sp-1 in human vascular endothelial cells. *J. Biol. Chem.* **2000**, *275*, 25781–25790. [CrossRef]
30. Fujiya, A.; Nagasaki, H.; Seino, Y.; Okawa, T.; Kato, J.; Fukami, A.; Himeno, T.; Uenishi, E.; Tsunekawa, S.; Kamiya, H.; et al. The role of S100B in the interaction between adipocytes and macrophages. *Obesity* **2014**, *22*, 371–379. [CrossRef]
31. Son, K.H.; Son, M.; Ahn, H.; Oh, S.; Yum, Y.; Choi, C.H.; Park, K.Y.; Byun, K. Age-related accumulation of advanced glycation end-products-albumin, S100β, and the expressions of advanced glycation end product receptor differ in visceral and subcutaneous fat. *Biochem. Biophys. Res. Commun.* **2016**, *477*, 271–276. [CrossRef] [PubMed]
32. Wu, L.-Z.; Xiao, X.-M. Evaluation of the effects of *Uncaria rhynchophylla* alkaloid extract on LPS-induced preeclamsia symptoms and inflammation in pregnant rat model. *Braz. J. Med. Biol. Res.* **2019**, *52*, e8273. [CrossRef] [PubMed]
33. Yamamoto, Y.; Harashima, A.; Saito, H.; Tsuneyama, K.; Munesue, S.; Motoyoshi, S.; Han, D.; Watanabe, T.; Asano, M.; Takasawa, S.; et al. Septic shock is associated with receptor for advanced glycation end products ligation of LPS. *J. Immunol.* **2011**, *186*, 3248–3257. [CrossRef] [PubMed]
34. Gasparotto, J.; Ribeiro, C.T.; Bortolin, R.C.; Somensi, N.; Fernandes, H.S.; Teixeira, A.A.; Guasselli, M.O.R.; Agani, C.A.J.O.; Souza, N.C.; Grings, M.; et al. Anti-RAGE antibody selectively blocks acute systemic inflammatory responses to LPS in serum, liver, CSF and striatum. *Brain Behav. Immun.* **2017**, *62*, 124–136. [CrossRef]
35. Ramsgaard, L.; Englert, J.M.; Manni, M.L.; Milutinovic, P.S.; Gefter, J.; Tobolewski, J.; Crum, L.; Coudriet, G.M.; Piganelli, J.; Zamora, R.; et al. Lack of the receptor for advanced glycation end-products attenuates *E. coli* pneumonia in mice. *PLoS ONE* **2011**, *6*, e20132. [CrossRef]
36. Rineiro, C.T.; Gasparotto, J.; Teixeira, A.A.; Portela, L.V.C.; Flores, V.N.L.; Moreira, J.C.F.; Gelain, D.P. Immune neutralization of the receptor for advanced glycation end products reduce liver oxidative damage induced by an acute systemic injection of lipopolysaccharide. *J. Biochem.* **2018**, *163*, 515–523.
37. Wang, L.; Wu, J.; Guo, X.; Huang, X.; Huang, Q. RAGE plays a role in LPS-induced NF-κB activation and endothelial hyperpermeability. *Sensors* **2017**, *17*, 722. [CrossRef]
38. Li, Y.; Wu, R.; Zhao, S.; Cheng, H.; Ji, P.; Yu, M.; Tian, Z. RAGE/NF-κB pathway mediates lipopolysaccharide-induced inflammation in alveolar type I epithelial cells isolated from neonate rats. *Inflammation* **2014**, *37*, 1623–1629. [CrossRef]
39. Umesawa, M.; Kobashi, G. Epidemiology of hypertensive disorders in pregnancy: Prevalence, risk factors, predictors and prognosis. *Hypertens. Res.* **2017**, *40*, 213–220. [CrossRef]
40. Wang, Z.; Wang, Z.; Wang, L.; Qiu, M.; Wang, Y.; Hou, X.; Guo, Z.; Wang, B. Hypertensive disorders during pregnancy and risk of type 2 diabetes in later life: a systematic review and meta-analysis. *Endocrine* **2017**, *55*, 809–821. [CrossRef]
41. Sohlberg, S.; Stephansson, O.; Cnattingius, S.; Wikström, A.-K. Maternal body mass index, height, and risks of preeclampsia. *Am. J. Hypertens.* **2012**, *25*, 120–125. [CrossRef] [PubMed]
42. Lim, C.C.; Mahmood, T. Obesity in pregnancy. *Best Pract. Res. Clin. Obstet. Gynaecol.* **2015**, *29*, 309–319. [CrossRef] [PubMed]
43. Lutsiv, O.; Mah, J.; Beyene, J.; McDonald, S.D. The effects of morbid obesity on maternal and neonatal health outcomes: a systematic review and meta-analyses. *Obes. Rev.* **2015**, *16*, 531–546. [CrossRef] [PubMed]
44. Mission, J.F.; Marshall, N.E.; Caughey, A.B. Pregnancy risks associated with obesity. *Obstet. Gynecol. Clin. North Am.* **2015**, *42*, 335–353. [CrossRef]
45. MacInnis, N.; Woolcott, C.G.; McDonald, S.; Kuhle, S. Population attributable risk fractions of maternal overweight and obesity for adverse perinatal outcomes. *Sci. Rep.* **2016**, *6*, 22895. [CrossRef]
46. Marchi, J.; Berg, M.; Dencker, A.; Olander, E.K.; Begley, C. Risks associated with obesity in pregnancy, for the mother and baby: a systematic review of reviews. *Obes. Rev.* **2015**, *16*, 621–638. [CrossRef]
47. Santangeli, L.; Sattar, N.; Huda, S.S. Impact of maternal obesity on perinatal and childhood outcomes. *Best Pract. Res. Clin. Obstet. Gynaecol.* **2015**, *29*, 438–448. [CrossRef]
48. Segovia, S.A.; Vickers, M.H.; Gray, C.; Reynolds, C.M. Maternal obesity, inflammation, and developmental programming. *BioMed Res. Int.* **2014**, *2014*, 418975. [CrossRef]

49. Khodabandehloo, H.; Gorgani-Firuzjaee, S.; Panahi, G.; Meshkani, R. Molecular and cellular mechanisms linking inflammation to insulin resistance and β-cell dysfunction. *Transl. Res.* **2016**, *167*, 228–256. [CrossRef]
50. Luo, Y.; Liu, M. Adiponectin: a versatile player of innate immunity. *J. Mol. Cell Biol.* **2016**, *8*, 120–128. [CrossRef]
51. Eder, K.; Baffy, N.; Falus, A.; Fulop, A.K. The major inflammatory mediator interleukin-6 and obesity. *Inflamm. Res.* **2009**, *58*, 727–736. [CrossRef] [PubMed]
52. Ouchi, N.; Parker, J.L.; Lugus, J.J.; Walsh, K. Adipokines in inflammation and metabolic disease. *Nat. Rev. Immunol.* **2011**, *11*, 85–97. [CrossRef] [PubMed]
53. Kulyté, A.; Belarbi, Y.; Lorente-Cebrián, S.; Bambace, C.; Arner, E.; Daub, C.O.; Hedén, P.; Rydén, M.; Mejhert, N.; Arner, P. Additive effects of microRNAs and transcription factors on CCL2 production in human white adipose tissue. *Diabetes* **2014**, *63*, 1248–1258. [CrossRef] [PubMed]
54. Sachs, U.J.; Chavakis, T.; Fung, L.; Lohrenz, A.; Bux, J.; Reil, A.; Ruf, A.; Santoso, S. Human alloantibody anti-Mart interferes with Mac-1-dependent leukocyte adhesion. *Blood* **2004**, *104*, 727–734. [CrossRef]
55. Masuda, N.; Tsujinaka, H.; Hirai, H.; Yamashita, M.; Ueda, T.; Ogata, N. Effects of concentration of amyloid β (Aβ) on viability of cultured retinal pigment epithelial cells. *BMC Ophthalmol.* **2019**, *19*, 70. [CrossRef]
56. Rong, L.L.; Gooch, C.; Szabolcs, M.; Herold, K.C.; Lalla, E.; Hays, A.P.; Yan, S.F.; Yan, S.S.; Schmidt, A.M. RAGE: a journey from the complications of diabetes to disorders of nervous system – striking a fine balance between injury and repair. *Restor. Neurol. Neurosci.* **2005**, *23*, 355–365.
57. Zhang, Z.; Yang, L.; Lei, L.; Chen, R.; Chen, H.; Zhang, H. Glucagon-like peptide-1 attenuates advanced oxidation protein product-mediated damage in islet microvascular endothelial cells partly through the RAGE pathway. *Int. J. Mol. Med.* **2016**, *38*, 1161–1169. [CrossRef]
58. Ruan, B.H.; Li, X.; Winkler, A.R.; Cunningham, K.M.; Kuai, J.; Greco, R.M.; Nocka, K.H.; Fitz, L.J.; Wright, J.F.; Pittman, D.D.; et al. Complement C3a, CpG oligos, and DNA/C3a complex stimulate IFN-α production in a receptor for advanced glycation end product-dependent manner. *J. Immunol.* **2010**, *185*, 4213–4222. [CrossRef]
59. He, M.; Kubo, H.; Morimoto, K.; Fujino, N.; Suzuki, T.; Takahasi, T.; Yamada, M.; Yamaya, M.; Maekawa, T.; Yamamoto, Y.; et al. Receptor for advanced glycation end products binds to phosphatidylserine and assists in the clearance of apoptotic cells. *EMBO Rep.* **2011**, *12*, 358–364. [CrossRef]
60. Yonekura, H.; Yamamoto, Y.; Sakurai, S.; Petrova, R.G.; Abedin, M.d.J.; Li, H.; Yasui, K.; Takeuchi, M.; Makita, Z.; Takasawa, S.; et al. Novel splice variants of the receptor for advance glycation end-products expressed in human vascular endothelial cells pericytes, and their putative roles in diabetes-induced vascular injury. *Biochem. J.* **2003**, *370*, 1097–1109. [CrossRef]
61. Harashima, A.; Yamamoto, Y.; Cheng, C.; Tsuneyama, K.; Myint, K.M.; Takeuchi, A.; Yoshimura, K.; Li, H.; Watanabe, T.; Takasawa, S.; et al. Identification of mouse orthologue of endogenous secretory receptor for advanced glycation end-products: structure, function and expression. *Biochem. J.* **2006**, *396*, 109–115. [CrossRef] [PubMed]
62. Kwon, J.-H.; Kim, Y.-H.; Kwon, J.-Y.; Park, Y.-W. Clinical significance of serum sRAGE and esRAGE in women with normal pregnancy and preeclampsia. *J. Perinat. Med.* **2011**, *39*, 507–513. [CrossRef] [PubMed]
63. Cooke, C.L.; Brockelsby, J.C.; Baker, P.N.; Davidge, S.T. The receptor for advanced glycation end products (RAGE) is elevated in women with preeclampsia. *Hypertens. Pregnancy* **2003**, *22*, 173–184. [CrossRef] [PubMed]
64. Xiao, W.; Hodge, D.R.; Wang, L.; Yang, X.; Zhang, X.; Farrar, W.L. Co-operative functions between nuclear factors NFκB and CCAT/enhancer-binding protein-β (C/EBP-β) regulate the IL-6 promoter in autocrine human prostate cancer cells. *Prostate* **2004**, *61*, 354–370. [CrossRef]
65. Rajaiya, J.; Sadeghi, N.; Chodosh, J. Specific NFκB subunit activation and kinetics of cytokine induction in adenoviral keratitis. *Mol. Vis.* **2009**, *15*, 2879–2889.
66. Kay, A.M.; Simpson, C.L.; Stewart, J., Jr. A. The role of AGE/RAGE signaling in diabetes–mediated vascular calcification. *J. Diabetes Res.* **2016**, *2016*, 6809703. [CrossRef]
67. Naruse, K.; Akasaka, J.; Shigemitsu, A.; Tsunemi, T.; Koike, N.; Yoshimoto, C.; Kobayashi, H. Involvement of visceral adipose tissue in immunological modulation of inflammatory cascade in preeclampsia. *Mediators Inflamm.* **2015**, *2015*, 325932. [CrossRef]
68. Uchiyama, T.; Ota, H.; Itaya-Hironaka, A.; Shobatake, R.; Yamauchi, A.; Sakuramoto-Tsuchida, S.; Makino, M.; Kimura, H.; Takeda, M.; Ohbayashi, C.; et al. Up-regulation of *selenoprotein P* and *HIP/PAP* mRNAs in

hepatocytes by intermittent hypoxia via down-regulation of miR-203. *Biochem. Biophys. Rep.* **2017**, *11*, 130–137. [CrossRef]
69. Ntambi, J.M.; Buhrow, S.A.; Kaestner, K.H.; Christy, R.J.; Sibley, E.; Kelly Jr., T.J.; Lane, M.D. Differentiation-induced gene expression in 3T3-L1 preadipocytes. Characterization of a differentially expressed gene encoding stearoyl-CoA desaturase. *J. Biol. Chem.* **1988**, *263*, 17291–17300.
70. Uchiyama, T.; Itaya-Hironaka, A.; Yamauchi, A.; Makino, M.; Sakuramoto-Tsuchida, S.; Shobatake, R.; Ota, H.; Takeda, M.; Ohbayashi, C.; Takasawa, S. Intermittent hypoxia up-regulates *CCL2*, RETN, and *TNFα* mRNAs in adipocytes via down-regulation of miR-452. *Int. J. Mol. Sci.* **2019**, *20*, 1960. [CrossRef]
71. Ota, H.; Tamaki, S.; Itaya-Hironaka, A.; Yamauchi, A.; Sakuramoto-Tsuchida, S.; Morioka, T.; Takasawa, S.; Kimura, H. Attenuation of glucose-induced insulin secretion by intermittent hypoxia via down-regulation of CD38. *Life Sci.* **2012**, *90*, 206–211. [CrossRef] [PubMed]
72. Ota, H.; Itaya-Hironaka, A.; Yamauchi, A.; Sakuramoto-Tsuchida, S.; Miyaoka, T.; Fujimura, T.; Tsujinaka, H.; Yoshimoto, K.; Nakagawara, K.; Tamaki, S.; et al. Pancreatic β cell proliferation by intermittent hypoxia via up-regulation of *Reg* family genes and *HGF* gene. *Life Sci.* **2013**, *93*, 664–672. [CrossRef] [PubMed]
73. Nakagawa, K.; Takasawa, S.; Nata, K.; Yamauchi, A.; Itaya-Hironaka, A.; Ota, H.; Yoshimoto, K.; Sakuramoto-Tsuchida, S.; Miyaoka, T.; Takeda, M.; et al. Prevention of Reg I-induced β-cell apoptosis by IL-6/dexamethasone through activation of *HGF* gene regulation. *Biochim Biophys Acta* **2013**, *1833*, 2988–2995. [CrossRef] [PubMed]
74. Yamauchi, A.; Itaya-Hironaka, A.; Sakuramoto-Tsuchida, S.; Takeda, M.; Yoshimoto, K.; Miyaoka, T.; Fujimura, T.; Tsujinaka, H.; Tsuchida, C.; Ota, H.; et al. Synergistic activations of *REG Iα* and *REG Iβ* promoters by IL-6 and glucocorticoids through JAK/STAT pathway in human pancreatic β cells. *J. Diabetes Res.* **2015**, *2015*, 173058. [CrossRef]
75. Fujimura, T.; Fujimoto, T.; Itaya-Hironaka, A.; Miyaoka, T.; Yoshimoto, K.; Yamauchi, A.; Sakuramoto-Tsuchida, S.; Kondo, S.; Takeda, M.; Tsujinaka, H.; et al. Interleukin-6/STAT pathway is responsible for the induction of gene expression of REG Iα, a new auto-antigen in Sjögren's syndrome patients, in salivary duct epithelial cells. *Biochem. Biophys. Rep.* **2015**, *2*, 69–74. [CrossRef]
76. Tsujinaka, H.; Itaya-Hironaka, A.; Yamauchi, A.; Sakuramoto-Tsuchida, S.; Ota, H.; Takeda, M.; Fujimura, T.; Takasawa, S.; Ogata, N. Human retinal pigment epithelial cell proliferation by the combined stimulation of hydroquinone and advanced glycation end-products via up-regulation of *VEGF* gene. *Biochem. Biophys. Rep.* **2015**, *2*, 123–131. [CrossRef]
77. Tsuchida, C.; Sakuramoto-Tsuchida, S.; Takeda, M.; Itaya-Hironaka, A.; Yamauchi, A.; Misu, M.; Shobatake, R.; Uchiyama, T.; Makino, M.; Pujol-Autonell, I.; et al. Expression of *REG* family genes in human inflammatory bowel diseases and its regulation. *Biochem. Biophys. Rep.* **2017**, *12*, 198–205. [CrossRef]
78. Tsujinaka, H.; Itaya-Hironaka, A.; Yamauchi, A.; Sakuramoto-Tsuchida, S.; Shobatake, R.; Makino, M.; Masuda, N.; Hirai, H.; Takasawa, S.; Ogata, N. Statins decrease vascular epithelial growth factor expression via down-regulation of receptor for advanced glycation end-products. *Heliyon* **2017**, *3*, e00401. [CrossRef]
79. Tohma, Y.; Dohi, Y.; Shobatake, R.; Uchiyama, T.; Takeda, M.; Takasawa, S.; Tanaka, Y.; Ohgushi, H. *Reg* gene expression in periosteum after fracture and its in vitro induction triggered by IL-6. *Int. J. Mol. Sci.* **2017**, *18*, 2257. [CrossRef]
80. Shobatake, R.; Takasawa, K.; Ota, H.; Itaya-Hironaka, A.; Yamauchi, A.; Sakuramoto-Tsuchida, S.; Uchiyama, T.; Makino, M.; Sugie, K.; Takasawa, S.; et al. Up-regulation of *POMC* and *CART* mRNAs by intermittent hypoxia via GATA transcription factors in human neuronal cells. *Int. J. Biochem. Cell Biol.* **2018**, *95*, 100–107. [CrossRef]
81. Kyotani, Y.; Itaya-Hironaka, A.; Yamauchi, A.; Sakuramoto-Tsuchida, S.; Makino, M.; Takasawa, S.; Yoshizumi, M. Intermittent hypoxia-induced epiregulin expression by IL-6 production in human coronary artery smooth muscle cells. *FEBS Open Bio* **2018**, *8*, 868–876. [CrossRef] [PubMed]
82. Takasawa, S.; Tsuchida, C.; Sakuramoto-Tsuchida, S.; Takeda, M.; Itaya-Hironaka, A.; Yamauchi, A.; Misu, M.; Shobatake, R.; Uchiyama, T.; Makino, M.; et al. Expression of human *REG* family genes in inflammatory bowel disease and their molecular mechanism. *Immunol. Res.* **2018**, *66*, 800–805. [CrossRef] [PubMed]
83. Yoshimoto, K.; Fujimoto, T.; Itaya-Hironaka, A.; Miyaoka, T.; Sakuramoto-Tsuchida, S.; Yamauchi, A.; Takeda, M.; Kasai, T.; Nakagawara, K.; Nonomura, A.; et al. Involvement of autoimmunity to REG, a regeneration factor, in patients with primary Sjögren's syndrome. *Clin. Exp. Immunol.* **2013**, *174*, 1–9. [CrossRef] [PubMed]

84. Murakami-Kawaguchi, S.; Takasawa, S.; Onogawa, T.; Nata, K.; Itaya-Hironaka, A.; Sakuramoto-Tsuchida, S.; Yamauchi, A.; Ota, H.; Takeda, M.; Kato, M.; et al. Expression of *Ins1* and *Ins2* genes in mouse fetal liver. *Cell Tissue Res.* **2014**, *355*, 303–314. [CrossRef]
85. Shobatake, R.; Itaya-Hironaka, A.; Yamauchi, A.; Makino, M.; Sakuramoto-Tsuchida, S.; Uchiyama, T.; Ota, H.; Takahashi, N.; Ueno, S.; Sugie, K.; et al. Intermittent hypoxia up-regulates gene expressions of *peptide YY (PYY)*, *glucagon-like peptide-1 (GLP-1)*, and *neurotensin (NTS)* in enteroendocrine cells. *Int. J. Mol. Sci.* **2019**, *20*, 1849. [CrossRef]

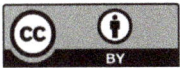

© 2019 by the authors. Licensee MDPI, Basel, Switzerland. This article is an open access article distributed under the terms and conditions of the Creative Commons Attribution (CC BY) license (http://creativecommons.org/licenses/by/4.0/).

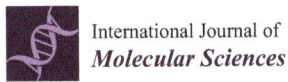

Article

Perinatal Micro-Bleeds and Neuroinflammation in E19 Rat Fetuses Exposed to Utero-Placental Ischemia

Ashtin B. Giambrone [1], Omar C. Logue [2], Qingmei Shao [1], Gene L. Bidwell III [1,2] and Junie P. Warrington [1,*]

1. Department of Neurology, University of Mississippi Medical Center, Jackson, MS 39216, USA
2. Department of Cell and Molecular Biology, University of Mississippi Medical Center, Jackson, MS 39216, USA
* Correspondence: jpwarrington@umc.edu; Tel.: +1-601-815-8969

Received: 14 July 2019; Accepted: 18 August 2019; Published: 20 August 2019

Abstract: Offspring of preeclampsia patients have an increased risk of developing neurological deficits and cognitive impairment. While low placental perfusion, common in preeclampsia and growth restriction, has been linked to neurological deficits, a causative link is not fully established. The goal of this study was to test the hypothesis that placental ischemia induces neuroinflammation and micro-hemorrhages *in utero*. Timed-pregnant Sprague Dawley rats were weight-matched for sham surgery (abdominal incision only) or induced placental ischemia (surgical reduction of utero-placental perfusion (RUPP)); n = 5/group on gestational day 14. Fetal brains (n = 1–2/dam/endpoint) were collected at embryonic day (E19). Placental ischemia resulted in fewer live fetuses, increased fetal demise, increased hematocrit, and no difference in brain water content in exposed fetuses. Additionally, increased cerebral micro-bleeds (identified with H&E staining), pro-inflammatory cytokines: IL-1β, IL-6, and IL-18, eotaxin (CCL11), LIX (CXCL5), and MIP-2 (CXCL2) were observed in RUPP-exposed fetuses. Microglial density in the sub-ventricular zone decreased in RUPP-exposed fetuses, with no change in cortical thickness. Our findings support the hypothesis that exposure to placental ischemia contributes to microvascular dysfunction (increased micro-bleeds), fetal brain inflammation, and reduced microglial density in proliferative brain areas. Future studies will determine whether *in utero* abnormalities contribute to long-term behavioral deficits in preeclampsia offspring through impaired neurogenesis regulation.

Keywords: micro-bleeds; cerebral cytokines; preeclampsia; microglia

1. Introduction

Preeclampsia (PE), a hypertensive disorder of pregnancy, is characterized by new onset hypertension with proteinuria, or in the absence of proteinuria, symptoms of other organ damage affecting kidney(s), the liver, or the brain [1]. Because PE is associated with increased risk of morbidity and mortality for the mother and offspring, PE contributes significantly to an increased public health burden. There is compelling evidence that exposure to PE has lasting effects on the offspring's cognitive abilities. Offspring of PE patients go on to have lower IQ scores at 3 years of age [2], have impaired working memory [3], and have other neurobehavioral impairments [4,5] that progressively exacerbate cognitive impairment into the geriatric years [6,7]. Even though the underlying pathophysiological mechanisms are not known, placental insufficiency is believed to play a critical role in these poor neurodevelopmental outcomes [8].

In addition to being the source of the maternal syndrome [9], the dysfunctional placenta fails to meet the metabolic demands of the developing brain [10], resulting in clinical manifestations of neurodevelopmental disorders [11]. Specifically, offspring of PE-complicated pregnancies have a 32% increased risk of autism spectrum disorders [12–14]. Moreover, PE is an independent risk factor for long-term neuropsychiatric morbidity in the offspring [15] demonstrating that exposure to maternal factors and/or maternal vascular malperfusion [16] have lasting impacts on learning and memory-function in the offspring. The underlying pathophysiological mechanisms are not fully known.

One potential mechanism could be reduced blood flow to the developing placenta and fetus, a finding in some PE-complicated pregnancies. Indeed, studies report increased expression of hyoxia-inducible factor 1 alpha (HIF-1α) mRNA in placentas from women with preeclampsia [17,18]. The rodent placental ischemia model, induced by surgically reducing utero-placental perfusion pressure (RUPP), is well characterized and shares numerous characteristics with the PE patient. For example, RUPP rats have increased mean arterial blood pressure, with or without proteinuria [19], increased inflammatory cytokines [20,21], and increased anti-angiogenic factors [22,23]. Studies from members of our group have shown that RUPP dams have evidence of cerebrovascular abnormalities [24,25]; however, the impact of placental ischemia on the developing fetal cerebrovasculature has not been investigated. Additionally, whether placental ischemia induces neuroinflammation in the developing brain is not known.

In this study, we induced and modeled placental malperfusion by using the well-established rat model of placental ischemia [26], and determined the effect of five days of ischemia on fetal cerebral micro-bleeds and neuroinflammation. We measured the number of micro-hemorrhages as a marker of micro-bleeds and vascular function, brain water content as a measure of cerebral edema, and cytokine levels and microglia changes to assess neuroinflammation in embryonic day (E19) rat brains.

2. Results

2.1. General Characteristics and Pregnancy Outcomes:

At gestational day (GD) 19, dams (n = 5 per group) subjected to placental ischemia had reduced body weight (266.5 ± 13.5 g) compared to sham-operated (control) pregnant rats (303.1 ± 9.1 g; p = 0.027; Figure 1A).

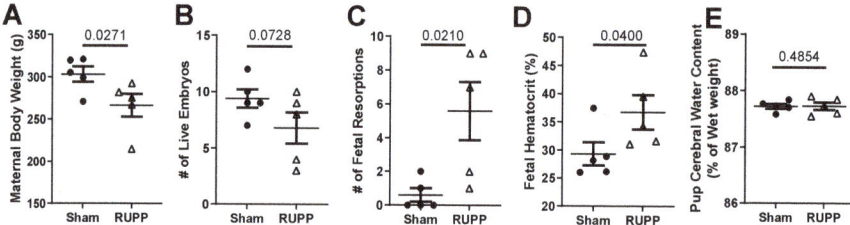

Figure 1. General characteristics of dams and fetuses subjected to placental ischemia. Dams had (**A**) reduced body weight, (**B**) reduced numbers of live fetuses, and (**C**) increased fetal demise at gestational day (GD) 19 compared to the sham controls. Fetuses subjected to placental ischemia had (**D**) increased hematocrits and (**E**) no change in brain water content. Values for individual rats (n = 5 dams per group) are shown along with the Mean ± SEM. Fetal hematocrit and pup brain water content represent the mean of 1–2 pups/dam (n = 5 dams). Differences between groups were analyzed using an unpaired t-test.

A key characteristic of placental ischemia, induced using the RUPP procedure, is fetal demise in the form of increased fetal resorptions [19]. We therefore counted the number of live versus resorbed fetuses present at GD 19. Dams subjected to placental ischemia had a trend for fewer live fetuses (7 ± 1 in RUPP group versus 9 ± 1 in the sham control; p = 0.073; Figure 1B) and more fetal resorptions (6 ± 2 in RUPP group versus 1 ± 0 in the sham control; p = 0.021; Figure 1C) compared to the sham controls. This demonstrates that we successfully induced placental ischemia in the dams. We then assessed the effect of placental ischemia on the developing fetus. Because placental ischemia leads to reduced blood flow to the fetal-placental unit, we hypothesized that fetuses would have evidence of systemic hypoxia. We, therefore, measured pups' hematocrits and found an increase in the hematocrits (36.7% ± 3.0% versus 29.3% ± 2.1% in sham) of fetuses exposed to placental ischemia ($p = 0.040$; Figure 1D). There was no difference in fetal brain water content between the groups (87.73% ± 0.04% in sham versus 87.73% ± 0.07% in RUPP-exposed; $p = 0.485$; Figure 1E), suggesting no cerebral edema. Additionally, in this cohort, we found no differences in maternal blood pressure between the groups (98 ± 4 mmHg in sham versus 99 ± 5 mmHg in RUPP; $p = 0.405$). Thus, our findings are due to utero-placental ischemia, independent of elevated blood pressure.

2.2. Micro-Hemorrhage in Fetal Brains

Using H&E staining, red blood cells can be visualized by their red staining in tissues. Figure 2A shows the location of brain slices used to quantify micro-bleeds. Figure 2B,C show representative micro-bleeds observed in the parenchyma (2B, cortex) and lateral and third ventricles (2C).

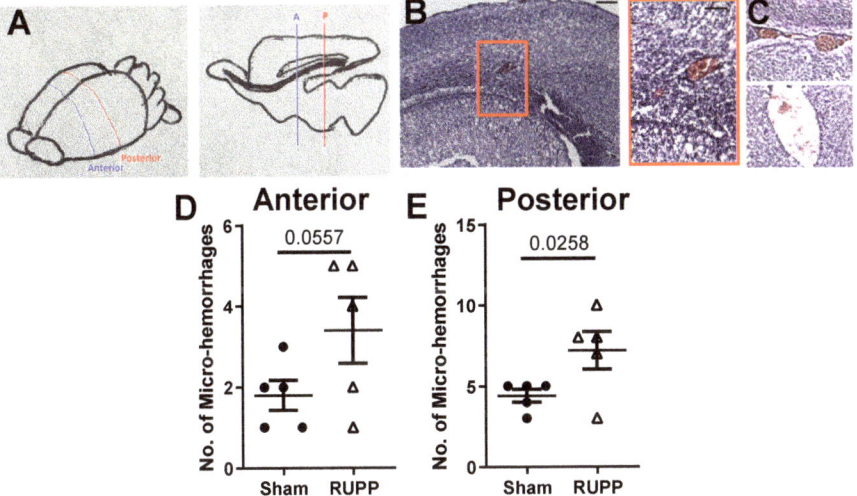

Figure 2. Placental ischemia exposure leads to increased number of micro-bleeds in brains of exposed fetuses. (**A**) Schematic of the regions where coronal sections were collected. (**B**) Representative images of fetal brains showing micro-bleeds in the cortex and (**C**) ventricles. Number of micro-bleeds in the (**D**) anterior (**E**) posterior slices of fetal brains. Points represent average micro-bleeds from 1–2 pups per dam (n = 5 dams per group). Mean ± SEM is also depicted. Data were analyzed using unpaired *t*-test and *p*-values are indicated.

We counted the number of micro-bleeds and found significantly higher numbers of micro-hemorrhages in the brains of fetuses exposed to placental ischemia in the posterior sections, and a trend for increased micro-bleeds in the anterior slices of the brain. In the anterior slices, RUPP-exposed fetuses had 3.4 ± 0.8 bleeds compared to the sham-exposed (1.8 ± 0.4 bleeds; $p = 0.056$; Figure 2D). In the posterior slices, sham-exposed fetuses had 4 ± 1 while RUPP-exposed fetuses had 7 ± 1 bleeds ($p = 0.026$, Figure 2E). Thus, exposure to placental ischemia almost doubled the incidence of fetal brain micro-bleeds *in utero*.

2.3. Inflammatory Profile in Fetal Brains

Due to placental ischemia inducing increased maternal, circulating and placental inflammatory cytokines [20,21,27], we hypothesized that the developing fetal brain may mirror the maternal pro-inflammatory environment. We therefore measured the levels of cytokines/chemokines in fetal brains exposed to normal pregnancy and placental ischemia. Out of 27 cytokines and chemokines, seven were undetectable or observed in only 1–2 fetal brains per group: EGF, G-CSF, GM-CSF, GRO/KC, IL-2, IL-5, and IL-13. We divided the remaining 20 cytokines/chemokines into pro-inflammatory/ cytotoxic, anti-inflammatory, and chemokines/growth factors [28]. The pro-inflammatory cytokines IL-1β, IL-6, and IL-18 increased significantly in fetal brains from placental ischemia-exposed pregnancies (Figure 3).

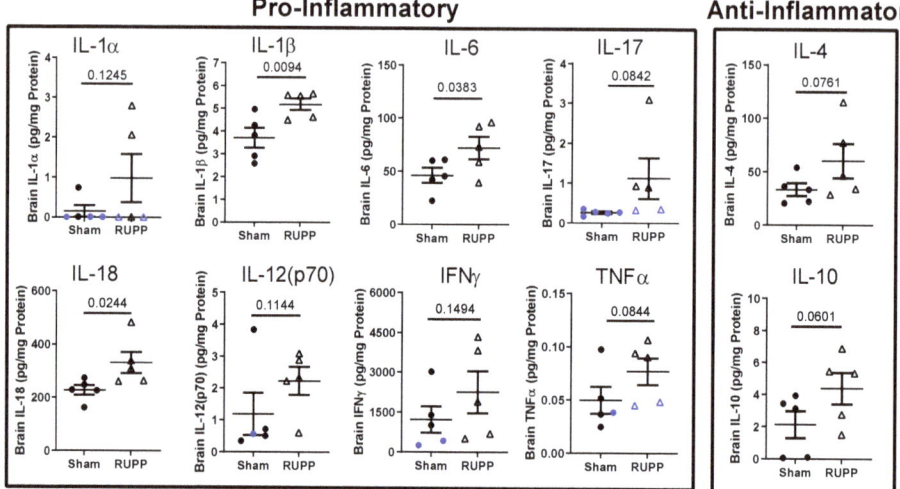

Figure 3. Placental ischemia leads to a shift towards a pro-inflammatory status in brains of exposed fetuses. A rat multiplex kit array of 27 cytokine/chemokine was used. Values were normalized to protein concentration. IL-1β, IL-6, and IL-18 increased significantly in fetal brains exposed to placental ischemia. Blue points represent extrapolated values (one value below the lowest detectable value and normalized to protein concentration). Not shown are: IL-2, IL-5, and IL-13. Values for individual rat fetuses (n = 5 fetuses per group) are shown along with the mean ± SEM. Only one fetal brain was collected per dam for cytokines/chemokines.

There was a trend toward increased anti-inflammatory cytokines, IL-4 and IL-10. Lastly, the chemokines/growth factors eotaxin (CCL11), LIX/CXCL5, and MIP-2/CXCL2 increased significantly in fetal brains exposed to placental ischemia compared to sham-exposed (Figure 4).

These data demonstrate that placental ischemia exposure induces a pro-inflammatory environment in fetal brains *in utero*. Whether the cerebral inflammatory profile persists in the postnatal period is unknown. Thus, future studies will determine whether the fetal cerebral pro-inflammatory status is unique to the *in utero* environment or whether it persists postnatally.

Because micro-hemorrhages are associated with a pro-inflammatory environment [29], we performed correlations to identify whether any factors were strongly associated with the number of micro-bleeds observed. Comparing fetuses from the same dam, we found that cerebral tissue IL-6 levels were positively associated with the number of micro-bleeds detected (Figure 5A; r = 0.673; p = 0.017). Surprisingly, although there were no differences in brain water content between the groups, fetal brain water content was negatively associated with the number of micro-bleeds (Figure 5B; r = −0.672; p = 0.017).

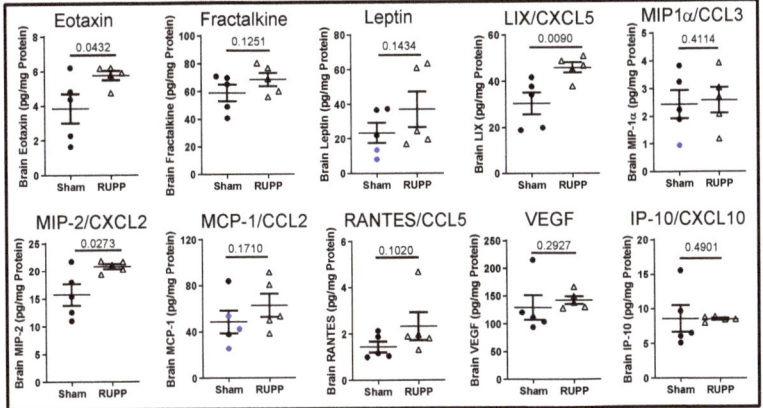

Figure 4. Changes in chemokines/growth factors in fetal brains. Placental ischemia exposure increased eotaxin, LIX, and MIP2 levels. Not shown are: EGF, G-CSF, GM-CSF, and GRO/KC. Blue points represent extrapolated values (one value below lowest detectable value and normalized to protein concentration). Values for individual fetuses ($n = 5$ fetuses per group) are shown along with the mean ± SEM. Data were analyzed using unpaired t-tests, and p-values are indicated.

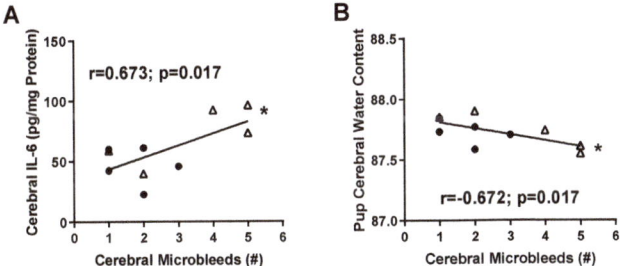

Figure 5. Correlation between number of micro-bleeds and IL-6 levels or brain water content. The number of micro-bleeds is (**A**) positively associated with fetal brain IL-6 levels and (**B**) negatively associated with fetal brain water content. Fetuses from same dam were used for the association analysis. Values for individual rats ($n = 5$ fetuses per group) are shown. Relationships between factors were analyzed using the Pearson correlation.

2.4. Microglia Changes in Fetal Brains

Microglia are key producers of cytokines in the brain, so we assessed changes in microglial density and morphology in the brains of exposed fetuses. As reviewed in [30], microglia migrate from the ventricles and meninges during development, making the sub-ventricular zone (SVZ) the ideal region to quantify changes in microglial density. Representative images of a brain section and the third ventricle from sham and placental ischemia-exposed fetuses are shown in Figure 6A, B. We found fewer Iba1 + cells in the SVZ of the third ventricle (40 ± 3 in shams versus 19 ± 4; $p = 0.003$), and this reduction was observed both in the open (23 ± 2 in sham versus 13 ± 4; $p = 0.036$) and closed (21 ± 1 in shams versus 9 ± 2; $p = 0.005$) portion of the third ventricle (Figure 6C). We further characterized the microglia based on morphology into primitive ramified or amoeboid microglia [31] (Figure 6D) and counted these separately. We found a significant decrease in primitive ramified microglia in fetuses exposed to RUPP (13 ± 4 versus 28 ± 2 in Sham, $p = 0.007$; Figure 6D) and no change in the number of amoeboid microglia (13 ± 4 in Sham versus 5 ± 2 in RUPP, $p = 0.089$). We found no significant difference in cortical plate thickness (a potential indicator of neuronal density) between the fetuses exposed to normal or placental ischemic pregnancies (Figure 6E,F).

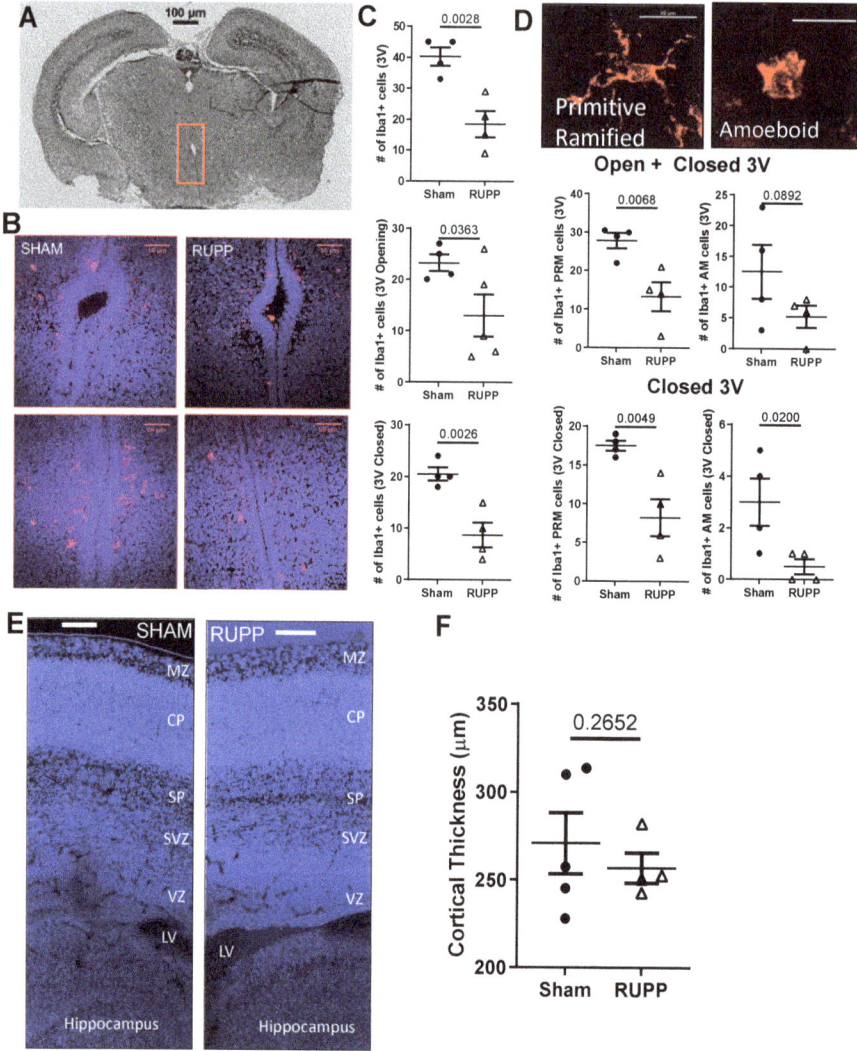

Figure 6. Changes in microglia at the proliferative areas (sub-ventricular zones—SVZ) of the 3rd Ventricle. (**A**) Representative image showing, at the brain-level, the section where the microglial analysis was conducted. Scale bar = 100 µm. (**B**) Representative images of Iba1 staining in the open region and closed region of the 3rd ventricle. Red—Iba1$^+$ cells; Blue—DAPI$^+$ nuclei. Scale bar represents 50 µm. (**C**) Decreased number of microglia in the SVZ of pups exposed to placental ischemia. (**D**) Examples of different microglia types observed (scale bar = 20 µm) and quantification of primitive ramified and amoeboid microglia in SVZ. (**E**) Representative images showing the different cortical layers in the embryonic day (E19) pup brain. Scale bar represents 100 µm. (**F**) Quantification of cortical plate thickness in fetuses exposed to sham or placental ischemia. Values from 1–2 pups were averaged per dam (n = 4–5 per group) and shown along with the mean ± SEM. Data were analyzed using unpaired t-tests, and p-values are indicated. MZ—marginal zone, CP—cortical plate, SP—subcortical plate, SVZ—sub-ventricular zone, VZ—ventricular zone, and LV—lateral ventricle.

3. Discussion

Offspring born to preeclampsia patients have an increased risk of developing several neurological complications, including neurobehavioral abnormalities, cerebral palsy, cognitive impairment, and perinatal stroke [32–34]—the underlying mechanisms of which are not fully known. Here, we tested the hypothesis that utero-placental ischemia leads to *in utero* cerebrovascular changes, including micro-hemorrhages, which may contribute to future neurological complications. We found that indeed, placental ischemia in the pregnant female rat induces an increased number of cerebral micro-bleeds, a more pro-inflammatory cerebral-tissue environment, and decreased microglial density in the sub-ventricular zone of fetal brains *in utero*.

Like previous findings, the RUPP procedure led to decreased maternal body weight and increased fetal demise, demonstrating successful induction of placental ischemia [19,35]. Because we did not see an increase in blood pressure in this small cohort of rats, our findings are attributable to placental ischemia, independent of hypertension. We hypothesized that as a result of reduced blood flow to the fetus, surviving fetuses would have evidence of hypoxia. We found significant increases in the hematocrits of fetuses exposed to placental ischemia, suggesting systemic hypoxia. Whether the increased fetal hematocrits were associated with increased angiogenesis through vascular endothelial growth factor (VEGF) in our model is not known. While this possibility cannot be ruled out, our finding of no difference in VEGF levels in the brain homogenates of exposed fetuses suggests that cerebral angiogenesis may not be different between the groups. VEGF also increases vascular permeability and could increase vessel leakage, causing extravasation of plasma proteins. Thus, as a measure of vascular dysfunction, we quantified micro-bleeds within tissue slices.

The incidence of cerebral micro-bleeds was significantly higher in the placental ischemia-exposed group compared to the sham control group. Micro-bleeds are thought to occur when blood vessels are structurally damaged [36]. Thus, an increased incidence of micro-bleeds is consistent with ongoing vascular damage in the brains of exposed fetuses. Cerebral micro-bleeds can lead to long-term neurological damage, including cognitive and motor deficits [36]. Vascular damage and increased blood-brain barrier permeability can result in increases in brain water content; therefore, we hypothesized that fetuses exposed to placental ischemia would have increased cerebral water content, a crude marker of cerebral edema. Contrary to our hypothesis, we found no difference in brain water content between fetuses exposed to normal pregnancy and those exposed to placental ischemia. Even more interesting is the finding of a negative association between the number of cerebral micro-bleeds and brain water content. A recent study reported that micro-bleeds are observed in high-altitude-induced injury long after cerebral edema has resolved [31]. Thus, our finding of no difference in brain water content even in the presence of micro-bleeds could be an indication of a resolution of edema. We do not know whether different fetal or postnatal time-points would yield similar results and this is an area for future investigation. Additionally, we assessed water content in the entire fetal brain and could have missed regional changes in water content as a result.

Maternal inflammation and cerebral micro-bleeds are associated with increases in neuroinflammation. Therefore, we assessed the levels of different cytokines/chemokines in brain homogenates of exposed fetuses. We found increases in the pro-inflammatory cytokines, IL-1β, IL-6, and IL-18, and a trend for increased levels of TNFα and IL-17 in brains of fetuses exposed to placental ischemia. Additionally, IL-10 and IL-4 levels tended to increase in brains of fetuses exposed to placental ischemia. Those data suggest two possibilities. The first possibility is that there is an increased transfer of maternal inflammatory factors across the placental barrier into the fetal circulation. This is plausible since preeclampsia patients have increased circulating levels of tumor necrosis factor alpha (TNFα) [20], interleukin (IL)-2 [37,38], IL-6 [21], and IL-17 [39–41]. Placental ischemic rats also have increased levels of inflammatory cytokines in the circulation and cerebrospinal fluid [20,21,27,42,43]. We have not assessed changes in placental barrier permeability in the RUPP model of placental ischemia, and this is an area of ongoing investigation. The second possibility is that there is increased local production of these cytokines in the fetal brains following exposure to placental ischemia.

A key finding in this study is that exposure to placental ischemia leads to increased cerebral levels of the pro-inflammatory cytokine, IL-1β in utero. There is evidence that placentas from preeclampsia patients secrete more IL-1β compared to normotensive placentas [44]. Additionally, infusion of IL-1β into the brains of young rats induces blood-brain barrier breakdown [45]. Taken together, increased tissue levels of IL-1β may play a deleterious role at the blood-brain barrier, contributing to structural damage and subsequent cerebral micro-bleeds. Whether increased IL-1β has a causal role in increased cerebral micro-bleeds in placental ischemia-exposed fetuses will be assessed in future studies.

Our multi-plex cytokine analysis also revealed increased levels of IL-6 and IL-18 in the brains of exposed fetuses. Not only was cerebral IL-6 increased in response to placental ischemia, but fetal brain IL-6 levels positively correlated to the number of cerebral micro-bleeds. Our findings are consistent with reports that serum levels of both IL-6 and IL-18 are higher in patients with cerebral micro-bleeds compared to those without [46]. Another study found that in patients with ischemic cerebrovascular disease, IL-6 was associated with an increased risk for cerebral micro-bleeds in an elderly, community-based cohort [47]. Furthermore, in the developing brain, micro-bleeds were observed in pups exposed to lipopolysaccharide, coupled with intrauterine ischemia, mainly if they were vaginally delivered [48], suggesting that *in utero* insults make blood vessels more susceptible to injury. Taken together, those studies and our current findings support the hypothesis that maternal inflammation, induced by placental ischemia, contributes to weakened cerebral vessels, making them more susceptible to blood-brain barrier (BBB) disruption and cerebral micro-bleeds.

Previously, we reported that eotaxin (CCL11) is increased in the cerebrospinal fluid of placental ischemic dams [42,49]. In the current study, we found increased levels of eotaxin in the brains of fetuses exposed to placental ischemia. The consequences and source of fetal brain eotaxin levels were not directly investigated in this study, although eotaxin has been shown to promote glutamate-induced neurotoxicity [50]. Importantly, CCL11 has been shown to directly regulate neurogenesis [51], such that increased circulating eotaxin was associated with reduced neurogenesis in aged mice and infusion of CCL11 into young mice resulted in decreased neurogenesis and cognitive impairment. Thus, increased eotaxin levels in the brains of fetuses exposed to placental ischemia suggest that neurogenesis may be impaired.

Microglia are essential during normal brain development and have important roles in pruning synapses, phagocytizing excess neuronal progenitor cells, and regulating the number of neurons at each stage of development [52]. Thus, changes in microglial numbers at late gestation could predict later neurological function. Microglia are also involved in secreting pro-inflammatory cytokines; thus, increased density of microglia could contribute to increases in local tissue inflammation. Following strokes, immune cells (microglia and macrophages) are activated by cytokines and chemokines, and migrate to damaged areas to remove dead neural cells. Those immune cells, induced by a chronic inflammatory environment, may become over-activated and produce large amounts of pro-inflammatory cytokines, disrupting neurogenesis and the BBB [53]. The presence of a pro-inflammatory environment and vascular damage in the brains of fetuses exposed to placental ischemia suggest that microglia may be activated. We therefore hypothesized that brains from exposed fetuses would have an increased density of microglia. Contrary to our hypothesis, we found that placental ischemia exposed fetuses had a decreased density of microglia in the SVZ of the third ventricle. Microglia in that region are vital for neurogenesis and oligodendrogenesis during fetal development and throughout life [52]. Reduced microglial density in the SVZ of placental ischemia-exposed fetuses may predict deficits in neurogenesis and oligodendrogenesis affecting the central nervous system long term. This possibility is a subject of ongoing investigation.

There is evidence that in both rats and mice, microglia protect neonatal brains from injury after ischemic stroke, and that depletion of microglia led to worse outcomes [54]. Thus, increased cerebral micro-hemorrhages, as occurred in exposed fetuses, coupled with fewer microglia, may indicate more severe damage/outcomes. During development, microglia can be disturbed by cytokines and chemokines released under conditions of maternal inflammation [55] seen in placental ischemia.

To our knowledge, this is the first study reporting the impact of placental ischemia on cerebral micro-bleed incidence and neuroinflammation in the offspring in utero. The inclusion of male and female offspring in all analyses is a strength of the current study; however, we were unable to assess sex differences in our endpoints. Ongoing and future studies are now utilizing genotyping for sex to specifically assess sex differences. Additionally, this study utilized only one time-point (E19) and we are therefore unable to extend our findings to the postnatal period. Because we used brain homogenates to assess the inflammatory status, we were unable to address regional changes in expression of the different cytokines, chemokines, and growth factors assessed. We limited our microglial analysis to the SVZ associated with the third ventricle for this study; however, analysis of microglial changes in other brain regions will be important.

In conclusion, the rat placental ischemia model induces increased cerebral micro-hemorrhages in the developing brain in utero and may be a good model to assess the etiology of cerebral micro-hemorrhages associated with preeclampsia-complicated pregnancies. Our data suggest that a hypoxic environment in the fetus, induced by reducing maternal utero-placental perfusion, induces abnormalities in cerebrovascular structure, increased blood-brain barrier disruption and micro-bleeds in the developing fetal brain. This is associated with a pro-inflammatory environment and reduced microglial density in proliferative brain regions, and may underlie the increased neurodevelopmental abnormalities observed in offspring born to preeclampsia patients. Additional studies are required to elucidate the underlying causes of these observations and to establish whether there are time-dependent differences in the outcome measures.

4. Materials and Methods

4.1. Animals

Female timed-pregnant Sprague Dawley rats were obtained from Harlan Laboratories and arrived on gestational day (GD) 11. For timed pregnant rats from Harlan Laboratories, the day of vaginal plug detection was considered gestational day 0. Pregnant rats were housed singly after surgery (GD 14) and had continuous access to standard rodent chow and tap water. One to two (1–2) fetuses per dam per endpoint were randomly selected at E19 from 5 dams per group. Both male and female fetuses were included in all analyses; however, the sex of individual fetuses was not determined. Rats were maintained on a 12 h light and 12 h dark cycle. All animal procedures were approved by the University of Mississippi Medical Center's Institutional Animal Care and Use Committee before animal procedures commenced (1379A, June 16 2016).

4.2. Placental Ischemia Induction

On GD 14, rats were anesthetized using isoflurane and an abdominal incision was made. The utero-placental unit was exteriorized and a silver clip (0.203 mm) was placed on the abdominal aorta (below the kidneys and above the bifurcation). Silver clips (0.1 mm) were also placed on both uterine artery branches between the ovaries and the first pup. This procedure induces placental ischemia by reducing utero-placental perfusion pressure (RUPP). Pregnant rats in the sham group were treated similarly, in that, an abdominal incision was made, the uterine horn was exteriorized, and vessels were manipulated without clip placement. Carprofen (5 mg/kg) was used as an analgesic in both groups.

4.3. Carotid Surgery and Blood Pressure Measurement

On GD18, rats were anesthetized using isoflurane anesthesia and the left carotid artery was isolated and cannulated using pre-made saline-filled catheters. Catheters were secured and exteriorized at the nape of the neck. The incision was closed and secured using Vetbond. The following morning, rats were placed in restrainer cages and catheters were connected to a pressure transducer. After

30 min of acclimation, blood pressure was recorded for 30 min using LabChart software. The mean arterial pressure was calculated for the duration of 30 min.

4.4. Harvest and Collection of Tissues

On GD 19, pregnant rats were anesthetized using isoflurane, and an abdominal incision was made. After exteriorization of the fetal-placental unit, maternal blood was collected from the abdominal aorta. Dams were euthanized by removal of the heart. The number of live and resorbed pups were counted. Fetuses were euthanized by decapitation. Trunk blood was collected from fetuses using micro-capillary tubes and hematocrit was noted. Fetal heads were processed differently depending on endpoints. For brain water content, brains were removed, weighed, and then dried for 48 h at 60 °C. Brain water content was calculated as a percentage ((wet weight − dry weight)/ wet weight). Brains for molecular analyses were removed and flash frozen in liquid nitrogen, followed by storage in a −80 °C freezer until processing. Brains for immunofluorescence staining or histology were kept within the skull and placed in 4% paraformaldehyde at 4 °C overnight. The following day, brains were removed from the skull and placed back in 4% paraformaldehyde overnight. Brains were then transferred to a 30% sucrose solution at 4 °C for 72 h and then embedded in Cryogel, and frozen at −80 °C until sectioning (1–2 fetal brains per mold). Brains were sectioned at 20 μm thickness, transferred directly to slides, and stored at −20 °C until staining.

4.5. Micro-Bleed Detection

Slides were washed and stained using hematoxylin and eosin following the manufacturer's directions. Slides were then cover-slipped and imaged using light microscopy. Micro-bleeds were identified as red cells within the parenchyma and outside of the blood vessel lumen or within the ventricles. Micro-bleeds were counted by an investigator blinded to the groups (ABG) in sections from the anterior and posterior part of the brain (Figure 2A). The number of micro-bleeds from two slices per region was averaged per fetus and further averaged per dam.

4.6. Fetal Brain Multiplex Array

To determine the cerebral inflammatory profile of exposed fetuses, a separate group of brains ($n = 1$ pup per dam) were homogenized in RIPA buffer, and protein concentration was measured using the BCA kit. Equal volumes (25 μL) of sample were loaded into 96 well-plates and incubated with magnetic beads, pre-mixed to detect 27 cytokine/chemokines (Rat multiplex kit, Millipore Sigma, Burlington, MA, USA). Samples were run alongside standards and kit controls in duplicate. The observed concentration was calculated using the standard curve generated and normalized to the protein concentration of the sample. Cytokine/chemokine concentration is, therefore, presented as pg/mg protein.

4.7. Analysis of Microglia

Slides were washed and then blocked using normal donkey serum followed by rabbit anti-Iba1 polyclonal antibody (1:500; Wako; 019-19741) overnight at 4 °C. This Iba1 antibody recognizes the carboxy-terminal of the Iba1 protein and is specific to microglia/macrophages. Slides were washed and incubated for 2 h in donkey anti-rabbit TRITC (JacksonImmuno, West Grove, PA, USA; 131591) at room temperature. After washing, slides were mounted using Vectashield Mounting Media with DAPI and placed on coverslips. Images were captured using confocal microscopy with a 40X objective. Iba1$^+$ cells were counted in the sub-ventricular zones (SVZ) associated with the third ventricle. A total of 2 sections per fetus were used for microglial assessment. Images of the third ventricle's open and closed regions were captured from each fetal brain. Microglia totals from 1–2 pups were averaged per dam. Counting was done in a blind fashion. At E19, microglia have a different morphology from those in the adult brain; and amoeboid and primitive ramified microglia are most commonly observed [31]. We therefore counted the number of amoeboid and primitive ramified microglia in the SVZ. Image analysis was done using ImageJ (version 1.51j8; NIH). Cortical images were captured using a 10X objective, and the thickness of the cortical plate was analyzed using NIS Elements' Analysis software (Nikon Instruments Inc., Melville, NY, USA; version 5.10.01). A total of 6 measurements per pup brain were obtained within the cortical plate and averaged per pup, and further averaged per dam.

4.8. Statistical Analysis

All statistical analyses were conducted using GraphPad Prism software (version 7). Differences between the sham-exposed and placental ischemia-exposed dams and fetuses were calculated using unpaired *t*-tests. For analyses where variances were different, we used Welch's *t*-test with corrections for unequal variance. Pearson's correlations were calculated to determine the association between various factors. Outlier tests (ROUT, Q = 1%) were conducted when visible outliers were suspected. For the microglia density data, two outliers (fetuses from the same dam from the sham-exposed group) were removed from analysis and are not shown. All graphs depict values for individual animals along with the mean ± SEM. The threshold for statistical difference was set at $p < 0.05$.

5. Conclusions

Placental ischemia, a common finding in preeclampsia-complicated pregnancies, leads to increased pro-inflammatory cytokines, increased micro-bleeds, and reduced microglia in proliferative zones of E19 fetal brains. Thus, our findings support the hypothesis that neuroinflammation, micro-vascular damage, and impaired microglia function may partly explain cognitive deficits that occur in offspring of preeclamptic pregnancies.

Author Contributions: Study design, J.P.W., G.L.B., and O.C.L.; collection of data, J.P.W., O.C.L., Q.S., and A.B.G.; drafting the manuscript, A.B.G. and J.P.W.; critically reviewing the manuscript, J.P.W., A.B.G., and G.L.B.; approving the final draft of manuscript A.B.G, O.C.L., Q.S., G.L.B., and J.P.W..

Funding: This research was funded by a COBRE pilot grant from the National Institutes of Health (P20GM104357) and a K99/R00 award to JPW (HL129192). Fluorescence images were captured using a confocal microscope from the Imaging Core, funded through an Institutional Development Award (IDeA) from the National Institute of General Medical Sciences of the NIH, under grant number P30GM103328. The APC was funded by NIH HL129192.

Conflicts of Interest: The authors declare no conflict of interest. The funders had no role in the design of the study; in the collection, analyses, or interpretation of data; in the writing of the manuscript, or in the decision to publish the results.

Abbreviations

PE	Preeclampsia
RUPP	Reduced Uterine Perfusion Pressure
SVZ	Sub-ventricular zone
GD	Gestational day
BBB	Blood-brain barrier

References

1. Roberts, J.M.; August, P.A.; Bakris, G.; Barton, J.R.; Bernstein, I.M.; Druzin, M.; Gaiser, R.R.; Granger, J.P.; Jeyabalan, A.; Johnson, D.D.; et al. Hypertension in pregnancy. Report of the American College of Obstetricians and Gynecologists' Task Force on Hypertension in Pregnancy. *Obs. Gynecol* **2013**, *122*, 1122–1131. [CrossRef]
2. Many, A.; Fattal, A.; Leitner, Y.; Kupferminc, M.J.; Harel, S.; Jaffa, A. Neurodevelopmental and cognitive assessment of children born growth restricted to mothers with and without preeclampsia. *Hypertens Pregnancy* **2003**, *22*, 25–29. [CrossRef] [PubMed]
3. Rätsep, M.T.; Hickman, A.F.; Maser, B.; Pudwell, J.; Smith, G.N.; Brien, D.; Stroman, P.W.; Adams, M.A.; Reynolds, J.N.; Croy, B.A.; et al. Impact of preeclampsia on cognitive function in the offspring. *Behav. Brain Res.* **2016**, *302*, 175–181. [CrossRef] [PubMed]

4. Muñoz-Moreno, E.; Fischi-Gomez, E.; Batalle, D.; Borradori-Tolsa, C.; Eixarch, E.; Thiran, J.P.; Gratacós, E.; Hüppi, P.S. Structural Brain Network Reorganization and Social Cognition Related to Adverse Perinatal Condition from Infancy to Early Adolescence. *Front. Neurosci.* **2016**, *10*, 560. [CrossRef] [PubMed]
5. Chen, J.; Chen, P.; Bo, T.; Luo, K. Cognitive and Behavioral Outcomes of Intrauterine Growth Restriction School-Age Children. *Pediatrics* **2016**, *137*. [CrossRef] [PubMed]
6. Tuovinen, S.; Aalto-Viljakainen, T.; Eriksson, J.G.; Kajantie, E.; Lahti, J.; Pesonen, A.K.; Heinonen, K.; Lahti, M.; Osmond, C.; Barker, D.J.; et al. Maternal hypertensive disorders during pregnancy: Adaptive functioning and psychiatric and psychological problems of the older offspring. *BJOG* **2014**, *121*, 1482–1491. [CrossRef] [PubMed]
7. Raikkonen, K.; Kajantie, E.; Pesonen, A.K.; Heinonen, K.; Alastalo, H.; Leskinen, J.T.; Nyman, K.; Henriksson, M.; Lahti, J.; Lahti, M.; et al. Early life origins cognitive decline: Findings in elderly men in the Helsinki Birth Cohort Study. *PLoS ONE* **2013**, *8*, e54707. [CrossRef] [PubMed]
8. Kaukola, T.; Räsänen, J.; Herva, R.; Patel, D.D.; Hallman, M. Suboptimal neurodevelopment in very preterm infants is related to fetal cardiovascular compromise in placental insufficiency. *Am. J. Obs. Gynecol.* **2005**, *193*, 414–420. [CrossRef]
9. Chaiworapongsa, T.; Chaemsaithong, P.; Yeo, L.; Romero, R. Pre-eclampsia part 1: Current understanding of its pathophysiology. *Nat. Rev. Nephrol.* **2014**, *10*, 466–480. [CrossRef]
10. Lo, J.O.; Roberts, V.H.J.; Schabel, M.C.; Wang, X.; Morgan, T.K.; Liu, Z.; Studholme, C.; Kroenke, C.D.; Frias, A.E. Novel Detection of Placental Insufficiency by Magnetic Resonance Imaging in the Nonhuman Primate. *Reprod. Sci.* **2018**, *25*, 64–73. [CrossRef]
11. Maher, G.M.; O'Keeffe, G.W.; Kearney, P.M.; Kenny, L.C.; Dinan, T.G.; Mattsson, M.; Khashan, A.S. Association of Hypertensive Disorders of Pregnancy With Risk of Neurodevelopmental Disorders in Offspring: A Systematic Review and Meta-analysis. *Jama Psychiatry* **2018**, *75*, 809–819. [CrossRef] [PubMed]
12. Dachew, B.A.; Mamun, A.; Maravilla, J.C.; Alati, R. Pre-eclampsia and the risk of autism-spectrum disorder in offspring: Meta-analysis. *Br. J. Psychiatry* **2018**, *212*, 142–147. [CrossRef] [PubMed]
13. Walker, C.K.; Krakowiak, P.; Baker, A.; Hansen, R.L.; Ozonoff, S.; Hertz-Picciotto, I. Preeclampsia, placental insufficiency, and autism spectrum disorder or developmental delay. *Jama Pediatr* **2015**, *169*, 154–162. [CrossRef] [PubMed]
14. Curran, E.A.; O'Keeffe, G.W.; Looney, A.M.; Moloney, G.; Hegarty, S.V.; Murray, D.M.; Khashan, A.S.; Kenny, L.C. Exposure to Hypertensive Disorders of Pregnancy Increases the Risk of Autism Spectrum Disorder in Affected Offspring. *Mol. Neurobiol* **2018**, *55*, 5557–5564. [CrossRef] [PubMed]
15. Nahum Sacks, K.; Friger, M.; Shoham-Vardi, I.; Sergienko, R.; Spiegel, E.; Landau, D.; Sheiner, E. Long-term neuropsychiatric morbidity in children exposed prenatally to preeclampsia. *Early Hum. Dev.* **2019**, *130*, 96–100. [CrossRef]
16. Parks, W.T. Manifestations of Hypoxia in the Second and Third Trimester Placenta. *Birth Defects Res.* **2017**, *109*, 1345–1357. [CrossRef] [PubMed]
17. Harati-Sadegh, M.; Kohan, L.; Teimoori, B.; Mehrabani, M.; Salimi, S. The association of the placental Hypoxia-inducible factor1-alpha polymorphisms and HIF1-alpha mRNA expression with preeclampsia. *Placenta* **2018**, *67*, 31–37. [CrossRef]
18. Wang, S.; Wang, X.; Weng, Z.; Zhang, S.; Ning, H.; Li, B. Expression and role of microRNA 18b and hypoxia inducible factor-1alpha in placental tissues of preeclampsia patients. *Exp. Med.* **2017**, *14*, 4554–4560. [CrossRef]
19. Alexander, B.T.; Kassab, S.E.; Miller, M.T.; Abram, S.R.; Reckelhoff, J.F.; Bennett, W.A.; Granger, J.P. Reduced uterine perfusion pressure during pregnancy in the rat is associated with increases in arterial pressure and changes in renal nitric oxide. *Hypertension* **2001**, *37*, 1191–1195. [CrossRef]
20. LaMarca, B.B.; Bennett, W.A.; Alexander, B.T.; Cockrell, K.; Granger, J.P. Hypertension produced by reductions in uterine perfusion in the pregnant rat: Role of tumor necrosis factor-alpha. *Hypertension* **2005**, *46*, 1022–1025. [CrossRef]
21. Gadonski, G.; LaMarca, B.B.; Sullivan, E.; Bennett, W.; Chandler, D.; Granger, J.P. Hypertension produced by reductions in uterine perfusion in the pregnant rat: Role of interleukin 6. *Hypertension* **2006**, *48*, 711–716. [CrossRef]
22. Gilbert, J.S.; Gilbert, S.A.; Arany, M.; Granger, J.P. Hypertension produced by placental ischemia in pregnant rats is associated with increased soluble endoglin expression. *Hypertension* **2009**, *53*, 399–403. [CrossRef]

23. Gilbert, J.S.; Babcock, S.A.; Granger, J.P. Hypertension produced by reduced uterine perfusion in pregnant rats is associated with increased soluble fms-like tyrosine kinase-1 expression. *Hypertension* **2007**, *50*, 1142–1147. [CrossRef]
24. Warrington, J.P.; Fan, F.; Murphy, S.R.; Roman, R.J.; Drummond, H.A.; Granger, J.P.; Ryan, M.J. Placental ischemia in pregnant rats impairs cerebral blood flow autoregulation and increases blood-brain barrier permeability. *Physiol. Rep.* **2014**, *2*. [CrossRef]
25. Warrington, J.P.; Drummond, H.A.; Granger, J.P.; Ryan, M.J. Placental Ischemia-induced Increases in Brain Water Content and Cerebrovascular Permeability: Role of TNFα. *Am. J. Physiol. Regul. Integr. Comp. Physiol.* **2015**, *309*, R1425–R1431. [CrossRef]
26. Granger, J.P.; LaMarca, B.B.; Cockrell, K.; Sedeek, M.; Balzi, C.; Chandler, D.; Bennett, W. Reduced uterine perfusion pressure (RUPP) model for studying cardiovascular-renal dysfunction in response to placental ischemia. *Methods Mol. Med.* **2006**, *122*, 383–392.
27. LaMarca, B.; Wallukat, G.; Llinas, M.; Herse, F.; Dechend, R.; Granger, J.P. Autoantibodies to the angiotensin type I receptor in response to placental ischemia and tumor necrosis factor alpha in pregnant rats. *Hypertension* **2008**, *52*, 1168–1172. [CrossRef]
28. Chhor, V.; Moretti, R.; Le Charpentier, T.; Sigaut, S.; Lebon, S.; Schwendimann, L.; Oré, M.V.; Zuiani, C.; Milan, V.; Josserand, J.; et al. Role of microglia in a mouse model of paediatric traumatic brain injury. *Brain Behav. Immun.* **2017**, *63*, 197–209. [CrossRef]
29. Ahn, S.J.; Anrather, J.; Nishimura, N.; Schaffer, C.B. Diverse Inflammatory Response After Cerebral Microbleeds Includes Coordinated Microglial Migration and Proliferation. *Stroke* **2018**, *49*, 1719–1726. [CrossRef]
30. Menassa, D.A.; Gomez-Nicola, D. Microglial Dynamics During Human Brain Development. *Front. Immunol.* **2018**, *9*, 1014. [CrossRef]
31. Dalmau, I.; Finsen, B.; Tønder, N.; Zimmer, J.; González, B.; Castellano, B. Development of microglia in the prenatal rat hippocampus. *J. Comp. Neurol.* **1997**, *377*, 70–84. [CrossRef]
32. Luo, L.; Chen, D.; Qu, Y.; Wu, J.; Li, X.; Mu, D. Association between hypoxia and perinatal arterial ischemic stroke: A meta-analysis. *PLoS ONE* **2014**, *9*, e90106. [CrossRef]
33. Lee, J.; Croen, L.A.; Backstrand, K.H.; Yoshida, C.K.; Henning, L.H.; Lindan, C.; Ferriero, D.M.; Fullerton, H.J.; Barkovich, A.J.; Wu, Y.W. Maternal and infant characteristics associated with perinatal arterial stroke in the infant. *JAMA* **2005**, *293*, 723–729. [CrossRef]
34. Wu, Y.W.; March, W.M.; Croen, L.A.; Grether, J.K.; Escobar, G.J.; Newman, T.B. Perinatal stroke in children with motor impairment: A population-based study. *Pediatrics* **2004**, *114*, 612–619. [CrossRef]
35. Li, J.; Lamarca, B.; Reckelhoff, J.F. A Model of Pre-eclampsia in Rats: The Reduced Uterine Perfusion Pressure (RUPP) Model. *Am. J. Physiol. Heart Circ. Physiol.* **2012**, *303*, H1–H8.
36. Martinez-Ramirez, S.; Greenberg, S.M.; Viswanathan, A. Cerebral microbleeds: Overview and implications in cognitive impairment. *Alzheimers Res.* **2014**, *6*, 33. [CrossRef]
37. Molvarec, A.; Szarka, A.; Walentin, S.; Beko, G.; Karádi, I.; Prohászka, Z.; Rigó, J. Serum leptin levels in relation to circulating cytokines, chemokines, adhesion molecules and angiogenic factors in normal pregnancy and preeclampsia. *Reprod. Biol. Endocrinol.* **2011**, *9*, 124. [CrossRef]
38. Szarka, A.; Rigó, J.; Lázár, L.; Beko, G.; Molvarec, A. Circulating cytokines, chemokines and adhesion molecules in normal pregnancy and preeclampsia determined by multiplex suspension array. *BMC Immunol.* **2010**, *11*, 59. [CrossRef]
39. Darmochwal-Kolarz, D.; Kludka-Sternik, M.; Tabarkiewicz, J.; Kolarz, B.; Rolinski, J.; Leszczynska-Gorzelak, B.; Oleszczuk, J. The predominance of Th17 lymphocytes and decreased number and function of Treg cells in preeclampsia. *J. Reprod. Immunol.* **2012**, *93*, 75–81. [CrossRef]
40. Toldi, G.; Rigó, J.; Stenczer, B.; Vásárhelyi, B.; Molvarec, A. Increased prevalence of IL-17-producing peripheral blood lymphocytes in pre-eclampsia. *Am. J. Reprod. Immunol.* **2011**, *66*, 223–229. [CrossRef]
41. Martínez-García, E.A.; Chávez-Robles, B.; Sánchez-Hernández, P.E.; Núñez-Atahualpa, L.; Martín-Máquez, B.T.; Muñoz-Gómez, A.; González-López, L.; Gámez-Nava, J.I.; Salazar-Páramo, M.; Dávalos-Rodríguez, I.; et al. IL-17 increased in the third trimester in healthy women with term labor. *Am. J. Reprod. Immunol.* **2011**, *65*, 99–103. [CrossRef]
42. Warrington, J.P. Placental ischemia increases seizure susceptibility and cerebrospinal fluid cytokines. *Physiol. Rep.* **2015**, *3*. [CrossRef]

43. LaMarca, B.B.; Cockrell, K.; Sullivan, E.; Bennett, W.; Granger, J.P. Role of endothelin in mediating tumor necrosis factor-induced hypertension in pregnant rats. *Hypertension* **2005**, *46*, 82–86. [CrossRef]
44. Amash, A.; Holcberg, G.; Sapir, O.; Huleihel, M. Placental secretion of interleukin-1 and interleukin-1 receptor antagonist in preeclampsia: Effect of magnesium sulfate. *J. Interferon Cytokine Res.* **2012**, *32*, 432–441. [CrossRef]
45. Anthony, D.; Dempster, R.; Fearn, S.; Clements, J.; Wells, G.; Perry, V.H.; Walker, K. CXC chemokines generate age-related increases in neutrophil-mediated brain inflammation and blood-brain barrier breakdown. *Curr. Biol.* **1998**, *8*, 923–926. [CrossRef]
46. Miwa, K.; Tanaka, M.; Okazaki, S.; Furukado, S.; Sakaguchi, M.; Kitagawa, K. Relations of blood inflammatory marker levels with cerebral microbleeds. *Stroke* **2011**, *42*, 3202–3206. [CrossRef]
47. Gu, Y.; Gutierrez, J.; Meier, I.B.; Guzman, V.A.; Manly, J.J.; Schupf, N.; Brickman, A.M.; Mayeux, R. Circulating inflammatory biomarkers are related to cerebrovascular disease in older adults. *Neurol. Neuroimmunol. Neuroinflamm.* **2019**, *6*, e521. [CrossRef]
48. Theriault, B.C.; Woo, S.K.; Karimy, J.K.; Keledjian, K.; Stokum, J.A.; Sarkar, A.; Coksaygan, T.; Ivanova, S.; Gerzanich, V.; Simard, J.M. Cerebral microbleeds in a neonatal rat model. *PLoS ONE* **2017**, *12*, e0171163. [CrossRef]
49. Zhang, L.W.; Warrington, J.P. Magnesium Sulfate Prevents Placental Ischemia-Induced Increases in Brain Water Content and Cerebrospinal Fluid Cytokines in Pregnant Rats. *Front. Neurosci.* **2016**, *10*, 561. [CrossRef]
50. Parajuli, B.; Horiuchi, H.; Mizuno, T.; Takeuchi, H.; Suzumura, A. CCL11 enhances excitotoxic neuronal death by producing reactive oxygen species in microglia. *Glia* **2015**, *63*, 2274–2284. [CrossRef]
51. Villeda, S.A.; Luo, J.; Mosher, K.I.; Zou, B.; Britschgi, M.; Bieri, G.; Stan, T.M.; Fainberg, N.; Ding, Z.; Eggel, A.; et al. The ageing systemic milieu negatively regulates neurogenesis and cognitive function. *Nature* **2011**, *477*, 90–94. [CrossRef]
52. Shigemoto-Mogami, Y.; Hoshikawa, K.; Goldman, J.E.; Sekino, Y.; Sato, K. Microglia enhance neurogenesis and oligodendrogenesis in the early postnatal subventricular zone. *J. Neurosci.* **2014**, *34*, 2231–2243. [CrossRef]
53. Xiong, X.Y.; Liu, L.; Yang, Q.W. Functions and mechanisms of microglia/macrophages in neuroinflammation and neurogenesis after stroke. *Prog. Neurobiol.* **2016**, *142*, 23–44. [CrossRef]
54. Fernández-López, D.; Faustino, J.; Klibanov, A.L.; Derugin, N.; Blanchard, E.; Simon, F.; Leib, S.L.; Vexler, Z.S. Microglial Cells Prevent Hemorrhage in Neonatal Focal Arterial Stroke. *J. Neurosci.* **2016**, *36*, 2881–2893. [CrossRef]
55. Thion, M.S.; Ginhoux, F.; Garel, S. Microglia and early brain development: An intimate journey. *Science* **2018**, *362*, 185–189. [CrossRef]

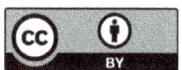

© 2019 by the authors. Licensee MDPI, Basel, Switzerland. This article is an open access article distributed under the terms and conditions of the Creative Commons Attribution (CC BY) license (http://creativecommons.org/licenses/by/4.0/).

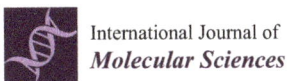

Article

Disturbed Cardiorespiratory Adaptation in Preeclampsia: Return to Normal Stress Regulation Shortly after Delivery?

Helmut K. Lackner [1],*, Ilona Papousek [2], Karin Schmid-Zalaudek [1], Mila Cervar-Zivkovic [3], Vassiliki Kolovetsiou-Kreiner [3], Olivia Nonn [4], Miha Lucovnik [5], Isabella Pfniß [3] and Manfred G. Moertl [6],*

[1] Division of Physiology, Otto Loewi Research Center, Medical University of Graz, 8010 Graz, Austria
[2] Department of Psychology, Biological Psychology Unit, University of Graz, 8010 Graz, Austria
[3] Department of Obstetrics and Gynecology, Medical University of Graz, 8036 Graz, Austria
[4] Division of Cell Biology, Histology and Embryology, Gottfried Schatz Research Center, Medical University of Graz, 8010 Graz, Austria
[5] Department of Perinatology, Division of Obstetrics and Gynecology, University Medical Centre Ljubljana, 1000 Ljubljana, Slovenia
[6] Department of Obstetrics and Gynecology, Clinical Center, 9020 Klagenfurt, Austria
* Correspondence: helmut.lackner@medunigraz.at (H.K.L.); manfred.moertl@kabeg.at (M.G.M.); Tel.: +43-316-385-73863 (H.K.L.); +43-463-538-39603 (M.G.M.)

Received: 27 May 2019; Accepted: 24 June 2019; Published: 27 June 2019

Abstract: Women with pregnancies complicated by preeclampsia appear to be at increased risk of metabolic and vascular diseases in later life. Previous research has also indicated disturbed cardiorespiratory adaptation during pregnancy. The aim of this study was to follow up on the physiological stress response in preeclampsia several weeks postpartum. A standardized laboratory test was used to illustrate potential deviations in the physiological stress responding to mildly stressful events of the kind and intensity in which they regularly occur in further everyday life after pregnancy. Fifteen to seventeen weeks postpartum, 35 women previously affected by preeclampsia (19 mild, 16 severe preeclampsia), 38 women after uncomplicated pregnancies, and 51 age-matched healthy controls were exposed to a self-relevant stressor in a standardized stress-reactivity protocol. Reactivity of blood pressure, heart rate, stroke index, and systemic vascular resistance index as well as baroreceptor sensitivity were analyzed. In addition, the mutual adjustment of blood pressure, heart rate, and respiration, partitioned for influences of the sympathetic and the parasympathetic branches of the autonomic nervous system, were quantified by determining their phase synchronization. Findings indicated moderately elevated blood pressure levels in the nonpathological range, reduced stroke volume, and elevated systemic vascular resistance in women previously affected by preeclampsia. Despite these moderate abnormalities, at the time of testing, women with previous preeclampsia did not differ from the other groups in their physiological response patterns to acute stress. Furthermore, no differences between early, preterm, and term preeclampsia or mild and severe preeclampsia were observed at the time of testing. The findings suggest that the overall cardiovascular responses to moderate stressors return to normal in women who experience a pregnancy with preeclampsia a few weeks after delivery, while the operating point of the arterial baroreflex is readjusted to a higher pressure. Yet, their regulation mechanisms may remain different.

Keywords: pregnancy complications; vagal withdrawal; baroreflex sensitivity; blunted cardiac response; cardiovascular adaptations; autonomic nervous system

1. Introduction

Preeclampsia is a pregnancy-specific disorder characterized by sudden onset of hypertension with either proteinuria or end-organ dysfunction, or both, after the 20th week of gestation in a previously normotensive woman, occurring in 3–5% of pregnancies in industrialized countries [1,2].

The pathogenesis of preeclampsia remains poorly understood, even though preeclampsia has been recognized for at least 100 years [3]. In the last 20 years, multiple theories about the ultimate cause of preeclampsia have been developed with little agreement, except for the conclusion that preeclampsia is a multifactorial disease [4,5].

Many approaches have been developed for predicting preeclampsia at an early stage and promising insights have been discovered [5–8]. Nevertheless, the etiology of preeclampsia remains incompletely understood, although the placenta has been identified as the central organ in the pathogenesis of preeclampsia. Impaired placentation and placental function in early pregnancy remains the leading hypothesis [9–12], while emerging hypotheses focus on the maternal cardiovascular susceptibility to preeclampsia and pregnancy adaptions [13]. Structural and functional cardiovascular changes were found in women 1 year after preeclamptic pregnancies [14], where the involvement of angiogenic factors such as soluble fms-like tyrosine kinase-1 (sFlt-1) and placental growth factor (PlGF) and placental factors such as placental protein 13 (PP13) and the dysbalance thereof may be used to predict severity and long-term cardiovascular complications of preeclampsia [15,16].

While the identification of etiological factors is without doubt an important task, the management of adverse concomitant effects and consequences of preeclampsia may be even more relevant. Women with pregnancies complicated by preeclampsia appear to be at increased risk of metabolic and cardiovascular diseases in later life, and pregnancy complications and coronary heart disease may have common disease mechanisms [17,18]. As cardiovascular disease (CVD) is a leading cause of death, earlier recognition of those at risk seems vital. Therefore, the diagnosis of preeclampsia, or adverse pregnancy more generally, could be an opportunity for the implementation of primary prevention strategies [17,19–21].

Pregnancy is associated with huge cardiovascular and metabolic changes and can be considered as a "stress test" of the somatic and cardiovascular system, suggesting that preeclampsia manifesting in pregnancy is akin to a "failed stress test". "Failing the stress-test", that is, absence of the typical autonomically regulated cardiovascular and cardiorespiratory adaptations to pregnancy, may be predictive of cardiovascular disorders in later life, when the system is put under similar strain [21,22].

The autonomic nervous system plays a central role in cardiovascular and cardiorespiratory adaptation to pregnancy-related hemodynamic changes [23–25]. Previous research has shown that the increases in peripheral vascular resistance and blood pressure that characterize preeclampsia are mediated, at least in part, by a substantial increase in sympathetic vasoconstrictor activity [26,27]. Autonomic nervous system functioning during pregnancy can be noninvasively assessed by analyzing continuous measures of cardiovascular variables, baroreceptor reflex sensitivity (BRS), and the mutual adjustment of blood pressure, heart rate, and respiration, partitioned for influences of the sympathetic and the parasympathetic branch of the autonomic nervous system [28–31]. Now, if we can determine abnormalities in blood pressure regulation in affected women at a time at which their preeclampsia is no longer present by definition (i.e., from 12 weeks after delivery onwards) by use of a simple and time-efficient test in the laboratory, this test may be used to evaluate the effectiveness of pharmacological or behavioral interventions for reducing affected women's cardiovascular risk. Therefore, the aim of this study was to follow up on the regulation of the physiological response to everyday stressful events in preeclampsia several weeks postpartum.

2. Results

2.1. Cardiovascular and Hemodynamic Variables

The groups differed in their blood pressure levels and related variables at rest (baseline; mean arterial pressure (MAP), $F(2,121) = 5.1$, $p < 0.01$; systolic blood pressure (SBP), $F(2,121) = 3.1$, $p < 0.05$; diastolic blood pressure (DBP), $F(2,121) = 4.7$, $p < 0.05$, stroke index ($F(2,121) = 6.1$, $p < 0.01$), systemic vascular resistance index (SVRI), $F(2,121) = 7.3$, $p < 0.01$). Bonferroni-corrected post-hoc tests indicated moderately elevated blood pressure levels in the nonpathological range, reduced stroke volume, and elevated systemic vascular resistance in women previously affected by preeclampsia. Group means can be obtained from Table 1.

Table 1. Hemodynamic variables (mean ± SD) of participants, and statistical results for group differences in response to the stress manipulation. CO: women without gestation during the last three years; UP: women with uncomplicated pregnancies; PE: women with a history of preeclampsia; BP: blood pressure; SVRI: systemic vascular resistance index.

	Baseline	Anticipation	Task	Post-Task	F-Statistics	
Mean Arterial BP (mmHg)						
CO	86.9 ± 9.4	89.7 ± 9.7	94.8 ± 10.5	90.3 ± 9.3	period	$F_{(1.7,207.2)} = 2.3$, $p = 0.108$
UP	84.9 ± 8.4	87.0 ± 8.5	94.0 ± 9.4	89.5 ± 8.2	period x group	$F_{(3.5,207.2)} = 1.7$, $p = 0.149$
PE	91.6 ± 10.0	92.7 ± 8.9	100.1 ± 10.7	95.5 ± 9.0		
Systolic BP (mmHg)						
CO	109.3 ± 11.0	112.8 ± 11.8	119.1 ± 12.7	113.3 ± 12.0	period	$F_{(1.2,200.7)} = 1.2$, $p = 0.307$
UP	107.0 ± 9.6	109.6 ± 10.2	118.7 ± 12.0	112.2 ± 9.5	period x group	$F_{(3.5,200.7)} = 1.4$, $p = 0.243$
PE	113.3 ± 11.8	115.2 ± 10.5	123.7 ± 12.6	118.2 ± 11.1		
Diastolic BP (mmHg)						
CO	70.9 ± 9.1	73.3 ± 8.8	77.5 ± 9.8	73.8 ± 8.5	period	$F_{(1.8,216.8)} = 3.5$, $p < 0.05$
UP	69.0 ± 8.2	71.2 ± 7.9	76.8 ± 8.6	73.2 ± 7.6	period x group	$F_{(3.6,216.8)} = 1.9$, $p = 0.124$
PE	75.4 ± 9.8	76.1 ± 8.9	82.6 ± 10.5	78.8 ± 8.3		
Heart Rate (bpm)						
CO	71.0 ± 10.9	73.6 ± 12.0	83.9 ± 15.0	72.1 ± 10.9	period	$F_{(1.3,153.2)} = 1.6$, $p = 0.208$
UP	72.6 ± 7.6	74.2 ± 8.8	83.5 ± 10.5	75.5 ± 8.7	period x group	$F_{(2.6,153.2)} = 5.5$, $p < 0.01$
PE	72.4 ± 9.3	74.5 ± 9.5	80.7 ± 11.7	74.9 ± 9.9		
Stroke Index (mL/m^2)						
CO	43.0 ± 8.9	42.9 ± 8.6	42.4 ± 9.4	42.6 ± 8.2	period	$F_{(1.8,218.0)} = 1.7$, $p = 0.183$
UP	41.6 ± 6.4	41.1 ± 6.2	40.0 ± 6.2	40.1 ± 6.5	period x group	$F_{(3.6,218.0)} = 0.8$, $p = 0.489$
PE	38.2 ± 7.0	37.7 ± 7.0	37.3 ± 7.1	37.2 ± 6.9		
SVRI (dyn·s·m^2/cm^5)						
CO	2267 ± 541	2325 ± 548	2223 ± 589	2400 ± 561	period	$F_{(1.7,208.9)} = 2.3$, $p = 0.438$
UP	2251 ± 514	2292 ± 506	2292 ± 524	2377 ± 534	period x group	$F_{(3.5,208.9)} = 1.7$, $p < 0.05$
PE	2692 ± 650	2680 ± 614	2743 ± 660	2788 ± 625		

The analyses of group differences in the time course of cardiovascular changes across the stress manipulation revealed differences between groups in changes of heart rate and systemic vascular resistance (significant interactions period x group). The different time courses are illustrated in Figure 1 (heart rate) and Figure 2 (SVRI). While women without previous pregnancy showed the typical pattern of activation and recovery, women with uncomplicated pregnancies and, even more so, women with former preeclampsia showed blunted responses during the memory task. No significant differences were found for stress-induced changes in blood pressure variables and stroke index. Details of the statistical findings can be found in Table 1.

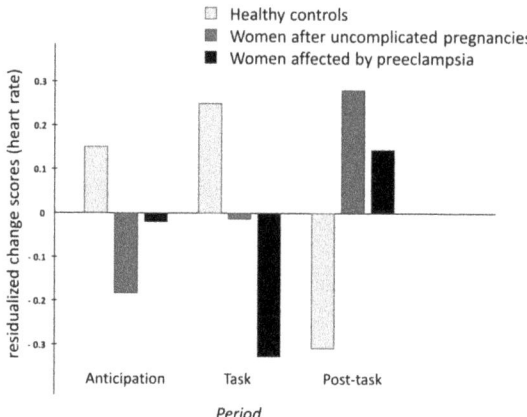

Figure 1. Barplot of the standardized residualized change scores for heart rate (HR).

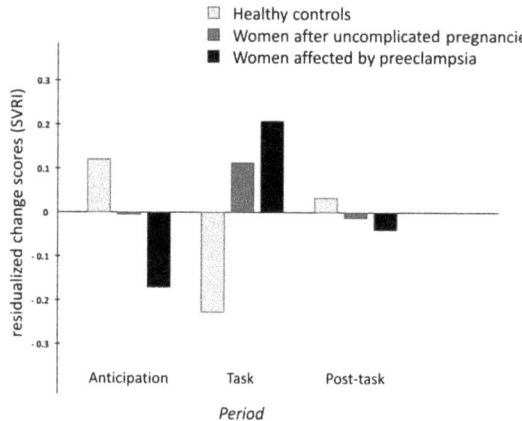

Figure 2. Barplot of the standardized residualized change scores for the systemic vascular resistance index (SVRI).

Women with mild vs. severe preeclampsia did not differ in HR and SVRI levels in resting conditions (baseline; all p values >0.504), and no differences were seen among women with early preeclampsia (<34 weeks), preterm preeclampsia (<37 weeks), and women with term preeclampsia (baseline; all p values >0.185) Neither did the time courses of changes across the stress manipulation differ between women with mild vs. severe preeclampsia (period x PE-group, all p values >0.123; period, all p values >0.191), nor were differences seen between early, preterm, and term preeclampsia (period x PE-time, all p values >0.221; period, all p values >0.144).

2.2. Respiration Rate and Baroreflex Sensitivity

The three groups did not differ in respiration rate ($F(2,121) = 2.3$, $p = 0.107$) and BRS ($F(2,121) = 0.7$, $p = 0.501$) in resting conditions (baseline). Changes of respiration rate and baroreflex sensitivity across the stress manipulation did not differ between groups (interactions period x group not significant; for details, see Table 2).

Table 2. Respiration rate and baroreflex sensitivity (mean ± SD) of participants, and statistical results for group differences in response to the stress manipulation. CO: women without gestation during the last three years; UP: women with uncomplicated pregnancies; PE: women with a history of preeclampsia.

	Baseline	Anticipation	Task	Post-Task	F-Statistics	
	Respiration Rate (breath/min)					
CO	14.7 ± 3.8	14.9 ± 3.5	17.4 ± 3.3	15.4 ± 4.1	period	$F_{(1.7, 205.9)} = 14.3, p < 0.001$
UP	15.9 ± 3.2	16.4 ± 2.5	18.0 ± 2.8	16.0 ± 2.8	period x group	$F_{(3.4, 205.9)} = 0.7, p = 0.565$
PE	16.4 ± 4.2	16.4 ± 2.6	17.8 ± 2.4	16.2 ± 2.6		
	Baroreflex Sensitivity (ms/mmHg)					
CO	14.4 ± 4.0	14.1 ± 3.8	11.9 ± 3.4	13.4 ± 3.8	period	$F_{(2, 240)} = 1.7, p = 0.177$
UP	13.4 ± 4.0	12.6 ± 3.1	11.8 ± 2.7	12.3 ± 3.2	period x group	$F_{(4, 240)} = 2.1, p = 0.088$
PE	14.0 ± 4.0	13.3 ± 3.4	11.7 ± 2.9	12.2 ± 4.2		

Respiration rate and BRS at rest did not differ between women with mild vs. severe preeclampsia, nor for women with early, preterm, or term preeclampsia (baseline; all p values >0.332 and all p values >0.665, respectively). Differences between mild and severe preeclampsia in the time courses of changes across the stress manipulation were also nonsignificant (interaction period x PE-group, all p values >0.317; main effect period, respiration rate: $(F(1.5, 49.0) = 6.0, p < 0.01$; BRS: $(F(2, 64) = 4.3, p < 0.05))$. Differences between early, preterm, and term preeclampsia in the time courses of changes across the stress manipulation were also nonsignificant (interaction period x PE-time, all p values >0.330; main effect period, respiration rate: $(F(1.6, 48.6) = 5.5, p < 0.05$; BRS: $(F(2, 62) = 4.6, p < 0.05))$.

2.3. Adjustment of Blood Pressure, R–R Intervals, and Respiration

2.3.1. Low-Frequency Components

The adjustment of blood pressure and R–R intervals (the interval between consecutive heart beats; RRI) in the low-frequency domain mainly represents the sympathetically modulated mutual interrelation between the two. There were no group differences in resting levels of the synchronization variables $\gamma_{SBPxRRI,LF}$, $\gamma_{DBPxRRI,LF}$, and $\gamma_{SBPxDBP,LF}$ (baseline; $F(2, 121) = 0.8, p = 0.461$; $F(2, 121) = 0.7, p = 0.516$; $F(2, 121) = 0.6, p = 0.567$). Furthermore, the groups did not differ in their stress responses in these variables (Table 3).

Table 3. Phase synchronization indices of the low-frequency (LF) components (mean ± SD) of participants, and statistical results for group differences in response to the stress manipulation. CO: women without gestation during the last three years; UP: women with uncomplicated pregnancies; PE: women with a history of preeclampsia; γ: synchronization index; SBP: systolic blood pressure, DBP: diastolic blood pressure; RRI: R–R intervals.

	Baseline	Anticipation	Task	Post-Task	F-Statistics	
	$\gamma_{SBPxRRI,LF}$ (–)					
CO	0.41 ± 0.21	0.48 ± 0.18	0.34 ± 0.13	0.41 ± 0.19	period	$F_{(2, 240)} = 0.4, p = 0.675$
UP	0.39 ± 0.17	0.41 ± 0.18	0.37 ± 0.15	0.42 ± 0.18	period x group	$F_{(4, 240)} = 2.3, p = 0.058$
PE	0.36 ± 0.17	0.39 ± 0.16	0.37 ± 0.16	0.38 ± 0.16		
	$\gamma_{DBPxRRI,LF}$ (–)					
CO	0.40 ± 0.19	0.45 ± 0.17	0.32 ± 0.13	0.40 ± 0.17	period	$F_{(2, 240)} = 0.2, p = 0.821$
UP	0.38 ± 0.15	0.38 ± 0.15	0.32 ± 0.13	0.40 ± 0.15	period x group	$F_{(4, 240)} = 1.0, p = 0.428$
PE	0.36 ± 0.15	0.40 ± 0.16	0.31 ± 0.16	0.36 ± 0.14		
	$\gamma_{SBPxDBP,LF}$ (–)					
CO	0.75 ± 0.13	0.79 ± 0.11	0.73 ± 0.13	0.75 ± 0.12	period	$F_{(1.9, 226.3)} = 0.7, p = 0.481$
UP	0.79 ± 0.12	0.78 ± 0.14	0.70 ± 0.17	0.78 ± 0.12	period x group	$F_{(3.8, 226.3)} = 1.7, p = 0.219$
PE	0.75 ± 0.13	0.79 ± 0.11	0.68 ± 0.15	0.74 ± 0.12		

Women with mild vs. severe preeclampsia did not differ in these variables (baseline, all p values >0.768; period x PE-group, all p values >0.271; period, all p values >0.446). No significant results were seen for women with early, preterm, and term preeclampsia (baseline, all p values >0.460; period x PE-time, all p values >0.098; period, all p values >0.591) either.

2.3.2. High-Frequency Components

The adjustment of blood pressure, R–R intervals, and respiration in the high-frequency domain represents the parasympathetically modulated mutual interrelations. In resting conditions, the groups did not differ in the synchronization variables $\gamma_{SBPxRRI,HF}$, $\gamma_{DBPxRRI,HF}$, $\gamma_{RESPxRRI,HF}$, $\gamma_{RESPxSBP,HF}$, and $\gamma_{RESPxDBP,LF}$ (baseline, $F(2,121) = 0.9$, $p = 0.43$; $F(2,121) = 0.5$, $p = 0.624$; $F(2,121) = 0.1$, $p = 0.917$, $F(2,121) = 0.2$, $p = 0.795$; $F(2,121) = 0.7$, $p = 0.523$). No significant differences were observed in the changes of these variables during the stress manipulation (Table 4). However, some statistical trends emerged for the adjustment of respiration and blood pressure, which seemed to be attributed to the women affected by preeclampsia.

Table 4. Phase synchronization indices of the high-frequency (HF) components (mean ± SD) of participants, and statistical results for group differences in response to the stress manipulation. CO: women without gestation during the last three years; UP: women with uncomplicated pregnancies; PE: women with a history of preeclampsia; γ: synchronization index; SBP: systolic blood pressure, DBP: diastolic blood pressure; RRI: R–R intervals; RESP: respiration.

	Baseline	Anticipation	Task	Post-Task	F-Statistics	
	$\gamma_{SBPxRRI,HF}$ (−)					
CO	0.60 ± 0.19	0.50 ± 0.20	0.33 ± 0.17	0.50 ± 0.25	period	$F_{(2,240)} = 0.6, p = 0.550$
UP	0.63 ± 0.22	0.52 ± 0.21	0.33 ± 0.15	0.52 ± 0.22	period x group	$F_{(4,240)} = 1.0, p = 0.408$
PE	0.66 ± 0.17	0.53 ± 0.19	0.29 ± 0.13	0.54 ± 0.20		
	$\gamma_{DBPxRRI,HF}$ (−)					
CO	0.40 ± 0.26	0.37 ± 0.20	0.29 ± 0.12	0.36 ± 0.23	period	$F_{(2,240)} = 8.4, p < 0.001$
UP	0.36 ± 0.22	0.30 ± 0.20	0.29 ± 0.15	0.33 ± 0.17	period x group	$F_{(4,240)} = 1.3, p = 0.258$
PE	0.37 ± 0.21	0.31 ± 0.21	0.22 ± 0.13	0.31 ± 0.20		
	$\gamma_{RESPxRRI,HF}$ (−)					
CO	0.71 ± 0.19	0.62 ± 0.18	0.39 ± 0.19	0.62 ± 0.22	period	$F_{(2,240)} = 0.5, p = 0.591$
UP	0.69 ± 0.22	0.57 ± 0.20	0.33 ± 0.18	0.55 ± 0.26	period x group	$F_{(4,240)} = 0.5, p = 0.736$
PE	0.70 ± 0.23	0.57 ± 0.25	0.32 ± 0.18	0.58 ± 0.22		
	$\gamma_{RESPxSBP,HF}$ (−)					
CO	0.67 ± 0.22	0.55 ± 0.20	0.30 ± 0.18	0.58 ± 0.24	period	$F_{(1.9,223.4)} = 1.1, p = 0.342$
UP	0.70 ± 0.22	0.58 ± 0.19	0.27 ± 0.16	0.53 ± 0.26	period x group	$F_{(3.7,223.4)} = 2.2, p = 0.080$
PE	0.68 ± 0.23	0.54 ± 0.24	0.22 ± 0.15	0.57 ± 0.25		
	$\gamma_{RESPxDBP,HF}$ (−)					
CO	0.33 ± 0.25	0.26 ± 0.18	0.18 ± 0.13	0.24 ± 0.19	period	$F_{(2,240)} = 3.0, p = 0.053$
UP	0.33 ± 0.20	0.24 ± 0.15	0.17 ± 0.12	0.24 ± 0.16	period x group	$F_{(4,240)} = 2.2, p = 0.065$
PE	0.28 ± 0.18	0.20 ± 0.19	0.11 ± 0.09	0.24 ± 0.19		

Women with mild vs. severe preeclampsia did not differ in these variables (baseline, all p values >0.199; period x PE-group, all p values >0.712 except for adjustment of respiration and R–R intervals, $p = 0.084$, and for respiration and systolic blood pressure, $p = 0.100$; period, all p values >0.199). Women with early, preterm, and term preeclampsia did not differ in these variables (baseline, all p values >0.649; period x PE-time, all p values > 0.162; period, all p values > 0.571).

2.4. Supplementary Analyses

No differences in chronic stress experience were seen between women with a history of preeclampsia (PE), women with uncomplicated pregnancies (UP), and age-matched women without gestation (CO) ($F(2,121) = 0.7, p = 0.507$). The rating of how difficult and how stressful the participants had perceived the task to be showed no differences between the groups (difficult, $F(2,211) = 0.1$, $p = 0.932$; stressful, $F(2,211) = 0.2, p = 0.802$). Furthermore, no differences in depressive symptoms were seen ($F(2,121) = 0.2, p = 0.784$).

3. Discussion

The results of the present study showed that the short-term blood pressure regulation in women previously affected by preeclampsia returns to normal several weeks postpartum. However, heart rate and systemic vascular resistance responses in women previously affected by preeclampsia indicated impaired ability to flexibly respond to moderate stress; this indicates that their overarching regulation mechanisms may be altered after all.

In the healthy organism, physiological mechanisms of blood pressure regulation maintain the arterial blood pressure at a largely constant level even in stressful conditions, ensuring adequate tissue perfusion throughout. However, the intense hemodynamic modifications during pregnancy result in a decrease of baroreceptor sensitivity; this is even more pronounced in preeclampsia, and it jeopardizes the proper adjustment of the physiological factors regulating the arterial blood pressure [29,32]. Impaired baroreceptor sensitivity can still be observed after pregnancy, depending on the time since delivery. Walther et al. reported reduced baroreflex sensitivity four days after delivery and concluded that the maternal cardiovascular system is still affected by pregnancy at that time [33]. With greater distance since delivery, BRS returns to levels recorded at the beginning of pregnancy [28,34]. The present findings indicate that this similarly applies to women who have had preeclampsia. Fifteen to seventeen weeks after delivery, the BRS of women with pregnancies complicated by preeclampsia did not differ from that of mothers with uncomplicated pregnancies, and neither did it differ from the BRS of women who did not give birth. Thus, persistently impaired BRS does not seem to explain the increased cardiovascular risk in later life of women who have had preeclampsia.

The assessment of BRS provides some indication of the regulatory activity of the autonomic nervous system in stressful conditions, but for more specific information, more profound analysis of the regulating factors is required. Important additional information is provided by more fine-grained analysis of the variations of the state of the complex regulatory system over time. Phase synchronization indexes, which indicate mutual adjustments of blood pressure, R–R intervals, and respiration across time, supply this information [35,36]. However, in the present study, mutual adjustment of the mainly sympathetically modulated low-frequency variations of heart rate and systolic blood pressure did not differ between groups, thus basically confirming the findings obtained from the BRS.

Nevertheless, the conclusion that blood pressure regulation has entirely returned to normal several weeks postpartum is still premature. From the mathematical approach for the estimation of BRS alone, it follows that baroreceptor sensitivity decreases with increasing levels of heart rate. While some heart rate acceleration during demanding conditions is adaptive, not all individuals may show this adaptation to the same extent. In other words, it is vital to also consider the contributing factors when interpreting the presence or absence of differences in baroreceptor sensitivity between groups (i.e., heart rate, stroke volume, and systemic vascular resistance).

To maintain a constant arterial blood pressure—the primary regulated variable in stressful situations—increases of heart rate (or stroke volume) must be compensated by decreased vascular resistance in line with the fundamental Darcy's law (or Ohm's law) of hemodynamics. In preeclamptic women, factors such as PP13, responsible for vasodilation and decreased vascular resistance, are reduced early in gestation [37]. Their dysregulation may thus not only be involved in endothelial dysfunction during pregnancy, but markers such as PlGF and sFlt-1 may also function as predictors for long-term cardiovascular health [38]. Later in pregnancy, PP13 is massively increased and returns to basal levels within two weeks in healthy women, while it takes more than eight weeks until it returns to normal levels in women who experienced preeclampsia [39]. Since the effects of PP13 last even after its disappearance, PP13 might still influence the maternal vascular system months after pregnancy [37]. Maybe only then do the true effects of preeclampsia on the maternal system become obvious.

In the present study, heart rate markedly increased and vascular resistance decreased accordingly in response to the stress manipulation only in women without previous pregnancy. By contrast, women who were pregnant, and in particular women with former preeclampsia, hardly showed any heart rate responses at all. Hence, in women recovering from preeclampsia, there was no necessity for short-term blood pressure regulation via activation of baroreceptors and subsequent adaptation of vascular resistance. From this, it follows that the similar outcomes in healthy women and women with preeclampsia in terms of baroreceptor sensitivity and maintenance of largely constant arterial blood pressure levels during brief periods of stress do not justify the conclusion that blood pressure regulation is unimpaired after preeclampsia. Instead, it appears to be that blunted cardiac responses in affected women did not make blood pressure regulation necessary to the same extent as in healthy women.

In women without previous pregnancy, the flexible cardiac response to the active performance task, which provides adaptive energy mobilization and oxygen supply, indicates proper functioning of their autonomic nervous system-mediated cardiovascular regulation [40]. In contrast, the blunted heart rate response in women previously affected by preeclampsia may be related to their generally elevated levels of systemic vascular resistance, and the more rigid vasoadaptation associated with this. This idea is fueled by the elevated systemic vascular resistance levels in women with a history of preeclampsia observed at baseline, which is in line with previous research [41].

Various proinflammatory factors, such as TNF-alpha, IL-10, IL-6, leptin, and CX3CL1, are elevated in preeclamptic women [42–44] and are also known to mediate cardiovascular remodeling outside of pregnancy, in crosstalk with reactive oxygen species, angiotensin II, and other proinflammatory cytokines [45–49]. In pregnancy, vascular remodeling may also be induced by an elevated maternal inflammatory profile. TNF-alpha induces collagen I deposition in the maternal vasculature, and MMP1 and -7 activity induce extracellular matrix degradation [50], while CYP2J2, elevated in preeclampsia, may also be involved in uteroplacental and vascular remodeling [51].

Thus, the blunted cardiac responses in women with former preeclampsia may arise from an attempt by the organism to protect itself against undue elevations of arterial blood pressure, which would occur as a result of the failure to lower the systemic vascular resistance synchronously with the rising heart rate (and/or stroke volume). With more severe stress as well as in later life when, due to normal aging alone, vasoadaptation becomes even more rigid, this compensatory mechanism may not suffice to prevent harmful elevations of blood pressure. One factor that may account for basally elevated levels of systemic vascular resistance in preeclampsia is the influence of endothelium-derived vasoconstrictors [20], which are linked to endothelial dysfunction and may be key components in the etiology of preeclampsia [52,53]. Impaired endothelial nitric oxide synthase (eNOS) function and decreased NO action, and on the other hand, overrepresentation of inflammatory and antiangiogenic factors, contribute to a preeclamptic phenotype. Restoring this balance is currently in focus for new therapeutic approaches such as capturing or silencing sFLt-1, and although still inconclusive, evidence also shows that the NO donor and vasodilator pentaerythritol tetranitrate (PETN) reduces the incidence of preeclampsia in a high-risk study population [54–56]. The vasoconstrictor angiotensin II mediates stimulation of factors such as human placental lactogen and sFlt-1, as well as transcription of inflammatory cytokines through angiotensin II type 1 receptor activation (AT1R) [57,58]. Increased agonistic autoantibodies against AT1R (AT1-AA) in preeclampsia [59,60] also contribute to AT1R activation, whereas AT1-AA blockade was shown to reduce preeclamptic symptoms in rats [61]. Other endothelium-derived factors promote monocyte adhesion and migration by monocyte chemotactic protein-1 (MCP-1) and intercellular adhesion molecule-1 (ICAM-1) expression, for example, contributing to vascular inflammation [62]. Hypertension-induced shear stress can induce endothelium-derived vasoconstrictors such as endothelin-1 and angiotensin II [63,64]. These do not only regulate the vascular tone, but also vascular smooth muscle cell (VSMC) growth and migration into the intima [65,66], where they proliferate in response to cytokines and growth factors such as platelet-derived growth factor (PDGF) [67]. Angiotensin II, endothelin-1, and other cytokines lead to VSMC dedifferentiation to a migratory proliferative type that is fundamental to vascular pathogenesis and remodeling [65,68], which eventually leads to collagen and elastin deposition by VSMCs into the intima and increased vascular rigidity [69].

When looking more closely at the contribution of the autonomic nervous system, it is important to note that scientists primarily focus on sympathetic nervous system control, although parasympathetic regulation appears to play an important role in pregnancy [70]. Moreover, as heart rate levels remain below the intrinsic heart rate, moderate active performance stressors such as the one used in the present study primarily trigger parasympathetically mediated cardiorespiratory adaptation, i.e., fast vagal withdrawal [29,35]. Another plausible explanation for the blunted heart rate responses to stress in women with former preeclampsia is impaired adaptation to changing demands through vagal withdrawal, brought about by subordinate functioning of the parasympathetic branch of the autonomic nervous system. This notion is corroborated by the present finding that the mutual adjustments of respiration and heart rate as well as the mutual adjustments of respiration and blood pressure during the stress manipulation tended to be lower in women with previous preeclampsia compared to healthy women. In line with that, previous research has shown that sympathetically mediated regulation prevails during pregnancy, and it has been suggested that impaired parasympathetic regulation along with sympathetic overactivity may contribute to the pathophysiology of preeclampsia [23,26,71].

Taken together, arterial blood pressure was maintained at a largely constant level throughout the stress manipulation in healthy women as well as in women with history of preeclampsia; however, different reasons seemed to have accounted for this outcome.

No differences were observed between women with severe compared to mild preeclampsia. However, while severity of preeclampsia was defined in the current study by recommended criteria, these criteria used to differentiate severe from mild preeclampsia are currently a subject of debate [12]. A further limitation may be that on average, women with preeclampsia had greater body mass, which is an important determinant of cardiovascular function. However, it should be noted that stroke volume and systemic vascular resistance were calculated relative to body surface area, thus mitigating the potential confoundment, and results remained unchanged if the variables were adjusted for body mass index (BMI). Nevertheless, possible effects of body mass cannot be completely ruled out. On the other hand, body mass did not differ between women with preeclampsia and women with uncomplicated pregnancies. The groups did not differ in parity either, which may also impact the development of blood pressure in later life [72]. In addition, the fact that we have no information about the women's stress responses in the time before they became pregnant and the relatively small sample size should also be considered as important limitations of this study. As the risk factors for preeclampsia are the same as those predisposing to cardiovascular disease and might have the same effect on stress responses, problems may already precede pregnancy and then persist after delivery. The latter to some extent limits the interpretation of the analysis, especially within the women with preeclampsia. Due to the relatively small sample size, some analyses are at the lower limit with regard to the statistical power, in particular those analyzing differences between subtypes of preeclampsia. We hope that reporting these results nevertheless may encourage other researchers to use similar methods in larger cohorts of women with former preeclampsia, while separating women according to the subtypes of preeclampsia. Furthermore, there are a variety of excellent methods for the description of important metabolic and vascular changes during pregnancy and beyond which the present study did not include. Lack of such variables without doubt limits the overall explanatory power of the study. However, the point of the present study was to introduce a different approach that represents a novel addition to these metabolic and vascular variables. The approach of the present study provides new and additional information that is not easily gained from metabolic and vascular variables, particularly with regard to the functionality of the neuro-regulation of cardiovascular adaptation on a short-term basis.

Recent longitudinal assessment of preeclampsia has suggested masked hypertension at 12 weeks postpartum [73]. In line with this observation, the present findings indicated moderately elevated blood pressure levels in women who were previously affected by preeclampsia. This suggests that the operating point of the arterial baroreflex may remain readjusted to a (slightly) higher pressure several weeks after delivery, although all blood pressure levels in the present study were in the nonpathological range. More importantly, the present study highlights that the identification of altered regulation mechanisms and impaired functioning of specific elements of the cardiovascular regulatory circuit in women with history of preeclampsia may be of greater scientific and finally clinical prognostic value than the monitoring of blood pressure levels and baroreceptor functioning alone. As preeclampsia has become a well-recognized risk factor for life-threatening cardiovascular complications in later life, several attempts have been made to include obstetric history in routine screening of cardiovascular risk. In the future, standardized stress response testing may significantly add to the identification of risk. Given the relatively novel stress parameters evaluated here, it appears that according to such novel lab testing to evaluate increased risk of developing cardiovascular complications (with or without relevant symptoms for metabolic syndrome), the risk is not clearly established early after delivery in women who experience preeclampsia during their pregnancy. Further studies are warranted to verify these findings and also to identify when such stress measures tested here become indicative of future cardiovascular complications for women who experienced preeclampsia. Finally, to date, very little guidance exists on the use of tailored prevention strategies in women with history of preeclampsia.

4. Materials and Methods

4.1. Participants

The study sample included 35 women with a history of preeclampsia (PE), 38 women with uncomplicated pregnancies (UP), and 51 age-matched women without gestation during the last three years (CO). Women with preceding pregnancy (PE and UP groups) were asked to participate in the study 13–15 weeks postpartum and were tested 15–17 weeks after delivery.

For twenty-one women with an uncomplicated pregnancy (UP), it was their first child (while in PE, $n = 22$); for 14, it was their second child (in PE, $n = 10$); for two, it was their third child (in PE, $n = 3$); and for one woman, it was her fourth child. Parity did not differ between women with uncomplicated pregnancies and women with a history of preeclampsia ($\chi^2 = 1.9$, $p = 0.59$). Of the 35 PE pregnancies, 19 were diagnosed with mild PE and 16 had symptoms of severe PE. In 6 PE pregnancies, gestation was terminated before 34 weeks (early PE), between weeks 34 and 37 (preterm preeclampsia) in 14 PE pregnancies, and 15 children were delivered after 37 weeks (term PE). One woman with a history of preeclampsia, two women with uncomplicated pregnancies, and 15 women without gestation were smokers. All women were of Caucasian ethnicity. Characteristics of the study sample are presented in Table 5.

Table 5. Characteristics of the participants (mean ± SD, range), and statistical differences.

	PE ($n = 35$)	UP ($n = 38$)	CO ($n = 51$)	p-Value
Age (years)	33.7 ± 4.8, 25–42	32.4 ± 4.0, 26–44	32.4 ± 5.3, 25–44	$p = 0.41$
Height (cm)	168.2 ± 6.8, 153–182	167.5 ± 5.8, 157.5–179	168.4 ± 5.6, 156–180	$p = 0.78$
Weight (kg)	77.9 ± 15.7 [3], 48.9–121.9	68.7 ± 11.5, 49.1–97.7	65.3 ± 10.5 [1], 45–93	$p < 0.001$
BMI (kg/m^2)	27.8 ± 5.9 [2,3], 20.7–44.2	24.6 ± 4.6 [1], 17–36.3	23.0 ± 3.2 [1], 16.9–30.9	$p < 0.001$
Delivery (day)	253 ± 21, 197–287	278 ± 10, 254–291	–	$p < 0.001$
Baby height (cm)	46.9 ± 5.1, 31–57	51.3 ± 1.8, 47–56	–	$p < 0.001$
Baby weight (g)	2568 ± 853, 800–3940	3404 ± 341, 2780–4010	–	$p < 0.001$

[1,2,3] Denotes a significant difference between PE ([1]), UP ([2]), and CO ([3]) based on Bonferroni-corrected post-hoc tests. BMI: body mass index.

Preeclampsia was confirmed using the recommendations of the American College of Obstetricians and Gynecologists Task Force on Hypertension in Pregnancy (2013) [74]. Inclusion criteria were: Systolic blood pressure ≥140 mmHg and/or diastolic blood pressure ≥90 mmHg, presenting at ≥20 weeks gestation and returning to normotensive values within 12 weeks postpartum, blood pressure measured twice and at least 4 h apart. Proteinuria: either protein ≥300 mg per 24 h urine collection, or protein/creatinine ratio ≥0.3, or protein ≥30 mg/dL or 1+ on urine dipstick. Severe preeclampsia was confirmed in the same way as preeclampsia, as defined above, except one of the following had to be present and proteinuria was not required: (1) systolic blood pressure ≥160 mmHg, measured twice at least 15 min apart; (2) diastolic blood pressure ≥110 mmHg, measured twice at least 15 min apart; (3) thrombocytopenia: platelet count <100,000/microliter; (4) impaired liver function: AST or ALT

≥70 units/L or twice the normal concentration; (5) renal insufficiency: serum creatinine ≥1.1 mg/dL or doubled from baseline values; (6) pulmonary edema; or (7) symptoms indicating possible cerebral or neurologic involvement: headache or visual changes (e.g., flashing, blurring, visual loss, blindness). Participants with uncomplicated pregnancies had singleton pregnancies with term delivery. Exclusion criteria in both groups with preceding pregnancy and the age-matched women without gestation were: diabetes mellitus, renal disease, chronic hypertension, antiphospholipid antibody syndrome, kidney transplant, hypothyroidism, thyroid antibodies, pre-existing cardiovascular problems, and seizures. Women with multiple gestations or substance abuse (alcohol, tobacco, illegal drugs) were also excluded.

Written informed consent was provided for all participants included in the study. The study was approved by the authorized ethics committee, Medical University Graz, Austria (No. 27-515 ex 14/15, *Pregnancy complications: challenge and/or chance for further cardiovascular risk in later life?*, date of approval: 14 September 2015) and the Ethics committee Carinthia, Austria (No. A16/15, *Pregnancy complications: challenge and/or chance for further cardiovascular risk in later life?*, date of approval: 10 September 2015)

4.2. Experimental Procedure

The experiment started with an approximately 30 min period in which the participating women could adapt and settle down. In this period, general questions were asked, electrodes were attached, and the electrophysiological signals were checked. The fully automated study protocol including highly synchronously transmitted physiological signals started with the perceived stress questionnaire, to measure chronic stress experience, and the depression scale (CES-D), as well as some other questionnaires that are not relevant to this paper [75,76]. After a 5 min resting period in which the participants were asked to remain seated, not to speak, and to relax, the memory task was explained using a prerecorded auditory instruction backed by corresponding information on a computer screen. To increase the self-relevance of the task and hence its stressful character, participants were told that their test performance would be evaluated by colleagues from the psychiatry department who would determine whether their mnemonic abilities corresponded to their age or if they indicated premature aging of the brain. The task was to recall as many words as they could from a list of words taken from a standardized memory test [77]. After the participants had confirmed that they had understood the instruction, the memory task was provided in a fully automated manner. Following completion of the memory task, there was another 5 min relaxation period, and participants subsequently rated how difficult and how stressful they had perceived the task to be, on two 17-point rating scales (ranging from "not difficult at all" to "extremely difficult" and from "not stressful at all" to "extremely stressful" [78–80]. Participants remained seated during the entire study protocol.

4.3. Data Acquisition and Preprocessing

Continuous hemodynamic monitoring of blood pressure (BP), heart rate (HR), and thoracic impedance was carried out with the Task Force Monitor® (TFM®; CNSystems, Graz, Austria) throughout the entire test procedure. HR (3-lead electrocardiography; sampling rate = 1 kHz) and thoracic impedance (sampling rate = 50 Hz) were recorded using specific CNSystems electrodes placed at the neck and the thoracic region, the latter specifically at the midclavicular line at the xiphoid process level. Continuous BP (sampling rate = 100 Hz) was derived from the finger using a refined version of the vascular unloading technique and corrected to absolute values with oscillometric BP measurement on the contralateral upper arm [81]. For analyzing the cardiovascular regulation, software-tools developed in MATLAB® (MathWorks, Natick, MA, USA) were used [29,82].

To obtain R–R intervals (RRI) and blood pressure time series with equidistant time steps, the beat-to-beat values were resampled at 4 Hz, using piecewise cubic spline interpolation after semiautomatic artifact correction. Single artifacts were replaced by interpolation [82]. Furthermore, the respiratory signal was derived from the thoracic impedance and downsampled to 4 Hz to obtain corresponding sampling times as RRI and BP.

The sequence technique was used for the assessment of baroreceptor reflex sensitivity (BRS) [83]. This technique is based on identifying consecutive cardiac beats in which an increase in systolic blood pressure is accompanied by an increase in RRI, or in which a decrease in systolic blood pressure is accompanied by a decrease in RRI. The regression line between the systolic blood pressure and RRI produces an estimate of BRS. We defined an equivalent change in heart rate and systolic blood pressure for at least three consecutive cardiac cycles as a regulatory event if the following criteria were fulfilled: RRI variations >4 ms and systolic blood pressure changes >1 mmHg [31].

4.4. Analysis Procedure Using Phase Synchronization

The analysis of synchronization, e.g., of R–R intervals and systolic blood pressure, is based upon the weak coupling of two different systems, which can be analyzed using the concept of analytic signals [29,35,84]. For this purpose, a phase (but not its amplitude) needs to be defined for a time series that contains oscillations in a narrow frequency band. That is, the adjustments of the rhythms of the R–R intervals, blood pressure, and respiration were partitioned for the sympathetic and the parasympathetic branches of the autonomic nervous system [29]. To permit a clear physical interpretation, we used the Hilbert transform to compute the so-called discrete-time analytic signal X_D, with $X_D = X_R + i \cdot X_I$ such that X_I is the Hilbert transform of the real vector X_R, from the band-pass filtered time series. Subsequently, the phase of the resulting signals $X_{D1}(t_i)$ and $X_{D2}(t_i)$ at every time point t_i and the difference between these two given phase vectors for the interpolated bivariate data series, e.g., between heart rate and respiration, was calculated.

The time series are defined as synchronized if the phase difference $\Psi(t_i)$ is constant over time. In case of synchronization, the distribution of the phase difference, quantified by the synchronization index $\gamma = \{\cos(\Psi(t_i))\}^2 + \{\sin(\Psi(t_i))\}^2$, shows a definite maximum. Theoretically, if the synchronization index $\gamma = 1$, then both time series are completely synchronized in a statistical sense, while in the case of $\gamma = 0$, both time series are completely desynchronized. Thus, the analysis of phase synchronization provides a quantitative indicator of the coordinated behavior of pairs of systems (i.e., in this case, R–R intervals and systolic blood pressure, partitioned for the sympathetic and the parasympathetic branches of the autonomic nervous system).

4.5. Statistical Analysis

To evaluate the main research question, analyses of variance were performed with period (anticipation, task, post-task) as the within-subjects factor, group (PE, UP, CO) as the between-subjects factor, and the respective cardiovascular variable as the dependent variable. Scores obtained at baseline were entered as covariates. That way, changes of cardiovascular variables produced by the stress manipulation were adjusted for baseline levels, ensuring that the analyzed residual scores were due to the acute stress, and not to individual differences in baseline levels. A further advantage of this approach, compared to simple change scores or the inclusion of baseline in the within-subjects factor, is that it controls for measurement error inherent in the use of repeated measures of the same kind [85–87]. If necessary, Greenhouse–Geisser corrections were used to adjust for nonsphericity of the variance–covariance matrices. In addition, the described statistical analyses were done within the group with a history of preeclampsia, with mild and severe as well as early, preterm, and term preeclampsia as the between-subjects factor. For graphical representation of the different time courses, standardized residualized change scores were calculated by linear regressions using the baseline period to predict the variables during the following periods, respectively [88,89]. These scores best represent those constituting the statistical results in the analyses of variance; i.e., they are adjusted for differences in baseline levels. One-way analyses of variance was performed to explore potential differences between the three groups in age, BMI, chronic stress, depression, and hemodynamic levels in resting conditions (at baseline). Further supplementary analyses were done to explore potential differences between groups in day of gestation, baby weight and height (independent *t*-tests), and parity (Chi-square test).

Author Contributions: Conceptualization, H.K.L., I.P. (Ilona Papousek), and M.G.M; Methodology, H.K.L. and I.P. (Ilona Papousek); Software, H.K.L.; Validation, I.P. (Ilona Papousek), M.L. and M.G.M.; Formal analysis, H.K.L. and I.P. (Ilona Papousek); Investigation, K.S.-Z. and I.P. (Isabella Pfniß); Resources, H.K.L. and M.G.M.; Data curation, I.P. (Isabella Pfniß), K.S.-Z. and V.K.-K.; Writing—original draft preparation, H.K.L., I.P. (Ilona Papousek), M.L., M.C.-Z., V.K.-K., O.N., and M.G.M.; Writing—review and editing, H.K.L., I.P. (Ilona Papousek), M.L., O.N., and M.G.M.; Visualization, H.K.L. and I.P. (Ilona Papousek); Supervision, M.G.M., M.C.-Z., and M.L.; Project administration, H.K.L. and K.S.Z.; Funding acquisition, H.K.L., I.P. (Ilona Papousek), and M.G.M.

Funding: Supported by funds of the Oesterreichische Nationalbank (Austrian Central Bank, Anniversary Fund, project number: 16426).

Acknowledgments: We wish to thank Anja Nischelwitzer, Kathrin Hilgarter, Jakob Riedl, Martina Rokov, Claudia Gruber, and Daniel Varga for their help in data collection. Furthermore, we wish to thank Trent Haigh for proofreading.

Conflicts of Interest: The authors declare no conflict of interest.

Abbreviations

BP	Blood pressure
BRS	Baroreflex reflex sensitivity
CO	Women without gestation during the last three years
DBP	Diastolic blood pressure
MAP	Mean arterial pressure
PE	Women with a history of preeclampsia
SBP	Systolic blood pressure
SI	Stroke index
SVRI	Systemic vascular resistance index
UP	Women with uncomplicated pregnancies

References

1. Abalos, E.; Cuesta, C.; Grosso, A.L.; Chou, D.; Say, L. Global and regional estimates of preeclampsia and eclampsia: A systematic review. *Eur. J. Obstet. Gynecol. Reprod. Biol.* **2013**, *170*, 1–7. [CrossRef] [PubMed]
2. Ananth, C.V.; Keyes, K.M.; Wapner, R.J. Pre-eclampsia rates in the United States, 1980–2010: Age-period-cohort analysis. *BMJ* **2013**, *347*, f6564. [CrossRef] [PubMed]
3. Roberts, J.M.; Bell, M.J. If we know so much about preeclampsia, why haven't we cured the disease? *J. Reprod Immunol.* **2013**, *99*, 1–9. [CrossRef] [PubMed]
4. Nelson, D.B.; Ziadie, M.S.; McIntire, D.D.; Rogers, B.B.; Leveno, K.J. Placental pathology suggesting that preeclampsia is more than one disease. *Am. J. Obstet. Gynecol.* **2014**, *210*, 66.e1–66.e7. [CrossRef] [PubMed]
5. Pennington, K.A.; Schlitt, J.M.; Jackson, D.L.; Schulz, L.C.; Schust, D.J. Preeclampsia: Multiple approaches for a multifactorial disease. *Dis. Model. Mech.* **2012**, *5*, 9–18. [CrossRef] [PubMed]
6. Lakovschek, I.C.; Ulrich, D.; Jauk, S.; Csapo, B.; Kolovetsiou-Kreiner, V.; Mayer-Pickel, K.; Stern, C.; Lang, U.; Obermayer-Pietsch, B.; Cervar-Zivkovic, M. Risk assessment for preterm preeclampsia in first trimester: Comparison of three calculation algorithms. *Eur. J. Obstet. Gynecol. Reprod. Biol.* **2018**, *231*, 241–247. [CrossRef] [PubMed]
7. Nzelu, D.; Dumitrascu-Biris, D.; Nicolaides, K.H.; Kametas, N.A. Chronic hypertension: First-trimester blood pressure control and likelihood of severe hypertension, preeclampsia, and small for gestational age. *Am. J. Obstet. Gynecol.* **2018**, *218*, 337.e1–337.e7. [CrossRef] [PubMed]
8. Powe, C.E.; Levine, R.J.; Karumanchi, S.A. Preeclampsia, a disease of the maternal endothelium: The role of antiangiogenic factors and implications for later cardiovascular disease. *Circulation* **2011**, *123*, 2856–2869. [CrossRef] [PubMed]
9. Huppertz, B. Placental origins of preeclampsia: Challenging the current hypothesis. *Hypertension* **2008**, *51*, 970–975. [CrossRef]
10. Palei, A.C.; Spradley, F.T.; Warrington, J.P.; George, E.M.; Granger, J.P. Pathophysiology of hypertension in pre-eclampsia: A lesson in integrative physiology. *Acta Physiol.* **2013**, *208*, 224–233. [CrossRef]

11. Sohlberg, S.; Mulic-Lutvica, A.; Lindgren, P.; Ortiz-Nieto, F.; Wikström, A.K.; Wikström, J. Placental perfusion in normal pregnancy and early and late preeclampsia: A magnetic resonance imaging study. *Placenta* **2014**, *35*, 202–206. [CrossRef]
12. Steegers, E.A.; von Dadelszen, P.; Duvekot, J.J.; Pijnenborg, R. Pre-eclampsia. *Lancet* **2010**, *376*, 631–644. [CrossRef]
13. Perry, H.; Khalil, A.; Thilaganathan, B. Preeclampsia and the cardiovascular system: An update. *Trends Cardiovasc. Med.* **2018**, *28*, 505–513. [CrossRef] [PubMed]
14. Melchiorre, K.; Sutherland, G.R.; Baltabaeva, A.; Liberati, M.; Thilaganathan, B. Maternal cardiac dysfunction and remodeling in women with preeclampsia at term. *Hypertension* **2011**, *57*, 85–93. [CrossRef] [PubMed]
15. Duhig, K.E.; Myers, J.; Seed, P.T.; Sparkes, J.; Lowe, J.; Hunter, R.M.; Shennan, A.H.; Chappell, L.C.; PARROT trial group. Placental growth factor testing to assess women with suspected pre-eclampsia: A multicentre, pragmatic, stepped-wedge cluster-randomised controlled trial. *Lancet* **2019**, *393*, 1807–1818. [CrossRef]
16. Ciobanu, A.; Wright, A.; Panaitescu, A.; Syngelaki, A.; Wright, D.; Nicolaides, K.H. Prediction of imminent preeclampsia at 35–37 weeks gestation. *Am. J. Obstet. Gynecol.* **2019**. [CrossRef]
17. Sattar, N.; Greer, I.A. Pregnancy complications and maternal cardiovascuar risk: Opportunities for intervention and prevention. *BMJ* **2002**, *325*, 157–160. [CrossRef] [PubMed]
18. Wu, P.; Haththotuwa, R.; Kwok, C.S.; Babu, A.; Kotronias, R.A.; Rushton, C.; Zaman, A.; Fryer, A.A.; Kadam, U.; Chew-Graham, C.A.; et al. Preeclampsia and Future Cardiovascular Health: A Systematic Review and Meta-Analysis. *Circ. Cardiovasc. Qual. Outcomes.* **2017**, *10*. [CrossRef]
19. Sattar, N.; Ramsay, J.; Crawford, L.; Cheyne, H.; Greer, I.A. Classic and novel risk factor parameters in women with a history of preeclampsia. *Hypertension* **2003**, *42*, 39–42. [CrossRef]
20. Thilaganathan, B.; Kalafat, E. Cardiovascular System in Preeclampsia and Beyond. *Hypertension* **2019**, *73*, 522–531. [CrossRef] [PubMed]
21. Ying, W.; Catov, J.M.; Ouyang, P. Hypertensive Disorders of Pregnancy and Future Maternal Cardiovascular Risk. *J. Am. Heart Assoc.* **2018**, *7*, e009382. [CrossRef] [PubMed]
22. Lugue, O.C.; George, E.M.; Bidwell, G.L. Preeclampsia and the brain: Neural control of cardiovascular changes during pregnancy and neurological outcomes of preeclampsia. *Clin. Sci.* **2016**, *130*, 1417–1434. [CrossRef] [PubMed]
23. Ekholm, E.M.; Erkkola, R.U. Autonomic cardiovascular control in pregnancy. *Eur. J. Obstet. Gynecol. Reprod. Biol.* **1996**, *64*, 29–36. [CrossRef]
24. Fu, Q.; Levine, B.D. Autonomic circulatory control during pregnancy in humans. *Semin. Reprod. Med.* **2009**, *27*, 330–337. [CrossRef] [PubMed]
25. Van Oppen, A.C.; Stigter, R.H.; Bruinse, H.W. Cardiac output in normal pregnancy: A critical review. *Obstet. Gynecol.* **1996**, *87*, 310–318. [CrossRef]
26. Schobel, H.; Fischer, T.; Heuszer, K.; Geiger, H.; Schmieder, R. Preeclampsia—A state of sympathetic overactivity. *N. Engl. J. Med.* **1996**, *335*, 1480–1485. [CrossRef] [PubMed]
27. Yang, C.; Chao, T.; Kuo, T.; Yin, C.; Chen, H. Preeclamptic pregnancy is associated with increased sympathetic and decreased parasympathetic control of HR. *Am. J. Physiol. Heart Circ. Physiol.* **2000**, *278*, 1269–1273. [CrossRef]
28. Kolovetsiou-Kreiner, V.; Moertl, M.G.; Papousek, I.; Schmid-Zalaudek, K.; Lang, U.; Schlembach, D.; Cervar-Zivkovic, M.; Lackner, H.K. Maternal cardiovascular and endothelial function from first trimester to postpartum. *PLoS ONE* **2018**, *13*, e0197748. [CrossRef]
29. Moertl, M.G.; Lackner, H.K.; Papousek, I.; Roessler, A.; Hinghofer-Szalkay, H.; Lang, U.; Kolovetsiou-Kreiner, V.; Schlembach, D. Phase synchronization of hemodynamic variables at rest and after deep breathing measured during the course of pregnancy. *PLoS ONE* **2013**, *8*, e60675. [CrossRef]
30. Voss, A.; Malberg, H.; Schumann, A.; Wessel, N.; Walther, T.; Stepan, H.; Faber, R. Baroreflex sensitivity, heart rate, and blood pressure variability in normal pregnancy. *Am. J. Hypertens.* **2000**, *13*, 1218–1225. [CrossRef]
31. Weber, T.M.; Lackner, H.K.; Roessler, A.; Papousek, I.; Kolovetsiou-Kreiner, V.; Lucovnik, M.; Schmid-Zalaudek, K.; Lang, U.; Moertl, M.G. Heart rate variability and baroreceptor reflex sensitivity in early- versus late-onset preeclampsia. *PLoS ONE* **2017**, *12*, e0186521. [CrossRef] [PubMed]
32. Faber, R.; Baumert, M.; Stepan, H.; Wessel, N.; Voss, A.; Walther, T. Baroreflex sensitivity, heart rate, and blood pressure variability in hypertensive pregnancy disorders. *J. Hum. Hypertens.* **2004**, *18*, 707–712. [CrossRef] [PubMed]

33. Walther, T.; Voss, A.; Baumert, M.; Truebner, S.; Till, H.; Stepan, H.; Wessel, N.; Faber, R. Cardiovascular variability before and after delivery: Recovery from arterial stiffness in women with preeclampsia 4 days post partum. *Hypertens. Pregnancy* **2014**, *33*, 1–14. [CrossRef] [PubMed]
34. Visontai, Z.; Lenard, Z.; Studinger, P.; Rigo Jr, J.; Kollai, M. Impaired baroreflex function during pregnancy is associated with stiffening of the carotid artery. *Ultrasound Obstet Gynecol.* **2002**, *20*, 364–369. [CrossRef] [PubMed]
35. Lackner, H.K.; Papousek, I.; Batzel, J.J.; Roessler, A.; Scharfetter, H.; Hinghofer-Szalkay, H. Phase synchronization of hemodynamic variables and respiration during mental challenge. *Int. J. Psychophysiol.* **2011**, *79*, 401–409. [CrossRef]
36. Schaefer, C.; Rosenblum, M.G.; Abel, H.H.; Kurths, J. Synchronization in the human cardiorespiratory system. *Phys. Rev. E Stat. Phys. Plasmas Fluids Relat. Interdiscip. Topics* **1999**, *60*, 857–870. [CrossRef]
37. Drobnjak, T.; Gizurarson, S.; Gokina, N.I.; Meiri, H.; Mandalá, M.; Huppertz, B.; Osol, G. Placental protein 13 (PP13)-induced vasodilation of resistance arteries from pregnant and nonpregnant rats occurs via endothelial-signaling pathways. *Hypertens. Pregnancy* **2017**, *36*, 186–195. [CrossRef]
38. Benschop, L.; Schalekamp-Timmermans, S.; Broere-Brown, Z.A.; Roeters van Lennep, J.E.; Jaddoe, V.W.V.; Roos-Hesselink, J.W.; Ikram, M.K.; Steegers, E.A.P.; Roberts, J.M.; Gandley, R.E. Placental Growth Factor as an Indicator of Maternal Cardiovascular Risk After Pregnancy. *Circulation* **2019**, *139*, 1698–1709. [CrossRef]
39. Huppertz, B.; Sammar, M.; Chefetz, I.; Neumaier-Wagner, P.; Bartz, C.; Meiri, H. Longitudinal determination of serum placental protein 13 during development of preeclampsia. *Fetal Diagn. Ther.* **2008**, *24*, 230–236. [CrossRef]
40. Shapiro, P.A.; Loan, R.P.; Horn, E.M.; Myers, M.M.; Gorman, J.M. Effect of innervation on heart rate response to mental stress. *Arch. Gen. Psychiatry* **1993**, *50*, 275–279. [CrossRef]
41. Lucovnik, M.; Lackner, H.K.; Papousek, I.; Schmid-Zalaudek, K.; Schulter, G.; Roessler, A.; Moertl, M.G. Systemic vascular resistance and endogenous inhibitors of nitric oxide synthesis in early- compared to lateonset preeclampsia: Preliminary findings. *Hypertens. Pregnancy* **2017**, *36*, 276–281. [CrossRef] [PubMed]
42. Herse, F.; Youpeng, B.; Staff, A.C.; Yong-Meid, J.; Dechend, R.; Rong, Z. Circulating and uteroplacental adipocytokine concentrations in preeclampsia. *Reprod. Sci.* **2009**, *16*, 584–590. [CrossRef] [PubMed]
43. Taylor, B.D.; Ness, R.B.; Olsen, J.; Hougaard, D.M.; Skogstrand, K.; Roberts, J.M.; Haggerty, C.L. Serum leptin measured in early pregnancy is higher in women with preeclampsia compared with normotensive pregnant women. *Hypertension* **2015**, *65*, 594–599. [CrossRef] [PubMed]
44. Lau, S.Y.; Guild, S.J.; Barrett, C.J.; Chen, Q.; McCowan, L.; Jordan, V.; Chamley, L.W. Tumor necrosis factor-alpha, interleukin-6, and interleukin-10 levels are altered in preeclampsia: A systematic review and meta-analysis. *Am. J. Reprod. Immunol.* **2013**, *70*, 412–427. [CrossRef] [PubMed]
45. Peraçoli, M.T.; Bannwart, C.F.; Cristofalo, R.; Borges, V.T.; Costa, R.A.; Witkin, S.S.; Peraçoli, J.C. Increased Reactive Oxygen Species and Tumor Necrosis Factor-Alpha Production by Monocytes are Associated with Elevated Levels of Uric Acid in Pre-Eclamptic Women. *Am. J. Reprod. Immunol.* **2011**, *66*, 460–467. [CrossRef] [PubMed]
46. Brassard, P.; Amiri, F.; Schiffrin, E.L. Combined angiotensin II type 1 and type 2 receptor blockade on vascular remodeling and matrix metalloproteinases in resistance arteries. *Hypertension* **2005**, *46*, 598–606. [CrossRef] [PubMed]
47. Forrester, S.J.; Elliott, K.J.; Kawai, T.; Obama, T.; Boyer, M.J.; Preston, K.J.; Yan, Z.; Eguchi, S.; Rizzo, V. Caveolin-1 Deletion Prevents Hypertensive Vascular Remodeling Induced by Angiotensin II. *Hypertension* **2017**, *69*, 79–86. [CrossRef] [PubMed]
48. Patel, V.B.; Zhong, J.C.; Fan, D.; Basu, R.; Morton, J.S.; Parajuli, N.; McMurtry, M.S.; Davidge, S.T.; Kassiri, Z.; Oudit, G.Y. Angiotensin-converting enzyme 2 is a critical determinant of angiotensin II-induced loss of vascular smooth muscle cells and adverse vascular remodeling. *Hypertension* **2014**, *64*, 157–164. [CrossRef]
49. Zhang, Z.Z.; Cheng, Y.W.; Jin, H.Y.; Chang, Q.; Shang, Q.H.; Xu, Y.L.; Chen, L.X.; Xu, R.; Song, B.; Zhong, J.C. The sirtuin 6 prevents angiotensin II-mediated myocardial fibrosis and injury by targeting AMPK-ACE2 signaling. *Oncotarget* **2017**, *8*, 72302–72314. [CrossRef]
50. Cui, N.; Li, W.; Mazzuca, M.Q.; Khalil, R.A.; Mata, K.M. Increased vascular and uteroplacental matrix metalloproteinase-1 and -7 levels and collagen type I deposition in hypertension in pregnancy: Role of TNF-α. *Am. J. Physiol. Circ. Physiol.* **2017**, *313*, H491–H507. [CrossRef]

51. Herse, F.; Lamarca, B.; Hubel, C.A.; Kaartokallio, T.; Lokki, A.I.; Ekholm, E.; Laivuori, H.; Gauster, M.; Huppertz, B.; Sugulle, M.; et al. Cytochrome P450 subfamily 2J polypeptide 2 expression and circulating epoxyeicosatrienoic metabolites in preeclampsia. *Circulation* **2012**, *126*, 2990–2999. [CrossRef] [PubMed]
52. Boeldt, D.S.; Bird, I.M. Vascular adaptation in pregnancy and endothelial dysfunction in preeclampsia. *J. Endocrinol.* **2017**, *232*, R27–R44. [CrossRef] [PubMed]
53. Possomato-Vieira, J.S.; Khalil, R.A. Mechanisms of Endothelial Dysfunction in Hypertensive Pregnancy and Preeclampsia. *Adv. Pharmacol.* **2016**, *77*, 361–431. [CrossRef] [PubMed]
54. Robertson, S.A. Preventing Preeclampsia by Silencing Soluble Flt-1? *N. Engl. J. Med.* **2019**, *380*, 1080–1082. [CrossRef]
55. Meher, S.; Duley, L. Nitric oxide for preventing pre-eclampsia and its complications. *Cochrane Database Syst. Rev.* **2007**, CD006490. [CrossRef] [PubMed]
56. Groten, T.; Fitzgerald, J.; Lehmann, T.; Schneider, U.; Kähler, C.; Schleussner, E. Reduction of preeclampsia related complications with with the NO-donor penterythriltetranitrat (petn) in risk pregnancies—A prospective randomized doubleblind placebo pilot study. *Pregnancy Hypertens.* **2012**, *2*, 181. [CrossRef] [PubMed]
57. Pan, P.; Fu, H.; Zhang, L.; Huang, H.; Luo, F.; Wu, W.; Guo, Y.; Liu, X. Angiotensin II upregulates the expression of placental growth factor in human vascular endothelial cells and smooth muscle cells. *BMC Cell Biol.* **2010**, *11*, 36. [CrossRef]
58. Zhou, C.C.; Ahmad, S.; Mi, T.; Xia, L.; Abbasi, S.; Hewett, P.W.; Sun, C.; Ahmed, A.; Kellems, R.E.; Xia, Y. Angiotensin II induces soluble fms-like tyrosine kinase-1 release via calcineurin signaling pathway in pregnancy. *Circ. Res.* **2007**, *100*, 88–95. [CrossRef]
59. Xia, Y.; Kellems, R.E. Angiotensin receptor agonistic autoantibodies and hypertension: Preeclampsia and beyond. *Circ. Res.* **2013**, *113*, 78–87. [CrossRef]
60. Parrish, M.R.; Wallace, K.; Tam Tam, K.B.; Herse, F.; Weimer, A.; Wenzel, K.; Wallukat, G.; Ray, L.F.; Arany, M.; Cockrell, K.; et al. Hypertension in response to AT1-AA: Role of reactive oxygen species in pregnancy-induced hypertension. *Am. J. Hypertens.* **2011**, *24*, 835–840. [CrossRef]
61. Cunningham, M.W., Jr.; Castillo, J.; Ibrahim, T.; Cornelius, D.C.; Campbell, N.; Amaral, L.; Vaka, V.R.; Usry, N.; Williams, J.M.; LaMarca, B. AT1-AA (angiotensin II type 1 receptor agonistic autoantibody) blockade prevents preeclamptic symptoms in placental ischemic rats. *Hypertension* **2018**, *71*, 886–893. [CrossRef] [PubMed]
62. Liang, B.; Wang, X.; Zhang, N.; Yang, H.; Bai, R.; Liu, M.; Bian, Y.; Xiao, C.; Yang, Z. Angiotensin-(1-7) attenuates angiotensin II-induced ICAM-1, VCAM-1, and MCP-1 expression via the MAS receptor through suppression of P38 and NF-κB pathways in HUVECs. *Cell Physiol. Biochem.* **2015**, *35*, 2472–2482. [CrossRef] [PubMed]
63. White, S.J.; Hayes, E.M.; Lehoux, S.; Jeremy, J.Y.; Horrevoets, A.J.; Newby, A.C. Characterization of the differential response of endothelial cells exposed to normal and elevated laminar shear stress. *J. Cell Physiol.* **2011**, *226*, 2841–2848. [CrossRef] [PubMed]
64. Ramkhelawon, B.; Rivas, D.; Lehoux, S. Shear stress activates extracellular signal-regulated kinase 1/2 via the angiotensin II type 1 receptor. *FASEB J.* **2013**, *27*, 3008–3016. [CrossRef] [PubMed]
65. Planas-Rigol, E.; Terrades-Garcia, N.; Corbera-Bellalta, M.; Lozano, E.; Alba, M.A.; Segarra, M.; Espígol-Frigolé, G.; Prieto-González, S.; Hernández-Rodríguez, J.; Preciado, S.; et al. Endothelin-1 promotes vascular smooth muscle cell migration across the artery wall: A mechanism contributing to vascular remodelling and intimal hyperplasia in giant-cell arteritis. *Ann. Rheum. Dis.* **2017**, *76*, 1624–1634. [CrossRef] [PubMed]
66. Atef, M.E.; Anand-Srivastava, M.B. Enhanced expression of Gqα and PLC-β1 proteins contributes to vascular smooth muscle cell hypertrophy in SHR: Role of endogenous angiotensin II and endothelin-1. *Am. J. Physiol. Cell Physiol.* **2014**, *307*, C97–C106. [CrossRef] [PubMed]
67. Azahri, N.S.; Di Bartolo, B.A.; Khachigian, L.M.; Kavurma, M.M. Sp1, acetylated histone-3 and p300 regulate TRAIL transcription: Mechanisms of PDGF-BB-mediated VSMC proliferation and migration. *J. Cell Biochem.* **2012**, *113*, 2597–2606. [CrossRef] [PubMed]
68. Das, S.; Zhang, E.; Senapati, P.; Amaram, V.; Reddy, M.A.; Stapleton, K.; Leung, A.; Lanting, L.; Wang, M.; Chen, Z.; et al. A novel angiotensin II-induced long noncoding RNA giver regulates oxidative stress, inflammation, and proliferation in vascular smooth muscle cells. *Circ. Res.* **2018**, *123*, 1298–1312. [CrossRef]

69. Jover, E.; Silvente, A.; Marín, F.; Martínez-González, J.; Orriols, M.; Martinez, C.M.; Puche, C.M.; Valdés, M.; Rodriguez, C.; Hernández-Romero, D. Inhibition of enzymes involved in collagen cross-linking reduces vascular smooth muscle cell calcification. *FASEB J.* **2018**, *32*, 4459–4469. [CrossRef]
70. Spradley, F.T. Sympathetic nervous system control of vascular function and blood pressure during pregnancy and preeclampsia. *J. Hypertens.* **2019**, *37*, 476–487. [CrossRef]
71. Riedl, M.; Suhrbier, A.; Stepan, H.; Kurths, J.; Wessel, N. Short-term couplings of the cardiovascular system in pregnant women suffering from pre-eclampsia. *Philos. Transact. A Math. Phys. Eng. Sci.* **2010**, *368*, 2237–2250. [CrossRef] [PubMed]
72. Haug, E.B.; Horn, J.; Markovitz, A.R.; Fraser, A.; Macdonald-Wallis, C.; Tilling, K.; Romundstad, P.R.; Rich-Edwards, J.W.; Åsvold, B.O. The impact of parity on life course blood pressure trajectories: The HUNT study in Norway. *Eur. J. Epidemiol.* **2018**, *33*, 751–761. [CrossRef] [PubMed]
73. Ditisheim, A.; Wuerzner, G.; Ponte, B.; Vial, Y.; Irion, O.; Burnier, M.; Boulvain, M.; Pechère-Bertschi, A. Prevalence of Hypertensive Phenotypes After Preeclampsia: A Prospective Cohort Study. *Hypertension* **2018**, *71*, 103–109. [CrossRef] [PubMed]
74. American College of Obstetricians and Gynecologists. Hypertension in pregnancy. Report of the American College of Obstetricians and Gynecologists' Task Force on Hypertension in Pregnancy. *Obstet. Gynecol.* **2013**, *122*, 1122–1131. [CrossRef]
75. Fliege, H.; Rose, M.; Arck, P.; Walter, O.B.; Kocalevent, R.D.; Weber, C.; Klapp, B.F. The Perceived Stress Questionnaire (PSQ) reconsidered: Validation and reference values from different clinical and healthy adult samples. *Psychosom. Med.* **2005**, *67*, 78–88. [CrossRef] [PubMed]
76. Hautzinger, M.; Bailer, M. *ADS: Allgemeine Depressions Skala*; Beltz: Weinheim, Germany, 1993. [CrossRef]
77. Niemann, H.; Sturm, W.; Thöne-Otto, A.I.; Willmes, K. *California Verbal Learning Test, German Adaptation*; Hogrefe: Boston, MA, USA, 2008.
78. Lackner, H.K.; Gramer, M.; Paechter, M.; Wimmer, S.; Hinghofer-Szalkay, H.; Papousek, I. Academic goal orientation and cardiovascular reactivity in a performance situation. *Appl. Psychophysiol. Biofeedback* **2015**, *40*, 189–200. [CrossRef] [PubMed]
79. Papousek, I.; Paechter, M.; Lackner, H.K. Delayed psychophysiological recovery after self-concept-inconsistent negative performance feedback. *Int. J. Psychophysiol.* **2011**, *82*, 275–282. [CrossRef] [PubMed]
80. Papousek, I.; Paechter, M.; Weiss, E.M.; Lackner, H.K. The tendency to ruminate and the dynamics of heart rate recovery after an ordinary, mildly stressful performance situation. *Pers. Individ. Dif.* **2017**, *104*, 150–154. [CrossRef]
81. Fortin, J.; Marte, W.; Grüllenberger, R.; Hacker, A.; Habenbacher, W.; Heller, A.; Wagner, C.; Wach, P.; Skrabal, F. Continuous non-invasive blood pressure monitoring using concentrically interlocking control loops. *Comput. Biol. Med.* **2006**, *36*, 941–957. [CrossRef]
82. Lackner, H.K.; Batzel, J.J.; Rössler, A.; Hinghofer-Szalkay, H.; Papousek, I. Multi-time scale perspective in analyzing cardiovascular data. *Physiol. Res.* **2014**, *63*, 439–456.
83. Parati, G.; Omboni, S.T.; Frattola, A.; di Rienzo, M.; Zanchetti, A.G. Dynamic evaluation of the baroreflex in ambulant subject. In *Blood Pressure and Heart Rate Variability*; Rienzo, M., Mancia, G., Parati, G., Pedotti, A., Zanchetti, A., Eds.; IOS Press: Amsterdam, The Netherlands, 1992; pp. 123–137.
84. Cysarz, D.; von Bonin, D.; Lackner, H.; Heusser, P.; Moser, M.; Bettermann, H. Oscillations of heart rate and respiration synchronize during poetry recitation. *Am. J. Physiol. Heart Circ. Physiol.* **2004**, *287*, H579–H587. [CrossRef] [PubMed]
85. Dimitrov, D.M.; Rumrill, P.D. Pretest-posttest designs and measurement of change. *Work* **2003**, *20*, 159–165. [PubMed]
86. Linden, W.; Earle, L.; Gerin, W.; Christenfeld, N. Physiological stress reactivity and recovery: Conceptual siblings separated at birth? *J. Psychosom. Res.* **1997**, *42*, 117–135. [CrossRef]
87. Steketee, G.S.; Chambless, D.L. Methodological issues in prediction of treatment outcome. *Clin. Psychol. Rev.* **1992**, *12*, 387–400. [CrossRef]

88. Papousek, I.; Weiss, E.M.; Schulter, G.; Fink, A.; Reiser, E.M.; Lackner, H.K. Prefrontal EEG alpha asymmetry changes while observing disaster happening to other people: Cardiac correlates and prediction of emotional impact. *Biol. Psychol.* **2014**, *103*, 184–194. [CrossRef] [PubMed]
89. Papousek, I.; Aydin, N.; Rominger, C.; Feyaerts, K.; Schmid-Zalaudek, K.; Lackner, H.K.; Fink, A.; Schulter, G.; Weiss, E.M. DSM-5 personality trait domains and withdrawal versus approach motivational tendencies in response to the perception of other people's desperation and angry aggression. *Biol. Psychol.* **2018**, *132*, 106–115. [CrossRef]

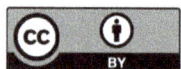

© 2019 by the authors. Licensee MDPI, Basel, Switzerland. This article is an open access article distributed under the terms and conditions of the Creative Commons Attribution (CC BY) license (http://creativecommons.org/licenses/by/4.0/).

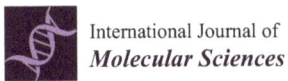

Article

Preeclampsia Is Associated with Sex-Specific Transcriptional and Proteomic Changes in Fetal Erythroid Cells

Zahra Masoumi [1,*], Gregory E. Maes [2,3], Koen Herten [2,4], Álvaro Cortés-Calabuig [4], Abdul Ghani Alattar [5,6], Eva Hanson [1], Lena Erlandsson [1], Eva Mezey [7], Mattias Magnusson [6], Joris R Vermeesch [2,3,4], Mary Familari [8,†] and Stefan R Hansson [9,†]

1. Division of Obstetrics and Gynecology, Department of Clinical Sciences Lund, Lund University, Klinikgatan 28, 22184 Lund, Sweden; eva.hanson@med.lu.se (E.H.); lena.erlandsson@med.lu.se (L.E.)
2. Laboratory for Cytogenetics and Genome Research, Center for Human Genetics, KU Leuven, Herestraat 49, 3000 Leuven, Belgium; gregory.maes@kuleuven.be (G.E.M.); koen.herten@kuleuven.be (K.H.); joris.vermeesch@uzleuven.be (J.R.V.)
3. Department of Human Genetics, Centre for Human Genetics, University Hospital Leuven, KU Leuven, Herestraat 49, 3000 Leuven, Belgium
4. Genomics Core, UZ Leuven, Herestraat 49, 3000 Leuven, Belgium; alvaro.cortes@uzleuven.be
5. Department of Hematology and Transfusion Medicine, Lund University, Klinikgatan 28, 22184 Lund, Sweden; abdul_ghani.alattar@med.lu.se
6. Department of Molecular Medicine and Gene Therapy, Lund University, Sölvegatan 17, 22184 Lund, Sweden; mattias.magnusson@med.lu.se
7. Adult Stem Cell Section, National Institute of Dental and Craniofacial Research, National Institutes of Health, 9000 Rockville Pike, Bethesda, MD 20892, USA; MezeyE@nidcr.nih.gov
8. School of Biosciences, Bldg 4, University of Melbourne, Parkville 3010, Australia; m.familari@unimelb.edu.au
9. Lund University, Skåne University Hospital, Obstetrics and Gynecology, Department of Clinical Sciences Lund, Klinikgatan 28, 22184 Lund, Sweden; stefan.hansson@med.lu.se
* Correspondence: zahra.masoumi@med.lu.se; Tel.: +46-(46)-222-30-27
† These authors contributed equally to this work.

Received: 14 March 2019; Accepted: 17 April 2019; Published: 25 April 2019

Abstract: Preeclampsia (PE) has been associated with placental dysfunction, resulting in fetal hypoxia, accelerated erythropoiesis, and increased erythroblast count in the umbilical cord blood (UCB). Although the detailed effects remain unknown, placental dysfunction can also cause inflammation, nutritional, and oxidative stress in the fetus that can affect erythropoiesis. Here, we compared the expression of surface adhesion molecules and the erythroid differentiation capacity of UCB hematopoietic stem/progenitor cells (HSPCs), UCB erythroid profiles along with the transcriptome and proteome of these cells between male and female fetuses from PE and normotensive pregnancies. While no significant differences were observed in UCB HSPC migration/homing and in vitro erythroid colony differentiation, the UCB HSPC transcriptome and the proteomic profile of the in vitro differentiated erythroid cells differed between PE vs. normotensive samples. Accordingly, despite the absence of significant differences in the UCB erythroid populations in male or female fetuses from PE or normotensive pregnancies, transcriptional changes were observed during erythropoiesis, particularly affecting male fetuses. Pathway analysis suggested deregulation in the mammalian target of rapamycin complex 1/AMP-activated protein kinase (mTORC1/AMPK) signaling pathways controlling cell cycle, differentiation, and protein synthesis. These results associate PE with transcriptional and proteomic changes in fetal HSPCs and erythroid cells that may underlie the higher erythroblast count in the UCB in PE.

Keywords: preeclampsia; hematopoietic stem/progenitor cells; umbilical cord blood; erythropoiesis

1. Introduction

Preeclampsia (PE) is a pregnancy related disorder that remains a major cause of maternal and fetal mortality by affecting 3% to 8% of pregnancies worldwide [1]. Although it is diagnosed after 20 weeks of gestation, based on the maternal symptoms, such as high blood pressure and proteinuria [2], the events leading to PE may be triggered during trophoblast invasion and embryonic implantation [3]. Insufficient trophoblast invasion into the decidua and the spiral arteries leads to dysfunctional placentation, altered placental blood flow, subsequent hypoxia, and cell senescence [4–8]. Changes in cellular metabolism, increased placental oxidative stress, and placental barrier damage lead to leakage of placental and fetal factors into the maternal circulation [5,9]. One of these factors is free fetal hemoglobin (HbF), which is found to be elevated in the maternal circulation as early as the first trimester in women who later develop PE [10]. Free hemoglobin triggers inflammation, vasoconstriction, and tissue damage [11], and particularly impairs the placenta barrier [12].

The negative consequences of a PE pregnancy affect the mother as well as the developing fetus [13–16]. Our group has previously demonstrated higher levels of total hemoglobin in the arterial and venous UCB [17], suggesting possible accelerated fetal erythropoiesis. Higher erythroblast count in the UCB is a common observation in PE pregnancies [18–21] that has been linked to elevated erythropoiesis induced by hypoxia and enhanced fetal erythropoietin (EPO) levels [22–25]. However, previous studies investigating in vitro colony formation of UCB HSPCs have not demonstrated any significant differences in the erythroid differentiation capacity of the cells obtained from PE vs. normotensive pregnancies [26,27]. This suggests that a mechanism other than hypoxia-induced EPO-dependent enhanced fetal erythropoiesis may affect erythroid maturation, underlying the higher erythroblast count documented in the UCB of PE pregnancies. For instance, levels of glucose, glucose/insulin ratio [28,29], lactic acid [30], and inflammatory cytokines, such as tumor necrosis factorα (TNFα) [31], are reported to be altered in the fetuses from PE pregnancies. All these factors are significant in regulating erythropoiesis and erythroid maturation [32–36]. However, the effects of these changes on the molecular pathways that control HSPC differentiation and late erythroid maturation in the fetus have not been investigated in detail.

Another important factor in regulating fetal hemoglobin levels is fetal sex [37,38], which also determines the onset of the disease and severity of maternal symptoms in PE [39,40] as well as maternal adaptation to pregnancy [41]. Sex-specific fetal responses in PE have been assessed in both an animal model [42] and in humans [43–46]. However, these studies are limited to comparing clinical parameters, such as blood pressure, height, and weight, indicating the importance of further analysis to investigate the molecular changes.

The focus of this study was to evaluate any changes in the migration/homing or differentiation capacity of fetal HSPCs by analyzing the expression of surface adhesion molecules (SAMs), the transcriptome, and the erythroid differentiation capacity of UCB hematopoietic stem/progenitor cells (HSPCs) in fetuses from PE pregnancies. Moreover, the proteomic profile of in vitro differentiated erythroid cells was studied to explore possible differences in erythroid maturation. Finally, using an established flow cytometry analysis [47], the profile of terminally differentiating erythroblasts in the UCB was compared between PE and normotensive pregnancies to explore any alterations in fetal erythroid populations. In addition, transcriptome analysis on isolated erythroid cells was performed, with particular attention to sex-specific differences, using SE50bp RNA sequencing.

2. Results

2.1. Preeclampsia Does Not Alter Migration/Homing or Differentiation Capacity of UCB HSPCs

To study the effect of PE on migration/homing of fetal HSPCs, the expression of known surface adhesion molecules (SAMs) was analyzed on the UCB CD34$^+$ CD45$^+$ cells (Figure 1A). The expression of CD49d, CD49e, CD184 (CXCR4), and CD11a (the upper panel Figure 1B) as well as CD44 and CD62L (L-selectin) (the lower panel Figure 1B) were not significantly different between the PE and normotensive groups (flow cytograms demonstrated in Supplementary Figure S1). In addition, the frequency of viable hematopoietic stem cell-enriched cells (HSCs) expressing specific markers (Table 1) was determined using flow cytometry (Figure 1C). The number of CD34$^+$ cells or the HSCs per mL of UCB obtained from each sample was not significantly different between the PE and normotensive samples.

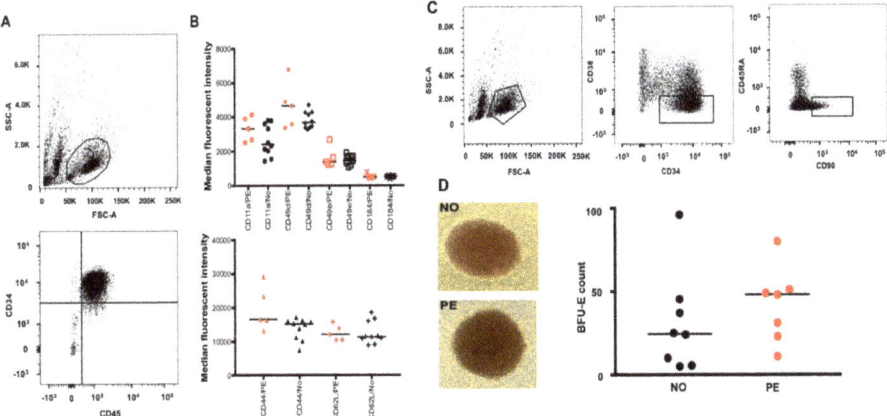

Figure 1. Flow cytometry analysis and isolation of UCB HSPCs and HSCs as well as assessment of surface adhesion molecules (SAMs) and in vitro erythroid differentiation capacity of the cells isolated from PE vs. normotensive (NO) pregnancies. (**A**) Flow cytometry analysis showing the UCB HSPC population gated based on size and granularity (FSC-A and SSC-A) and CD34$^+$ CD45$^+$ expression. (**B**) Demonstrating the median fluorescent intensity (MFI) for various SAMs in red (PE, $n = 5$) and black (NO, $n = 10$); despite large differences in some MFI values, the differences were not statistically significant. (**C**) Flow cytometry analysis of the HSC population from UCB samples; the population was gated (from left to right) based on size and granularity followed by CD34$^+$, CD38^{lo}, and CD45RA$^-$, CD90$^+$ expression. As previously reported by others, the CD34$^+$ CD38^{lo} population was very small in the majority of our samples. This specific individual sample with a large CD34$^+$ CD38^{lo} population was particularly chosen for specifically visualizing a clearly distinct CD34$^+$ CD38^{lo} CD45RA$^-$ and CD90$^+$ population in the figure. (**D**) Example of BFU-Es in culture (10× magnification) from normotensive ($n = 8$) and PE ($n = 7$) samples after the UCB CD34$^+$ cells were cultured for 14 days. No significant difference was observed BFU-E count comparison between PE and normotensive groups.

Table 1. The markers used in flow cytometry analyses.

To Recognize	Markers/Profile
Hematopoietic stem/progenitor cells (HSPCs)	CD34$^+$ (clone 581) CD45$^+$ (clone HI30)
Surface adhesion molecules (SAMs)	CD44 (clone 515) CD49d (clone 9F10) CD49e (clone IIA1) CD184 (clone 12G5) CD11a (clone HI111) CD62L (polyclonal)
Hematopoietic stem cells (HSCs)	CD34$^+$ (clone 581) CD38^{lo} (clone HIT2) CD45RA$^-$ (clone HI100) CD90$^+$ (clone 5E10)
Erythroid cells (Flow cytometry) from proerythroblasts to mature erythrocytes	CD45$^-$ (clone HI30) GPA$^+$ (clone HIR2) Band 3 (clone BRIC6) CD49d (clone 9F10)

To investigate whether PE altered the erythroid differentiation capacity of fetal HSPCs, resulting in enhanced erythropoiesis and UCB erythroblast count, CD34+ cells from normotensive and PE UCB samples were isolated and used in a colony formation assay. Despite a large difference in the median values between the groups, the number of burst forming units-erythroid (BFU-Es) showed no significant difference (Figure 1D).

2.2. Preeclampsia Affects the Gene Expression in UCB HSPCs

Since there was no difference in the migration/homing or erythroid differentiation capacity of the UCB HSPCs (CD34+ CD45+ cells) that could explain the higher UCB erythroblast count documented in PE [18–21], cDNA subtractive hybridization was carried out to elucidate possible gene expression differences that might affect the maturation of erythroblasts. To perform cDNA subtractive hybridization, CD34+ CD45+ cells from normotensive and PE UCB samples were used as driver and tester groups, respectively. Sequencing of the differential fragments resulted in 26 protein-coding genes (Figure 2). Predictions by String suggested that the eukaryotic translation elongation factor 1 alpha 1 (EEF1A1) interacted with glyceraldehyde 3-phosphate dehydrogenase (GAPDH) as well as several ribosomal proteins (RPs). The pathways of significance based on GSEA are presented in Supplementary Table S1. The RPs were also associated with significant hematological phenotypes, such as increased mean corpuscular volume, macrocytic anemia, persistence of HbF, and reticulocytopenia, as determined by ToppFun (false discovery rate (FDR) < 0.01).

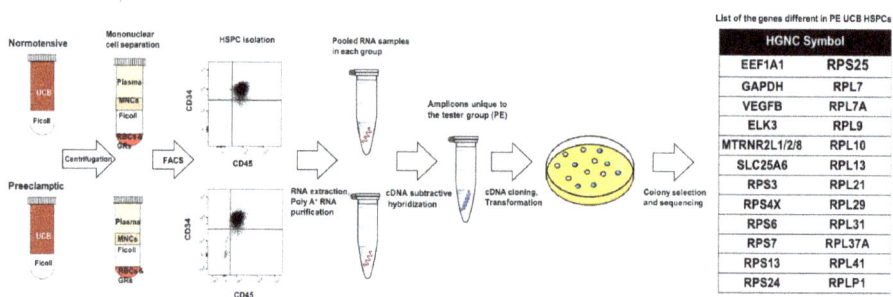

Figure 2. Gene expression analysis in the UCB HSPCs using cDNA subtractive hybridization. The procedure is demonstrated from separating mononuclear cells (MNCs) from the umbilical cord blood (UCB) and isolating hematopoietic stem/progenitor cells (HSPCs) to the final list of genes that were found to be different in PE. The HSPCs (CD34+ CD45+) were sorted during SAM analysis and were used in this experiment (PE, $n = 5$ and NO, $n = 10$).

2.3. Preeclampsia Is Associated with Changes in Metabolic and Protein Synthesis Pathways of In Vitro Differentiated Erythroid Cells

To investigate whether changes in ribosomal and metabolic pathways in the HSPCs affected late erythroid maturation steps in fetuses from PE pregnancies, proteomics analysis was performed using TMT-mass spectrometry on in vitro differentiated erythroid cells. After mapping the peptide sequences to proteins, 6222 proteins were detected (FDR ≤0.01) (Supplementary Table S2). At a threshold of fold change ≥20% and p value ≤0.05, a total of 90 proteins were increased and 14 proteins were decreased in PE vs. normotensive in vitro differentiated erythroid cells (Supplementary Table S2). The heat map of the differentially expressed proteins and the enriched pathways predicted by GSEA are presented in Figure 3. The protein–protein interaction network and the connection between the enriched pathways are presented in Supplementary Figure S2. The affected pathways were mainly related to ATP production (oxidative phosphorylation and the TCA cycle), as well as protein synthesis, transport, and metabolism (Figure 3).

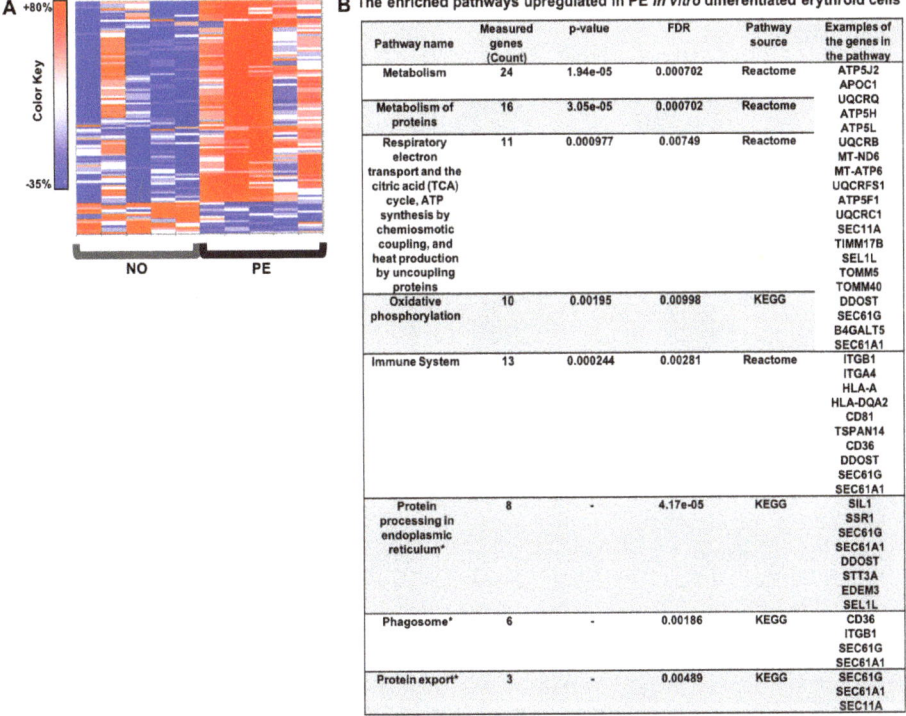

Figure 3. The proteomics analysis heat map and the enriched pathways in the in vitro differentiated erythroid colonies. (**A**) The heat map for the significantly differentially expressed proteins in PE ($n = 5$) vs. normotensive ($n = 5$) in vitro differentiated erythroid cells. (**B**) The enrichment analysis in the gene set analysis in CPDB human network was performed based on the protein average fold ratio in PE and normotensive samples.

2.4. Preeclampsia Does Not Alter the UCB Profile of Terminally Differentiating Erythroblasts

Considering that the in vitro analyses indicated no changes in molecular pathways rather than erythroid cell production, the frequency of various stages of terminally differentiating erythroid cells was investigated in the UCB erythroblasts between male and female fetuses from PE and normotensive pregnancies. The viable single cells were gated based on GPA and CD45 expression. The $CD45^-$, GPA^+ erythroid population was analyzed for surface expression of CD49d and Band 3 to evaluate the terminal erythroid differentiation stages of the UCB erythroblasts (Figure 4A). The erythroid precursors present in the samples were predominately basophilic erythroblasts II to orthochromatic erythroblasts. Comparing the erythroid profile of the samples, no significant differences were observed between the venous or arterial UCB from PE or normotensive pregnancies in male nor female fetuses (Figure 4B).

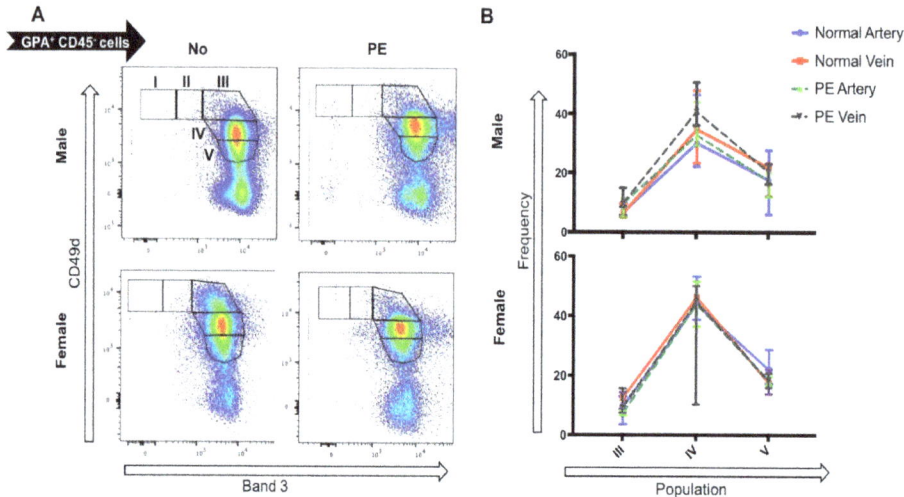

Figure 4. Comparison of the erythroid progenitor profile in the umbilical cord blood (UCB) from PE ($n = 6$) and normotensive ($n = 7$) pregnancies. (**A**) The flow cytometry profile of CD45$^-$ GPA$^+$ cells expressing CD49d (Integrin α4) and Band 3 protein during their maturation from proerythrocytes (CD49d$^+$ Band 3$^-$) to mature erythrocytes (Cd49d$^-$ Band 3$^+$). (**B**) No significant differences were observed between arterial or venous UCB from male or female in PE vs. normotensive pregnancies.

2.5. Gene Expression Differences between Male vs. Female Samples Are Irrespective of Pregnancy Outcome

The absence of a significant increase in the frequency of immature erythroid cells in PE UCB samples was in line with the results from the in vitro differentiation cultures. Therefore, further RNA-sequencing analysis was performed to explore possible changes in the molecular pathways that may explain the higher erythroblast count. Gene expression of arterial vs. venous erythroid cells did not differ significantly (Supplementary Figure S3). Sample clustering by principal component analysis (PCA) indicated a major difference in gene expression in the male vs. female erythroid cells irrespective of pregnancy outcome (Figure 5A). A total of 35 genes were determined by EdgeR and Deseq2 to be differentially expressed (DE) in male vs. female fetuses, affecting pathways, such as RNA transcription (Supplementary Table S3) (Figure 5B). A more distinct clustering of PE vs. normotensive samples was observed in the samples from male fetuses (Figure 5A). Based on the DE genes confirmed by Deseq2 and EdgeR, 40 genes that affected metabolism and protein processing in endoplasmic reticulum (ER)/vesicle trafficking were downregulated in PE (Figure 5C). In addition, 21 genes that were involved in pathways, such as heat shock response and protein kinase activation by RHO GTPases, were upregulated (Figure 5C).

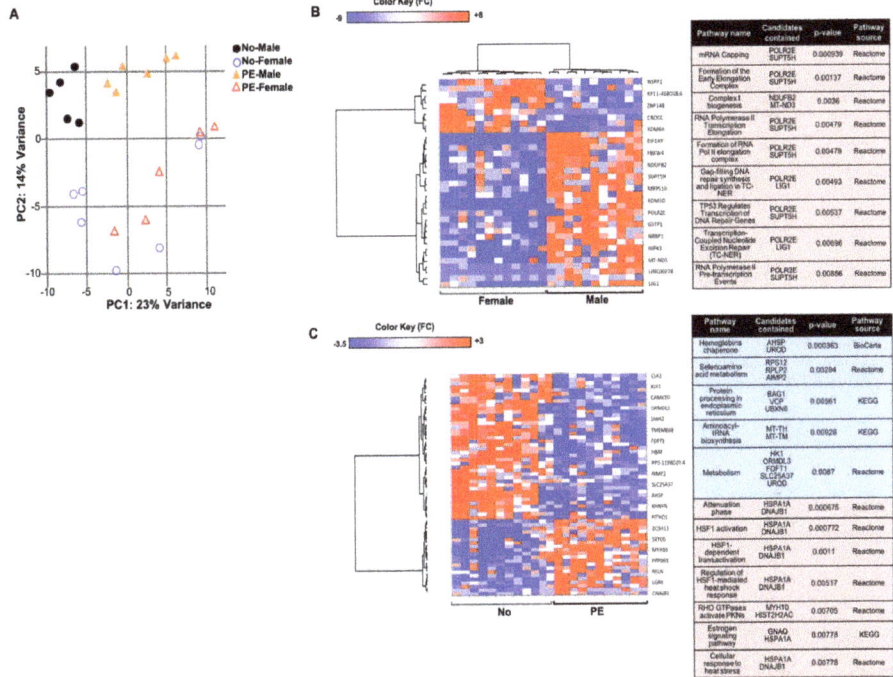

Figure 5. Primary gene expression analysis of the UCB erythroid progenitors. (**A**) A distinct clustering was observed between male and female samples in the principal component analysis (PCA) plot. Also, among the PE (*n* = 6) and normotensive (*n* = 7) samples, a clearer clustering was observed in the male compared to female fetuses. The heat maps of the differentially expressed genes and the related pathways are presented when comparing (**B**) male vs. female and (**C**) PE vs. normotensive samples. Shades of blue and red indicates down- or up-regulated genes/pathways, respectively.

2.6. Effects of PE on Gene Expression in UCB Erythroid Cells Are Sex-Specific

Taking into account the sex-specific clustering of the samples from the RNA-sequencing analysis, the effect of PE on male and female samples was analyzed separately. In the males, a total of 40 DE genes were determined in PE vs. normotensive groups by Deseq2 and EdgeR (Supplementary Table S3). The affected pathways included endocytosis, protein ubiquitination, regulation of cell cycle, and convergent extension, i.e., the process of cell lengthening and narrowing along one axis (Figure 6A). Among the females, a total of 21 DE genes were confirmed in the PE group using Deseq2 and EdgeR (Supplementary Table S3). The altered pathways included metabolism, mTOR signaling, and cellular response to stress (via heat shock proteins) (Figure 6B).

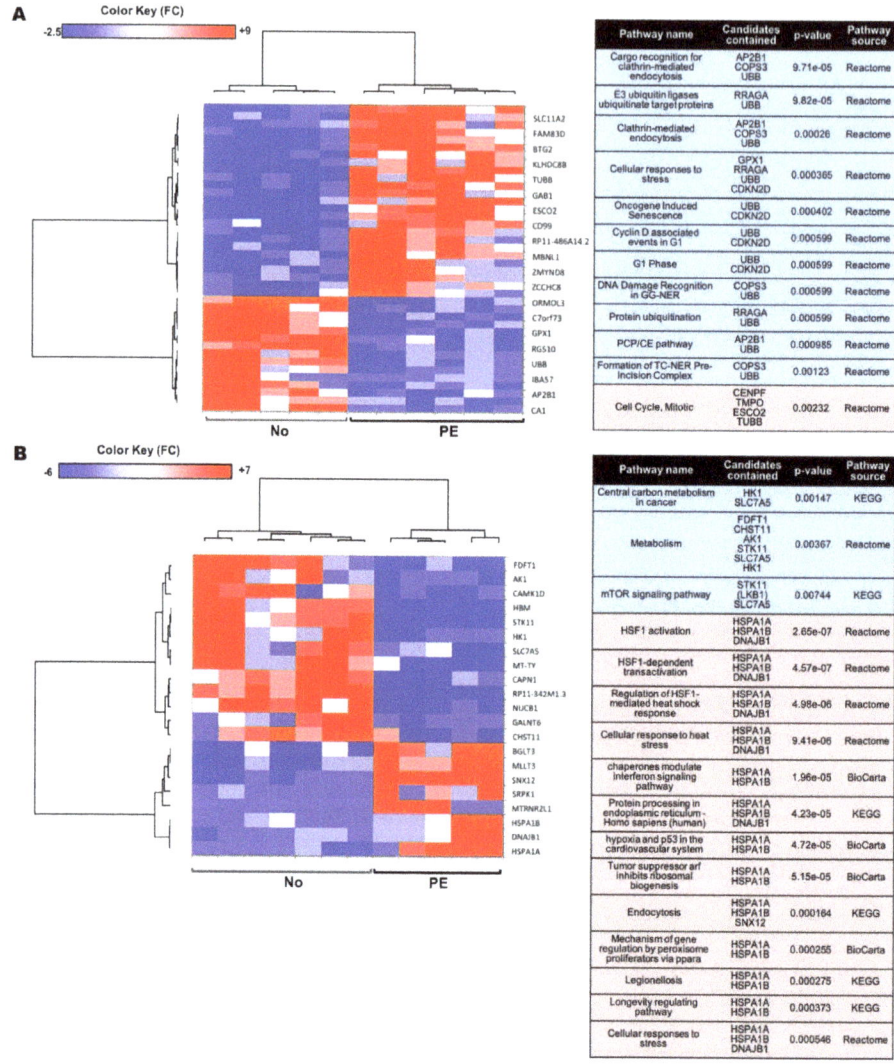

Figure 6. Sex-specific transcriptome comparison in the UCB erythroid progenitors from PE vs. normotensive pregnancies. (**A**,**B**) The heat maps of the differentially expressed genes and the related pathways are presented when comparing PE vs. normotensive sample from (**A**) male and (**B**) female fetuses. Shades of blue and red indicate down- or up-regulated genes/pathways, respectively.

2.7. Data Archiving

All data generated or analyzed during this study are included in this published article (and its Supplementary Information files). All the datasets generated during the current study are available on European Nucleotide Archive (https://www.ebi.ac.uk/ena) under accession number PRJEB27744 and PRIDE archive (https://www.ebi.ac.uk/pride/archive) under accession number PXD010364.

3. Discussion

This study focused on analyzing the changes in the molecular pathways regulating HSPCs and erythroid differentiation in fetuses from PE pregnancies. Our results were in agreement with previous reports [27,48] demonstrating no significant differences in the frequency of UCB HSPCs or the expression of the SAMs on these cells, despite originating from PE or normotensive pregnancies. In addition, the absence of significant differences in the number of BFU-Es produced during in vitro differentiation of the UCB CD34$^+$ cells from PE and normotensive groups in our samples was in accordance with previous reports [26,27]. Interestingly, both function and expression of SAMs on HSPCs are precisely regulated during embryonic development [49–51] as well as lineage differentiation [47,52,53]. Thus, the absence of significant differences in SAM expression and colony formation imply that PE may not cause significant changes in fetal HSPC migration/homing or intrinsic differentiation capacity.

Investigation of transcriptional changes demonstrated differences in gene expression in UCB HSPCs in PE vs. normotensive pregnancies. Many of the detected mRNAs were those of ribosomal proteins (RPs), important in proliferating cells [54,55] and primarily known to play a role in the maturation of ribosomal RNAs, ribosome biogenesis, and polysome formation [56,57]. However, ribosomal dysfunction can also trigger apoptosis, autophagy, cell cycle arrest as well as cellular senescence [58–62] and has been related to several hematological disorders, such as Diamond-Blackfan anemia [63,64]. These results prompted us to explore whether PE might be associated with changes in gene expression that adversely affect erythropoiesis and erythroid maturation. Analyzing the proteomics of the in vitro differentiated erythroid cells suggested changes in pathways important in the metabolism, immune system, protein processing, and export as well as phagosomes. Considering that efficient erythroid differentiation and maturation requires a synchronized regulation of iron, amino acid, and glucose metabolism [34], as well as various signaling pathways [65,66], alterations in these pathways could lead to intracellular changes and ineffective erythroid maturation.

To investigate if the results obtained in our in vitro analyses translated into changes in vivo, we compared the UCB erythroid profiles in PE vs. normotensive pregnancies. No significant differences were observed in the erythroid populations from arterial or venous UCB of male or female fetuses in either group. This observation was in agreement with our earlier results and suggested that disruption of erythroid maturation may contribute to a higher erythroblast count in the UCB from PE pregnancies independent of fetal hypoxia-induced EPO-dependent erythropoiesis [18–21,24]. It is also important to consider that fetal hypoxia in pregnancy is chronic, rather than acute, and hemolysis is not commonly observed in the fetuses born to PE. Thus, the release of immature erythroblasts into the UCB may have explanations other than those suggested for acute hypoxia or hemolytic anemia [67].

To confirm any mechanisms that could affect fetal erythroid maturation and enucleation in PE, the transcriptome of UCB erythroid cells were analyzed. Clustering of the male and female erythroid cells based on transcriptome analysis indicated that the expression of some genes located on both autosomal and sex chromosomes varied between the sexes, specifically upregulating the RNA transcription pathway and several mitochondrial factors in the male fetuses. Comparing the male fetuses among the PE and the normotensive groups indicated a decrease in DNA repair, convergent extension, protein ubiquitination, and vesicle trafficking, as well as deregulation in the cell cycle. For instance, lower CDKN2D (p19) and RRAGA, two regulators of cell cycle G1 progression [68], and amino acid-dependent mTORC1 activity [69,70] were associated with increased BTG2 and WRINP1 that regulate G1/S transition [71] and G1/S or G2/M arrest [72], respectively. Along with these changes, inhibitors of RNA transcription and several genes important in cell cycle S and mitosis phases were upregulated (Supplementary Table S3). Interestingly, KLHDC8B, a factor that safeguards the cell against mitotic errors and nuclear abnormalities, was also increased [73,74]. Due to the absence of significant differences in UCB erythroid populations between PE and normotensive male fetuses, the changes in gene expression could not be explained by elevated late basophilic or polychromatic erythroblasts [75], which express high levels of mitosis-related genes. Thus, the gene expression alterations observed in PE samples from male fetuses may be related to regulation of the cell cycle via mammalian target of rapamycin (mTOR) and AMP-activated protein kinase (AMPK) pathways [76] (Figure 7). Considering their role in regulating cell division, growth, or autophagy [77], altered phosphorylation and imbalance in AMPK/mTOR pathways can lead to a defective cell cycle and also erythroid maturation [78–81].

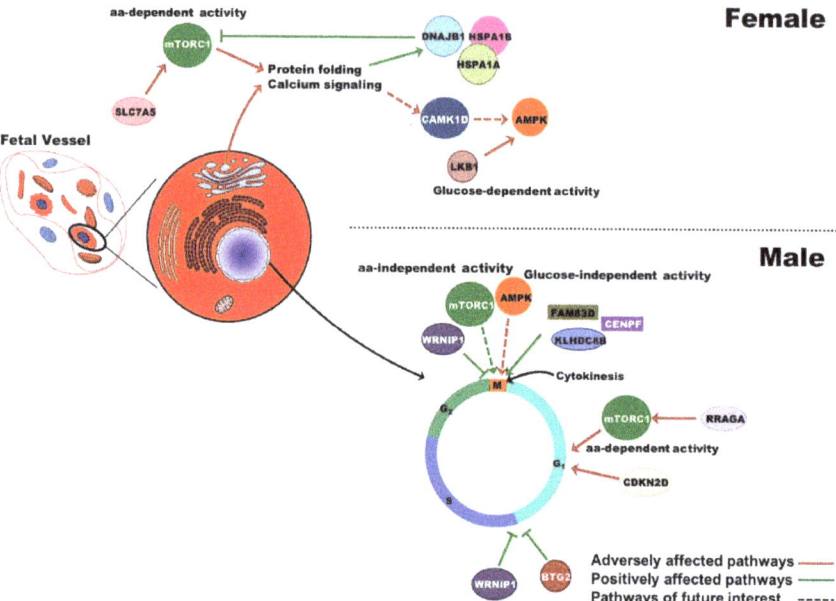

Figure 7. Sex-specific disruption of fetal erythropoiesis in PE. The interplay of the intracellular pathways that could disrupt fetal erythroid maturation has been demonstrated. A magnified erythroid cell with various organelles is used to illustrate the altered pathways in detail. aa: amino acid; SLC7A5 (LAT1): solute carrier family 7 member 5; DNAJB1: DnaJ heat shock protein family (Hsp40) member B1; HSPA1A: heat shock protein family A (Hsp70) member 1A; HSPA1A: heat shock protein family A (Hsp70) member 1B; CAMK1D (CKLiK): calcium/calmodulin dependent protein kinase ID; LKB1 (STK11): serine/threonine kinase 11; AMPK: AMP-activated protein kinase; mTORC1: mammalian target of rapamycin complex1; WRNIP1: Werner helicase interacting protein 1; FAM83D: family with sequence similarity 83 member D; CENPF: centromere protein F; KLHDC8B: kelch domain containing 8B; RRAGA: Ras related GTP binding A; CDKN2D: cyclin dependent kinase inhibitor 2D; BTG2: BTG anti-proliferation factor 2.

Among the female fetuses, decreased metabolism and increased cellular response to stress were the major pathways altered in the PE UCB erythroid cells. Genes that were important in protein processing and calcium homeostasis in Golgi, as well as calcium/calmodulin-dependent protein kinase 1D (CAMK1D) were downregulated in PE. The CAMK1D has been shown to control calcium-induced apoptosis in serum-deprived erythroleukemia cells in vitro [82]. Also, an upstream inducer of AMPK (STK11/LKB1) and amino acid-transporter required for mTORC1 activity (SLC7A5) [83] were lower in UCB erythroid cells from female fetuses born to PE pregnancies. These results along with the upregulated heat shock proteins imply a disturbance in protein processing that might affect cell maturation and survival (Figure 7). Considering that the activity of mTOR and AMPK proteins are regulated by phosphorylation at protein levels, future experiments are required to confirm and evaluate possible phosphorylation changes in erythroblasts in both male and female fetuses from PE pregnancies to indicate any sex-specific associations.

Interestingly, a surface glycoprotein was differentially expressed in each sex group in PE vs. normotensive UCB erythroid cells. Among the male fetuses, the expression of CD99, a glycoprotein associated with the Xg blood group, was upregulated in PE cases. While CD99 is located on the pseudoautosomal areas of sex chromosomes, its level of expression varies during development and based on sex [84]. On the other hand, the female fetuses from PE pregnancies indicated a significant decrease in expressing RP11-342M1.3, which is an antisense to erythroblast membrane associated protein (ERMAP), the surface glycoprotein known for the Scianna blood group [84]. Gene regulation by antisense expression can take place at different layers [85]. Considering that the expression of ERMAP was not significantly different between female PE vs. normotensive erythroid cells, it seems very likely that RP11-342M1.3 has a trans-regulatory effect on ERMAP mRNA. Other candidate genes for future studies include SLC25A6, MTRNR2L1, and CD36 that were determined in various analyses to be differentially expressed in PE and in a sex-specific manner. Further studies are required to confirm the possible sex-specific effects and outcomes of particular changes in fetal erythropoiesis in PE pregnancies.

There is a rising interest in evaluating the effect of various pregnancy complications on fetal development. Long-term analyses of PE pregnancies demonstrate several health problems among the offspring [86], with behavioral and cognitive dysfunction [87] having been a main focus. On the other hand, more studies are shedding light on the significance of fetal sex in regulating various aspects of a pregnancy, from maternal adaptation [41] to placental and fetal gene expression [88,89] and metabolism [90]. Sex-specificity of the placenta function and structure [91] as well as fetal and placental metabolism [90] have been suggested to underlie the higher vulnerability of male fetuses to pregnancy complications, such as obesity or PE [46,92]. The data in this study suggests that besides the nervous system, PE also affects the development of the fetal hematopoietic system. This is mainly through the triggering of transcriptional and proteomic changes in fetal HSPCs and erythroblasts that may disrupt erythroid maturation, explaining the higher UCB erythroblast count in these pregnancies. Our work also suggests that the changes observed in the molecular pathways are more severe among the male compared to the female fetuses. This is in line with higher adverse outcomes in pregnancies with male fetuses [39,40], as well as an increased risk of diseases of the blood and blood-forming organs, such as anemia, among the male children born to PE mothers [93].

4. Materials and Methods

4.1. Ethical Approval and Sample Collection

The study with identification number Dnr 2014/191 was approved on 24 April 2014 by the Lund Regional Ethics Committee Review Board (EPN) for studies on human subjects at Lund University and Skåne University Hospital, Lund, Sweden. Collection of UCB from normotensive and PE pregnancies was performed following both Caesarean and vaginal deliveries at Skåne University Hospital, after written informed consent from patients. All the experiments were performed in accordance with relevant guidelines and regulations. Preeclampsia was defined as blood pressure ≥140/90 mmHg and proteinuria ≥300 mg/L according to ISSHP definition [2]. A summary of the clinical condition of the patients included in this study and the subsequent experiments performed is available in Table 2 (details in Supplementary Table S4). The UCB was collected in flasks containing 10 mL Dulbecco's Modified Eagle's Medium, 10% fetal bovine serum (FBS), 100 IU/mL penicillin, 100 µg/mL streptomycin (Gibco®, Stockholm, Sweden) and 25 IU/mL heparin (Vianex S.A., Athens, Greece). The samples were stored at 4 °C and processed within 4 h after sampling.

Table 2. Clinical characterization of all the included patients with respect to the experiments.

Analysis	N	Pregnancy Condition	Gestational Age (Weeks)	Comments
SAM expression on UCB HSPCs	10	Normotensive	36–42	These samples were also used for cDNA subtractive hybridization.
	5	PE	36–39	
Colony formation assay	8	Normotensive	38–40	Performed in two sets of individual experiments, with three technical replicates in each set.
	7	PE	30–41	

Table 2. Cont.

Analysis	N	Pregnancy Condition	Gestational Age (Weeks)	Comments
Quantitative proteomic analysis	5	Normotensive	38–40	The colonies were obtained from the colony formation assay.
	5	PE	37–41	
UCB erythroid profile and transcriptome analysis	7	Normotensive	36–40	
	6	PE	36–40	

4.2. Mononuclear Cell Isolation from the UCB

Total mononuclear cells (MNCs) were isolated from UCB using the density centrifugation media Ficoll-Paque PLUS (GE Healthcare Life Sciences, Uppsala, Sweden) according to the manufacturer's protocol. In brief, the total UCB was mixed 1:1 (*w/v*) with wash buffer containing 1× phosphate buffered saline (PBS), 2% FBS and 2 mM EDTA. Each sample was carefully laid upon Ficoll-Paque PLUS before centrifugation at 400× *g* for 30 min at room temperature (RT). After the centrifugation, the interphase layer containing the MNCs was retrieved and mixed with ice-cold Iscove's Modified Dulbecco's Medium (IMDM), 10% FBS in 1:2 (*w/v*) (Gibco®). The MNC suspension was centrifuged and rinsed in wash buffer for erythroid profile analysis or $CD34^+$ cell isolation.

4.3. Isolation of UCB $CD34^+$ Cells

Using the human CD34 MicroBead Kit (Miltenyi Biotec, Lund, Sweden), the UCB $CD34^+$ cells were isolated according to the manufacturer's protocol. In summary, the MNCs were incubated with FcR Blocking Reagent and CD34 MicroBeads at 4 °C for 30 min followed by rinse and centrifugation at 300× *g* at 4 °C for 10 min. The cell suspension was filtered at 40 µm and $CD34^+$ cells were magnetically selected on LS columns (Miltenyi Biotec, Lund, Sweden). The $CD34^+$ cells were either resuspended in 10% Dimethyl sulfoxide (DMSO) freezing medium, stored at −80 °C for at least 24 h and transferred to liquid nitrogen tank for later in vitro cell culture assays, or were stained and analyzed for surface adhesion molecules using flow cytometry.

4.4. Flow Cytometric Analysis of SAM Expression on UCB HSPCs

The UCB HSPCs were detected by flow cytometry as $CD34^+$ $CD45^+$ cells and the expression of 6 different SAMs was analyzed using phycoerythrin-conjugated mouse anti-human antibodies (Table 1) [49,94–97]. Six separate suspensions of $CD34^+$-enriched cells were prepared and each was incubated for 30 min on ice with appropriate amounts of antibodies (1:25) specific for CD34 (CD34-phycoerythrin/Cy7) and CD45 (CD45-FITC) in combination with one of the SAMs. After rinse in wash buffer, the cells were analyzed using a BD FACSAria™ I. Spectral compensation was carried out using VersaComp Antibody Capture Beads kit (Beckman Coulter, Bromma, Sweden) and the gates were set based on unstained and fluorescent minus one controls. 7AAD at 10 µg/mL (Sigma Aldrich, Stockholm, Sweden) was used as a viability marker. All viable $CD34^+$ $CD45^+$ cells from each sample were sorted into a tube and used for RNA extraction. Data analysis was performed using FlowJo (V.10.0.8. Ashland, OR, US).

4.5. Flow Cytometric Analysis of UCB Stem Cells and Colony Formation Assay

Frozen $CD34^+$ enriched cells were thawed and stored with FcR Blocking Reagent (Miltenyi Biotec) at 4 °C for 30 min. The cells were then stained as described above, with the following antibodies: CD34-phycoerythrin/Cy7, CD38-APC, CD45RA-FITC, and CD90-BV421 (1:25, BD Biosciences, San Jose, CA, US). After performing spectral compensation and setting the gates as mentioned earlier, the UCB HSC population was analyzed by flow cytometry (Table 1) and a total of 15000 viable $CD34^+$ cells were collected from each sample using fluorescent activated cell sorting (FACS). The cells were mixed with Cell Resuspension Solution (R&D Systems, Oxon, Sweden) and Human Methylcellulose Complete Media containing EPO, Granulocyte macrophage colony-stimulating factor (GM-CSF),

Interlukin-3 (IL-3), and Stem Cell Factor (SCF) (HSC003, R&D Systems). 500 cells/well were plated in triplicate in 6-well plates and placed in a humid chamber incubated at 37 °C with 5% CO2. Burst forming units-erythroid (BFU-Es) were counted in each well after 14 days of culture as indicated by R&D Systems (https://www.rndsystems.com/resources/protocols/human-colony-forming-cell-cfc-assay-using-methylcellulose-based-media).

4.6. RNA Extraction and cDNA Subtractive Hybridization

The sorted viable $CD34^+$ $CD45^+$ cells from aforementioned SAM expression analysis were used for total RNA extraction was performed by lysing the cells in Trizol (Ambion, Naugatuck, CT, US). Following addition of chloroform to the lysate, the aqueous phase was mixed with 70% ethanol and transferred to RNeasy Mini spin columns (Qiagen, Hilden, Germany). Total RNA preparation was completed according to the manufacturer's protocol. Poly A^+ RNA purification was performed using Oligotex Direct mRNA mini kit (Qiagen) following the manufacturer's instructions. Subtractive hybridization was carried out using the Clontech® PCR-Select™ Differential Screening kit (Takara Bio USA, Inc., Mountain View, CA 94043, USA) according to the manufacturer's protocol. The poly A^+ RNA from PE and normotensive groups were respectively used as tester and driver for cDNA synthesis. Enriched tester-specific amplicons from the second round of subtraction were ligated into pGEM-T Easy Vector System I (Promega, Madison, WI, US) for insert sequencing (Beckman Coulter Genomics, Bishop's Stortford, United Kingdom). All retrieved sequences representing genes unique to the tester (PE) population compared to the normotensive population were blasted using BLAST analysis on NCBI (https://blast.ncbi.nlm.nih.gov/Blast.cgi).

4.7. Quantitative Proteomic Analysis

Proteomic analysis was performed at the Proteomics Core Facility at Sahlgrenska Academy, University of Gothenburg. For this purpose, the in vitro differentiated erythroid colonies were collected from the colony formation assay. The colonies were rinsed in PBS twice to remove any residues from the culture. The cell pellets were stored at −70 °C prior to lysis and protein extraction. The sample preparation and liquid chromatography-mass spectrometry process were carried out as explained in the Supplementary Materials and Methods [98]. Data analysis was performed using Proteome Discoverer version 1.4 (Thermo Fisher Scientific, Stockholm, Sweden) against the Human Swissprot Database version March 2017 (Swiss Institute of Bioinformatics, Switzerland). Mascot 2.5 (Matrix Science, London, UK) was used as a search engine with precursor mass tolerance of 5 ppm and fragment mass tolerance of 200 mmu. Tryptic peptides were accepted with zero missed cleavage and variable modifications of methionine oxidation, cysteine alkylation and fixed modifications of N-terminal TMT-label and lysine TMT-label were selected. The detected peptide threshold in the software was set to false discovery rate (FDR) ≤0.01 by searching against a reversed database. Identified proteins were grouped by sharing the same sequences to minimize redundancy. Reporter ion intensities were quantified in MS2 spectra at Minimum Quan Value Threshold set to 2000. The resulting ratios were normalized in the Proteome Discoverer 1.4 on the median protein value of 1.0 in each sample. Heat maps were generated using XLSTAT software.

4.8. Fluorescent-Activated Sorting of Erythroblasts from the UCB

To block Fc receptors, the isolated MNCs were incubated with FcR Blocking Reagent (Miltenyi Biotec) at 4 °C for 30 min. The cells were rinsed and pelleted 300× g at 4 °C. After resuspension and filtering through a 50 μm cup-shaped filter (BD Biosciences), the cells were stained for different surface markers using the following mouse anti-human antibody (ab)-conjugation set: CD45-FITC [1:25], CD235a/Glycophorin A (GPA)-BV421 [1:100] (BD Biosciences), CD49d/Integrin alpha 4-phycoerythrin/Cy7 [1:300] (BioLegend, Täby, Sweden) and CD233/Band 3-phycoerythrin [1:300] (Bristol Institute for Transfusion Sciences). After 30 min incubation on ice, the cells were rinsed and analyzed by a BD FACSAria™ I. 7AAD (Sigma Aldrich, Stockholm, Sweden) at a final concentration of

10 µg/mL was used as a viability marker. Spectral compensation was carried out using VersaComp Antibody Capture Beads kit (Beckman Coulter) and the gates were set based on unstained and fluorescent minus one controls. The data analysis was performed using FlowJo (version 10.0.8).

Considering the few numbers of the early-stage erythroid precursors, all the cells from proerythroblasts (CD45$^-$ GPA$^+$ CD49d^{hi} Band 3$^-$) to reticulocytes (CD45$^-$ GPA$^+$ CD49d^{lo} Band 3$^+$) were pooled together for each arterial and venous UCB sample. A total of 10^6 cells were sorted and collected for each sample. The cells were centrifuged at 300× g for 10 min, lysed in 350 µL of Buffer RLT from AllPrep DNA/RNA/Protein Mini Kit (Qiagen) according to the manufacturer's protocol and stored at −80 °C until later processing.

4.9. RNA Extraction, Library Preparation and Quality Check

All samples were thawed on ice and processed for RNA extraction using AllPrep DNA/RNA/Protein Mini (Qiagen) according to manufacturer's instructions. All centrifugations were performed at RT at 9000× g and the RNA was eluted in 50 µL RNase-free water. RNA samples were frozen at −80 °C and thawed for quality check and library preparation. RNA integrity was analyzed using Agilent RNA 600 Nano Kit (Agilent Technologies, Santa Clara, CA, US) on a Bioanalyzer 2100 (Agilent™, Santa Clara, CA, US) according to the manufacturer's instructions. All the samples indicated an RNA integrity number (RIN) ≥ 9 and were used for library preparation and amplification by the QuantSeq 3′ mRNA kit (Lexogen™, Vienna, Austria) according to the manufacturer's protocol. Quality and sequence length of the libraries were assessed by Fragment analyzer using the High sensitivity NGS fragment analysis kit (Advanced Analytical Technologies, Inc., Heidelberg, Germany), while concentration evaluation was performed by BioTek™ Synergy™ 2 (BioTek Instruments, Inc., Winooski, VT, US) microplate reader using Quant-iT™ PicoGreen™ dsDNA Assay Kit (Invitrogen™, Carlsbad, CA, US) for a low-range assay. The RNA library was sequenced in SE50bp mode on an Illumina HiSeq 2500 (Illumina, San Diego, CA, US).

4.10. Bioinformatics Analysis

Using random primers, the Lexogen Quantseq kit (Lexogen) generates fragments that end with a poly A tail. Since this random primer may introduce mistakes, the first 11bp of all reads were trimmed. Poly A tails and adapters at the end of each read were trimmed, along with basic quality trimming. Only reads longer than 20 bps were kept for further processing. All trimming and filtering steps were done using bbduk of bbtools 36.84 [99]. Reads were mapped to the Human genome (hg38) using STAR 2.5 [100]. Bam file modifications were done using elprep 2.5 [101]. Htseq 0.6.1p1 [102] was used to count the number of mapped reads per known gene. The gene definitions of Ensembl 87 were used. Reads were only considered in the counting process if the mapping quality was equal to or higher than 10, the strand of the read was the same strand as the gene and the read was not mapped in overlapping gene definitions (the union option). Differential expression analysis was performed using tools DESeq2 [103] and EdgeR [104,105]. The results of these tools were merged. Only genes that were significant with an FDR <0.1 in both tools were considered for further pathway analysis.

4.11. Pathway Analysis

Protein-protein interaction prediction and gene set enrichment analysis (GSEA) were performed by String (V.10.0) [106] and ConsensusPathDB (CPDB) [107] on UCB HSPCs and in vitro differentiated erythroid cells. The link between the genes, human phenotype and diseases were evaluated by performing functional gene list enrichment using ToppFun analysis from ToppGene Suite [108]. Gene ontologies were recovered from Gene, NCBI (https://www.ncbi.nlm.nih.gov/gene/).

4.12. Statistical Analysis

To calculate the protein fold change percentage (FC%), the average value of the normalized protein ratio of the PE group was divided over that of the normotensive samples. Also, the normalized protein ratios were used in the Student's *t*-test to calculate the statistical significance of the observed FC. Considering the low variability and high sensitivity of the TMT-MS, a FC ≥ 20% and *p* value ≤ 0.05 was determined as a significant difference in protein expression between PE and normotensive samples.

GraphPad Prism (version 7, San Diego, CA, US) was used to perform Mann Whitney U Test and to prepare the graphs.

5. Conclusions

In conclusion, our results indicate that the intrinsic migration and differentiation capacity of fetal HSPCs does not alter significantly in PE pregnancies. However, PE is associated with transcriptional and proteomic changes in fetal erythroid cells that may disrupt erythroid maturation, particularly in male fetuses.

Supplementary Materials: Supplementary materials can be found at http://www.mdpi.com/1422-0067/20/8/2038/s1. Reference [109] is cited in the supplementary materials.

Author Contributions: Conceptualization, Z.M. and S.R.H.; Investigation and validation, Z.M., E.H., M.F. and A.G.A.; Formal analysis, Z.M., G.E.M., K.H., Á.C.-C., A.G.A.; Project administration, Z.M., G.E.M.; Supervision, L.E., E.M., M.M., J.R.V., M.F. and S.R.H.; Writing—original draft preparation and visualization, Z.M.; All the authors reviewed and revised the manuscript; funding acquisition: M.F., S.R.H.

Funding: This project was supported by Erasmus + Program of the European Union (Framework agreement number: 2013-0040).

Acknowledgments: We specifically thank Per Anders Bertilsson (Flow Cytometry Core Facility, Clinical Research Center, Lund University) and Vanessa Brys (Genomics Core, UZ Leuven) for their excellent skillful technical assistance. We appreciate Annika Thorsell and Carina Sihbom's help with the TMT-mass spectrometry (Proteomics Core Facility, Sahlgrenska Academy, University of Gothenburg). We are grateful to the staff at Skåne University Hospital for assisting with sample collection.

Conflicts of Interest: S.R.H. holds patent related to diagnosis and treatment of preeclampsia and is co-founder of A1M Pharma and Preelumina Diagnostics (www.a1m.se). All the other authors declare no competing interests.

Abbreviations

PE	Preeclampsia/preeclamptic
UCB	Umbilical cord blood
HS(P)Cs	Hematopoietic stem (progenitor) cells
SAM	Surface adhesion molecule
mTORC1	mammalian target of rapamycin complex 1
AMPK	AMP-activated protein kinase
FDR	False discovery rate
DE	Differentially expressed

References

1. WHO. *WHO Recommendations for Prevention and Treatment of Pre-Eclampsia and Eclampsia*; World Health Organization: Geneva, Switzerland, 2011.
2. Davey, D.A.; MacGillivray, I. The classification and definition of the hypertensive disorders of pregnancy. *Am. J. Obstet. Gynecol.* **1988**, *158*, 892–898. [CrossRef]
3. Redman, C.W.; Sargent, I.L. Latest advances in understanding preeclampsia. *Science* **2005**, *308*, 1592–1594. [CrossRef] [PubMed]
4. Kingdom, J.C.; Kaufmann, P. Oxygen and placental villous development: Origins of fetal hypoxia. *Placenta* **1997**, *18*, 613–621. [CrossRef]
5. Redman, C.W.; Sargent, I.L. Placental stress and pre-eclampsia: A revised view. *Placenta* **2009**, *30*, S38–S42. [CrossRef] [PubMed]
6. Browne, V.A.; Julian, C.G.; Toledo-Jaldin, L.; Cioffi-Ragan, D.; Vargas, E.; Moore, L.G. Uterine artery blood flow, fetal hypoxia and fetal growth. *Philos. Trans R Soc. Lond. B Biol. Sci.* **2015**, *370*, 20140068. [CrossRef] [PubMed]

7. Soleymanlou, N.; Jurisica, I.; Nevo, O.; Ietta, F.; Zhang, X.; Zamudio, S.; Post, M.; Caniggia, I. Molecular evidence of placental hypoxia in preeclampsia. *J. Clin. Endocrinol. Metab.* **2005**, *90*, 4299–4308. [CrossRef]
8. Sultana, Z.; Maiti, K.; Aitken, J.; Morris, J.; Dedman, L.; Smith, R. Oxidative stress, placental ageing-related pathologies and adverse pregnancy outcomes. *Am. J. Reprod. Immunol.* **2017**, *77*, e1265. [CrossRef]
9. Tannetta, D.; Sargent, I. Placental disease and the maternal syndrome of preeclampsia: Missing links? *Curr. Hypertens. Rep.* **2013**, *15*, 590–599. [CrossRef]
10. Anderson, U.D.; Olsson, M.G.; Rutardottir, S.; Centlow, M.; Kristensen, K.H.; Isberg, P.E.; Thilaganathan, B.; Akerstrom, B.; Hansson, S.R. Fetal hemoglobin and alpha1-microglobulin as first- and early second-trimester predictive biomarkers for preeclampsia. *Am. J. Obstet. Gynecol.* **2011**, *204*, e521–e525. [CrossRef]
11. Winterbourn, C.C. Oxidative reactions of hemoglobin. *Methods Enzymol.* **1990**, *186*, 265–272.
12. May, K.; Rosenlof, L.; Olsson, M.G.; Centlow, M.; Morgelin, M.; Larsson, I.; Cederlund, M.; Rutardottir, S.; Siegmund, W.; Schneider, H.; et al. Perfusion of human placenta with hemoglobin introduces preeclampsia-like injuries that are prevented by alpha1-microglobulin. *Placenta* **2011**, *32*, 323–332. [CrossRef] [PubMed]
13. Cheng, S.W.; Chou, H.C.; Tsou, K.I.; Fang, L.J.; Tsao, P.N. Delivery before 32 weeks of gestation for maternal pre-eclampsia: Neonatal outcome and 2-year developmental outcome. *Early Hum. Dev.* **2004**, *76*, 39–46. [CrossRef] [PubMed]
14. Backes, C.H.; Markham, K.; Moorehead, P.; Cordero, L.; Nankervis, C.A.; Giannone, P.J. Maternal preeclampsia and neonatal outcomes. *J. Pregnancy* **2011**, *2011*, 214365. [CrossRef]
15. Williams, D. Long-term complications of preeclampsia. *Semin. Nephrol.* **2011**, *31*, 111–122. [CrossRef] [PubMed]
16. Ratsep, M.T.; Paolozza, A.; Hickman, A.F.; Maser, B.; Kay, V.R.; Mohammad, S.; Pudwell, J.; Smith, G.N.; Brien, D.; Stroman, P.W.; et al. Brain Structural and Vascular Anatomy Is Altered in Offspring of Pre-Eclamptic Pregnancies: A Pilot Study. *AJNR Am. J. Neuroradiol.* **2016**, *37*, 939–945. [CrossRef] [PubMed]
17. Masoumi, Z.; Familari, M.; Kallen, K.; Ranstam, J.; Olofsson, P.; Hansson, S.R. Fetal hemoglobin in umbilical cord blood in preeclamptic and normotensive pregnancies: A cross-sectional comparative study. *PLoS ONE* **2017**, *12*, e0176697. [CrossRef] [PubMed]
18. Akercan, F.; Cirpan, T.; Saydam, G. Nucleated red blood cells in infants of women with preterm labor and pre-eclampsia. *Int. J. Gynaecol. Obstet.* **2005**, *90*, 138–139. [CrossRef]
19. Catarino, C.; Rebelo, I.; Belo, L.; Rocha-Pereira, P.; Rocha, S.; Bayer Castro, E.; Patricio, B.; Quintanilha, A.; Santos-Silva, A. Erythrocyte changes in preeclampsia: Relationship between maternal and cord blood erythrocyte damage. *J. Perinat. Med.* **2009**, *37*, 19–27. [CrossRef] [PubMed]
20. Hebbar, S.; Misha, M.; Rai, L. Significance of maternal and cord blood nucleated red blood cell count in pregnancies complicated by preeclampsia. *J. Pregnancy* **2014**, *2014*, 496416. [CrossRef]
21. Aali, B.S.; Malekpour, R.; Sedig, F.; Safa, A. Comparison of maternal and cord blood nucleated red blood cell count between pre-eclamptic and healthy women. *J. Obstet. Gynaecol. Res.* **2007**, *33*, 274–278. [CrossRef]
22. Hermansen, M.C. Nucleated red blood cells in the fetus and newborn. *Arch. Dis. Child Fetal Neonatal. Ed.* **2001**, *84*, F211–F215. [CrossRef]
23. Teramo, K.A.; Widness, J.A. Increased fetal plasma and amniotic fluid erythropoietin concentrations: Markers of intrauterine hypoxia. *Neonatology* **2009**, *95*, 105–116. [CrossRef]
24. Thilaganathan, B.; Athanasiou, S.; Ozmen, S.; Creighton, S.; Watson, N.R.; Nicolaides, K.H. Umbilical cord blood erythroblast count as an index of intrauterine hypoxia. *Arch. Dis. Child Fetal Neonatal. Ed.* **1994**, *70*, F192–F194. [CrossRef] [PubMed]
25. Korst, L.M.; Phelan, J.P.; Ahn, M.O.; Martin, G.I. Nucleated red blood cells: An update on the marker for fetal asphyxia. *Am. J. Obstet. Gynecol.* **1996**, *175*, 843–846. [CrossRef]
26. Santillan, D.A.; Hamilton, W.; Christensen, A.; Talcott, K.; Gravatt, L.; Santillan, M.K.; Hunter, S.K. The effects of preeclampsia on signaling to hematopoietic progenitor cells. *Proc. Obstet. Gynecol.* **2013**, *3*, 11. [CrossRef]
27. Surbek, D.V.; Danzer, E.; Steinmann, C.; Tichelli, A.; Wodnar-Filipowicz, A.; Hahn, S.; Holzgreve, W. Effect of preeclampsia on umbilical cord blood hematopoietic progenitor-stem cells. *Am. J. Obstet. Gynecol.* **2001**, *185*, 725–729. [CrossRef]
28. Keele, D.K.; Kay, J.L. Plasma free fatty acid and blood sugar levels in newborn infants and their mothers. *Pediatrics* **1966**, *37*, 597–604.

29. Sahasrabuddhe, A.; Pitale, S.; Raje, D.; Sagdeo, M.M. Cord blood levels of insulin and glucose in full-term pregnancies. *J. Assoc. Phys. India* **2013**, *61*, 378–382.
30. Yang, J.M.; Wang, K.G. Relationship between acute fetal distress and maternal-placental-fetal circulations in severe preeclampsia. *Acta Obstet. Gynecol. Scand.* **1995**, *74*, 419–424. [CrossRef]
31. Guillemette, L.; Lacroix, M.; Allard, C.; Patenaude, J.; Battista, M.C.; Doyon, M.; Moreau, J.; Menard, J.; Ardilouze, J.L.; Perron, P.; et al. Preeclampsia is associated with an increased pro-inflammatory profile in newborns. *J. Reprod. Immunol.* **2015**, *112*, 111–114. [CrossRef]
32. Luo, S.T.; Zhang, D.M.; Qin, Q.; Lu, L.; Luo, M.; Guo, F.C.; Shi, H.S.; Jiang, L.; Shao, B.; Li, M.; et al. The Promotion of Erythropoiesis via the Regulation of Reactive Oxygen Species by Lactic Acid. *Sci. Rep.* **2017**, *7*, 38105. [CrossRef]
33. Morceau, F.; Dicato, M.; Diederich, M. Pro-inflammatory cytokine-mediated anemia: Regarding molecular mechanisms of erythropoiesis. *Mediators Inflamm.* **2009**, *2009*, 405016. [CrossRef]
34. Oburoglu, L.; Romano, M.; Taylor, N.; Kinet, S. Metabolic regulation of hematopoietic stem cell commitment and erythroid differentiation. *Curr. Opin. Hematol.* **2016**, *23*, 198–205. [CrossRef]
35. Oburoglu, L.; Tardito, S.; Fritz, V.; de Barros, S.C.; Merida, P.; Craveiro, M.; Mamede, J.; Cretenet, G.; Mongellaz, C.; An, X.; et al. Glucose and glutamine metabolism regulate human hematopoietic stem cell lineage specification. *Cell Stem Cell* **2014**, *15*, 169–184. [CrossRef]
36. Prince, O.D.; Langdon, J.M.; Layman, A.J.; Prince, I.C.; Sabogal, M.; Mak, H.H.; Berger, A.E.; Cheadle, C.; Chrest, F.J.; Yu, Q.; et al. Late stage erythroid precursor production is impaired in mice with chronic inflammation. *Haematologica* **2012**, *97*, 1648–1656. [CrossRef] [PubMed]
37. Galacteros, F.; Guilloud-Bataille, M.; Feingold, J. Sex, gestational age, and weight dependancy of adult hemoglobin concentration in normal newborns. *Blood* **1991**, *78*, 1121–1124.
38. Burman, D. Haemoglobin levels in normal infants aged 3 to 24 months, and the effect of iron. *Arch. Dis. Child* **1972**, *47*, 261–271. [CrossRef]
39. Elsmen, E.; Kallen, K.; Marsal, K.; Hellstrom-Westas, L. Fetal gender and gestational-age-related incidence of pre-eclampsia. *Acta Obstet. Gynecol. Scand.* **2006**, *85*, 1285–1291. [CrossRef] [PubMed]
40. Global Pregnancy, C.; Schalekamp-Timmermans, S.; Arends, L.R.; Alsaker, E.; Chappell, L.; Hansson, S.; Harsem, N.K.; Jalmby, M.; Jeyabalan, A.; Laivuori, H.; et al. Fetal sex-specific differences in gestational age at delivery in pre-eclampsia: A meta-analysis. *Int. J. Epidemiol.* **2016**, *46*, 632–642. [CrossRef]
41. Brown, R.N. Maternal adaptation to pregnancy is at least in part influenced by fetal gender. *BJOG* **2015**, *123*, 1087–1095. [CrossRef] [PubMed]
42. Lu, F.; Bytautiene, E.; Tamayo, E.; Gamble, P.; Anderson, G.D.; Hankins, G.D.; Longo, M.; Saade, G.R. Gender-specific effect of overexpression of sFlt-1 in pregnant mice on fetal programming of blood pressure in the offspring later in life. *Am. J. Obstet. Gynecol.* **2007**, *197*, e411–e415. [CrossRef]
43. Higgins, M.; Keller, J.; Moore, F.; Ostrander, L.; Metzner, H.; Stock, L. Studies of blood pressure in Tecumseh, Michigan. I. Blood pressure in young people and its relationship to personal and familial characteristics and complications of pregnancy in mothers. *Am. J. Epidemiol.* **1980**, *111*, 142–155. [CrossRef]
44. Langford, H.G.; Watson, R.L. Prepregnant blood pressure, hypertension during pregnancy, and later blood pressure of mothers and offspring. *Hypertension* **1980**, *2*, 130–133. [CrossRef]
45. Palti, H.; Rothschild, E. Blood pressure and growth at 6 years of age among offsprings of mothers with hypertension of pregnancy. *Early Hum. Dev.* **1989**, *19*, 263–269. [CrossRef]
46. Spinillo, A.; Montanari, L.; Gardella, B.; Roccio, M.; Stronati, M.; Fazzi, E. Infant sex, obstetric risk factors, and 2-year neurodevelopmental outcome among preterm infants. *Dev. Med. Child Neurol.* **2009**, *51*, 518–525. [CrossRef]
47. Hu, J.; Liu, J.; Xue, F.; Halverson, G.; Reid, M.; Guo, A.; Chen, L.; Raza, A.; Galili, N.; Jaffray, J.; et al. Isolation and functional characterization of human erythroblasts at distinct stages: Implications for understanding of normal and disordered erythropoiesis in vivo. *Blood* **2013**, *121*, 3246–3253. [CrossRef]
48. Wisgrill, L.; Schuller, S.; Bammer, M.; Berger, A.; Pollak, A.; Radke, T.F.; Kogler, G.; Spittler, A.; Helmer, H.; Husslein, P.; et al. Hematopoietic stem cells in neonates: Any differences between very preterm and term neonates? *PLoS ONE* **2014**, *9*, e106717. [CrossRef]
49. Timeus, F.; Crescenzio, N.; Basso, G.; Ramenghi, U.; Saracco, P.; Gabutti, V. Cell adhesion molecule expression in cord blood CD34+ cells. *Stem Cells* **1998**, *16*, 120–126. [CrossRef]

50. Roy, V.; Verfaillie, C.M. Expression and function of cell adhesion molecules on fetal liver, cord blood and bone marrow hematopoietic progenitors: Implications for anatomical localization and developmental stage specific regulation of hematopoiesis. *Exp. Hematol.* **1999**, *27*, 302–312. [CrossRef]
51. Surbek, D.V.; Steinmann, C.; Burk, M.; Hahn, S.; Tichelli, A.; Holzgreve, W. Developmental changes in adhesion molecule expressions in umbilical cord blood CD34 hematopoietic progenitor and stem cells. *Am. J. Obstet. Gynecol.* **2000**, *183*, 1152–1157. [CrossRef]
52. Kohn, L.A.; Hao, Q.L.; Sasidharan, R.; Parekh, C.; Ge, S.; Zhu, Y.; Mikkola, H.K.; Crooks, G.M. Lymphoid priming in human bone marrow begins before expression of CD10 with upregulation of L-selectin. *Nat. Immunol.* **2012**, *13*, 963–971. [CrossRef]
53. Gunji, Y.; Nakamura, M.; Hagiwara, T.; Hayakawa, K.; Matsushita, H.; Osawa, H.; Nagayoshi, K.; Nakauchi, H.; Yanagisawa, M.; Miura, Y.; et al. Expression and function of adhesion molecules on human hematopoietic stem cells: CD34+ LFA-1- cells are more primitive than CD34+ LFA-1+ cells. *Blood* **1992**, *80*, 429–436.
54. Chen, F.W.; Ioannou, Y.A. Ribosomal proteins in cell proliferation and apoptosis. *Int. Rev. Immunol.* **1999**, *18*, 429–448. [CrossRef]
55. Shama, S.; Avni, D.; Frederickson, R.M.; Sonenberg, N.; Meyuhas, O. Overexpression of initiation factor eIF-4E does not relieve the translational repression of ribosomal protein mRNAs in quiescent cells. *Gene Expr. Patt.* **1995**, *4*, 241–252.
56. Robledo, S.; Idol, R.A.; Crimmins, D.L.; Ladenson, J.H.; Mason, P.J.; Bessler, M. The role of human ribosomal proteins in the maturation of rRNA and ribosome production. *RNA* **2008**, *14*, 1918–1929. [CrossRef]
57. Zhou, X.; Liao, W.J.; Liao, J.M.; Liao, P.; Lu, H. Ribosomal proteins: Functions beyond the ribosome. *J. Mol. Cell Biol.* **2015**, *7*, 92–104. [CrossRef]
58. Bieging, K.T.; Mello, S.S.; Attardi, L.D. Unravelling mechanisms of p53-mediated tumour suppression. *Nat. Rev. Cancer* **2014**, *14*, 359–370. [CrossRef]
59. Blagosklonny, M.V. Geroconversion: Irreversible step to cellular senescence. *Cell Cycle* **2014**, *13*, 3628–3635. [CrossRef]
60. Green, D.R.; Kroemer, G. Cytoplasmic functions of the tumour suppressor p53. *Nature* **2009**, *458*, 1127–1130. [CrossRef]
61. Levine, B.; Abrams, J. p53: The Janus of autophagy? *Nat. Cell Biol.* **2008**, *10*, 637–639. [CrossRef]
62. Scherz-Shouval, R.; Weidberg, H.; Gonen, C.; Wilder, S.; Elazar, Z.; Oren, M. p53-dependent regulation of autophagy protein LC3 supports cancer cell survival under prolonged starvation. *Proc. Natl. Acad. Sci. USA* **2010**, *107*, 18511–18516. [CrossRef]
63. Raiser, D.M.; Narla, A.; Ebert, B.L. The emerging importance of ribosomal dysfunction in the pathogenesis of hematologic disorders. *Leuk. Lymphoma* **2014**, *55*, 491–500. [CrossRef]
64. Flygare, J.; Karlsson, S. Diamond-Blackfan anemia: Erythropoiesis lost in translation. *Blood* **2007**, *109*, 3152–3154. [CrossRef]
65. Zhang, J.; Wu, K.; Xiao, X.; Liao, J.; Hu, Q.; Chen, H.; Liu, J.; An, X. Autophagy as a regulatory component of erythropoiesis. *Int. J. Mol. Sci.* **2015**, *16*, 4083–4094. [CrossRef]
66. Steelman, L.S.; Abrams, S.L.; Whelan, J.; Bertrand, F.E.; Ludwig, D.E.; Basecke, J.; Libra, M.; Stivala, F.; Milella, M.; Tafuri, A.; et al. Contributions of the Raf/MEK/ERK, PI3K/PTEN/Akt/mTOR and Jak/STAT pathways to leukemia. *Leukemia* **2008**, *22*, 686–707. [CrossRef]
67. Constantino, B.T.; Cogionis, b. Nucleated RBCs—Significance in the Peripheral Blood Film. *Lab. Med.* **2000**, *31*, 223–229. [CrossRef]
68. Roussel, M.F. The INK4 family of cell cycle inhibitors in cancer. *Oncogene* **1999**, *18*, 5311–5317. [CrossRef]
69. Jin, G.; Lee, S.W.; Zhang, X.; Cai, Z.; Gao, Y.; Chou, P.C.; Rezaeian, A.H.; Han, F.; Wang, C.Y.; Yao, J.C.; et al. Skp2-Mediated RagA Ubiquitination Elicits a Negative Feedback to Prevent Amino-Acid-Dependent mTORC1 Hyperactivation by Recruiting GATOR1. *Mol. Cell* **2015**, *58*, 989–1000. [CrossRef]
70. Kalaitzidis, D.; Lee, D.; Efeyan, A.; Kfoury, Y.; Nayyar, N.; Sykes, D.B.; Mercier, F.E.; Papazian, A.; Baryawno, N.; Victora, G.D.; et al. Amino acid-insensitive mTORC1 regulation enables nutritional stress resilience in hematopoietic stem cells. *J. Clin. Investig.* **2017**, *127*, 1405–1413. [CrossRef]
71. Lim, I.K. TIS21 (/BTG2/PC3) as a link between ageing and cancer: Cell cycle regulator and endogenous cell death molecule. *J. Cancer Res. Clin. Oncol.* **2006**, *132*, 417–426. [CrossRef]

72. Kanu, N.; Zhang, T.; Burrell, R.A.; Chakraborty, A.; Cronshaw, J.; DaCosta, C.; Gronroos, E.; Pemberton, H.N.; Anderton, E.; Gonzalez, L.; et al. RAD18, WRNIP1 and ATMIN promote ATM signalling in response to replication stress. *Oncogene* **2016**, *35*, 4020. [CrossRef]
73. Krem, M.M.; Luo, P.; Ing, B.I.; Horwitz, M.S. The kelch protein KLHDC8B guards against mitotic errors, centrosomal amplification, and chromosomal instability. *J. Biol. Chem.* **2012**, *287*, 39083–39093. [CrossRef] [PubMed]
74. Yan, H.; Wang, Y.; Qu, X.; Li, J.; Hale, J.; Huang, Y.; An, C.; Papoin, J.; Guo, X.; Chen, L.; et al. Distinct roles for TET family proteins in regulating human erythropoiesis. *Blood* **2017**, *129*, 2002–2012. [CrossRef]
75. An, X.; Schulz, V.P.; Li, J.; Wu, K.; Liu, J.; Xue, F.; Hu, J.; Mohandas, N.; Gallagher, P.G. Global transcriptome analyses of human and murine terminal erythroid differentiation. *Blood* **2014**, *123*, 3466–3477. [CrossRef] [PubMed]
76. Cuyas, E.; Corominas-Faja, B.; Joven, J.; Menendez, J.A. Cell cycle regulation by the nutrient-sensing mammalian target of rapamycin (mTOR) pathway. *Methods Mol. Biol.* **2014**, *1170*, 113–144. [CrossRef]
77. Kim, J.; Kundu, M.; Viollet, B.; Guan, K.L. AMPK and mTOR regulate autophagy through direct phosphorylation of Ulk1. *Nat. Cell Biol.* **2011**, *13*, 132–141. [CrossRef] [PubMed]
78. Diekmann, F.; Rovira, J.; Diaz-Ricart, M.; Arellano, E.M.; Vodenik, B.; Jou, J.M.; Vives-Corrons, J.L.; Escolar, G.; Campistol, J.M. mTOR inhibition and erythropoiesis: Microcytosis or anaemia? *Nephrol. Dial Transpl.* **2012**, *27*, 537–541. [CrossRef]
79. Knight, Z.A.; Schmidt, S.F.; Birsoy, K.; Tan, K.; Friedman, J.M. A critical role for mTORC1 in erythropoiesis and anemia. *Elife* **2014**, *3*, e01913. [CrossRef]
80. Zhang, X.; Camprecios, G.; Rimmele, P.; Liang, R.; Yalcin, S.; Mungamuri, S.K.; Barminko, J.; D'Escamard, V.; Baron, M.H.; Brugnara, C.; et al. FOXO3-mTOR metabolic cooperation in the regulation of erythroid cell maturation and homeostasis. *Am. J. Hematol.* **2014**, *89*, 954–963. [CrossRef]
81. Mortensen, M.; Ferguson, D.J.; Edelmann, M.; Kessler, B.; Morten, K.J.; Komatsu, M.; Simon, A.K. Loss of autophagy in erythroid cells leads to defective removal of mitochondria and severe anemia in vivo. *Proc. Natl. Acad. Sci. USA* **2010**, *107*, 832–837. [CrossRef] [PubMed]
82. Yamada, T.; Suzuki, M.; Satoh, H.; Kihara-Negishi, F.; Nakano, H.; Oikawa, T. Effects of PU.1-induced mouse calcium-calmodulin-dependent kinase I-like kinase (CKLiK) on apoptosis of murine erythroleukemia cells. *Exp. Cell Res.* **2004**, *294*, 39–50. [CrossRef] [PubMed]
83. Chung, J.; Bauer, D.E.; Ghamari, A.; Nizzi, C.P.; Deck, K.M.; Kingsley, P.D.; Yien, Y.Y.; Huston, N.C.; Chen, C.; Schultz, I.J.; et al. The mTORC1/4E-BP pathway coordinates hemoglobin production with L-leucine availability. *Sci. Sig.* **2015**, *8*, ra34. [CrossRef] [PubMed]
84. Daniels, G. Xg blood group system. In *Human Blood Groups*, 2nd ed.; Blackwell Science Ltd.: Oxford, UK, 2002.
85. Pelechano, V.; Steinmetz, L.M. Gene regulation by antisense transcription. *Nat. Rev. Genet.* **2013**, *14*, 880–893. [CrossRef] [PubMed]
86. Goffin, S.M.; Derraik, J.G.B.; Groom, K.M.; Cutfield, W.S. Maternal pre-eclampsia and long-term offspring health: Is there a shadow cast? *Pregnancy Hypertens.* **2018**, *12*, 11–15. [CrossRef]
87. Figueiro-Filho, E.A.; Mak, L.E.; Reynolds, J.N.; Stroman, P.W.; Smith, G.N.; Forkert, N.D.; Paolozza, A.; Ratsep, M.T.; Croy, B.A. Neurological function in children born to preeclamptic and hypertensive mothers—A systematic review. *Pregnancy Hypertens.* **2017**, *10*, 1–6. [CrossRef]
88. Sood, R.; Zehnder, J.L.; Druzin, M.L.; Brown, P.O. Gene expression patterns in human placenta. *Proc. Natl. Acad. Sci. USA* **2006**, *103*, 5478–5483. [CrossRef]
89. Sedlmeier, E.M.; Brunner, S.; Much, D.; Pagel, P.; Ulbrich, S.E.; Meyer, H.H.; Amann-Gassner, U.; Hauner, H.; Bader, B.L. Human placental transcriptome shows sexually dimorphic gene expression and responsiveness to maternal dietary n-3 long-chain polyunsaturated fatty acid intervention during pregnancy. *BMC Genom.* **2014**, *15*, 941. [CrossRef] [PubMed]
90. Dearden, L.; Bouret, S.G.; Ozanne, S.E. Sex and gender differences in developmental programming of metabolism. *Mol. Metab.* **2018**, *15*, 8–19. [CrossRef] [PubMed]
91. Rosenfeld, C.S. Sex-Specific Placental Responses in Fetal Development. *Endocrinology* **2015**, *156*, 3422–3434. [CrossRef] [PubMed]
92. Reynolds, S.A.; Roberts, J.M.; Bodnar, L.M.; Haggerty, C.L.; Youk, A.O.; Catov, J.M. Newborns of preeclamptic women show evidence of sex-specific disparity in fetal growth. *Gend. Med.* **2012**, *9*, 424–435. [CrossRef]

93. Wu, C.S.; Nohr, E.A.; Bech, B.H.; Vestergaard, M.; Catov, J.M.; Olsen, J. Health of children born to mothers who had preeclampsia: A population-based cohort study. *Am. J. Obstet. Gynecol.* **2009**, *201*, e261–e269. [CrossRef]
94. Turner, M.L.; McIlwaine, K.; Anthony, R.S.; Parker, A.C. Differential expression of cell adhesion molecules by human hematopoietic progenitor cells from bone marrow and mobilized adult peripheral blood. *Stem Cells* **1995**, *13*, 311–316. [CrossRef] [PubMed]
95. Voermans, C.; van Hennik, P.B.; van der Schoot, C.E. Homing of human hematopoietic stem and progenitor cells: New insights, new challenges? *J. Hematother. Stem Cell Res.* **2001**, *10*, 725–738. [CrossRef]
96. Deguchi, T.; Komada, Y.; Sugiyama, K.; Zhang, X.L.; Azuma, E.; Yamamoto, H.; Sakurai, M. Expression of homing-associated cell adhesion molecule (H-CAM/CD44) on human CD34+ hematopoietic progenitor cells. *Exp. Hematol.* **1999**, *27*, 542–552. [CrossRef]
97. Yanai, N.; Sekine, C.; Yagita, H.; Obinata, M. Roles for integrin very late activation antigen-4 in stroma-dependent erythropoiesis. *Blood* **1994**, *83*, 2844–2850. [PubMed]
98. Wisniewski, J.R.; Zougman, A.; Nagaraj, N.; Mann, M. Universal sample preparation method for proteome analysis. *Nat. Methods* **2009**, *6*, 359–362. [CrossRef]
99. Bushnell, B. BBTools. Available online: http://jgi.doe.gov/data-and-tools/bbtools/ (accessed on 1 May 2017).
100. Dobin, A.; Davis, C.A.; Schlesinger, F.; Drenkow, J.; Zaleski, C.; Jha, S.; Batut, P.; Chaisson, M.; Gingeras, T.R. STAR: Ultrafast universal RNA-seq aligner. *Bioinformatics* **2013**, *29*, 15–21. [CrossRef]
101. Herzeel, C.; Costanza, P.; Decap, D.; Fostier, J.; Reumers, J. elPrep: High-Performance Preparation of Sequence Alignment/Map Files for Variant Calling. *PLoS ONE* **2015**, *10*, e0132868. [CrossRef] [PubMed]
102. Anders, S.; Pyl, P.T.; Huber, W. HTSeq—A Python framework to work with high-throughput sequencing data. *Bioinformatics* **2015**, *31*, 166–169. [CrossRef] [PubMed]
103. Love, M.I.; Huber, W.; Anders, S. Moderated estimation of fold change and dispersion for RNA-seq data with DESeq2. *Genome Biol.* **2014**, *15*, 550. [CrossRef] [PubMed]
104. Robinson, M.D.; McCarthy, D.J.; Smyth, G.K. edgeR: A Bioconductor package for differential expression analysis of digital gene expression data. *Bioinformatics* **2010**, *26*, 139–140. [CrossRef]
105. McCarthy, D.J.; Chen, Y.; Smyth, G.K. Differential expression analysis of multifactor RNA-Seq experiments with respect to biological variation. *Nucleic Acids Res.* **2012**, *40*, 4288–4297. [CrossRef] [PubMed]
106. Szklarczyk, D.; Franceschini, A.; Wyder, S.; Forslund, K.; Heller, D.; Huerta-Cepas, J.; Simonovic, M.; Roth, A.; Santos, A.; Tsafou, K.P.; et al. STRING v10: Protein-protein interaction networks, integrated over the tree of life. *Nucleic Acids Res.* **2015**, *43*, D447–D452. [CrossRef] [PubMed]
107. Kamburov, A.; Wierling, C.; Lehrach, H.; Herwig, R. ConsensusPathDB—A database for integrating human functional interaction networks. *Nucleic Acids Res.* **2009**, *37*, D623–D628. [CrossRef]
108. Chen, J.; Bardes, E.E.; Aronow, B.J.; Jegga, A.G. ToppGene Suite for gene list enrichment analysis and candidate gene prioritization. *Nucleic Acids Res.* **2009**, *37*, W305–W311. [CrossRef]
109. Niklasson, A.; Albertsson-Wikland, K. Continuous growth reference from 24th week of gestation to 24 months by gender. *BMC Pediatr.* **2008**, *8*, 8. [CrossRef]

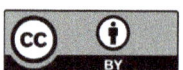

© 2019 by the authors. Licensee MDPI, Basel, Switzerland. This article is an open access article distributed under the terms and conditions of the Creative Commons Attribution (CC BY) license (http://creativecommons.org/licenses/by/4.0/).

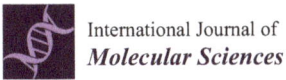

Article

Postnatal Expression Profile of microRNAs Associated with Cardiovascular and Cerebrovascular Diseases in Children at the Age of 3 to 11 Years in Relation to Previous Occurrence of Pregnancy-Related Complications

Ilona Hromadnikova [1,*], Katerina Kotlabova [1], Lenka Dvorakova [1], Ladislav Krofta [2] and Jan Sirc [2]

[1] Department of Molecular Biology and Cell Pathology, Third Faculty of Medicine, Charles University, 10000 Prague, Czech Republic; katerina.kotlabova@lf3.cuni.cz (K.K.); lenka.dvorakova@lf3.cuni.cz (L.D.)
[2] Institute for the Care of the Mother and Child, Third Faculty of Medicine, Charles University, 14700 Prague, Czech Republic; ladislav.krofta@upmd.eu (L.K.); jan.sirc@upmd.eu (J.S.)
* Correspondence: ilona.hromadnikova@lf3.cuni.cz; Tel.: +420-296511336

Received: 3 January 2019; Accepted: 30 January 2019; Published: 2 February 2019

Abstract: Children descending from pregnancies complicated by gestational hypertension (GH), preeclampsia (PE) or fetal growth restriction (FGR) have a lifelong cardiovascular risk. The aim of the study was to verify if pregnancy complications induce postnatal alterations in gene expression of microRNAs associated with cardiovascular/cerebrovascular diseases. Twenty-nine microRNAs were assessed in peripheral blood, compared between groups, and analyzed in relation to both aspects, the current presence of cardiovascular risk factors and cardiovascular complications and the previous occurrence of pregnancy complications with regard to the clinical signs, dates of delivery, and Doppler ultrasound examination. The expression profile of miR-21-5p differed between controls and children with a history of uncomplicated pregnancies with abnormal clinical findings. Abnormal expression profile of multiple microRNAs was found in children affected with GH (miR-1-3p, miR-17-5p, miR-20a-5p, miR-21-5p, miR-23a-3p, miR-26a-5p, miR-29a-3p, miR-103a-3p, miR-125b-5p, miR-126-3p, miR-133a-3p, miR-146a-5p, miR-181a-5p, miR-195-5p, and miR-342-3p), PE (miR-1-3p, miR-20a-5p, miR-20b-5p, miR-103a-3p, miR-133a-3p, miR-342-3p), and FGR (miR-17-5p, miR-126-3p, miR-133a-3p). The index of pulsatility in the ductus venosus showed a strong positive correlation with miR-210-3p gene expression in children exposed to PE and/or FGR. Any of changes in epigenome (up-regulation of miR-1-3p and miR-133a-3p) that were induced by pregnancy complications are long-acting and may predispose children affected with GH, PE, or FGR to later development of cardiovascular/cerebrovascular diseases. Novel epigenetic changes (aberrant expression profile of microRNAs) appeared in a proportion of children that were exposed to GH, PE, or FGR. Screening of particular microRNAs may stratify a highly risky group of children that might benefit from implementation of early primary prevention strategies.

Keywords: Body mass index (BMI); cardiovascular/cerebrovascular diseases; cardiovascular risk; children; echocardiography; microRNA expression; pregnancy complications; prehypertension/hypertension; primary prevention; screening

---

1. Introduction

There exists a progressive increase of data linking specific levels of risk factors in prenatal life with cardiovascular disease outcomes in children and adolescents. Recent epidemiologic and experimental data substantially indicate that children descending from pregnancies complicated by gestational hypertension (GH), preeclampsia (PE), or fetal growth restriction (FGR) have an unique, lifetime cardiovascular risk profile that is present from early life. Young offspring of pregnancies complicated by GH or PE already have increased body mass index (BMI) and wider waist circumference [1,2]. Systolic and/or diastolic blood pressures (BP) were also reported to be higher in offspring of mothers with GH or PE compared with offspring of mothers without hypertensive disorders of pregnancy [1–5]. These differences were even consistent till the age of 18 years, as the patterns of blood pressure change did not differ between children of hypertensive and normotensive pregnancies [6]. Offspring from pregnancies with early PE (onset < 34 weeks) had at the age of 6 to 13 years a higher systolic BP and higher nocturnal systolic and diastolic BP than those born to late onset PE [7]. Maternal central pulsatile BP components (systolic BP and pulse pressure) during pregnancy were associated with higher BP in the offspring of women with PE. This positive correlation was already evident at 3 years old children [8]. These results suggested a possible association between maternal hypertensive disorders of pregnancy and offspring BP that may be driven by genetics or familial non-genetic risk factors particular to BP [5]. In addition, PE leaves a persistent alteration in the systemic and the pulmonary circulation of the children. Pulmonary artery pressure was roughly 30% higher and flow-mediated dilation was 30% smaller in children of PE-affected mothers than in controls. This alteration predisposes children to exaggerated hypoxic pulmonary hypertension already during childhood and may cause premature cardiovascular disease in the systemic circulation at some time in the future [9].

Sarvari et al. [10] reported that FGR induced cardiac remodeling persists until preadolescence (8–12 years of age) with findings similar to those reported in their prenatal life and childhood. Echocardiography and three-dimensional shape computational analysis revealed a more spherical and smaller hearts, decreased longitudinal motion and impaired relaxation in children affected with FGR [10]. Yiallourou et al. [11] revealed that preterm FGR children aged 5–12 years had smaller left ventricular lengths, ascending aorta, and left ventricular outflow tract diameter and vascular compliance was positively correlated with gestational age. These findings result in the hypothesis of FGR caused primary cardiac programming for explaining the association between low birth weight and later cardiovascular risk [10].

Birth weight influences childhood BP as well, but the effects may vary depending on ethnic group. FGR and early gestational age were associated with higher BP in white but not African American children at the age of 5 years [12].

Altogether, childhood obesity, hypertension, diabetes, and cardiac remodeling are the most prevalent intermediate and long-standing health consequences of undernutrition of the fetus caused by insufficiency of the placenta [13,14].

Although, health factors such as lipid levels, BMI, and BP normally change with age, growth, and development, children affected by pregnancy complications including GH, PE, and FGR represent a population that would benefit from implementation of early primary prevention strategies. At least modification of diet and physical activity are first-line interventions. Appropriate pharmacological intervention may be also considered when lifestyle change is not successful [15].

The goal of the study was to evaluate an epigenetic profile for the detection of cardiovascular risk in whole peripheral blood of children at the age of 3 to 11 years born out of pregnancies complicated by GH, PE, and FGR. Postnatal epigenetic profiling of microRNAs playing a role in pathogenesis of diverse cardiovascular/cerebrovascular diseases (miR-1-3p, miR-16-5p, miR-17-5p, miR-20a-5p, miR-20b-5p, miR-21-5p, miR-23a-3p, miR-24-3p, miR-26a-5p, miR-29a-3p, miR-92a-3p, miR-100-5p, miR-103a-3p, miR-125b-5p, miR-126-3p, miR-130b-3p, miR-133a-3p, miR-143-3p, miR-145-5p, miR-146a-5p, miR-155-5p, miR-181a-5p, miR-195-5p, miR-199a-5p, miR-210-3p, miR-221-3p, miR-342-3p, miR-499a-5p, and miR-574-3p) was the subject of our interest. We focused mainly on those microRNAs known to be involved in the onset of dyslipidaemia [16,17], hypertension [18–20], vascular inflammation [21,22], insulin resistance and diabetes [23], atherosclerosis [24,25], angiogenesis [26,27], coronary artery disease [19,22,26,28], myocardial infarction and heart failure [18,29–32], stroke [33], intracranial aneurysm [34], pulmonary arterial hypertension [35], and peripartum cardiomyopathy [36].

MicroRNAs are the members of the family of small noncoding RNAs that regulate expression of genes at the posttranscriptional level by blocking translation or degrading of target messenger RNA [37]. MicroRNA analyses indicate that under pathological conditions a variety of tissues display diverse microRNA expression profiles, which may be used in clinical diagnostics [38]. Recent studies have demonstrated that GH, PE, and FGR are associated with alterations in microRNA expression in the maternal circulation, placenta, and umbilical cord blood [39–43].

To the best of our knowledge, any study on expression profiling of microRNAs associated with cardiovascular and cerebrovascular diseases in whole peripheral blood of children descending from GH, PE, and FGR affected pregnancies has not been carried out.

2. Results

2.1. Distribution of Children Descending from Normal Pregnancies into Groups Based on Clinical Examination and Consequent Findings

Children descending from normal pregnancies were divided into two groups based on the results of examination and clinical findings. Children already dispesarized in the department of pediatric cardiology ($n = 8$) and those ones indicated by the sonographer to have valve problems and heart defects tricuspid valve regurgitation ($n = 8$), mitral valve regurgitation ($n = 1$), pulmonary valve regurgitation ($n = 2$), bicuspid aortic valve regurgitation ($n = 1$), ventricular septum defect ($n = 1$), atrial septum defect ($n = 1$), foramen ovale apertum ($n = 5$), arrhythmia ($n = 1$) constituted particular group together with children confirmed over several visits to have a high BP ($n = 16$) (systolic blood pressure (SBP) and/or diastolic blood pressure (DBP) $\geq$ 90th percentile evaluated by the Age-Based Pediatric Blood Pressure Reference Charts calculator) and/or high BMI ($n = 9$) (BMI 85th percentile evaluated by the BMI Percentile Calculator for Child and Teens). Overall, this group consisted of 38 children (43.18%). The second group consisted from 50 children with normal anamnesis, normal BP, normal BMI, and normal reference values of echocardiographic measurements.

2.2. Up-Regulation of miR-21-5p in Children Descending from Normal Pregnancies that are Overweight/Obese, Prehypertensive/Hypertensive and/or have Abnormal Echocardiogram Findings

Since we identified within the group of children descending from normal pregnancies those ones with cardiac findings who were already dispesarized in the department of pediatric cardiology, or those ones who were overweight/obese, had prehypertension/hypertension, and/or abnormal echocardiogram findings, we compared the microRNA profile of this group to that one consisting of children with normal anamnesis, normal BP, normal BMI and normal reference values of echocardiographic measurements. The performance of receivers operating characteristic (ROC) curve analysis revealed that only miR-21-5p differentiated children descending from normal pregnancies in dependence on the presence or absence of postnatal abnormal clinical findings with a sensitivity of 28.95% at a specificity of 90.0% (Figure 1).

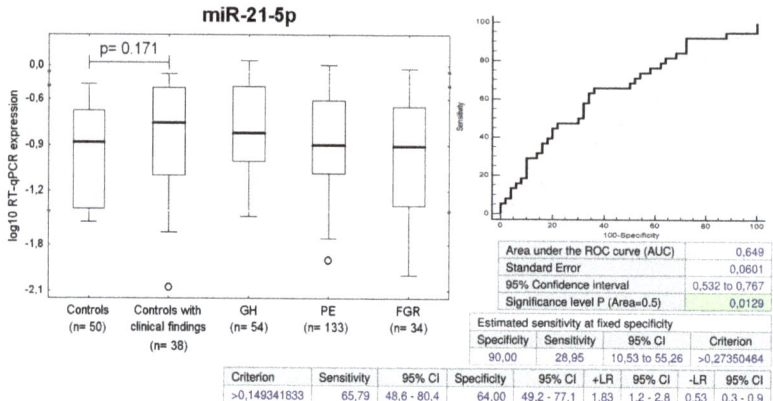

Figure 1. Up-regulation of miR-21-5p in children descending from normal pregnancies that are overweight/obese, prehypertensive/hypertensive and/or have abnormal echocardiogram findings. GH: gestational hypertension; PE: preeclampsia; FGR: fetal growth restriction; ROC: receivers operating characteristic; AUC: Area under the curve; +LR: likelihood ratio positive; −LR: likelihood ratio negative.

2.3. Dysregulation of Cardiovascular/Cerebrovascular Disease Associated microRNAs in Children Descending from Complicated Pregnancies

MicroRNA gene expression was compared between children descending from normal and complicated pregnancies (GH, PE, and FGR). MicroRNA gene expression was analyzed in relation to both aspects, the current presence of cardiovascular risk factors (overweight/obesity and/or prehypertension/hypertension) and cardiovascular complications (valve problems and heart defects) and the previous occurrence of pregnancy-related complications with respect to clinical signs (mild versus severe preeclampsia), dates of delivery (< and > 34 weeks in case of PE, < and > 32 weeks in case of FGR, respectively). The association between microRNA gene expression and Doppler ultrasonography parameters (pulsatility index (PI) in the umbilical artery, PI in the middle cerebral artery, the cerebroplacental ratio, PI in the uterine artery, PI in the ductus venosus, and the presence of unilateral or bilateral diastolic notch in the uterine artery) was analyzed in the group of complicated pregnancies (PE and/or FGR). Just the results that reached a statistical significance or displayed a trend toward aberrant microRNA expression profile in complicated cases are presented below.

2.4. Multiple microRNAs are Up-Regulated in Children Descending from GH Pregnancies

The ROC curve analysis revealed a significant up-regulation of miR-1-3p, miR-17-5p, miR-20a-5p, miR-21-5p, miR-23a-3p, miR-26a-5p, miR-29a-3p, miR-126-3p, miR-133a-3p, miR-146a-5p, and miR-181a-5p for children descending from GH pregnancies when the comparison to the controls was performed (Figure 2).

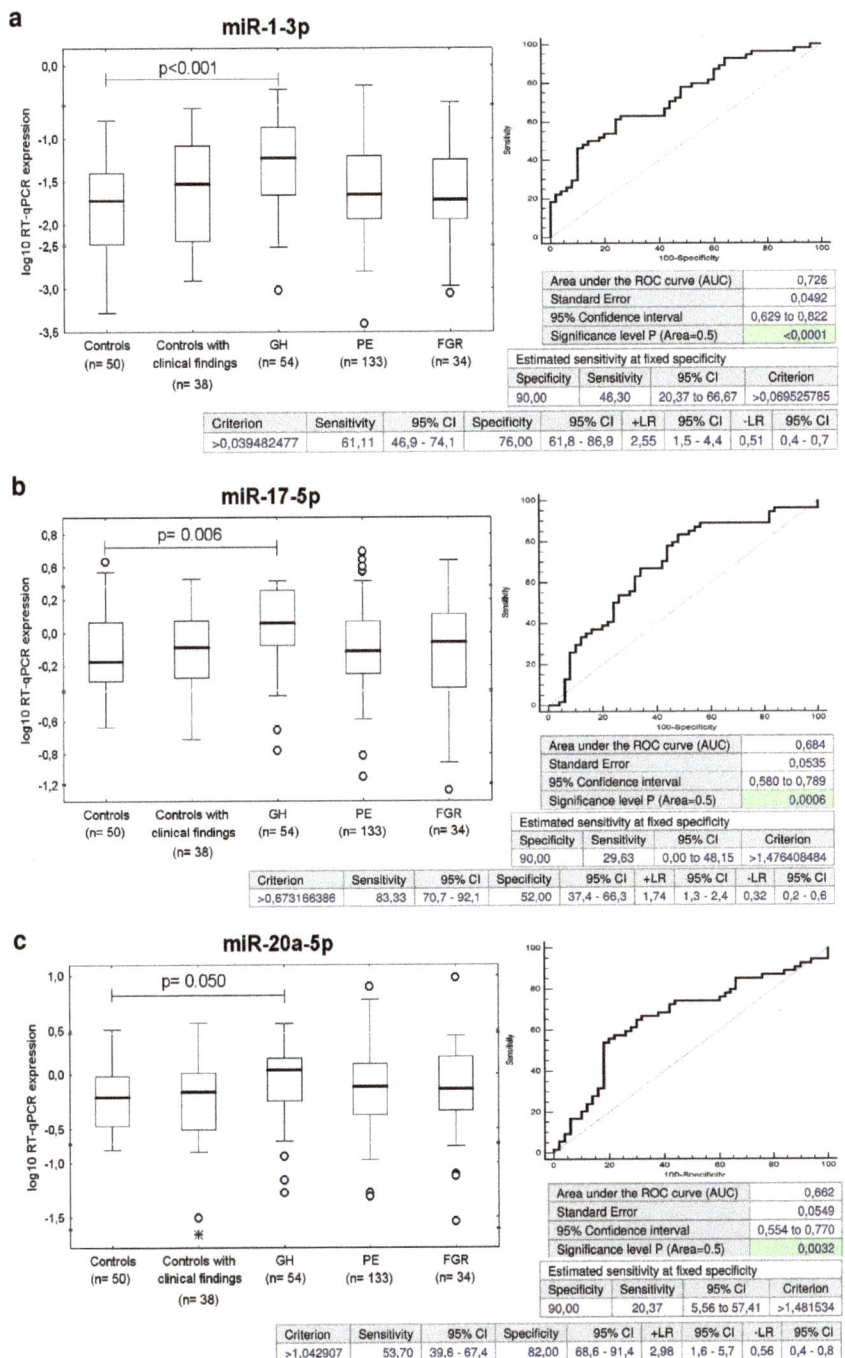

Figure 2. Cont.

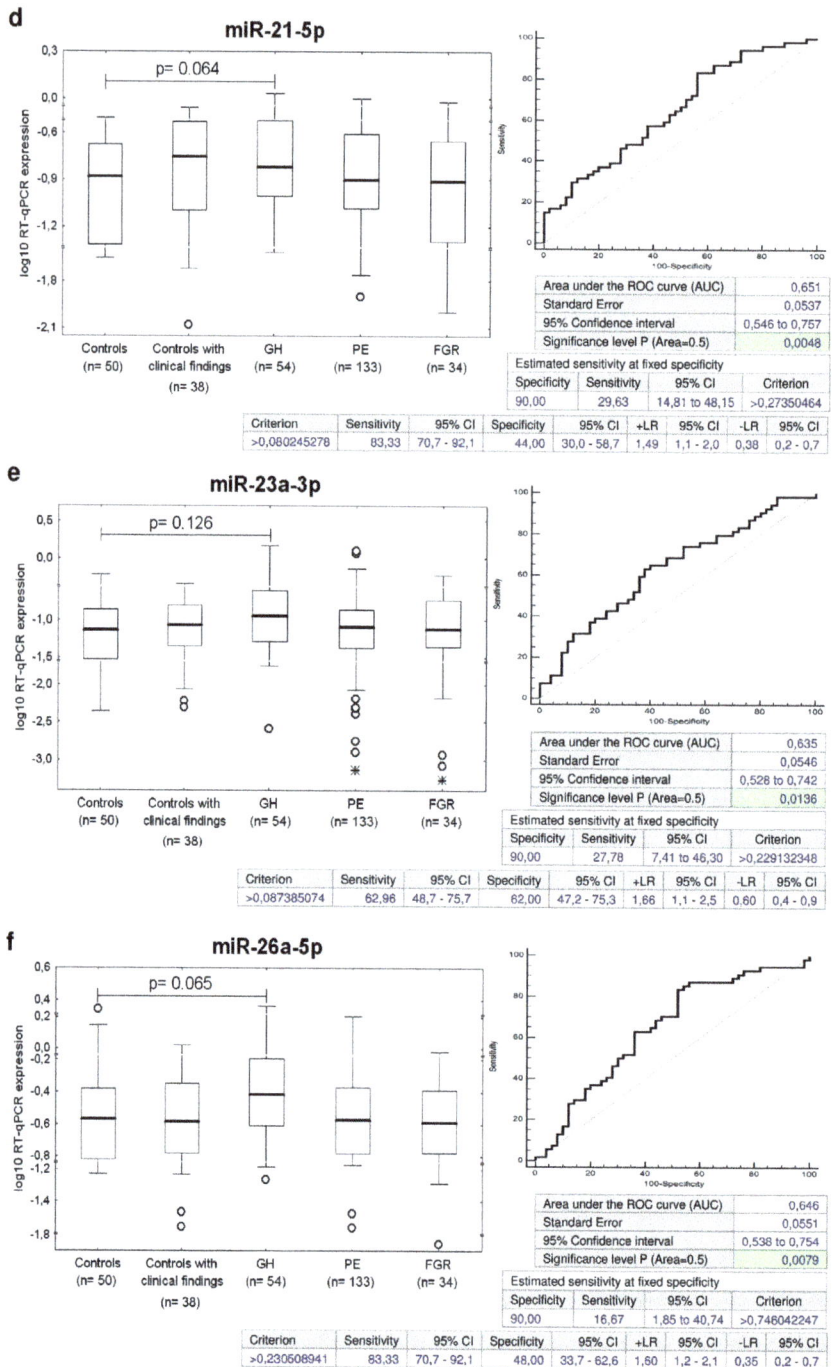

Figure 2. *Cont.*

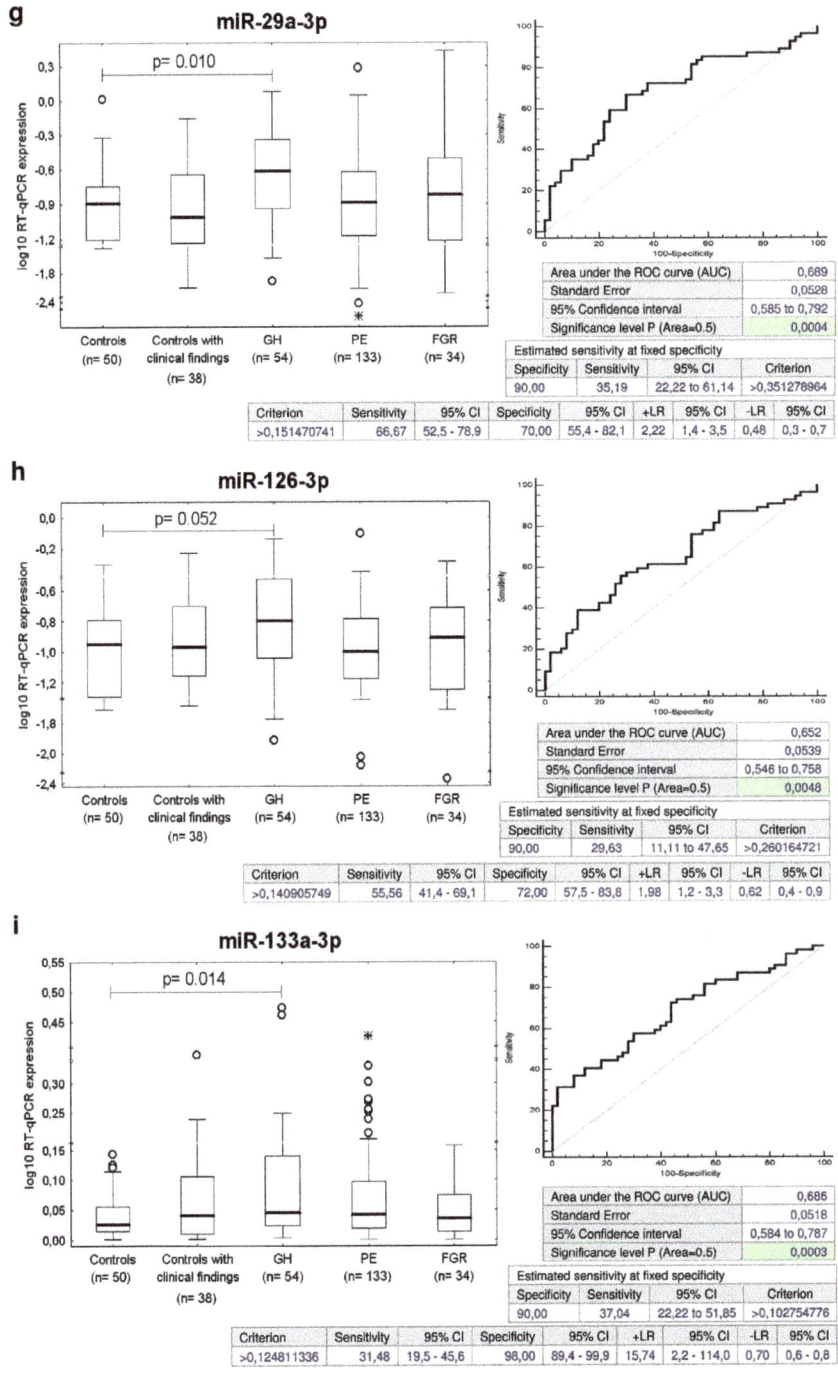

Figure 2. *Cont.*

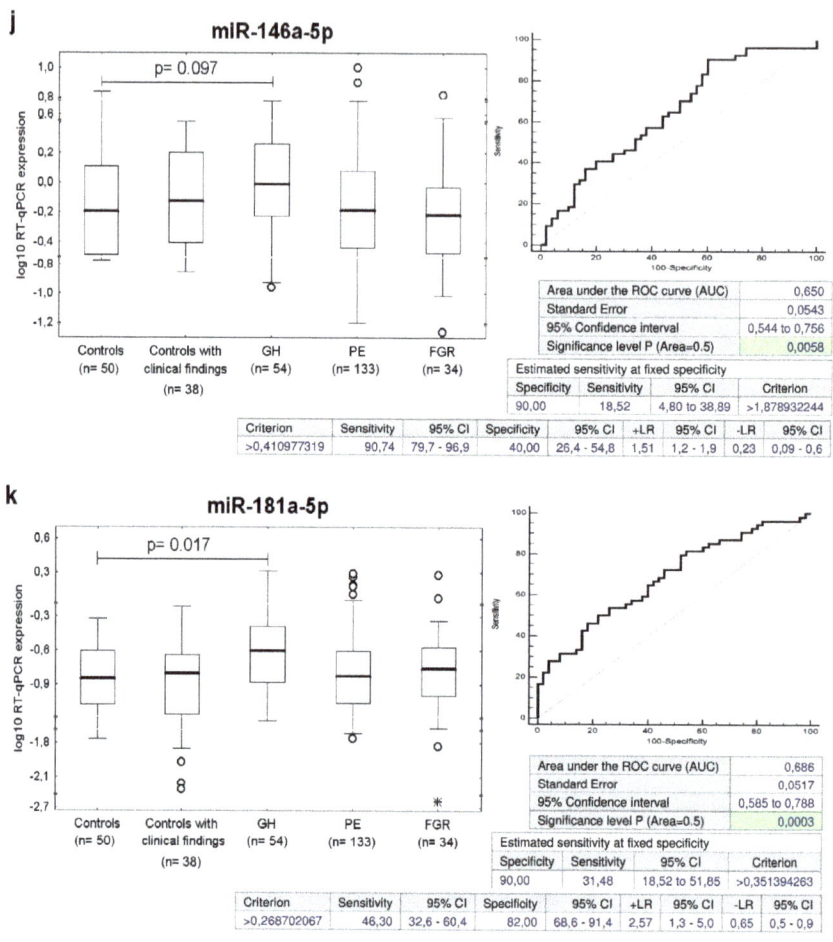

Figure 2. Postnatal microRNA expression profile in children descending from GH pregnancies. (**a–k**) Up-regulation of miR-1-3p, miR-17-5p, miR-20a-5p, miR-21-5p, miR-23a-3p, miR-26a-5p, miR-29a-3p, miR-126-3p, miR-133a-3p, miR-146a-5p, and miR-181a-5p was observed in children descending from GH pregnancies when the comparison to the controls was performed.

The sensitivity at 10.0% false positive rate (FPR) for miR-1-3p (46.3%), miR-17-5p (29.63%), miR-20a-5p (20.37%), miR-21-5p (29.63%), miR-23a-3p (27.78%), miR-26a-5p (16.67%), miR-29a-3p (35.19%), miR-126-3p (29.63%), miR-133a-3p (37.04%), miR-146a-5p (18.52%), and miR-181a-5p (31.48%) was found (Figure 2).

2.5. Up-Regulation of miR-21-5p, miR-23a-3p, miR-26a-5p, miR-103a-3p, miR-125b-5p, miR-195-5p, and miR-342-3p in Children with Normal Postnatal Clinical Findings Descending from GH Pregnancies

Concurrently, it was observed that the expression of miR-21-5p, miR-23a-3p, miR-26a-5p, miR-103a-3p, miR-125b-5p, miR-195-5p, and miR-342-3p differed significantly between the groups of children affected with GH with normal postnatal clinical findings and the controls (Figure 3). The sensitivity of individual microRNAs at 10.0% FPR was the following: miR-21-5p (39.13%), miR-23a-3p (34.78%), miR-26a-5p (21.74%), miR-103a-3p (30.43%), miR-125b-5p (47.83%), miR-195-5p (34.78%), and miR-342-3p (21.74%) (Figure 3).

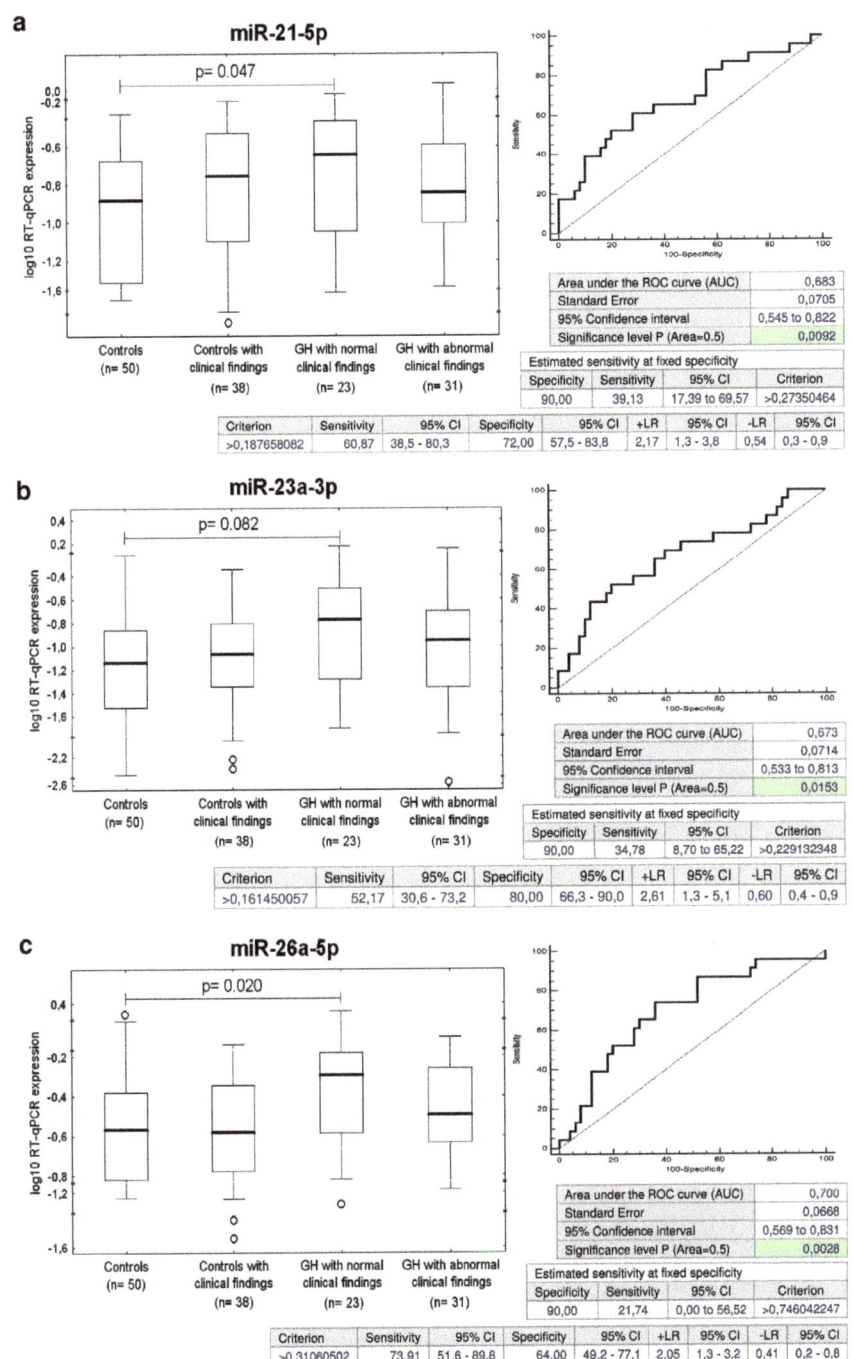

Figure 3. *Cont.*

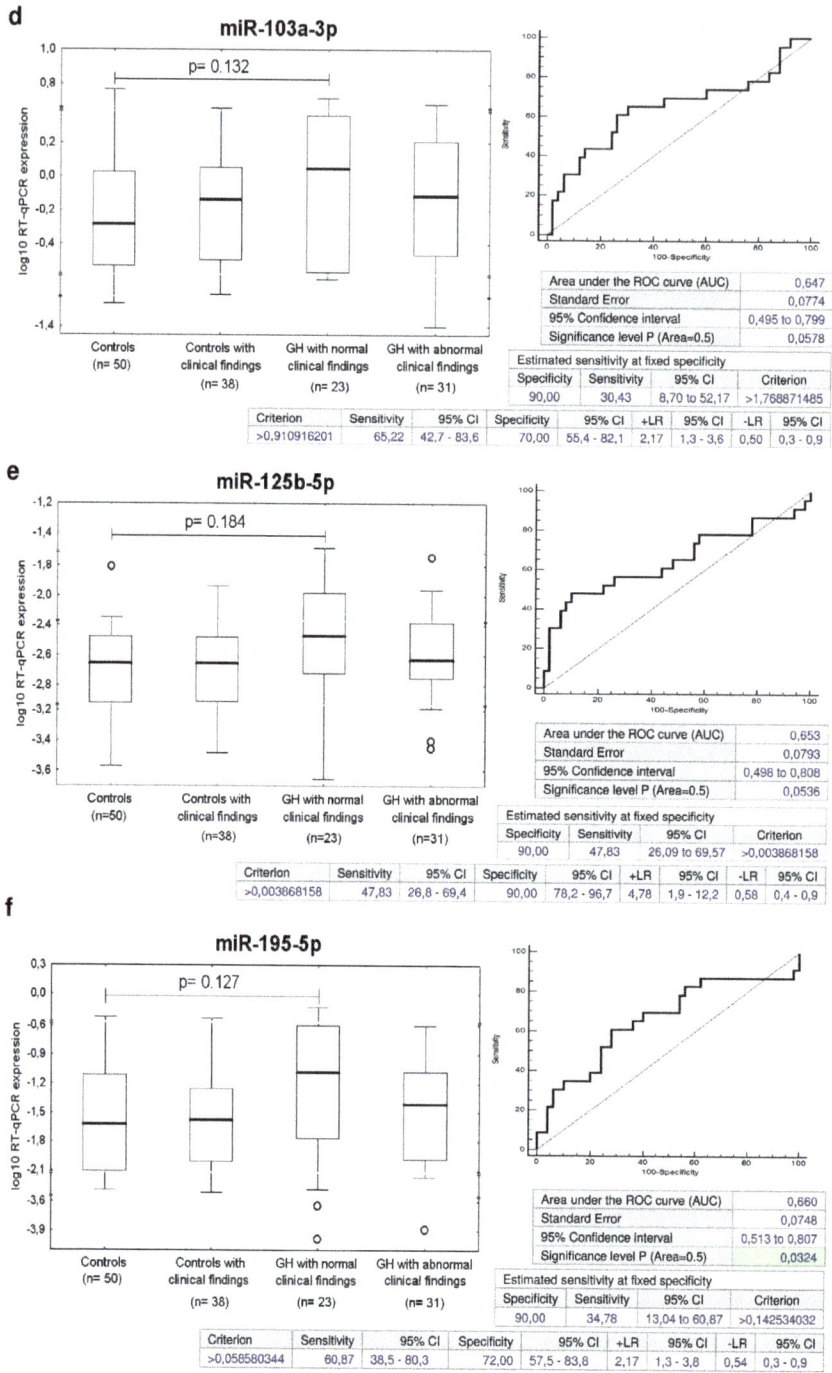

Figure 3. *Cont.*

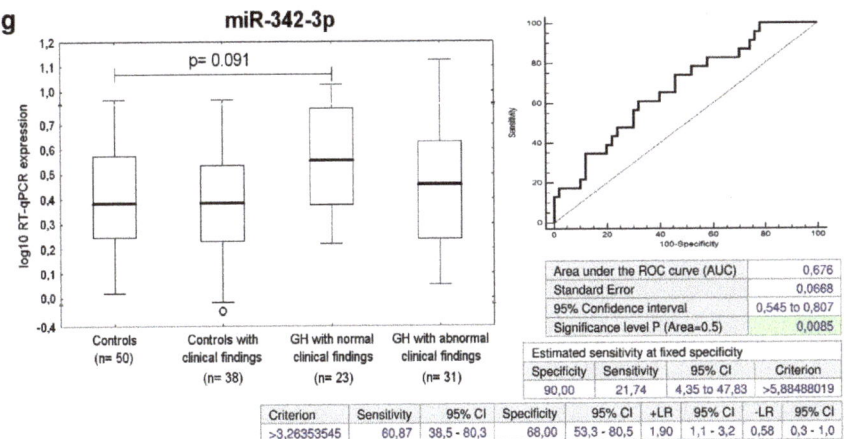

Figure 3. Postnatal microRNA expression profile in children with normal postnatal clinical findings descending from GH pregnancies. (**a–g**) Up-regulation of miR-21-5p, miR-23a-3p, miR-26a-5p, miR-103a-3p, miR-125b-5p, miR-195-5p and miR-342-3p was observed in children with normal postnatal clinical findings descending from GH pregnancies.

Screening based on the combination of miR-26a-5p and miR-195-5p showed the highest accuracy for children with normal clinical findings with a prior exposure to GH (AUC 0.717, $p = 0.001$, sensitivity 86.96%, specificity 52.0%, cut off > 0.246824). It was able to identify 34.78% children with an increased cardiovascular risk at 10.0% FPR (Figure 4).

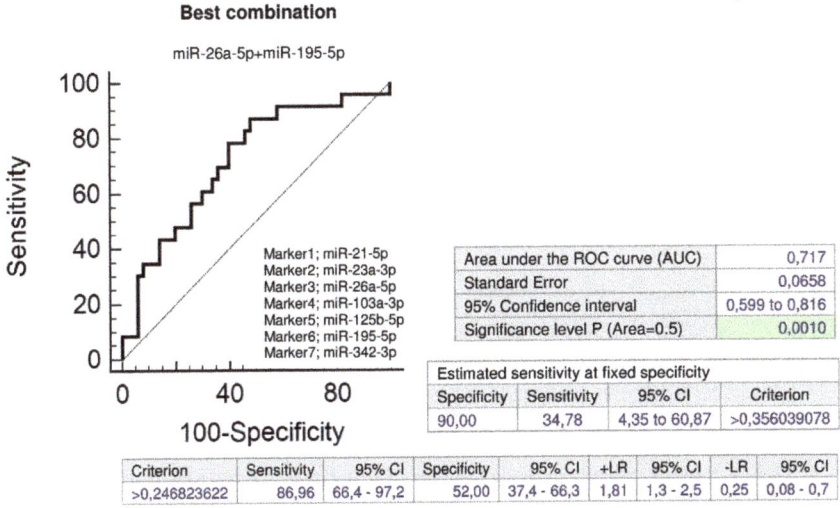

Figure 4. Combined postnatal screening of microRNAs in the identification of children with normal postnatal clinical findings descending from GH pregnancies. Postnatal combined screening of miR-26a-5p and miR-195-5p showed the highest accuracy for the identification of children with normal clinical findings with a prior exposure to GH at a higher risk of later development of cardiovascular/cerebrovascular diseases.

2.6. Up-Regulation of miR-20a-5p in Children with Abnormal Postnatal Clinical Findings Descending from GH Pregnancies

Overall, the group with abnormal postnatal clinical findings consisted of 31/54 children (57.41%) exposed to GH, 5 children already dispesarized in the department of pediatric cardiology, 12 children with abnormal echocardiographic findings (6 tricuspid valve regurgitation, 1 mitral valve regurgitation, 3 pulmonary valve regurgitation, 1 bicuspid aortic valve regurgitation, 1 ventricular septum defect, 2 foramen ovale apertum), 17 children with prehypertension/hypertension, and 3 children with high BMI. miR-20a-5p expression differed between the groups of children affected with GH with abnormal postnatal clinical findings and the controls. miR-20a-5p differentiated between the children descending from pregnancies affected with GH with abnormal postnatal clinical findings and the controls with a sensitivity of 25.81% at 10.0% FPR (Figure 5).

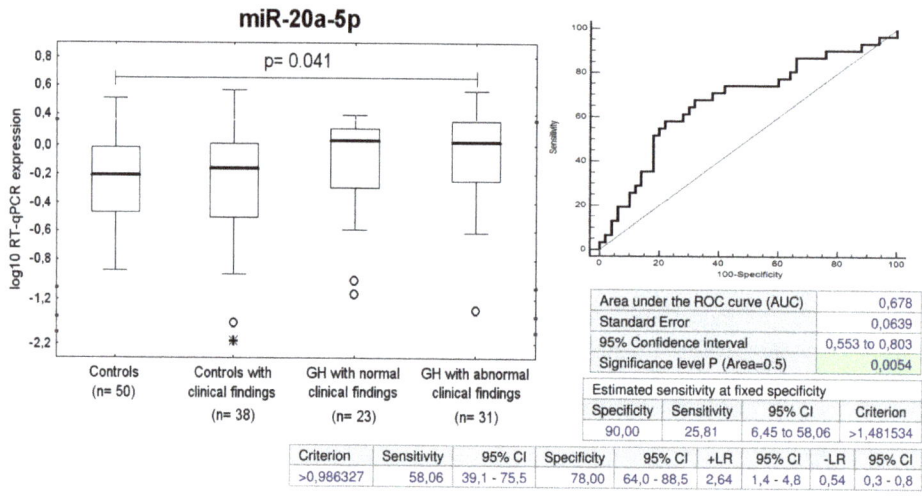

Figure 5. Increased expression of miR-20a-5p in children with abnormal postnatal clinical findings descending from GH pregnancies. Increased expression of miR-20a-5p was found in children with abnormal postnatal clinical findings descending from GH pregnancies.

2.7. Up-Regulation of miR-1-3p, miR-17-5p, miR-29a-3p, miR-126-3p, miR-133a-3p, miR-146a-5p, and miR-181a-5p in Children Descending from GH Pregnancies Irrespective of Postnatal Clinical Findings

The ROC curve analysis showed the difference in gene expression of miR-1-3p, miR-17-5p, miR-29a-3p, miR-126-3p, miR-133a-3p, miR-146a-5p, and miR-181a-5p between the controls and the group of children exposed to GH with postnatal normal clinical findings or children with a prior exposure to GH that already developed any cardiovascular complication (valve problems and heart defects) or were identified to be overweight/obese and/or prehypertensive/hypertensive (Figure 6). The sensitivity at 10.0% FPR for miR-1-3p (47.83% versus 45.16%) and miR-17-5p (30.43% versus 29.03%) for children descending from GH pregnancies with postnatal normal and abnormal clinical findings was approximately equal (Figure 6). The sensitivity at 10.0% FPR for miR-29a-3p (39.13% versus 32.26%), miR-126-3p (39.13% versus 22.58%), miR-133a-3p (43.48% versus 32.26%), miR-146a-5p (26.09% versus 12.9%), and miR-181a-5p (39.13% versus 25.81%) was slightly higher for children descending from GH pregnancies with postnatal normal clinical findings when compared to those ones with postnatal abnormal clinical findings (Figure 6).

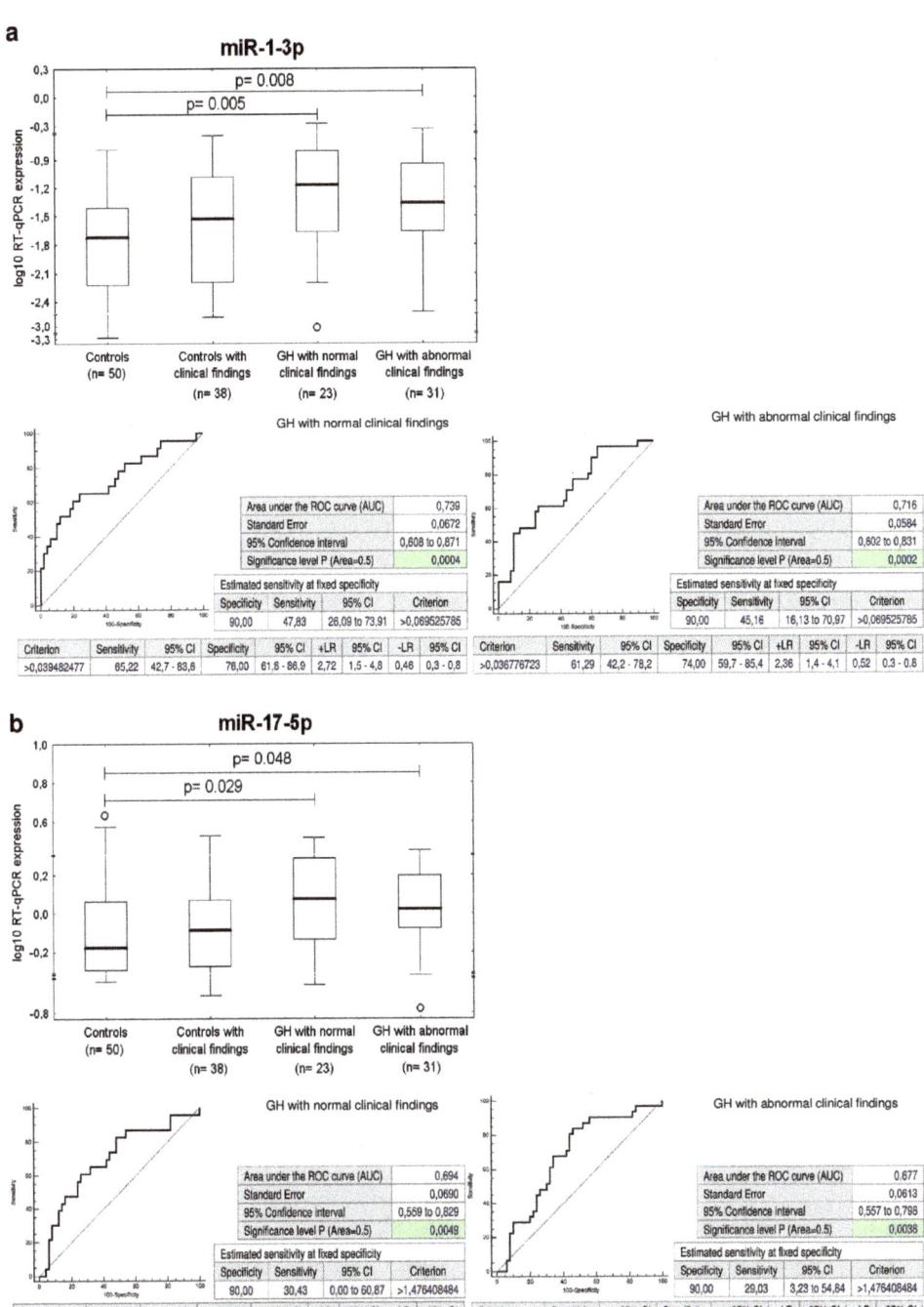

Figure 6. Cont.

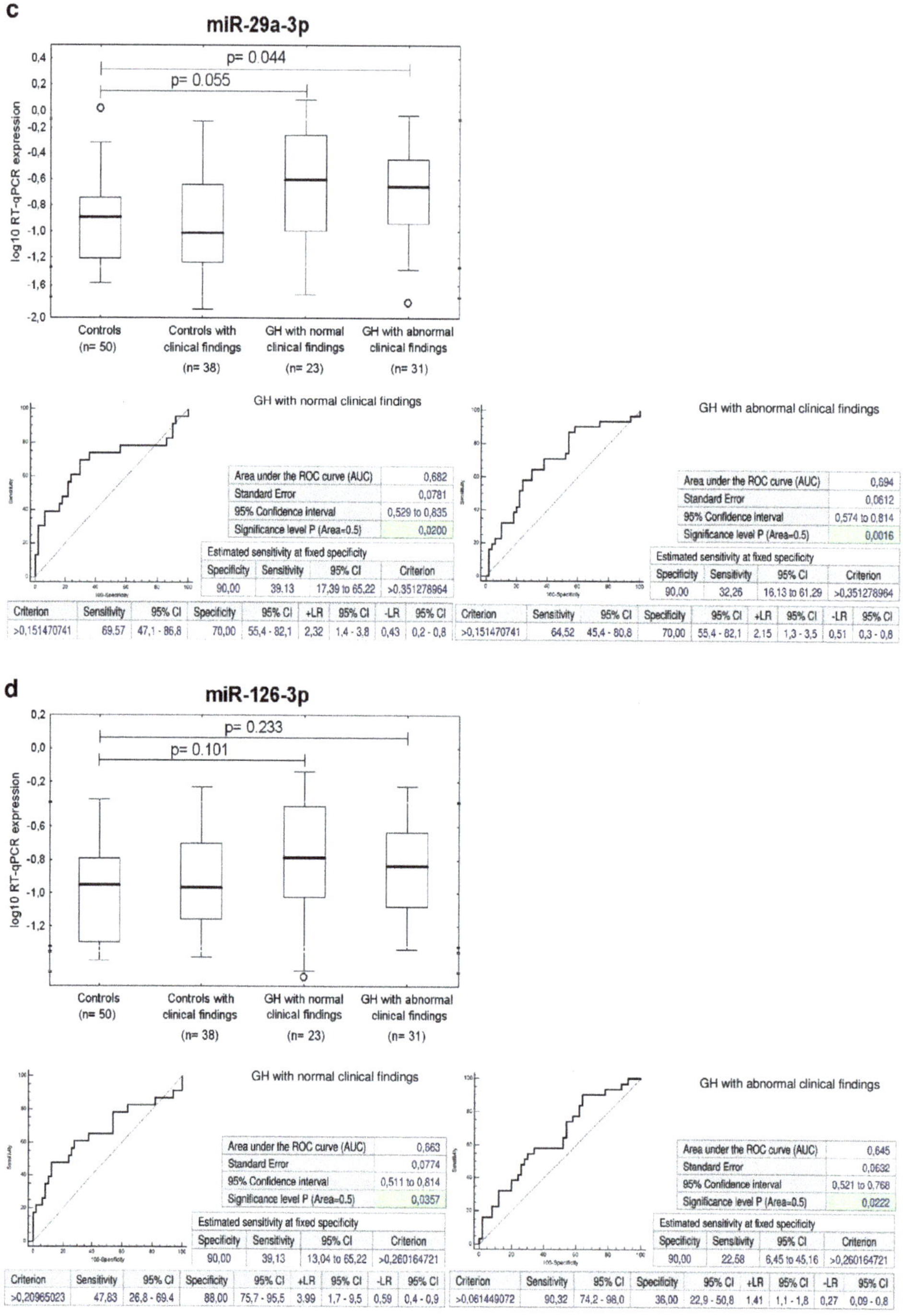

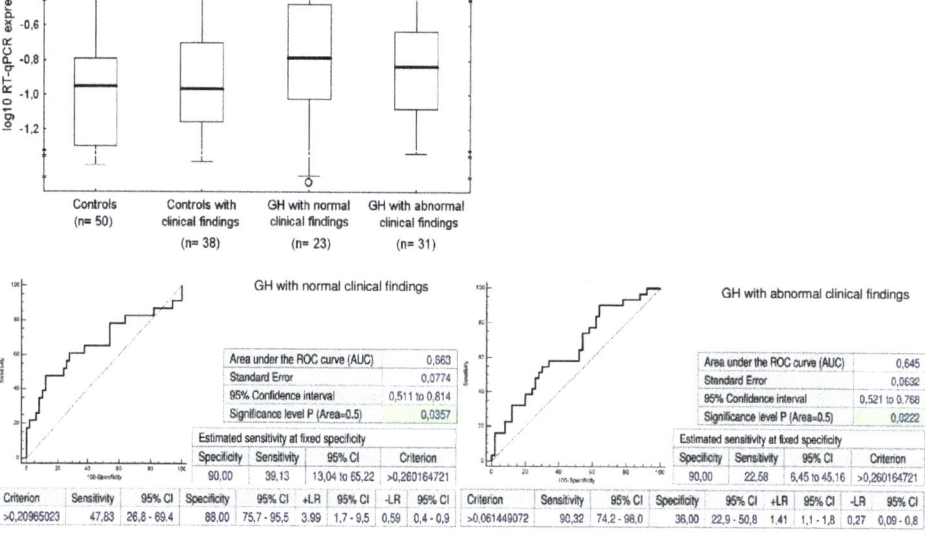

Figure 6. *Cont.*

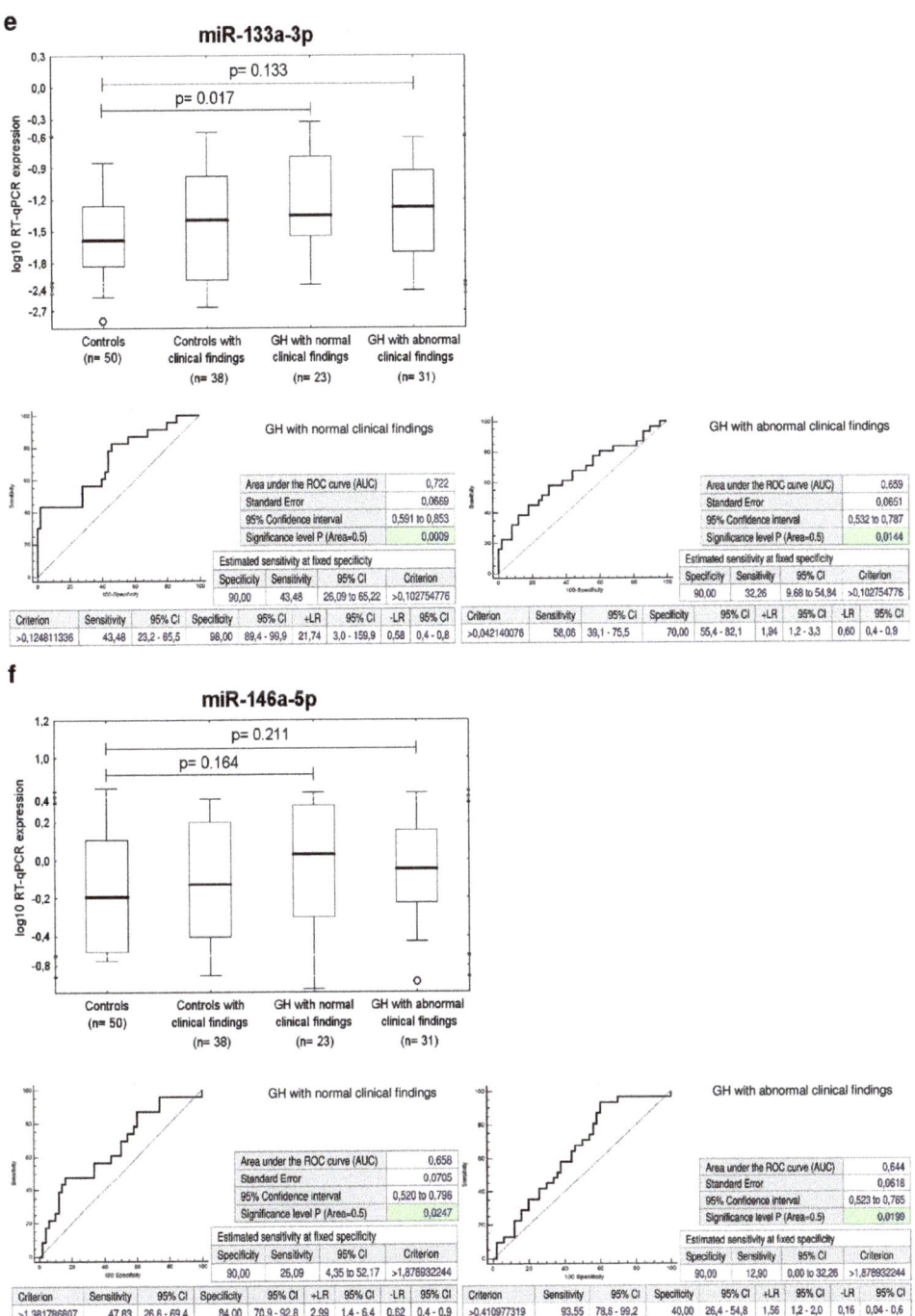

Figure 6. *Cont.*

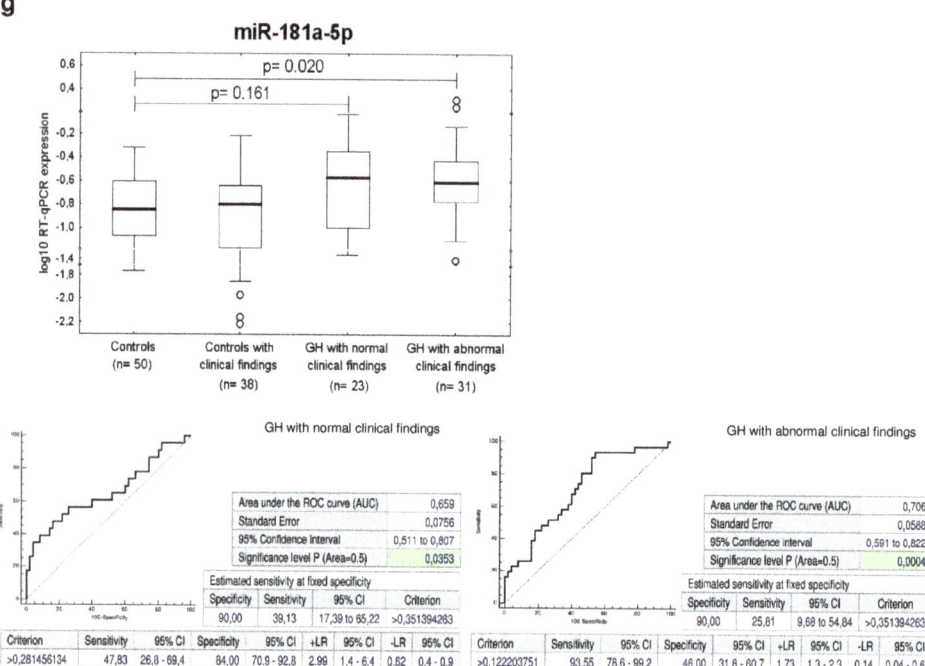

Figure 6. Postnatal microRNA expression profile in children descending from GH pregnancies irrespective of postnatal clinical findings. (**a–g**) Increased expression of miR-1-3p, miR-17-5p, miR-29a-3p, miR-126-3p, miR-133a-3p, miR-146a-5p, and miR-181a-5p was observed in children descending from GH pregnancies with normal or abnormal postnatal clinical findings. The ROC curve analysis showed the difference in microRNA gene expression between the controls and the group of children exposed to GH with postnatal normal clinical findings or children with a prior exposure to GH that already developed any cardiovascular complication (valve problems and heart defects) or were identified to be overweight/obese and/or prehypertensive/hypertensive.

Combined screening of miR-1-3p, miR-29a-3p, miR-126-3p, miR-133a-3p, and miR-181a-5p showed the highest accuracy for children with a prior exposure to GH with normal clinical findings (AUC 0.803, $p < 0.001$, sensitivity 82.61%, specificity 74.0%, cut off > 0.224754). It was able to identify 47.83% children with an increased cardiovascular risk at 10.0% FPR (Figure 7).

In addition, the combination of all seven microRNA biomarkers (miR-1-3p, miR-17-5p, miR-29a-3p, miR-126-3p, miR-133a-3p, miR-146a-5p, and miR-181a-5p) may be used to identify children with a prior exposure to GH with abnormal clinical findings (AUC 0.801, $p < 0.001$, sensitivity 70.97%, specificity 76.0%, cut off > 0.353483). It was able to identify 38.71% children with an increased cardiovascular risk at 10.0% FPR (Figure 8).

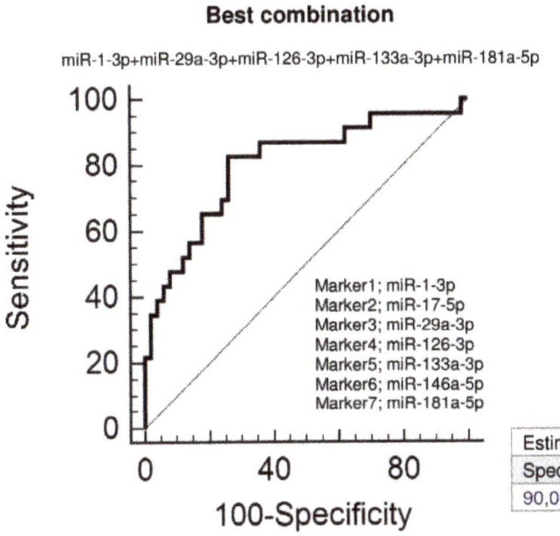

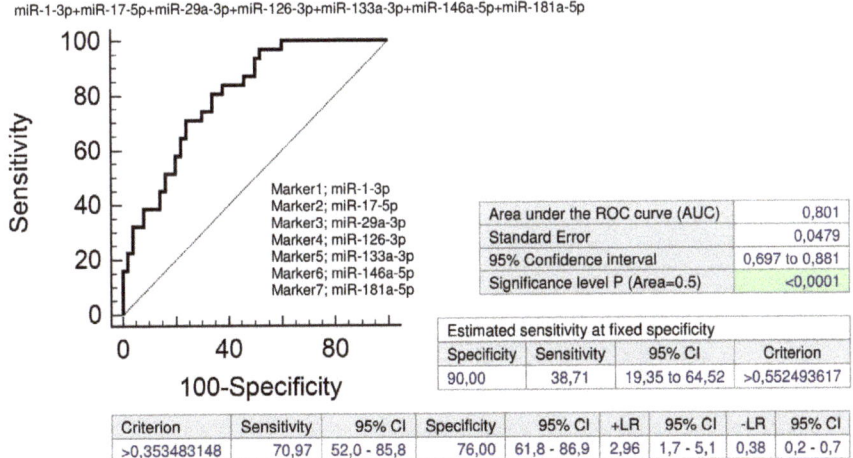

Figure 7. Combined postnatal screening of microRNAs in the identification of children with normal postnatal clinical findings descending from GH pregnancies. Postnatal combined screening of miR-1-3p, miR-29a-3p, miR-126-3p, miR-133a-3p and miR-181a-5p showed the highest accuracy for the identification of children with normal clinical findings with a prior exposure to GH at a higher risk of later development of cardiovascular/cerebrovascular diseases.

Figure 8. Combined postnatal screening of microRNAs in the identification of children with abnormal postnatal clinical findings descending from GH pregnancies. Postnatal combined screening of miR-1-3p, miR-17-5p, miR-29a-3p, miR-126-3p, mir-133a-3p, miR-146a-5p, and miR-181a-5p showed the highest accuracy for the identification of children with abnormal clinical findings with a prior exposure to GH at an increased risk of later onset of cardiovascular/cerebrovascular diseases.

2.8. Cardiovascular/Cerebrovascular Disease Associated microRNAs are Dysregulated in Children Descending from PE Pregnancies

Overall, the group with abnormal postnatal clinical findings consisted of 63/133 children (47.37%) exposed to PE 19 children already dispesarized in the department of pediatric cardiology, 18 children with abnormal echocardiographic findings (7 tricuspid valve regurgitation, 2 mitral valve regurgitation, 1 pulmonary valve regurgitation, 1 ventricular septum defect, 1 atrial septum defect, 1 hypertrophic ventricular septum, 9 foramen ovale apertum, and 1 arrhythmia), 36 children with prehypertension/hypertension and 5 children with high BMI. Abnormal clinical findings were found in 16/27 children affected with mild PE (59.3%), 47/106 children exposed to severe PE (44.3%), 26/49 children exposed to early PE (53.1%), and 37/84 children affected with late PE (44.0%).

2.9. Increased Expression of miR-133a-3p in Children Descending from PE Pregnancies

The ROC curve analysis was able to identify up-regulated expression profile of miR-133a-3p in 22.56% children affected with PE regardless of the severity of the disease and the delivery date at 10.0% FPR (Figure 9a).

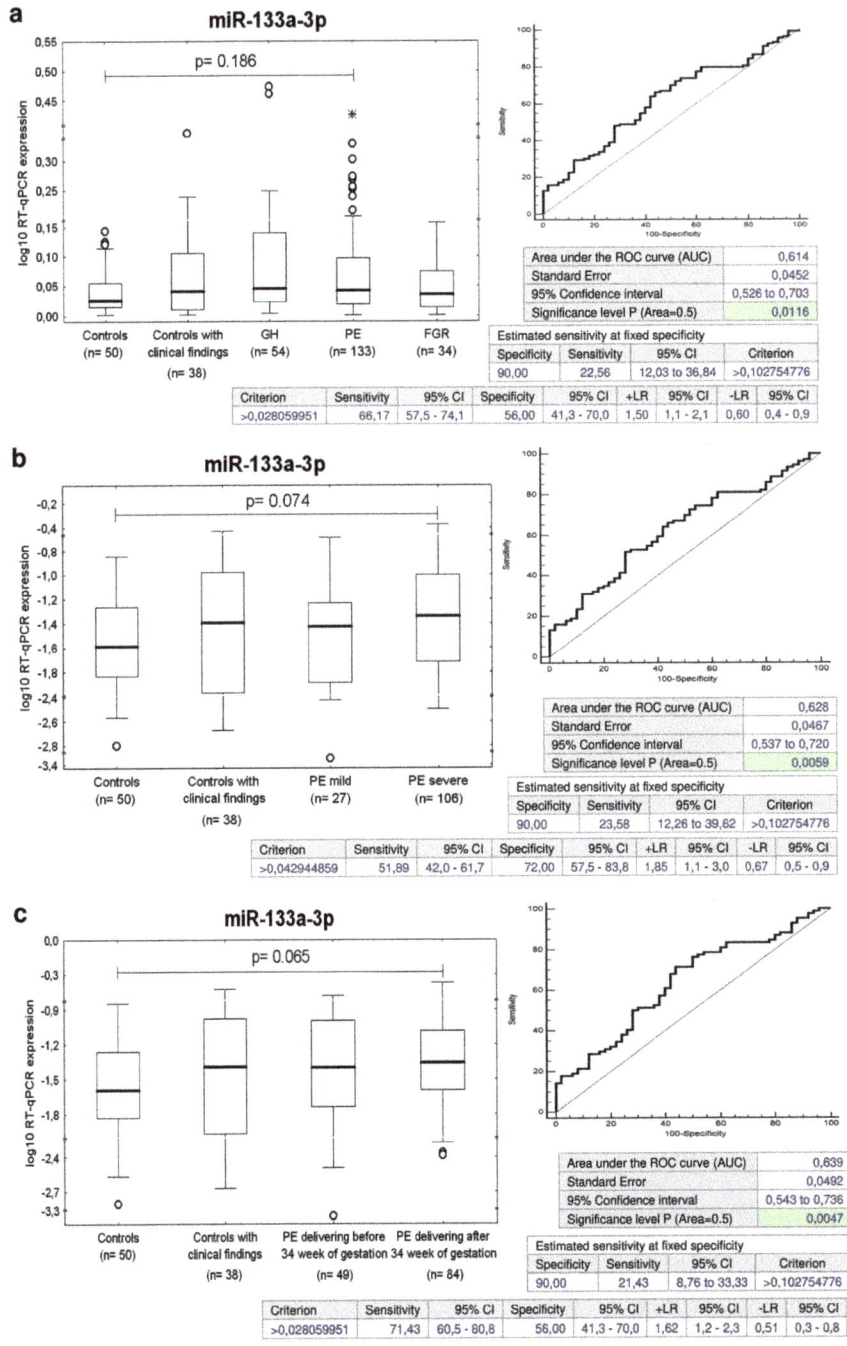

Figure 9. Cont.

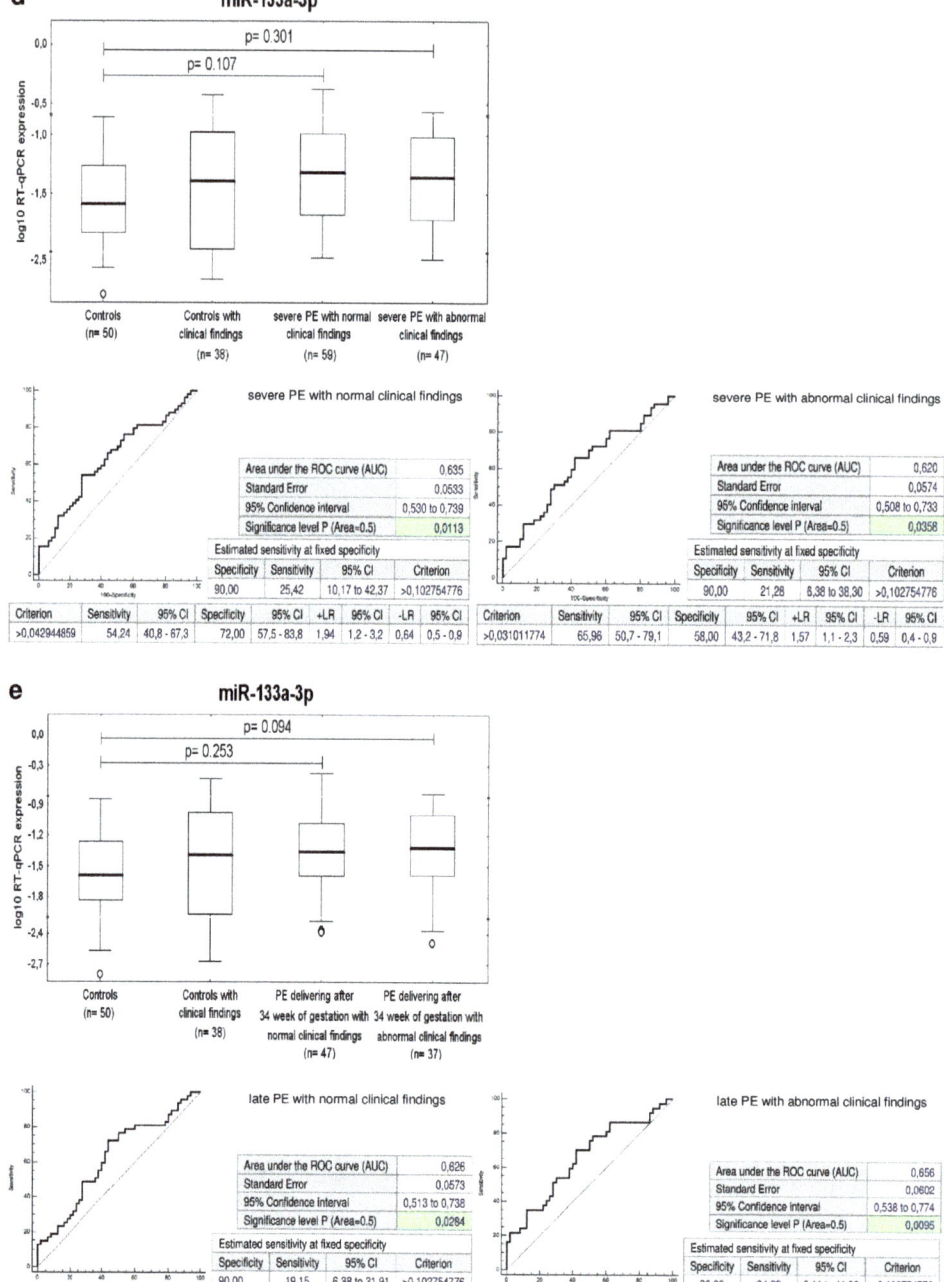

Figure 9. Cont.

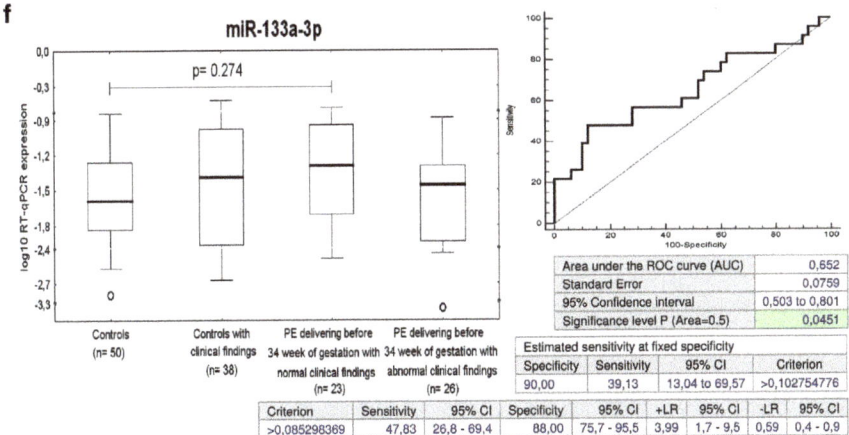

Figure 9. Increased expression of miR-133a-3p in children descending from PE pregnancies. (**a–c**) Increased expression of miR-133a-3p was observed in children descending from PE pregnancies regardless of the severity of the disease and delivery date, severe PE and late PE; (**d,e**) Increased expression of miR-133a-3p was found in children with both normal and abnormal postnatal clinical findings previously exposed to severe PE and late PE; (**f**) Increased expression of miR-133a-3p was found in children with normal postnatal clinical findings previously exposed to early PE.

Subsequently, miR-133a-3p differentiated between children affected with severe PE and controls with a sensitivity of 23.58% at a specificity of 90.0% (Figure 9b).

Parallel, miR-133a-3p was able to identify children exposed to late PE with a sensitivity of 21.43% at a specificity of 90.0% (Figure 9c).

In addition to that, the consecutive analysis showed that the accuracy of miR-133a-3p biomarker for severe PE affected children identified to have normal or abnormal clinical findings was 25.42% and 21.28% sensitivity at 10.0% FPR (Figure 9d).

Similarly, postnatal screening of miR-133a-3p was able to identify children with a history of late PE with either normal or abnormal clinical findings with a sensitivity of 19.15% and 24.32% at a specificity of 90.0% (Figure 9e).

Parallel, ROC curve analysis of miR-133a-3p identified a significant proportion of children with normal clinical findings exposed to early PE during gestation (a sensitivity of 39.13% at 10.0% FPR) (Figure 9f).

2.10. Increased Expression of miR-1-3p, miR-20a-5p, miR-103a-3p, and miR-342-3p in Children with Abnormal Clinical Findings Descending from PE Pregnancies

The sensitivity at 10.0% FPR for miR-1-3p for children exposed to late PE was 27.38% and miR-1-3p showed even a higher performance for children with abnormal postnatal clinical findings that were exposed to late PE (a sensitivity of 35.14% at a specificity of 90.0%) (Figure 10a).

Furthermore, at 10.0% FPR, miR-103a-3p was up-regulated in 12.77% and 13.51% children with abnormal clinical findings that were exposed to severe PE or late PE (Figure 10b,c).

In addition, miR-20a-5p was up-regulated in 13.51% children with abnormal clinical findings with a prior exposure to late PE (Figure 10d).

MiR-342-3p represented the unique marker, which was able to differentiate between the group of children with abnormal clinical findings that were exposed to early PE and the controls (a sensitivity of 26.92% at 10.0% FPR) (Figure 11).

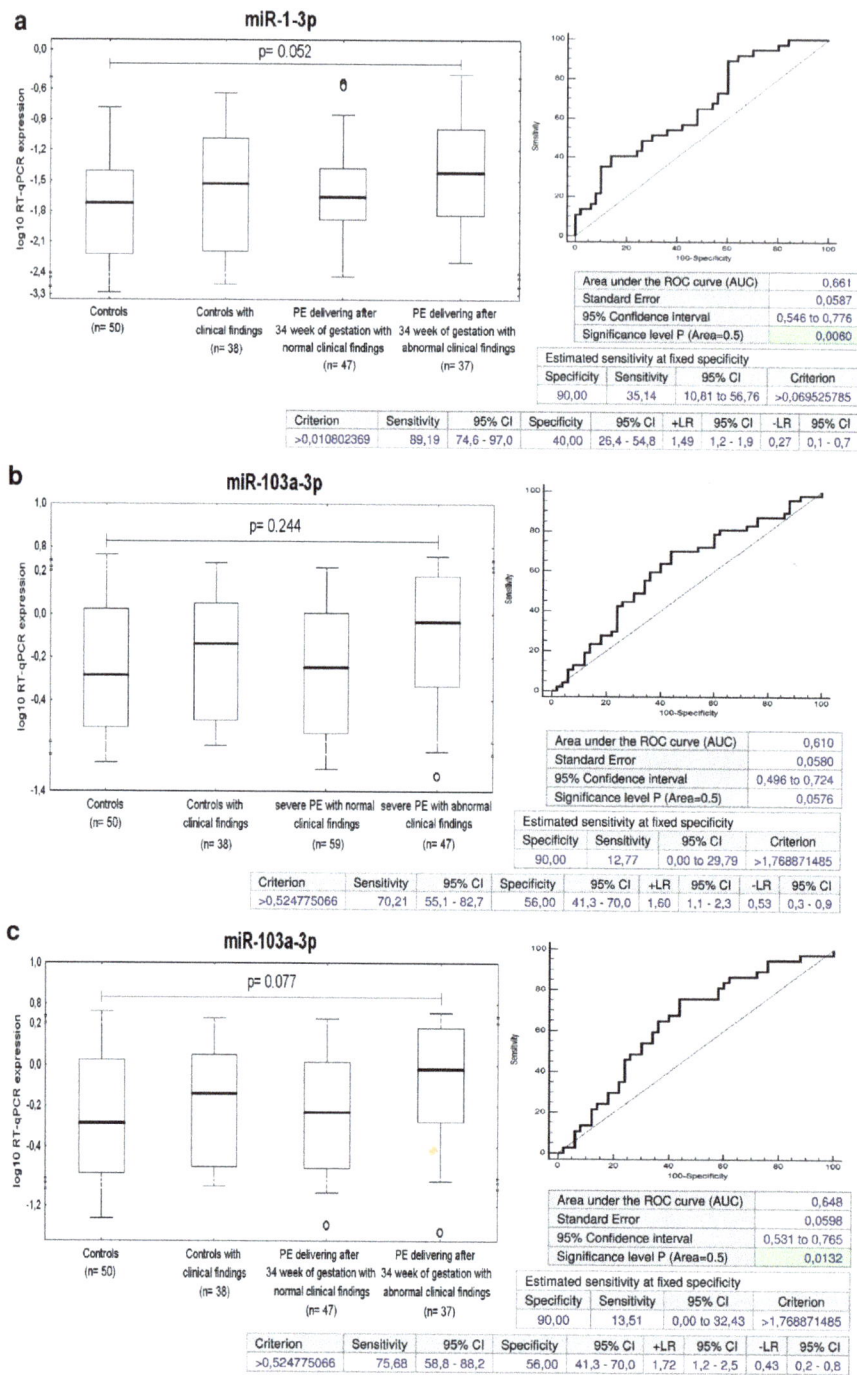

Figure 10. *Cont.*

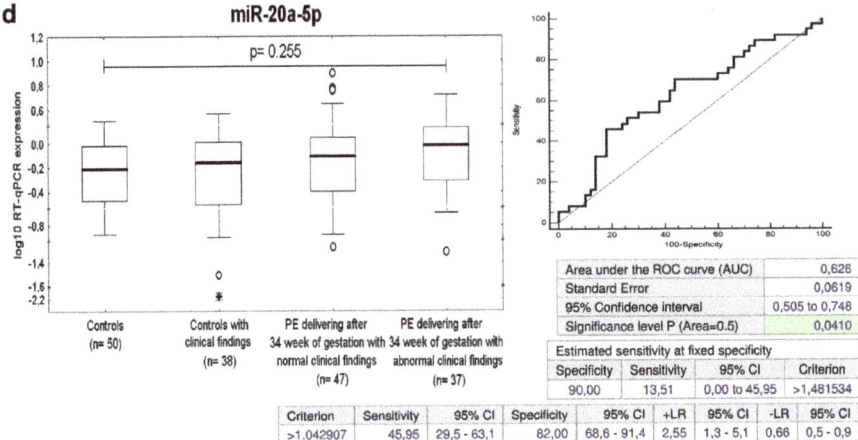

Figure 10. Postnatal microRNA expression profile in children with abnormal postnatal clinical findings descending from PE pregnancies. (**a**) Increased expression of miR-1-3p was found in children with abnormal postnatal clinical findings exposed to late PE; (**b**,**c**) Increased expression of miR-103a-3p was observed in children with abnormal postnatal clinical findings exposed to severe PE or late PE; (**d**) Increased expression of miR-20a-5p was found in children with abnormal postnatal clinical findings with a prior exposure to late PE.

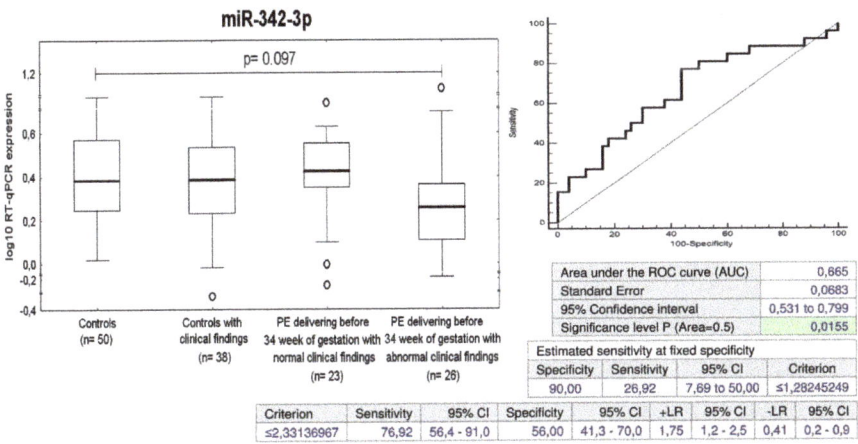

Figure 11. Decreased expression of miR-342-3p in children with abnormal postnatal clinical findings descending from early PE pregnancies.

The combination of miR-103a-3p and miR-133a-3p (AUC 0.637, p = 0.015, sensitivity 70.21%, specificity 56.0%, cut off > 0.429300) was superior over using only individual microRNA biomarkers, since it was able to identify at 10.0% FPR within the group of children with abnormal clinical findings previously exposed to severe PE 21.28% children with an increased cardiovascular risk (Figure 12).

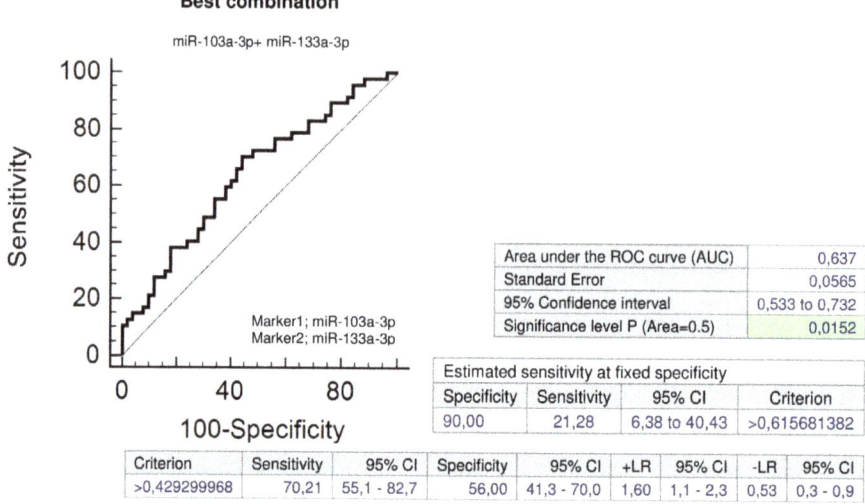

Figure 12. Combined postnatal screening of microRNAs in the identification of children with abnormal postnatal clinical findings descending from severe PE pregnancies. Postnatal combined screening of miR-103a-3p and miR-133a-3p showed the highest accuracy for the identification of children with abnormal clinical findings with a prior exposure to severe PE at a higher risk of later development of cardiovascular/cerebrovascular diseases.

Parallel, combined screening of four microRNAs (miR-1-3p, miR-20a-5p, miR-103a-3p, and miR-133a-3p) showed the highest accuracy for children with abnormal clinical findings with a prior exposure to late PE (AUC 0.701, $p < 0.001$, sensitivity 59.46%, specificity 72.0%, cut off > 0.391116). It was able to identify 32.43% children with an increased cardiovascular risk at 10.0% FPR (Figure 13).

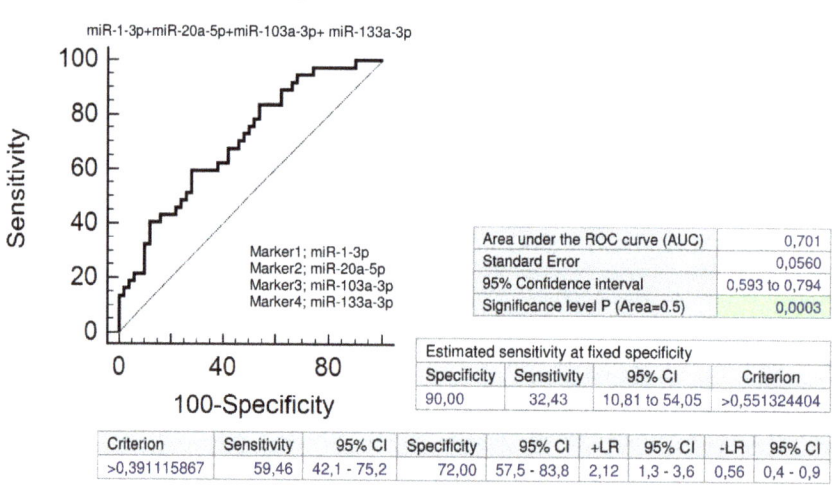

Figure 13. Combined postnatal screening of microRNAs in the identification of children with abnormal postnatal clinical findings descending from late PE pregnancies. Postnatal screening based on the combination of miR-1-3p, miR-20a-5p, miR-103a-3p, and miR-133a-3p showed the highest accuracy for the identification of children with abnormal clinical findings with a prior exposure to late PE at a higher risk of later development of cardiovascular/cerebrovascular diseases.

2.11. Up-Regulation of miR-20b-5p in Children with Normal Clinical Findings Descending from Mild PE Pregnancies

MiR-20b-5p was the only biomarker that differentiated between the group of children with normal clinical findings that were exposed to mild PE and the controls (a sensitivity of 36.36% at 10.0% FPR) (Figure 14).

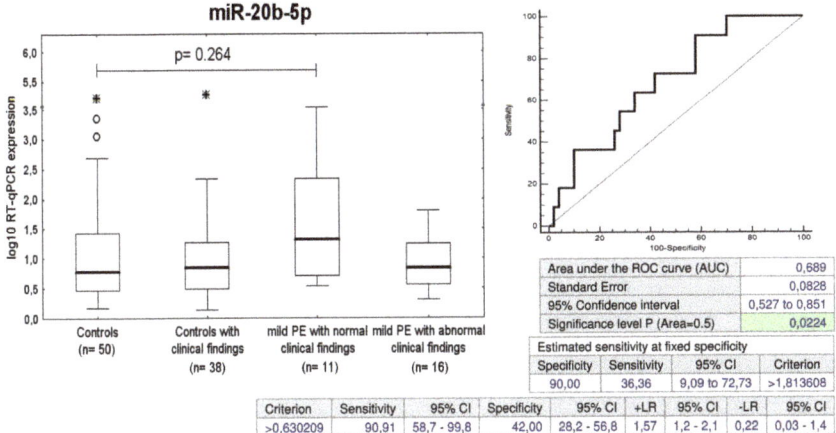

Figure 14. Increased expression of miR-20b-5p in children with normal postnatal clinical findings descending from mild PE pregnancies.

2.12. Dysregulation of Cardiovascular/Cerebrovascular Disease Associated microRNAs in Children Descending from FGR Pregnancies

Overall, the group with abnormal postnatal clinical findings consisted of 22/34 children (64.7%) exposed to FGR (9 children already dispesarized in the department of pediatric cardiology, 9 children with abnormal echocardiographic findings (4 tricuspid valve regurgitation, 3 pulmonary valve regurgitation, 1 atrial septum defect, 6 foramen ovale apertum), 9 children with prehypertension/hypertension and 1 child with high BMI). Abnormal clinical findings were found in 7/13 children affected with early FGR (53.85%), and in 15/21 children exposed to late FGR (71.43%).

2.13. Increased Expression of miR-17-5p, miR-126-3p and miR-133a-3p in Children with Abnormal Clinical Findings Descending from FGR Pregnancies

MiR-17-5p, miR-126-3p, and miR-133a-3p differentiated between the group of children with abnormal clinical findings that were affected with FGR and the controls with a sensitivity of 22.73 %, 31.82% and 31.82% at a specificity of 90.0% (Figure 15a–c).

The combination of all examined microRNAs (AUC 0.710, p = 0.002, sensitivity 63.64%, specificity 78.0%, cut off > 0.305781) was superior over using only individual microRNA biomarkers, since it was able to identify at 10.0% FPR within the group of children with abnormal clinical findings affected with FGR 40.91% children with an increased cardiovascular risk (Figure 16).

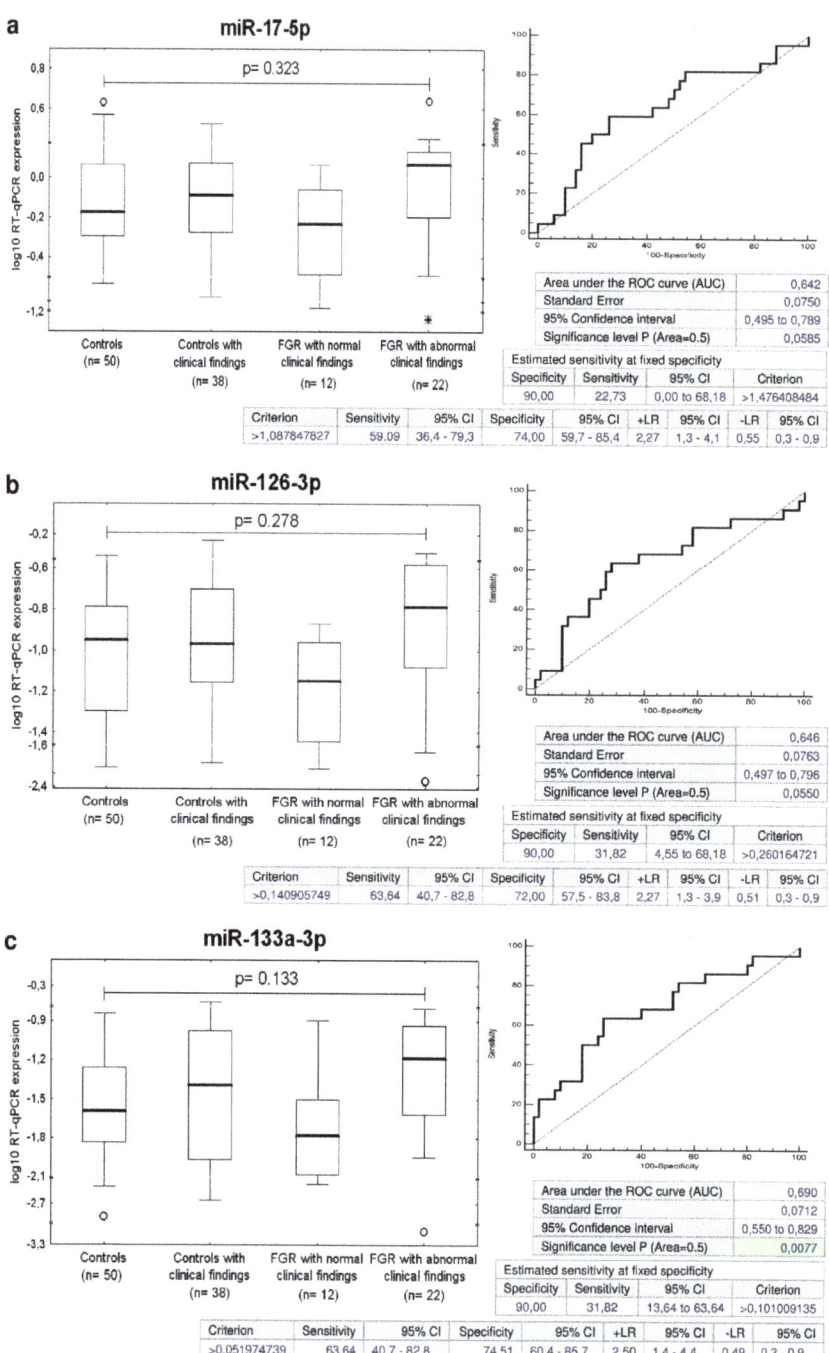

Figure 15. Postnatal microRNA expression profile in children with abnormal postnatal clinical findings descending from FGR pregnancies. (**a–c**) Increased expression of miR-17-5p, miR-126-3p, and miR-133a-3p was observed in children with abnormal postnatal clinical findings descending from FGR pregnancies.

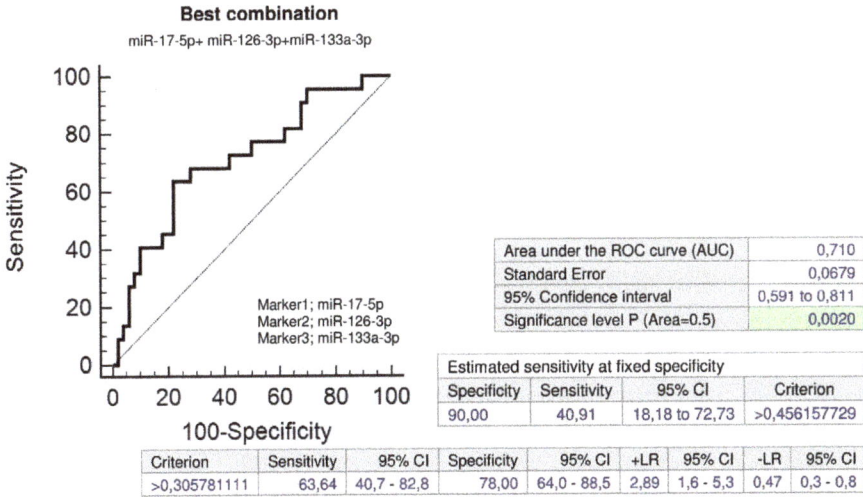

Figure 16. Combined postnatal screening of microRNAs in the identification of children with abnormal postnatal clinical findings descending from FGR pregnancies. Postnatal screening based on the combination of miR-17-5p, miR-126-3p and miR-133a-3p showed the highest accuracy for the identification of children with abnormal clinical findings with a prior exposure to FGR at a higher risk of later development of cardiovascular/cerebrovascular diseases.

2.14. The Association between Postnatal Expression of miR-210-3p and the Severity of PE and/or FGR with regard to Doppler Ultrasonography Parameters

The index of pulsatility in the ductus venosus (DV) showed a strong positive correlation with miR-210-3p gene expression in children with a history of PE and/or FGR (Figure 17). That means that children with prior findings of DV dilatation indicating poor outcome in severe FGR demonstrated increased postpartum levels of miR-210-3p.

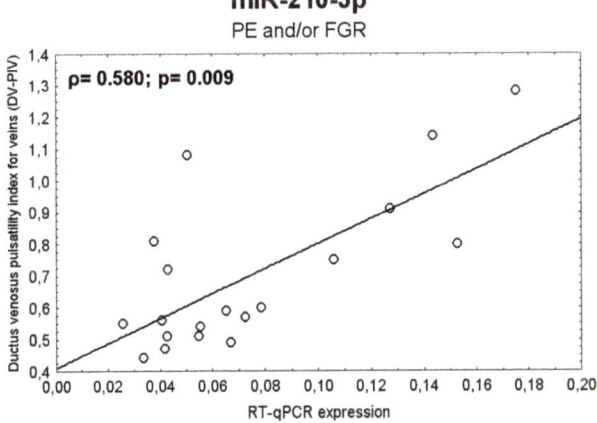

Figure 17. Association between postnatal miR-210-3p expression and the pulsatility index in the ductus venosus in PE and/or FGR patients. The pulsatility index in the ductus venosus showed a strong positive correlation with miR-210-3p gene expression in patients with a history of PE and/or FGR.

The results of aberrant expression profile of microRNAs in children descending from pregnancy-related complications are summarized in Table 1.

Table 1. Aberrant expression profile of microRNAs in children descending from pregnancy-related complications.

	MicroRNA Expression in Children Descending from Pregnancy-Related Complications		
miRBase ID	Gestational Hypertension (GH)	Preeclampsia (PE)	Fetal Growth Restriction (FGR)
hsa-miR-1-3p	↑ children with both normal and abnormal clinical findings	↑ late PE, only children with abnormal clinical findings	
hsa-miR-17-5p	↑ children with both normal and abnormal clinical findings		↑ only children with abnormal clinical findings
hsa-miR-20a-5p	↑ only children with abnormal clinical findings	↑ late PE, only children with abnormal clinical findings	
hsa-miR-20b-5p		↑ mild PE, only children with normal clinical findings	
hsa-miR-21-5p	↑ only children with normal clinical findings		
hsa-miR-23a-3p	↑ only children with normal clinical findings		
hsa-miR-26a-5p	↑ only children with normal clinical findings		
hsa-miR-29a-3p	↑ children with both normal and abnormal clinical findings		
hsa-miR-103a-3p		↑ severe PE, late PE, only children with abnormal clinical findings	
hsa-miR-125b-5p	↑ only children with normal clinical findings		
hsa-miR-126-3p	↑ children with both normal and abnormal clinical findings		↑ only children with abnormal clinical findings
hsa-miR-133a-3p	↑ children with both normal and abnormal clinical findings	↑ PE, severe PE, late PE children with both normal and abnormal clinical findings early PE, only children with normal clinical findings	↑ only children with abnormal clinical findings
hsa-miR-146a-5p	↑ children with both normal and abnormal clinical findings		
hsa-miR-181a-5p	↑ children with both normal and abnormal clinical findings		
hsa-miR-195-5p	↑ only children with normal clinical findings		
hsa-miR-210-3p		↑ children descending from PE and/or FGR complicated pregnancies with increased PI in the ductus venosus during gestation	
hsa-miR-342-3p		↓ early PE, only children with abnormal clinical findings	

↑ increased expression of microRNA, ↓ decreased expression of microRNA.

2.15. The Effect of Children Age on Particular microRNA Expression in Children Descending from Normal and Complicated Pregnancies

The effect of children age on particular microRNA expression in children descending from normal and complicated pregnancies is discussed in supplementary file (Figures S1–S4).

3. Discussion

Cardiovascular/cerebrovascular disease associated microRNA expression profile was assessed in children at the age of 3 to 11 years. Subsequently, epigenetic profile was compared between groups descending from pregnancies that had normal course of gestation or were complicated by GH, PE, and FGR, and correlated with the severity of the disease with regard to clinical signs (mild versus severe preeclampsia), dates of delivery (< and >34 weeks in case of PE, < and >32 weeks in case of FGR, respectively), and Doppler ultrasound parameters.

Initially, we collected the anamnesis at children and parents, performed medical examination (BP measurement, and BMI assessment) and utilized Doppler echocardiography to check the heart's anatomy and function and diagnose or rule out cardiac problems in the studied cohorts. That is the reason why the control group of children after normal pregnancies consisted just of those children who had normal BP, normal BMI, normal reference values of echocardiographic measurements and no cardiac findings in anamnesis. The second group of offspring born out of normal pregnancies consisted of children either already dispensarized in the department of pediatric cardiology, or those ones who were indicated during our medical examination to have valve problems and heart defects, abnormal BP or BMI. In general, the expression profile of microRNAs was equal between these two groups of children descending from uncomplicated pregnancies with an exception of miR-21-5p, which was up-regulated in a proportion of children with abnormal clinical findings (28.95%). According to our opinion, this group of children would benefit from dispensarization and implementation of primary prevention strategies, since it may be at higher risk of later development of cardiovascular diseases.

Since we identified a large proportion of children with abnormal clinical findings within groups descending from complicated pregnancies (57.41% children with a prior exposure to GH, 47.37% children exposed to PE, and 64.7% children affected with FGR), we analyzed also microRNA gene expression in relation to both aspects, the current presence or absence of cardiovascular risk factors (overweight/obesity and/or prehypertension/hypertension) and cardiovascular complications (valve problems and heart defects) and the previous occurrence of pregnancy-related complications.

As expected, the expression profile of microRNAs differed between children with a history of complicated pregnancies (GH, PE, and FGR) and controls. With respect to particular pregnancy-related complication subtypes, abnormal expression profile of multiple microRNAs was found in children affected with GH (15/29 studied microRNAs: miR-1-3p, miR-17-5p, miR-20a-5p, miR-21-5p, miR-23a-3p, miR-26a-5p, miR-29a-3p, miR-103a-3p, miR-125b-5p, miR-126-3p, miR-133a-3p, miR-146a-5p, miR-181a-5p, miR-195-5p, and miR-342-3p), clinically established PE (6/29 studied microRNAs: miR-1-3p, miR-20a-5p, miR-20b-5p, miR-103a-3p, miR-133a-3p, miR-342-3p) and FGR (3/29 studied microRNAs: miR-17-5p, miR-126-3p, miR-133a-3p).

Interestingly, a set of microRNAs associated with cardiovascular/cerebrovascular diseases (miR-1-3p, miR-17-5p, miR-29a-3p, miR-126-3p, miR-133a-3p, miR-146a-5p, and miR-181a-5p) was dysregulated in both groups of children with a prior exposure to GH regardless of the occurrence of postnatal clinical findings. Seven additional microRNAs (miR-21-5p, miR-23a-3p, miR-26a-5p, miR-103a-3p, miR-125b-5p, miR-195-5p, and miR-342-3p) were observed to be dysregulated in children affected with GH with normal postnatal clinical findings. In addition, higher expression levels of miR-20a-5p were detected in children with a prior exposure to GH, who were found to have abnormal clinical findings.

With regard to miR-133a-3p, a group of children exposed to PE produced similar findings to the group of children affected with GH. MiR-133a-3p up-regulation appeared in 37.04% and 22.56% children descending from GH or preeclamptic pregnancies irrespective of the postnatal clinical findings. Nevertheless, miR-133a-3p up-regulation was detected mainly in a group of children affected with severe PE (23.58%) and late PE (21.43%). On the other hand, up-regulation of miR-133a-3p appeared only in those children affected with FGR that were identified to have abnormal clinical findings (31.82%).

This study showed similar findings to our previous study [44], where we observed increased expression of miR-133a-3p in umbilical cord blood from patients with PE and/or FGR that had decreased values of the CPR indicating a protective reaction of the fetus against hypoxia. We suggest that the increased expression of miR-133a-3p found in a proportion of children previously exposed to GH, PE and/or FGR may be a long-term consequence of pregnancy-related complications. We suppose that up-regulation of miR-133a-3p may have rather compensatory than harmful effect, but postnatal miR-133a-3p screening may stratify a risky group of children predisposed to later cardiovascular disease development.

Interestingly, the data resulting from our previous studies [44,45] indicated that miR-1-3p was significantly up-regulated in placental tissues or umbilical cord blood of PE and/or FGR patients with an abnormal index of pulsatility in the umbilical artery or the signs of centralization of the fetal circulation, or in late PE, apparently as a consequence of an incapacity of maternal cardiovascular system to deal with the demands of an advanced pregnancy. That's why the increased expression of miR-1-3p present in circulation of children born out of pregnancies complicated with GH or late PE may also be associated with previous occurrence of hypertensive disorders of pregnancy. A large proportion of children with an up-regulated miR-1-3p profile with a prior exposure to GH (47.83% children with normal clinical findings and 45.16% children with abnormal clinical findings) or late PE (35.14% children with abnormal clinical findings) was identified. We suppose that children descending from complicated pregnancies with aberrant expression profile of miR-1-3p are at a higher risk of later onset of cardiovascular diseases, and should be carefully monitored in the long term.

This study demonstrated that the dysregulation of at least two microRNAs (miR-1-3p and miR-133a-3p) caused by pregnancy complications in placental tissues and/or umbilical cord blood is present as well in circulation of children with hindsight (3 to 11 years after the birth) after the exposure to GH, PE, or FGR. It is obvious that changes in epigenome induced by pregnancy complications in placental tissue and umbilical cord blood may cause later development of cardiovascular and cerebrovascular diseases in offspring. An impact of the environment on early life epigenetic programming might support the phenomena known as developmental programming and explain the developmental origins of diseases. It is well known that complex diseases, such as diabetes, obesity, and heart disease, result from the interaction between genetic and environmental factors. Alternatively, other explanations to the aberrant microRNA expression in pregnancy-related complications may be taken into consideration. For instance, it may be that complicated pregnancies induce changes in proportional representation of any of cell subpopulations including endothelial stem cells and immune cells, which may be the cause of different microRNA expression.

However, it is also evident that epigenetic profiles of other microRNAs have been changing with time by force of various circumstances, since several microRNAs which were up-regulated in children exposed to GH (miR-17-5p, miR-20a-5p, miR-21-5p, miR-23a-3p, miR-29a-3p, miR-146a-5p, and miR-181a-5p), PE (miR-20a-5p, and miR-20b-5p) or FGR (miR-17-5p) were not observed to be dysregulated in placental tissues and/or umbilical cord blood during the clinical manifestation of pregnancy-related complications [44,45].

In parallel, several microRNAs which were up-regulated in children exposed to GH (miR-26a-5p, miR-103a-3p, miR-125b-5p, miR-126-3p, miR-195-5p, and miR-342-3p), PE (miR-103a-3p, and miR-342-3p) or FGR (miR-126-3p) were observed to be down-regulated in placental tissues and/or umbilical cord blood during the clinical manifestation of pregnancy-related complications [44,45].

However, existing data suggests that these microRNAs play a role in the pathogenesis of cardiovascular/cerebrovascular diseases (Table 2) [21,23,25,29,39,46–138].

Table 2. The role of differentially expressed microRNAs in children descending from gestational hypertension, preeclampsia and/or fetal growth restriction complicated pregnancies in the pathogenesis of cardiovascular/cerebrovascular diseases.

miRBase ID	Gene Location on Chromosome	Expression	Role in the Pathogenesis of Cardiovascular/Cerebrovascular Diseases	Potential Therapeutic Target in Treatment of Cardiovascular Diseases
hsa-miR-1-3p	20q13.3 18q11.2 [46]	Cardiac and skeletal muscles, myocardium	Acute myocardial infarction, heart ischemia, post-myocardial infarction complications [47]	+ [48–50]
hsa-miR-17-5p	13q31.3 [51,52]	Endothelial cells, vascular smooth muscle cells [53]	Cardiac development [54], ischemia/reperfusion-induced cardiac injury [55], kidney ischemia-reperfusion injury [57], diffuse myocardial fibrosis in hypertrophic cardiomyopathy [58], acute ischemic stroke [59], coronary artery disease [60]	+ [55,56]
hsa-miR-20a-5p	13q31.3 [61]	Pulmonary arteries [62]	Pulmonary hypertension [62], gestational diabetes mellitus [63]	+ [62]
hsa-miR-20b-5p	Xq26.2 [61]		Hypertension-induced heart failure [64], small for gestational age foetuses [65]	
hsa-miR-21-5p	17q23.2 [66]	Cardiomyocytes	Homeostasis of the cardiovascular system [67], cardiac fibrosis and heart failure [68,70]	+ [68,69]
hsa-miR-23a-3p	19p13.12	Cardiomyocytes	Heart failure [71], coronary artery disease [72], cerebral ischemia-reperfusion [73]	
hsa-miR-26a-5p	3p22.2 12q14.1 [74]	Cardiac fibroblasts [75]	Heart failure, cardiac hypertrophy [75]	
hsa-miR-29a-3p	7q32.3	Heart	Ischemia/reperfusion-induced cardiac injury [76], cardiac cachexia, heart failure [77], atrial fibrillation [78], diffuse myocardial fibrosis in hypertrophic cardiomyopathy [58], gestational diabetes mellitus [63], T2DM [2,3,80]	+ [76]
hsa-miR-103a-3p	5q34 20p13 [81]	Heart Pulmonary arterial smooth muscle cells	Hypertension [82], hypoxia-induced pulmonary hypertension [84], myocardial ischemia/reperfusion injury, acute myocardial infarction [82], obesity, regulation of insulin sensitivity [85]	+ [83]

Table 2. Cont.

miRBase ID	Gene Location on Chromosome	Expression	Role in the Pathogenesis of Cardiovascular/Cerebrovascular Diseases	Potential Therapeutic Target in Treatment of Cardiovascular Diseases
hsa-miR-125b-5p	11q24.1 21q21.1 [86]	Endothelial cells [89], cardiomyocytes [90]	Acute ischemic stroke [87], acute myocardial infarction [88,90]	
hsa-miR-126-3p	9q34.3 [91]	Endothelial cells [21], vascular smooth muscle cells [95]	Acute myocardial infarction [93], T2DM [94]	+ [21,95]
hsa-miR-133a-3p	18q11.2 20q13.33 [96]	Heart	Heart failure [98], myocardial fibrosis in hypertrophic cardiomyopathy [58,97], arrhythmogenesis in the hypertrophic and failing hearts [99,100], coronary artery calcification [102]	+ [99,100]
hsa-miR-146a-5p	5q33.3 [103,104]	Myocardium, brain	Angiogenesis [105], hypoxia, ischemia/reperfusion-induced cardiac injury [107], coronary atherosclerosis, coronary heart disease in patients with subclinical hypothyroidism [108], acute ischemic stroke, acute cerebral ischemia [106]	+ [107]
hsa-miR-181a-5p	1q32.1 9q33.3 [109]	Monocytes, adipocytes, hepatocytes	Atherosclerosis [109], T1DM [113], T2DM [109,111], obesity [109–111], metabolic syndrome, coronary artery disease [110], insulin resistance [111], non-alcoholic fatty liver disease [112], ischaemic stroke, transient ischaemic attack, acute myocardial infarction [114,115]	
hsa-miR-195-5p	17p13.1 [116]	Aorta, abdominal aorta	Cardiac hypertrophy, heart failure [29,118], abdominal aortic aneurysms [119], aortic stenosis [120]	+ [29,118]
hsa-miR-210-3p	11p15.5	Endothelial cells, cardiomyocytes [125], skeletal muscle [124]	Hypoxia [39], atherosclerotic plaque formation [25,123,126], heart failure [127], cerebral ischemia [128]	
hsa-miR-342-3p	14q32.2	Endothelial cells	Obesity [129], T1DM [130,133], T2DM [130–132], GDM [130], endothelial dysfunction [134]	

+ Potential Therapeutic Target in Treatment of Cardiovascular Diseases.

MiR-1-3p is from the precursors for miR-1-1 and miR-1-2 encoded by distinct genes located on chromosome 20q13.3 and on chromosome 18q11.2 [46]. MiR-1 is abundantly expressed in cardiac and skeletal muscles, especially in myocardium. Extracellular miR-1 levels are significantly increased in patients with acute MI and highly correlate with circulating troponin T, a reliable marker of cardiac damage [47]. MiR-1 also represents a promising therapeutic target in treatment of cardiovascular diseases, heart ischemia, and post-MI complications. Inhibition of miR-1 with antisense oligonucleotides is cardioprotective, since it leads to reduction of apoptosis, increase of resistance to oxidative stress, and attenuation of spontaneous arrhythmogenic oscillations [48–50].

A large proportion of children with an up-regulated miR-1-3p profiles with a prior exposure to GH (47.83% children with normal clinical findings and 45.16% children with abnormal clinical findings) or late PE (35.14% children with abnormal clinical findings) was identified. We suppose that children descending from complicated pregnancies with aberrant expression profiles of miR-1-3p are at a higher risk of later onset of cardiovascular diseases, and should be carefully monitored in the long term.

MiR-17-5p, a member of miR-17-92 cluster, located on the human chromosome 13q31.3 [51,52], is overexpressed in endothelial cells and lowly expressed in vascular smooth muscle cells [53]. MiR-17p~92 microRNAs were found to play a major role in cardiac development, since the hearts of miR-17p~92 deficient mutant embryos presented a clear ventricular septal defect [54]. Moreover, multiple studies have also confirmed the involvement of miR-17-5p in regulating ischemia/reperfusion-induced cardiac injury (I/R-I). Up-regulation of miR-17-5p has been reported to promote apoptosis induced by oxidative stress via targeting Stat3 in in vivo I/R-I mouse model and in vitro cellular model of oxidative stress induced by H_2O_2 [55]. The inhibition of miR-17-5p by its specific inhibitors preserved cell survival and rescued cell death in both in in vivo I/R-I mouse and in vitro cellular oxidative stress models [55] and improved cardiac function after acute myocardial infarction via weakening of apoptosis in endothelial cells in SD rat model [56]. Kaucsar et al. reported that miR-17-5p was activated during kidney ischemia-reperfusion injury in mice [57]. In humans, circulating miR-17-5p represents one of the potential up-regulated biomarkers for diffuse myocardial fibrosis in hypertrophic cardiomyopathy [58], in patients with acute ischemic stroke [59], and for the severity of coronary artery disease [60]. Our data showed that miR-17-5p was overexpressed in a proportion of children with a prior exposure to GH, regardless of normal or abnormal clinical findings (30.43% versus 29.03%), and in children previously affected with FGR, however only with abnormal clinical findings (22.73%). In view of the fact that the overexpression of miR-17-5p is associated with a high cardiovascular risk, we suppose that children with aberrant expression profile of miR-17-5p need to be stratified as soon as possible to prevent them from later cardiovascular disease development.

MiR-20a-5p belongs to the miR-17 family and is also transcribed from the miR-17-92 cluster located on the human chromosome 13q31.3 [61]. MiR-20a is involved with inflammatory signaling in pulmonary hypertension [62]. Intraperitoneal injections of antagomiR-20a significantly down-regulated the expression levels of miR-20a-5p and restored functional levels of bone morphogenetic protein receptor type 2 (BMPR2) in pulmonary arteries in hypoxia-induced pulmonary hypertension mouse model [62]. A previous pilot study of Zhu et al. demonstrated increased plasma levels of miR-17-5p and miR-20a-5p also in patients diagnosed with gestational diabetes mellitus (GDM) at 16–19 weeks of gestation [63]. Our results support the involvement of miR-20a-5p in pathogenesis of pathologies enhancing a cardiovascular risk, since overexpression of miR-20a-5p was identified only in a proportion of children with abnormal clinical findings that were previously exposed to GH (25.81%) or preeclampsia terminated after 34 weeks of gestation (13.51%). The early identification of this risky group of children may improve their future cardiovascular health.

MiR-20b-5p also belongs to the miR-17 family, however is transcribed from the miR-106a-363 cluster located on chromosome Xq26.2 [61]. Recent study showed that increased plasmatic levels of miR-20b served as one of selected biomarkers in hypertension-induced heart failure in adult male Dahl salt-sensitive rats [64]. In addition, higher levels of miR-20b-5p were found in second trimester maternal sera of pregnancies with small-for-gestational age fetuses when compared with appropriate-for-gestational age fetuses [65]. In our study, mir-20b-5p represented a unique biomarker that was up-regulated in a proportion of children with contemporary normal clinical findings that were previously affected with mild preeclampsia (36.36%). Due to the lack of information on aberrant expression profile of miR-20b-5p in cardiovascular diseases, its role in children descending from complicated pregnancies remains for us unclear.

MiR-21-5p and miR-21-3p are encoded by the gene located on chromosome 17q23.2 [66] and mediate the homeostasis of the cardiovascular system [67]. Overexpression of miR-21 promotes cardiac fibrosis and development of heart failure with preserved left ventricular ejection fraction. Inhibition of miR-21 by miR-21 antagonists led to amelioration of cardiac atrophy and cardiac fibrosis [68]. MiR-21 is upregulated by HIF-1α under hypoxia in cardiomyocytes and silencing of HIF-1α and inhibition of miR-21 increase the apoptosis of hypoxic cardiomyocytes [69]. Extracellular miR-21 can be used as a biomarker for the diagnosis and prognosis of heart failure. Serum levels of miR-21 were higher in patients with heart failure than in controls, and correlated with ejection fraction and brain natriuretic peptide [70]. In our study miR-21-5p was up-regulated in a proportion of children descending from normal pregnancies with abnormal clinical findings (28.95%) and in children descending from GH pregnancies with normal clinical findings (39.13%). According to our opinion, this group of children would benefit from dispensarization and implementation of primary prevention strategies, since it may be at higher risk of later development of cardiovascular diseases.

MiR-23a, encoded by a gene located at chromosome 19p13.12, has two mature microRNAs: miR-23a-5p and miR-23a-3p. MiR-23a regulates cardiomyocyte apoptosis, a key pathogenesis factor of heart failure, by targeting manganese superoxide dismutase [71] and the vasculogenesis of coronary artery disease via targeting epidermal growth factor receptor [72]. Extracellular miR-23a may be a new biomarker for coronary artery disease, since increased levels of miR-23a may be used to predict the presence and severity of coronary lesions in patients with coronary artery disease [72]. MiR-23a-3p also suppressed oxidative stress injury in a mouse model of focal cerebral ischemia-reperfusion [73]. Since our study demonstrated overexpression of miR-23a-3p in a proportion of children with normal clinical findings born of GH complicated pregnancies only (34.78%), we suppose that compensatory effect of miR-23a-3p may appear more likely in these children to normalize cardiomyocyte state and vasculogenesis.

MiR-26a-5p is produced by miR-26a-1 and miR-26a-2, whose genes are located on chromosomes 3p22.2 and 12q14.1 [74]. MiR-26a-5p was demonstrated to regulate the autophagy in cardiac fibroblasts by targeting a key component of autophagy pathway, ULK1 (unc-51 like autophagy activating kinase 1). Overexpression of miR-26a-5p reduces the expression of ULK1 and decreases the activation of LC3-I to LC3-II (microtubule-associated protein 1 light chain) participating in the formation of autophagosome membranes during autophagy [75]. Autophagy plays a protective role in heart failure and cardiac hypertrophy by removing damaged proteins [65]. Nevertheless, in some cases inhibited autophagy may also improve cardiac function [75]. Since our study showed overexpression of miR-26a-5p in a proportion of children with normal clinical findings that were affected with GH (21.74%), we suggest that this phenomenon may have protective effect against potential development of cardiac fibrosis.

MiR-29a-3p, a member of miR-29 family, is encoded by a gene located on chromosome 7q32.3. Antagomirs against miR-29a significantly increased Mcl-2 expression and significantly reduced myocardial infarct size and apoptosis in rat hearts subjected to ischaemia-reperfusion injury [76]. Increased expression of miR-29a-3p was also observed in cardiac cachexia, a common complication of heart failure, in Wistar rat models [77]. In patients with atrial fibrillation, overexpression of miR-29a-3p found in the biopsies collected from the right atrial appendage during the general surgical procedure was associated with underexpression of calcium voltage-gated channel subunit alpha 1C (CACNA1C) [78]. Circulating miR-29a-3p represents one of potential up-regulated biomarkers for diffuse myocardial fibrosis in hypertrophic cardiomyopathy [58]. Previous pilot study of Zhu et al. demonstrated increased plasma levels of miR-29a-3p in GDM patients at 16–19 weeks of gestation [63].

Serum mir-29a-3p levels were also shown to be elevated in patients with recent diagnosis of type 2 diabetes mellitus (T2DM) [23]. Moreover, overexpression of miR-29a-3p was found in resistance arterioles obtained by biopsy from T2DM patients [79]. Our study indicated the presence of overexpression of miR-29a-3p in both groups of children with normal and abnormal clinical findings descending from pregnancies complicated by GH (39.13% versus 32.26%). We believe that this group of children is endangered by later development of cardiovascular diseases and would benefit from early prevention programs to decrease a cardiovascular risk.

MiR-103 and miR-107 are paralogous microRNAs binding the same target sites. MiR-103 is encoded by two different genes located on chromosomes 5q34 and 20p13 [80]. Both genes generate miR-103a-3p. MiR-103/107 regulate programmed necrosis and myocardial ischemia/reperfusion injury via targeting FADD (Fas-associated protein with death domain). Both miR-103 and miR-107 are overexpressed in the ischemic zone of ischemic heart. Plasma miR-103a concentration is also significantly elevated in patients with high blood pressure and acute myocardial infarction [81]. Injection of miR-103/107 antagomir led to a reduction of FADD and induced a reduction in the myocardial necrosis and myocardial infarct sizes [82]. MiR-103/107 is also involved in hypoxia-induced pulmonary hypertension through hypoxia-induced proliferation of pulmonary arterial smooth muscle cells via targeting HIF-1β. Nevertheless, in this model miR-103/107 induced overexpression led to inhibition of hypoxia induced pulmonary arterial smooth muscle cell proliferation and hypoxia-induced pulmonary hypertension [83]. In addition, miR-103/107 play the central importance in regulation of insulin sensitivity. Overexpression of miR-103/107 is present in obese mice and silencing of miR-103/miR-107 leads to the improvement of glucose homeostasis and insulin sensitivity [84]. Our data are similar to findings of Huang et al. [81] and Trajkovski et al. [84]. Since we identified overexpression of miR-103a-3p in a proportion of children with abnormal clinical findings who were exposed to severe preeclampsia (12.77%) and or preeclampsia developing after 34 weeks of gestation (13.51%), we consider up-regulation of miR-103-3p in circulation of children as a highly risky feature of potential development of cardiovascular diseases.

There are two paralogs, miR-125b-1 on chromosome 11q24.1 and miR-125b-2 on chromosome 21q21.1, both producing miR-125b-5p [85]. A set of upregulated circulating microRNAs including miR-125b-5p was identified to be associated with acute ischemic stroke [86] and acute myocardial infarction [87]. Overexpression of miR-125b-5p was shown to protect endothelial cells from apoptosis under oxidative stress via negative regulation of SMAD4 (SMAD family member 4) [88]. In addition, miR-125b-5p was identified as an ischemic stress-responsive protector against cardiomyocyte apoptosis. Cardiomyocytes overexpressing miR-125b-5p have increased prosurvival signaling and protected the heart from acute myocardial infarction by repressing pro-apoptotic bak1 and klf13 [89]. Our results are consistent with the data of Wei et al. [88] and Bayoumi et al. [89], since we observed overexpression of miR-125b-5p in a significant proportion of children with normal clinical findings that were previously affected with GH (47.83%). We suggest that a protective effect of miR-125-5p may be present just in children previously exposed to minor pregnancy-related complications, while in children exposed to severe pregnancy-related complications it apparently vanished.

MiR-126, producing miR-126-3p, is an intronic microRNA located in intron 7 of EGFL7 (epidermal growth factor-like protein 7) gene on chromosome 9q34.3 [90]. MiR-126 regulates endothelial expression of vascular cell adhesion molecule 1 (VCAM-1) and controls vascular inflammation. Overexpression of miR-126 decreases VCAM-1 expression and in opposite transfection of endothelial cells with miR-126 antagomirs increases TNFα-stimulated VCAM-1 expression [21]. MiR-126-3p was down-regulated in the sera derived from patients with acute myocardial infarction [91] and in the plasma of type 2 diabetes patients [92]. Recent experiments also demonstrated that intercellular transfer of miR-126-3p by endothelial microparticles reduced vascular smooth muscle cell proliferation and limited neointima formation via inhibition of LRP6 (LDL receptor related protein 6) [93]. It seems that compensatory role of miR-126-3p also appears in a proportion of children with both normal or abnormal clinical findings with a prior exposure to GH (39.13% versus 22.58%) or FGR (31.82%), most likely with the aim to induce suppression of cytokine activated endothelial cells and vascular smooth muscle cell proliferation.

MiR-133a-3p belongs to the miR-133 family. MiR-133a-1 gene is located on chromosome 18q11.2 and miR-133a-2 gene on chromosome 20q13.33, respectively. Both genes produce miR-133a-3p [94]. MiR-133 was down-regulated with hypertrophy [95], heart failure [96], and down-regulation of miR-133 also contributed to arrhythmogenesis in the hypertrophic and failing hearts. Induction of overexpression of miR-133 reduced hypertrophy as well as lead to correction of conduction abnormalities [97,98]. Furthermore, circulating miR-133a-3p provides one of up-regulated candidates as potential biomarkers for diffuse myocardial fibrosis in hypertrophic cardiomyopathy [58] and coronary artery calcification [99]. We suggest that the overexpression of miR-133a-3p observed in our study in a proportion of children previously exposed to GH, PE and/or FGR may be a long-term consequence of pregnancy-related complications and we believe that postnatal miR-133a-3p screening may stratify a risky group of children predisposed to later cardiovascular disease development.

The miR-146 family consists of 2 members, with nearly identical sequences, miR-146a-5p and miR-146b-5p [100]. MIR146A gene was found within a larger long noncoding RNA host gene, MIR3142HG, on chromosome 5q33.3 [101]. MiR-146a-5p is actively involved in multiple oncological processes such as antitumor immune suppression, metastasis, and angiogenesis [102]. MiR-146a-5p is an anti-inflammatory microRNA, since it functions as a negative regulator of inflammation by targeting interleukin-1 receptor-associated kinase 1 (IRAK1) and tumor necrosis factor (TNF) receptor associated factor 6 (TRAF6), resulting in inhibition of NF-κB activation [103]. Furthermore, miR-146a is one of the microRNAs that is most sensitive to hypoxia. It seems that miR-146a overexpression can protect the myocardium from I/R damage. Lentivirus expressing miR-146a transfected into mouse hearts decreased I/R-induced myocardial infarct size and prevented I/R-induced decreases in ejection fraction and fractional shortening [104]. Increased circulating plasma levels of miR-146a also correlated with the severity of coronary atherosclerosis in patients with subclinical hypothyroidism and have been suggested as good predictor for coronary heart disease development among individuals with elevated TSH levels [105]. Nevertheless, a significant reduction of miR-146a expression was observed in acute ischemic stroke. A down-regulation of miR-146a was suggested to be a self-protective response of the brain against the consequences of acute cerebral ischemia injury via the up-regulation of Fbxl10 expression, which protects neurons from ischemic death [103]. Since we observed the overexpression of miR-146a-5p in both groups of children with normal and abnormal clinical findings, whose pregnancies were complicated by GH only (26.09% versus 12.9%), we believe that a protective role of miR-146a-5p is applied at least at a lesser group of children with the aim to reduce inflammation and its negative consequences.

MiR-181a and miR-181b cluster together on chromosomes 1q32.1 and 9q33.3. MiR-181a generates several mature microRNAs involving miR-181a-5p, miR-181a-3p and miR-181a2-3p [106]. The miR-181 family plays a key role in both acute and chronic inflammatory disease states such as atherosclerosis, type 2 diabetes, and obesity [106]. Nevertheless, contradictory data are reported concerning expression levels of miR-181a in various pathological conditions. Decreased expression of miR-181a observed in monocytes of obese patients was associated with the metabolic syndrome and coronary artery disease [107]. However, another study reported that overexpression of miR-181a-5p in adipocytes upregulated insulin-stimulated AKT activation and reduced TNFα-induced insulin resistance [108]. Moreover, increased hepatic miR-181a impaired glucose and lipid homeostasis by silencing sirtuin 1 in non-alcoholic fatty liver disease [109]. Several contradictory data are also reported concerning serum levels of miR-181a in diabetic patients. While serum levels of miR-181a-5p were decreased in obese and diabetic patients [108], circulating levels of miR-181a were increased in type 1 diabetic children and adolescents [110]. Nevertheless, circulating miR-181a-5p levels were increased in patients with ischaemic stroke, transient ischaemic attack and acute myocardial infarction [111,112]. Our study revealed overexpression of miR-181a-5p in a proportion of children with both normal and abnormal clinical findings descending from GH pregnancies (39.13% and 25.81%). In view of the inconsistency between studies, the role of miR-181a-5p is not clear. Nevertheless, we believe that increased levels of miR-181a-5p in whole peripheral blood of children previously exposed to GH may predispose to later development of cardiovascular diseases.

MiR-195 gene is located on the chromosome 17p13.1 and generates two microRNAs, miR-195-5p and miR-195-3p [113]. MiR-195 is increasing in cardiac hypertrophy, and cardiac miR-195 overexpression results in heart failure [29,114]. MiR-195 is also a powerful regulator of the aortic extracellular matrix. Administration of miR-195 antagomirs led to significant elevation of elastin and collagens in the murine aorta, but has no effect on survival and aortic diameter size. Nevertheless, in plasma samples an inverse correlation between miR-195 and the presence of abdominal aortic aneurysms and aortic diameter was observed. Surprisingly, miR-195 plasma levels were decreased in abdominal aortic aneurysms [115]. On the other hand, aortic stenosis caused by leaflet calcification of the bicuspid aortic valve was associated with down-regulation of miR-195 [116]. The mechanism of miR-195 action is not completely understood. Since we observed overexpression of miR-195-5p in a proportion of children with normal clinical findings previously affected with GH only (34.78%), we suggest that overexpression of miR-195-5p may have rather protective role than harmful effect.

MiR-210-3p, encoded by a gene located on chromosome 11p15.5, is the most prominent microRNA consistently stimulated under hypoxic conditions. A significant increase of mir-210 levels was detected in placentas of women with preeclampsia, a condition that is characterized by hypoxia resulting from inadequate blood supply to the placenta [39]. Several microRNAs involving miR-210 were reported to be involved in atherosclerotic plaque formation through the regulation of endothelial apoptosis [25,117]. Nevertheless, some authors reported that up-regulated levels of miR-210 positively correlated with the level of endothelial cell apoptosis [117], while the others found that miR-210 blockage only led to induction of endothelial cell apoptosis and cell death in hypoxia [128]. Another study showed that up-regulation of miR-210 had cytoprotective effects, mainly in cardiomyocytes [119] and the skeletal muscle [118]. Increased serum levels of miR-210 may indicate early stages of atherosclerosis obliterans [120] and heart failure [121]. MiR-210 also regulates angiogenesis in response to ischemic injury to the brain. Overexpression of miR-210 may activate the Notch signaling pathway, which probably contributes to angiogenesis after cerebral ischemia [122]. In view of the fact that we observed a strong positive correlation between gene expression of miR-210-3p in whole peripheral blood of children with a history of preeclampsia and/or FGR and the pulsatility index in the ductus venosus, we believe that children descending from preeclampsia and/or FGR affected pregnancies who had high postnatal levels of miR-210-3p in their circulation represent a risky group, that is endangered by the onset of cardiovascular and cerebrovascular diseases in the future, since increased PI in the ductus venosus is a sign of a poor perinatological outcome.

MiR-342-3p is encoded by a gene located on chromosome 14q32.2. MiR-342-3p is considered as an obesity-associated microRNA, since it positively regulates adipogenesis of adipose-derived mesenchymal stem cells by suppressing CtBP2 and releasing the key adipogenic regulator C/EBPα from CtBP2 binding [123]. A set of up-regulated microRNAs expressed in peripheral blood mononuclear cells involving mir-342-3p was shared among patients with type 1 diabetes mellitus, type 2 diabetes mellitus and gestational diabetes mellitus [124]. Urinary exosomal miR-342 was also expressed at significantly elevated levels in type 2 diabetes mellitus patients [125]. However, miR-342-3p expression was significantly reduced in endothelial cells isolated from lung and heart tissues of type 2 diabetes mellitus mice and this inhibition blocked vasculogenesis in vivo by repressing endothelial proliferation and migration [126]. Decreased expression of miR-342 was also observed in T regulatory cells of patients with type 1 diabetes mellitus [127]. Moreover, plasma miR-342-3p was identified as a potential down-regulated biomarker of children aged 5–10 years with endothelial dysfunction [128]. Our study demonstrated decreased expression of miR-342-3p in a proportion of children with abnormal clinical findings that were previously exposed to early preeclampsia, which required the termination of gestation before 34 weeks (26.92%). Therefore, we suggest that this group of children is a highly risky group, which would benefit from implementation of early primary prevention strategies and long-term follow-up.

4. Materials and Methods

4.1. Participants

The study included prospectively collected cohort of Caucasian children born within 2007–2014 descending from pregnancies with GH ($n = 54$), PE ($n = 133$), FGR ($n = 34$), and children after normal course of gestation ($n = 88$) that were chosen on the basis of equal age. An in-person visit was conducted 3–11 years after the pregnancy ended. Of the 133 PE pregnancies, 27 were diagnosed with mild PE and 106 had symptoms of severe PE. In 49 PE pregnancies gestation was terminated before 34 weeks (early PE) and 84 children were delivered after 34 weeks (late PE). PE occurred mainly in normotensive patients (128 cases), or exceptionally was superimposed on prior hypertension (5 cases). Thirteen FGR fetuses required delivery <32 weeks (early FGR) and 21 cases were delivered >32 weeks (late FGR). Oligohydramnios and/or anhydramnios were present in 20 FGR fetuses and 19 PE cases.

Arterial Doppler examination showed an abnormal pulsatility index (PI) in the umbilical artery (PI > 95th percentile) in 9 PE and 20 FGR cases and in the middle cerebral artery (PI < 5th percentile) in 7 PE and 8 FGR cases. The cerebro-placental ratio (CPR) was 5th percentile in 15 PE and 21 FGR cases. The umbilical artery Doppler showed absent and/or zero diastolic flow in 2 PE and 4 FGR cases. The mean PI in the uterine artery >95th percentile was identified in 10 PE and 7 FGR pregnancies with the presence of unilateral or bilateral diastolic notch in 12 PE and 6 FGR cases. Ductus venosus examination revealed an absence of flow during atrial contraction (a wave) (deep a wave) in 1 FGR pregnancy. In addition, abnormal PI of ductus venosus (>1) was detected in 3 PE and/or FGR pregnancies.

The clinical characteristics of children descending from normal and complicated pregnancies are presented in Table 3.

Normal pregnancies were defined as those without medical, obstetrical, or surgical complications at the time of the study and who subsequently delivered full term, singleton healthy infants weighing >2500 g after 37 completed weeks of gestation.

Gestational hypertension usually develops after 20 weeks of gestation and is defined as high blood pressure (>140/90 mmHg) without the sign of proteinuria. On the other hand, preeclampsia is characterized as hypertension (blood pressure > 140/90 mmHg in two determinations 4 h apart) associated with proteinuria (>300 mg/24 h) that appears after the twentieth week of gestation [129].

Severe preeclampsia is defined by the presence of one or more of the following findings: 1) a systolic blood pressure over 160 mmHg or a diastolic blood pressure over 110 mmHg, 2) proteinuria (>5 g of protein in a 24-h sample), 3) very low urine output (<500 mL in 24 h), 4) signs of pulmonary oedema or cyanosis, 5) impairment of liver function, 6) signs of severe headache, visual disturbances, 7) pain in the epigastric area or right upper quadrant, 8) thrombocytopenia, and 9) the presence of severe FGR [129].

FGR fetuses are defined as those with the estimated fetal weight (EFW) < 3rd percentile or <10th percentile for the evaluated gestational age after the adjustments for the appropriate population standards of the Czech Republic (the Hadlock formula, Astraia Software GmbH). Early onset FGR was diagnosed when the EFW was less than the third percentile or absent and/or zero diastolic flow was present in the umbilical artery. In addition, early onset FGR was classified when fetal weight below the threshold of the 10th percentile was associated with an abnormal pulsatility index in the umbilical artery (>95th percentile) or an abnormal pulsatility index in the uterine artery (>95th percentile). Late onset FGR was determined by only one parameter (EWF below the third percentile) or by the combination of 2 parameters: EFW below the tenth percentile and the cerebro–placental ratio (CPR) below the fifth percentile. CPR is expressed as a ratio between the middle cerebral artery and the umbilical artery pulsatility indexes [130–132].

Table 3. Characteristics of cases and controls.

	Normal Pregnancies with Normal Clinical Findings (n = 50)	Normal Pregnancies with Abnormal Clinical Findings (n = 38)	PE (n = 133)	FGR (n = 34)	GH (n = 54)	p-Value [1]	p-Value [2]	p-Value [3]	p-Value [4]
At follow-up									
Age (years)	5 (3–11)	5 (3–11)	5 (3–11)	4 (3–10)	4.5 (3–10)	1.000	1.000	1.000	1.000
Height (cm)	115 (98–144.5)	118.5 (100–153)	114 (97–155)	106.5 (93–152)	111.5 (96–159.5)	1.000	1.000	**0.020**	1.000
Weight (kg)	20.35 (14–37)	22.3 (14.7–40.8)	19.4 (11.85–54.9)	16.25 (12–37)	19.6 (14–47.5)	1.000	1.000	**0.002**	1.000
BMI (kg/m^2)	15.43 (13.22–18.09)	15.87 (13.3–20)	14.91 (12.34–22.81)	14.18 (12.7–19.24)	15.35 (13.42–19.7)	1.000	1.000	**0.004**	1.000
Systolic BP (mmHg)	98 (84–115)	104 (89–123)	99 (84–132)	97 (82–123)	99 (80–129)	**0.001**	1.000	1.000	0.487
Diastolic BP (mmHg)	60 (38–68)	64.4 (43–81)	61 (41–88)	60 (42–75)	61.5 (49–83)	**0.028**	0.545	1.000	1.000
Heart rate (n/min)	90 (67–110)	90.5 (51–120)	92 (64–117)	96 (62–112)	94.5 (65–129)	1.000	1.000	1.000	1.000
During gestation									
Maternal age at delivery (years)	32.5 (26–40)	32 (25–43)	32 (21–44)	32 (22–41)	32 (27–51)	1.000	1.000	1.000	1.000
GA at delivery (weeks)	39.86 (37.71–41.57)	39.93 (37.86–41.86)	35.79 (26–41.72)	35.64 (28–41)	38.63 (33.43–41.28)	1.000	**<0.001**	**<0.001**	**0.002**
Mode of delivery						0.429	**<0.001**	**<0.001**	**<0.001**
Vaginal	46 (92.00%)	33 (68.84%)	8 (14.3 %)	7 (20.59%)	24 (44.44%)				
CS	4 (8.00 %)	5 (13.16%)	48 (85.7 %)	27 (79.41%)	30 (55.56%)				
Fetal birth weight (g)	3425 (2730–4220)	3295 (2530–4450)	2370 (660–4490)	1870 (650–3010)	3140 (1040–4310)	1.000	**<0.001**	**<0.001**	0.113
Fetal sex						0.217	0.055	0.470	0.414
Boy	29 (58.00%)	17 (44.74%)	56 (42.11%)	17 (50.00%)	27 (50.00%)				
Girl	21 (42.00 %)	21 (55.26%)	77 (57.89%)	17 (50.00%)	27 (50.00%)				
Primiparity						0.140	**0.001**	**<0.001**	0.362
Yes	29 (58.00%)	16 (42.11%)	108 (81.20%)	33 (97.06%)	36 (66.67 %)				
No	21 (42.00%)	22 (57.89%)	25 (18.80 %)	1 (2.94%)	18 (33.33 %)				

Table 3. *Cont.*

	Normal Pregnancies with Normal Clinical Findings (n = 50)	Normal Pregnancies with Abnormal Clinical Findings (n = 38)	PE (n = 133)	FGR (n = 34)	GH (n = 54)	*p*-Value [1]	*p*-Value [2]	*p*-Value [3]	*p*-Value [4]
Birth order of index pregnancy						0.158	0.168	**0.009**	0.602
1st	25 (50.00%)	12 (31.58%)	86 (64.66%)	28 (82.35)	28 (51.85%)				
2nd	18 (36.00%)	14 (36.84%)	27 (20.30%)	2 (5.88%)	14 (25.93%)				
3rd	5 (10.00%)	10 (26.32%)	13 (9.77 %)	2 (5.88%)	9 (16.66 %)				
4th+	2 (4.00 %)	2 (5.26%)	7 (5.26 %)	2 (5.88%)	3 (5.56 %)				
Infertility treatment						0.726	**0.001**	**0.007**	0.117
Yes	2 (4.00%)	1 (2.63%)	34 (25.56%)	8 (23.53 %)	7 (12.96%)				
No	48 (96.00%)	37 (97.37%)	99 (74.44%)	26 (76.47 %)	47 (87.04%)				

Data are presented as median (range) for continuous variables and as number (percent) for categorical variables. Statistically significant results are marked in bold. Continuous variables were compared using Kruskal-Wallis test. *p*-value [1]: the comparison among normal pregnancies with normal and abnormal postnatal clinical findings; *p*-value [2,3,4]: the comparison among normal pregnancies with normal postnatal clinical findings and preeclampsia, fetal growth restriction or gestational hypertension, respectively. Categorical variables were compared using a chi-square test.; GA, gestational age; BP, blood pressure; CS, Caesarean section.

The presence of absent and/or zero end-diastolic flow (AEDF) in the umbilical artery in mid to late pregnancy usually occurs as a result of placental insufficiency. Increased resistance (the mean PI > 95th percentile) in the uterine artery with or without the presence of unilateral or bilateral diastolic notch identifies pregnancies with a risk of placental failure. Centralization of the fetal circulation manifests itself in redistribution of the circulation in the brain, liver and heart at the expense of the flow reduction in the periphery and represents a protective reaction of the fetus against hypoxia [133,134]. Absence or reversal of flow during atrial contraction (a wave) (deep a wave in the ductus venosus) indicates failure of fetal circulatory compensation to supply well oxygenated blood to vital organ. The pulsatility index of DV more than 1 between the second trimester and term indicates of DV dilatation and poor outcome in severe fetal growth retardation.

Patients demonstrating other pregnancy-related complications such as premature rupture of membranes, in utero infections, fetal anomalies or chromosomal abnormalities, and fetal demise in utero or stillbirth were not involved in the study.

Written informed consent was provided for all participants included in the study. The study was approved by the Ethics Committee of the Institute for the Care of the Mother and Child, Prague, Czech Republic (grant no. AZV 16-27761A, Long-term monitoring of complex cardiovascular profile in the mother, fetus and offspring descending from pregnancy-related complications, date of approval: 28 May 2015) and by the Ethics Committee of the Third Faculty of Medicine, Prague, Czech Republic (grant no. AZV 16-27761A, Long-term monitoring of complex cardiovascular profile in the mother, fetus and offspring descending from pregnancy-related complications, date of approval: 27 March 2014).

4.2. BP Measurements

Standardized BP measurements were performed. BP was measured three times in the right arm after a 5-min rest period during which the participant seated using an automated device (OMRON M6W, Omron Healthcare Co., Kyoto, Japan) and cuff for arm circumference 17–22 cm (OMRON CS). The average of the last 2 systolic and diastolic BP was used for the data analyses.

Normal BP was characterized as systolic blood pressure (SBP) and diastolic blood pressure (DBP) that were below the 90th percentile for gender, age, and height. Hypertension was diagnosed when average SBP or DBP reached on at least 3 separate occasions ≥95th percentile for gender, age, and height. Average SBP or DBP levels that were within the range of ≥90th percentile and <95th percentile were designated as prehypertension [135].

4.3. BMI Assessment

Body weight was measured to the nearest 0.05–0.1 kg using an electronic scale and height was measured to the nearest 0.1 cm using a built-in stadiometer (calibrated balance scales, RADWAG WPT 100/200 OW, RADWAG, Czech Republic). The BMI Percentile Calculator was used to calculate BMI in children and teens (https://www.cdc.gov/healthyweight/assessing/bmi/childrens_bmi/about_childrens_bmi.html).

This calculator provides age- and sex-specific BMI. Normal or healthy weight children had BMI within the range of the 5th percentile and the 85th percentile. Children with BMI within the 85th percentile and the 95th percentile were in the overweight category. Children with BMI equal to or greater than the 95th percentile were in the obese category.

4.4. Echocardiography Measurements

Examinations were performed using Philips HD15 ultrasound machine (Philips Ultrasound, Bothell, WA, USA) with sector array transducer (3–8 MHz) incorporating color flow, pulse wave, and continuous wave Doppler measurements with adaptive technology. Children were calm and in supine position during ultrasound examination. A complete two-dimensional echocardiography was performed by a single investigator experienced with pediatric echocardiography. The transducer beam was kept as close as possible to the Doppler beam at <20% degrees to calculate valve regurgitation.

No angle correction of Doppler signal was applied. Children with abnormal findings were referred to pediatric cardiologist.

4.5. Processing of Samples

Homogenized cell lysates were prepared immediately after collection of whole peripheral blood samples (EDTA tubes, 200 µL) using QIAamp RNA Blood Mini Kit (Qiagen, Hilden, Germany, no: 52304).

Total RNA was extracted from homogenized cell lysates stored at $-80\ °C$ using a mirVana microRNA Isolation kit (Ambion, Austin, USA, no: AM1560) and followed by an enrichment procedure for small RNAs. To minimize DNA contamination, the eluted RNA was treated for 30 min at $37\ °C$ with 5 µL of DNase I (Thermo Fisher Scientific, CA, USA, no: EN0521). A RNA fraction highly enriched in short RNAs (<200 nt) was obtained. The concentration and quality of RNA was assessed using a NanoDrop ND-1000 spectrophotometer (NanoDrop Technologies, Wilmington, NC, USA). If the A(260/280) absorbance ratio of isolated RNA was 1.8–2.0 and the A(260/230) absorbance ratio was greater than 1.6, the RNA fraction was pure and used for the consecutive analysis.

4.6. Reverse Transcriptase Reaction

Individual microRNAs were reverse transcribed into complementary DNA (cDNA) in a total reaction volume of 10 µL using microRNA-specific stem-loop RT primers, components of TaqMan MicroRNA Assays (Table 5), and TaqMan MicroRNA Reverse Transcription Kit (Applied Biosystems, Branchburg, NJ, USA, no: 4366597). Reverse transcriptase reactions were performed with the following thermal cycling parameters: 30 min at $16\ °C$, 30 min at $42\ °C$, 5 min at $85\ °C$, and then held at $4\ °C$ using a 7500 Real-Time PCR system (Applied Biosystems, Branchburg, NJ, USA).

Table 4. Characteristics of microRNAs involved in the study.

Assay Name	miRBase ID	NCBI Location Chromosome	microRNA Sequence
hsa-miR-1	hsa-miR-1-3p	Chr20: 61151513-61151583 [+]	5′-UGGAAUGUAAAGAAGUAUGUAU-3′
hsa-miR-16	hsa-miR-16-5p	Chr13: 50623109-50623197 [−]	5′-UAGCAGCACGUAAAUAUUGGCG-3′
hsa-miR-17	hsa-miR-17-5p	Chr13: 92002859-92002942 [+]	5′-CAAAGUGCUUACAGUGCAGGUAG-3′
hsa-miR-20a	hsa-miR-20a-5p	Chr13: 92003319-92003389 [+]	5′-UAAAGUGCUUAUAGUGCAGGUAG-3′
hsa-miR-20b	hsa-miR-20b-5p	ChrX: 133303839-133303907 [−]	5′-CAAAGUGCUCAUAGUGCAGGUAG-3′
hsa-miR-21	hsa-miR-21-5p	Chr17: 57918627-57918698 [+]	5′-UAGCUUAUCAGACUGAUGUUGA-3′
hsa-miR-23a	hsa-miR-23a-3p	Chr19: 13947401-13947473 [−]	5′-AUCACAUUGCCAGGGAUUUCC-3′
hsa-miR-24	hsa-miR-24-3p	Chr19: 13947101-13947173 [−]	5′-UGGCUCAGUUCAGCAGGAACAG-3′
hsa-miR-26a	hsa-miR-26a-5p	Chr3: 38010895-38010971 [+]	5′-UUCAAGUAAUCCAGGAUAGGCU-3′
hsa-miR-29a	hsa-miR-29a-3p	Chr7: 130561506-130561569 [−]	5′-UAGCACCAUCUGAAAUCGGUUA-3′
hsa-miR-92a	hsa-miR-92a-3p	Chr13: 92003568-92003645 [+]	5′-UAUUGCACUUGUCCCGGCCUGU-3′
hsa-miR-100	hsa-miR-100-5p	Chr11: 122022937-122023016 [−]	5′-AACCCGUAGAUCCGAACUUGUG-3′
hsa-miR-103	hsa-miR-103a-3p	Chr20: 3898141-3898218 [+]	5′-AGCAGCAUUGUACAGGGCUAUGA-3′
hsa-miR-125b	hsa-miR-125b-5p	Chr21: 17962557-17962645 [+]	5′-UCCCUGAGACCCUAACUUGUGA-3′
hsa-miR-126	hsa-miR-126-3p	Chr9: 139565054-139565138 [+]	5′-UCGUACCGUGAGUAAUAAUGCG-3′
hsa-miR-130b	hsa-miR-130b-3p	Chr22: 22007593-22007674 [+]	5′-CAGUGCAAUGAUGAAAGGGCAU-3′
hsa-miR-133a	hsa-miR-133a-3p	Chr20: 61162119-61162220 [+]	5′-UUUGGUCCCCUUCAACCAGCUG-3′
hsa-miR-143	hsa-miR-143-3p	Chr5: 148808481-148808586 [+]	5′-UGAGAUGAAGCACUGUAGCUC-3′
hsa-miR-145	hsa-miR-145-5p	Chr5: 148810209-148810296 [+]	5′-GUCCAGUUUUCCCAGGAAUCCCU-3′
hsa-miR-146a	hsa-miR-146a-5p	Chr5: 159912359-159912457 [+]	5′-UGAGAACUGAAUUCCAUGGGUU-3′
hsa-miR-155	hsa-miR-155-5p	Chr21: 26946292-26946356 [+]	5′-UUAAUGCUAAUCGUGAUAGGGGU-3′
hsa-miR-181a	hsa-miR-181a-5p	Chr9: 127454721-127454830 [+]	5′-AACAUUCAACGCUGUCGGUGAGU-3′
hsa-miR-195	hsa-miR-195-5p	Chr17: 6920934-6921020 [−]	5′-UAGCAGCACAGAAAUAUUGGC-3′
hsa-miR-199a	hsa-miR-199a-5p	Chr19: 10928102-10928172 [−]	5′-CCCAGUGUUCAGACUACCUGUUC-3′
hsa-miR-210	hsa-miR-210-3p	Chr11: 568089-568198 [−]	5′-CUGUGCGUGUGACAGCGGCUGA-3′

Table 5. Characteristics of microRNAs involved in the study.

Assay Name	miRBase ID	NCBI Location Chromosome	microRNA Sequence
hsa-miR-221	hsa-miR-221-3p	ChrX: 45605585-45605694 [−]	5′-AGCUACAUUGUCUGCUGGGUUUC-3′
hsa-miR-342-3p	hsa-miR-342-3p	Chr14: 100575992-100576090 [+]	5′-UCUCACACAGAAAUCGCACCCGU-3′
mmu-miR-499	hsa-miR-499a-5p	Chr20: 33578179-33578300 [+]	5′-UUAAGACUUGCAGUGAUGUUU-3′
hsa-miR-574-3p	hsa-miR-574-3p	Chr4: 38869653-38869748 [+]	5′-CACGCUCAUGCACACACCCACA-3′

[+] A single strand of DNA sense (or positive (+)) if an RNA version of the same sequence is translated or translatable into protein. [−] Its complementary strand is called antisense (or negative (−) sense).

4.7. Relative Quantification of microRNAs by Real-Time PCR

3 µL of cDNA were mixed with specific TaqMan MGB probes and primers (TaqMan MicroRNA Assay, Applied Biosystems, Branchburg, NJ, USA), and the ingredients of the TaqMan Universal PCR Master Mix (Applied Biosystems, Branchburg, NJ, USA, no: 4318157). A total reaction volume was 15 µL. TaqMan PCR conditions were set up as described in the TaqMan guidelines for a 7500 Real-Time PCR system. All PCRs were performed in duplicates with the involvement of multiple negative controls such as NTC (water instead of cDNA sample), NAC (non-transcribed RNA samples), and genomic DNA (isolated from equal biological samples), which did not generate any signal during PCR reactions. The samples were considered positive if the amplification signal occurred at $Ct < 40$ (before the 40th threshold cycle).

The expression of particular microRNA was determined using the comparative Ct method [136] relative to normalization factor (geometric mean of two selected endogenous controls) [137]. Two non-coding small nucleolar RNAs (RNU58A and RNU38B) were optimal for qPCR data normalization in this setting. They demonstrated equal expression between children descending from normal and complicated pregnancies. RNU58A and RNU38B also served as positive controls for successful extraction of RNA from all samples and were used as internal controls for variations during the preparation of RNA, cDNA synthesis, and real-time PCR.

A reference sample, RNA fraction highly enriched for small RNAs isolated from the fetal part of one randomly selected placenta derived from gestation with normal course, was used throughout the study for relative quantification.

4.8. Statistical Analysis

Data normality was assessed using the Shapiro–Wilk test [138]. Since our experimental data did not follow a normal distribution, microRNA levels were compared between groups using the Kruskal–Wallis one-way analysis of variance with post-hoc test for the comparison among multiple groups. The significance level was established at a *p*-value of $p < 0.05$.

Receivers operating characteristic (ROC) curves were constructed to calculate the area under the curve (AUC) and the best cut-off point for particular microRNA was used in order to calculate the respective sensitivity at 90.0% specificity (MedCalc Software bvba, Ostend, Belgium). For every possible threshold or cut-off value, the MedCalc® v16.8.4 program reports the sensitivity, specificity, likelihood ratio positive (LR+), likelihood ratio negative (LR−).

To select the optimal combinations of microRNA biomarkers logistic regression was used (MedCalc® v16.8.4 program, MedCalc Software bvba, Ostend, Belgium). The logistic regression procedure allows to analyze the relationship between one dichotomous dependent variable and one or more independent variables. Another method to evaluate the logistic regression model makes use of ROC curve analysis. In this analysis, the power of the model's predicted values to discriminate between positive and negative cases is quantified by the area under the ROC curve (AUC). To perform a full ROC curve analysis the predicted probabilities are first saved and next used as a new variable in ROC curve analysis. The dependent variable used in logistic regression then acts as the classification variable in the ROC curve analysis dialog box.

Correlation between variables was calculated using the Spearman's rank correlation coefficient (ρ). Spearman's rank correlation coefficient, a nonparametric measure of rank correlation, assesses how well the relationship between two variables can be described using a monotonic function.

If the correlation coefficient value ranges within <0.5; 1.0>, there is a strong positive correlation. The significance level was established at a *p*-value of $p < 0.05$.

Box plots encompassing the median (dark horizontal line) of log-normalized gene expression values for particular microRNAs were generated using Statistica software (version 9.0; StatSoft, Inc., Tulsa, OK, USA). The upper and lower limits of the boxes represent the 75th and 25th percentiles, respectively. The upper and lower whiskers indicate the maximum and minimum values that are no more than 1.5 times the span of the interquartile range (range of the values between the 25th and the 75th percentiles). Outliers are marked by circles and extremes by asterisks.

5. Conclusions

In conclusion, epigenetic changes characteristic for cardiovascular/cerebrovascular diseases are also present in children descending from complicated pregnancies. Previous occurrence of GH, PE, or FGR may predispose to later development of cardiovascular/cerebrovascular diseases in offspring. Consecutive large scale studies including the children with a single clinical entity are needed to verify the findings resulting from this particular pilot study.

6. Patents

National Patent Application-Industrial Property Office, Czech Republic (PV 2018-595).

Supplementary Materials: Supplementary materials can be found at http://www.mdpi.com/1422-0067/20/3/654/s1.

Author Contributions: Conceptualization, I.H. and L.K.; methodology, I.H., K.K. and L.D.; software, I.H., K.K., J.S.; validation, I.H., L.K. and J.S.; formal analysis, I.H., K.K.; investigation, K.K., L.D. and J.S.; resources, L.D.; data curation, I.H., K.K. and L.D.; writing—original draft preparation, I.H., K.K. and J.S.; writing—review and editing, I.H. and K.K.; visualization, K.K.; supervision, I.H. and L.K.; project administration, I.H. and L.K.; funding acquisition, I.H. and L.K.

Funding: This research was funded by the Agency of Medical Research, Ministry of Health, Prague, Czech Republic, grant number AZV 16-27761A and by the Charles University, Prague, Czech Republic, grant number PROGRES Q34. All rights reserved.

Acknowledgments: All procedures were in accordance with the ethical standards of the responsible committee on human experimentation (institutional and national) and with the Helsinki Declaration of 1975, as revised in 2000. We thank to the staff of the Institute for the Care of Mother and child (Katerina Hamplova, Katerina Mackova, Radek Cabela and Adam Krasny) for assistance with collection of patients' anamnesis. We also thank to Jana Kumprichtova, Sarka Stranska, Bc. Veronika Marvanova and Bc. Andrea Semencova for assistance with biological sample collection and processing.

Conflicts of Interest: The authors declare no conflict of interest.

Abbreviations

PE	Preeclampsia
FGR	Fetal growth restriction
GH	Gestational hypertension
DV	Ductus venosus
CPR	Cerebro-placental ratio
PI	Pulsatility index
BMI	Body mass index

References

1. Davis, E.F.; Lazdam, M.; Lewandowski, A.J.; Worton, S.A.; Kelly, B.; Kenworthy, Y.; Adwani, S.; Wilkinson, A.R.; McCormick, K.; Sargent, I.; et al. Cardiovascular risk factors in children and young adults born to preeclamptic pregnancies: A systematic review. *Pediatrics* **2012**, *129*, e1552–e1561. [CrossRef]
2. Alsnes, I.V.; Vatten, L.J.; Fraser, A.; Bjørngaard, J.H.; Rich-Edwards, J.; Romundstad, P.R.; Åsvold, B.O. Hypertension in Pregnancy and Offspring Cardiovascular Risk in Young Adulthood: Prospective and Sibling Studies in the HUNT Study (Nord-Trøndelag Health Study) in Norway. *Hypertension* **2017**, *69*, 591–598. [PubMed]
3. Tenhola, S.; Rahiala, E.; Martikainen, A.; Halonen, P.; Voutilainen, R. Blood pressure, serum lipids, fasting insulin, and adrenal hormones in 12-year-old children born with maternal preeclampsia. *J. Clin. Endocrinol. Metab.* **2003**, *88*, 1217–1222. [CrossRef] [PubMed]

4. Øglaend, B.; Forman, M.R.; Romundstad, P.R.; Nilsen, S.T.; Vatten, L.J. Blood pressure in early adolescence in the offspring of preeclamptic and normotensive pregnancies. *J. Hypertens.* **2009**, *27*, 2051–2054. [CrossRef]
5. Fraser, A.; Nelson, S.M.; Macdonald-Wallis, C.; Sattar, N.; Lawlor, D.A. Hypertensive disorders of pregnancy and cardiometabolic health in adolescent offspring. *Hypertension* **2013**, *62*, 614–620. [CrossRef] [PubMed]
6. Staley, J.R.; Bradley, J.; Silverwood, R.J.; Howe, L.D.; Tilling, K.; Lawlor, D.A.; Macdonald-Wallis, C. Associations of blood pressure in pregnancy with offspring blood pressure trajectories during childhood and adolescence: Findings from a prospective study. *J. Am. Heart Assoc.* **2015**, *4*, e001422. [CrossRef]
7. Lazdam, M.; de la Horra, A.; Diesch, J.; Kenworthy, Y.; Davis, E.; Lewandowski, A.J.; Szmigielski, C.; Shore, A.; Mackillop, L.; Kharbanda, R.; et al. Unique blood pressure characteristics in mother and offspring after early onset preeclampsia. *Hypertension* **2012**, *60*, 1338–1345. [CrossRef]
8. Lim, W.Y.; Lee, Y.S.; Yap, F.K.; Aris, I.M.; Lek, N.; Meaney, M.; Gluckman, P.D.; Godfrey, K.M.; Kwek, K.; Chong, Y.S.; et al. Maternal Blood Pressure During Pregnancy and Early Childhood Blood Pressures in the Offspring: The GUSTO Birth Cohort Study. *Medicine (Baltimore)* **2015**, *94*, e1981. [CrossRef]
9. Jayet, P.Y.; Rimoldi, S.F.; Stuber, T.; Salmòn, C.S.; Hutter, D.; Rexhaj, E.; Thalmann, S.; Schwab, M.; Turini, P.; Sartori-Cucchia, C.; et al. Pulmonary and systemic vascular dysfunction in young offspring of mothers with preeclampsia. *Circulation* **2010**, *122*, 488–494. [CrossRef]
10. Sarvari, S.I.; Rodriguez-Lopez, M.; Nuñez-Garcia, M.; Sitges, M.; Sepulveda-Martinez, A.; Camara, O.; Butakoff, C.; Gratacos, E.; Bijnens, B.; Crispi, F. Persistence of Cardiac Remodeling in Preadolescents with Fetal Growth Restriction. *Circ. Cardiovasc. Imaging* **2017**, *10*, e005270. [CrossRef]
11. Yiallourou, S.R.; Wallace, E.M.; Whatley, C.; Odoi, A.; Hollis, S.; Weichard, A.J.; Muthusamy, J.S.; Varma, S.; Cameron, J.; Narayan, O.; et al. Sleep: A Window Into Autonomic Control in Children Born Preterm and Growth Restricted. *Sleep* **2017**, *40*. [CrossRef] [PubMed]
12. Rostand, S.G.; Cliver, S.P.; Goldenberg, R.L. Racial disparities in the association of foetal growth retardation to childhood blood pressure. *Nephrol. Dial. Transplant.* **2005**, *20*, 1592–1597. [CrossRef] [PubMed]
13. Libby, G.; Murphy, D.J.; McEwan, N.F.; Greene, S.A.; Forsyth, J.S.; Chien, P.W.; Morris, A.D.; DARTS/MEMO Collaboration. Pre-eclampsia and the later development of type 2 diabetes in mothers and their children: An intergenerational study from the Walker cohort. *Diabetologia* **2007**, *50*, 523–530. [CrossRef] [PubMed]
14. Tappia, P.S.; Gabriel, C.A. Role of nutrition in the development of the fetal cardiovascular system. *Expert Rev. Cardiovasc. Ther.* **2006**, *4*, 211–225. [CrossRef] [PubMed]
15. Lloyd-Jones, D.M.; Hong, Y.; Labarthe, D.; Mozaffarian, D.; Appel, L.J.; Van Horn, L.; Greenlund, K.; Daniels, S.; Nichol, G.; Tomaselli, G.F.; et al. Defining and setting national goals for cardiovascular health promotion and disease reduction: The American Heart Association's strategic Impact Goal through 2020 and beyond. *Circulation* **2010**, *121*, 586–613. [CrossRef]
16. Elmén, J.; Lindow, M.; Silahtaroglu, A.; Bak, M.; Christensen, M.; Lind-Thomsen, A.; Hedtjärn, M.; Hansen, J.B.; Hansen, H.F.; Straarup, E.M.; et al. Antagonism of microRNA-122 in mice by systemically administered LNA-antimiR leads to up-regulation of a large set of predicted target mRNAs in the liver. *Nucleic Acids Res.* **2008**, *36*, 1153–1162. [CrossRef]
17. Yang, K.; He, Y.S.; Wang, X.Q.; Lu, L.; Chen, Q.J.; Liu, J.; Sun, Z.; Shen, W.F. MiR-146a inhibits oxidized low-density lipoprotein-induced lipid accumulation and inflammatory response via targeting toll-like receptor 4. *FEBS Lett.* **2011**, *585*, 854–860. [CrossRef]
18. Thum, T.; Gross, C.; Fiedler, J.; Fischer, T.; Kissler, S.; Bussen, M.; Galuppo, P.; Just, S.; Rottbauer, W.; Frantz, S.; et al. MicroRNA-21 contributes to myocardial disease by stimulating MAP kinase signalling in fibroblasts. *Nature* **2008**, *456*, 980–984. [CrossRef]
19. Xin, M.; Small, E.M.; Sutherland, L.B.; Qi, X.; McAnally, J.; Plato, C.F.; Richardson, J.A.; Bassel-Duby, R.; Olson, E.N. MicroRNAs miR-143 and miR-145 modulate cytoskeletal dynamics and responsiveness of smooth muscle cells to injury. *Genes Dev.* **2009**, *23*, 2166–2178. [CrossRef]
20. Li, S.; Zhu, J.; Zhang, W.; Chen, Y.; Zhang, K.; Popescu, L.M.; Ma, X.; Lau, W.B.; Rong, R.; Yu, X.; et al. Signature microRNA expression profile of essential hypertension and its novel link to human cytomegalovirus infection. *Circulation* **2011**, *124*, 175–184. [CrossRef]

21. Harris, T.A.; Yamakuchi, M.; Ferlito, M.; Mendell, J.T.; Lowenstein, C.J. MicroRNA-126 regulates endothelial expression of vascular cell adhesion molecule 1. *Proc. Natl. Acad. Sci. USA* **2008**, *105*, 1516–1521. [CrossRef] [PubMed]
22. Wang, Y.S.; Wang, H.Y.; Liao, Y.C.; Tsai, P.C.; Chen, K.C.; Cheng, H.Y.; Lin, R.T.; Juo, S.H. MicroRNA-195 regulates vascular smooth muscle cell phenotype and prevents neointimal formation. *Cardiovasc. Res.* **2012**, *95*, 517–526. [CrossRef] [PubMed]
23. Kong, L.; Zhu, J.; Han, W.; Jiang, X.; Xu, M.; Zhao, Y.; Dong, Q.; Pang, Z.; Guan, Q.; Gao, L.; et al. Significance of serum microRNAs in pre-diabetes and newly diagnosed type 2 diabetes: A clinical study. *Acta Diabetol.* **2011**, *48*, 61–69. [CrossRef] [PubMed]
24. Ji, R.; Cheng, Y.; Yue, J.; Yang, J.; Liu, X.; Chen, H.; Dean, D.B.; Zhang, C. MicroRNA expression signature and antisense-mediated depletion reveal an essential role of MicroRNA in vascular neointimal lesion formation. *Circ. Res.* **2007**, *100*, 1579–1588. [CrossRef] [PubMed]
25. Raitoharju, E.; Lyytikäinen, L.P.; Levula, M.; Oksala, N.; Mennander, A.; Tarkka, M.; Klopp, N.; Illig, T.; Kähönen, M.; Karhunen, P.J.; et al. miR-21, miR-210, miR-34a, and miR-146a/b are up-regulated in human atherosclerotic plaques in the Tampere Vascular Study. *Atherosclerosis* **2011**, *219*, 211–217. [CrossRef] [PubMed]
26. Poliseno, L.; Tuccoli, A.; Mariani, L.; Evangelista, M.; Citti, L.; Woods, K.; Mercatanti, A.; Hammond, S.; Rainaldi, G. MicroRNAs modulate the angiogenic properties of HUVECs. *Blood* **2006**, *108*, 3068–3071. [CrossRef] [PubMed]
27. Doebele, C.; Bonauer, A.; Fischer, A.; Scholz, A.; Reiss, Y.; Urbich, C.; Hofmann, W.K.; Zeiher, A.M.; Dimmeler, S. Members of the microRNA-17-92 cluster exhibit a cell-intrinsic antiangiogenic function in endothelial cells. *Blood* **2010**, *115*, 4944–4950. [CrossRef] [PubMed]
28. Fichtlscherer, S.; De Rosa, S.; Fox, H.; Schwietz, T.; Fischer, A.; Liebetrau, C.; Weber, M.; Hamm, C.W.; Röxe, T.; Müller-Ardogan, M.; et al. Circulating microRNAs in patients with coronary artery disease. *Circ. Res.* **2010**, *107*, 677–684. [CrossRef]
29. van Rooij, E.; Sutherland, L.B.; Liu, N.; Williams, A.H.; McAnally, J.; Gerard, R.D.; Richardson, J.A.; Olson, E.N. A signature pattern of stress-responsive microRNAs that can evoke cardiac hypertrophy and heart failure. *Proc. Natl. Acad. Sci. USA* **2006**, *103*, 18255–18260. [CrossRef]
30. Ikeda, S.; Kong, S.W.; Lu, J.; Bisping, E.; Zhang, H.; Allen, P.D.; Golub, T.R.; Pieske, B.; Pu, W.T. Altered microRNA expression in human heart disease. *Physiol. Genom.* **2007**, *31*, 367–373. [CrossRef]
31. D'Alessandra, Y.; Devanna, P.; Limana, F.; Straino, S.; Di Carlo, A.; Brambilla, P.G.; Rubino, M.; Carena, M.C.; Spazzafumo, L.; De Simone, M.; et al. Circulating microRNAs are new and sensitive biomarkers of myocardial infarction. *Eur. Heart. J.* **2010**, *31*, 2765–2773. [CrossRef] [PubMed]
32. Beaumont, J.; López, B.; Hermida, N.; Schroen, B.; San José, G.; Heymans, S.; Valencia, F.; Gómez-Doblas, J.J.; De Teresa, E.; Díez, J.; et al. microRNA-122 down-regulation may play a role in severe myocardial fibrosis in human aortic stenosis through TGF-β1 up-regulation. *Clin. Sci. (Lond.)* **2014**, *126*, 497–506. [CrossRef] [PubMed]
33. Maitrias, P.; Metzinger-Le Meuth, V.; Nader, J.; Reix, T.; Caus, T.; Metzinger, L. The Involvement of miRNA in Carotid-Related Stroke. *Arterioscler. Thromb. Vasc. Biol.* **2017**, *37*, 1608–1617. [CrossRef] [PubMed]
34. Jiang, Y.; Zhang, M.; He, H.; Chen, J.; Zeng, H.; Li, J.; Duan, R. MicroRNA/mRNA profiling and regulatory network of intracranial aneurysm. *BMC Med. Genom.* **2013**, *6*, 36. [CrossRef] [PubMed]
35. Bienertova-Vasku, J.; Novak, J.; Vasku, A. MicroRNAs in pulmonary arterial hypertension: Pathogenesis, diagnosis and treatment. *J. Am. Soc. Hypertens.* **2015**, *9*, 221–234. [CrossRef] [PubMed]
36. Halkein, J.; Tabruyn, S.P.; Ricke-Hoch, M.; Haghikia, A.; Nguyen, N.Q.; Scherr, M.; Castermans, K.; Malvaux, L.; Lambert, V.; Thiry, M.; et al. MicroRNA-146a is a therapeutic target and biomarker for peripartum cardiomyopathy. *J. Clin. Investig.* **2013**, *123*, 2143–2154. [CrossRef] [PubMed]
37. Lai, E.C. Micro RNAs are complementary to 3′ UTR sequence motifs that mediate negative post-transcriptional regulation. *Nat. Genet.* **2002**, *30*, 363–364. [CrossRef]
38. Rosenfeld, N.; Aharonov, R.; Meiri, E.; Rosenwald, S.; Spector, Y.; Zepeniuk, M.; Benjamin, H.; Shabes, N.; Tabak, S.; Levy, A.; et al. MicroRNAs accurately identify cancer tissue origin. *Nat. Biotechnol.* **2008**, *26*, 462–469. [CrossRef]

39. Pineles, B.L.; Romero, R.; Montenegro, D.; Tarca, A.L.; Han, Y.M.; Kim, Y.M.; Draghici, S.; Espinoza, J.; Kusanovic, J.P.; Mittal, P.; et al. Distinct subsets of microRNAs are expressed differentially in the human placentas of patients with preeclampsia. *Am. J. Obstet. Gynecol.* **2007**, *196*, 261.e1–261.e6. [CrossRef]
40. Hu, Y.; Li, P.; Hao, S.; Liu, L.; Zhao, J.; Hou, Y. Differential expression of microRNAs in the placentae of Chinese patients with severe pre-eclampsia. *Clin. Chem. Lab. Med.* **2009**, *47*, 923–929. [CrossRef]
41. Maccani, M.A.; Padbury, J.F.; Marsit, C.J. miR-16 and miR-21 expression in the placenta is associated with fetal growth. *PLoS ONE* **2011**, *6*, e21210. [CrossRef] [PubMed]
42. Higashijima, A.; Miura, K.; Mishima, H.; Kinoshita, A.; Jo, O.; Abe, S.; Hasegawa, Y.; Miura, S.; Yamasaki, K.; Yoshida, A.; et al. Characterization of placenta-specific microRNAs in fetal growth restriction pregnancy. *Prenat. Diagn.* **2013**, *33*, 214–222. [CrossRef] [PubMed]
43. Xu, P.; Zhao, Y.; Liu, M.; Wang, Y.; Wang, H.; Li, Y.X.; Zhu, X.; Yao, Y.; Wang, H.; Qiao, J.; et al. Variations of microRNAs in human placentas and plasma from preeclamptic pregnancy. *Hypertension* **2014**, *63*, 1276–1284. [CrossRef] [PubMed]
44. Hromadnikova, I.; Kotlabova, K.; Ivankova, K.; Vedmetskaya, Y.; Krofta, L. Profiling of cardiovascular and cerebrovascular disease associated microRNA expression in umbilical cord blood in gestational hypertension, preeclampsia and fetal growth restriction. *Int. J. Cardiol.* **2017**, *249*, 402–409. [CrossRef] [PubMed]
45. Hromadnikova, I.; Kotlabova, K.; Hympanova, L.; Krofta, L. Cardiovascular and Cerebrovascular Disease Associated microRNAs Are Dysregulated in Placental Tissues Affected with Gestational Hypertension, Preeclampsia and Intrauterine Growth Restriction. *PLoS ONE* **2015**, *10*, e0138383. [CrossRef] [PubMed]
46. Li, J.; Dong, X.; Wang, Z.; Wu, J. MicroRNA-1 in Cardiac Diseases and Cancers. *Korean J. Physiol. Pharmacol.* **2014**, *18*, 359–363. [CrossRef] [PubMed]
47. Li, Y.Q.; Zhang, M.F.; Wen, H.Y.; Hu, C.L.; Liu, R.; Wei, H.Y.; Ai, C.M.; Wang, G.; Liao, X.X.; Li, X. Comparing the diagnostic values of circulating microRNAs and cardiac troponin T in patients with acute myocardial infarction. *Clinics (Sao Paulo)* **2013**, *68*, 75–80. [CrossRef]
48. Chistiakov, D.A.; Orekhov, A.N.; Bobryshev, Y.V. Cardiac-specific miRNA in cardiogenesis, heart function, and cardiac pathology (with focus on myocardial infarction). *J. Mol. Cell. Cardiol.* **2016**, *94*, 107–121. [CrossRef]
49. Tang, Y.; Zheng, J.; Sun, Y.; Wu, Z.; Liu, Z.; Huang, G. MicroRNA-1 regulates cardiomyocyte apoptosis by targeting Bcl-2. *Int. Heart J.* **2009**, *50*, 377–387. [CrossRef]
50. Terentyev, D.; Belevych, A.E.; Terentyeva, R.; Martin, M.M.; Malana, G.E.; Kuhn, D.E.; Abdellatif, M.; Feldman, D.S.; Elton, T.S.; Györke, S. miR-1 overexpression enhances Ca(2+) release and promotes cardiac arrhythmogenesis by targeting PP2A regulatory subunit B56alpha and causing CaMKII-dependent hyperphosphorylation of RyR2. *Circ. Res.* **2009**, *104*, 514–521. [CrossRef]
51. Mogilyansky, E.; Rigoutsos, I. The miR-17/92 cluster: A comprehensive update on its genomics, genetics, functions and increasingly important and numerous roles in health and disease. *Cell Death Differ.* **2013**, *20*, 1603–1614. [CrossRef] [PubMed]
52. Zhou, L.; Qi, R.Q.; Liu, M.; Xu, Y.P.; Li, G.; Weiland, M.; Kaplan, D.H.; Mi, Q.S. microRNA miR-17-92 cluster is highly expressed in epidermal Langerhans cells but not required for its development. *Genes Immun.* **2014**, *15*, 57–61. [CrossRef] [PubMed]
53. Bonauer, A.; Carmona, G.; Iwasaki, M.; Mione, M.; Koyanagi, M.; Fischer, A.; Burchfield, J.; Fox, H.; Doebele, C.; Ohtani, K.; et al. MicroRNA-92a controls angiogenesis and functional recovery of ischemic tissues in mice. *Science* **2009**, *324*, 1710–1713. [CrossRef] [PubMed]
54. Danielson, L.S.; Park, D.S.; Rotllan, N.; Chamorro-Jorganes, A.; Guijarro, M.V.; Fernandez-Hernando, C.; Fishman, G.I.; Phoon, C.K.; Hernando, E. Cardiovascular dysregulation of miR-17-92 causes a lethal hypertrophic cardiomyopathy and arrhythmogenesis. *FASEB J.* **2013**, *27*, 1460–1467. [CrossRef] [PubMed]
55. Du, W.; Pan, Z.; Chen, X.; Wang, L.; Zhang, Y.; Li, S.; Liang, H.; Xu, C.; Zhang, Y.; Wu, Y.; et al. By targeting Stat3 microRNA-17-5p promotes cardiomyocyte apoptosis in response to ischemia followed by reperfusion. *Cell. Physiol. Biochem.* **2014**, *34*, 955–965. [CrossRef] [PubMed]
56. Yang, S.; Fan, T.; Hu, Q.; Xu, W.; Yang, J.; Xu, C.; Zhang, B.; Chen, J.; Jiang, H. Downregulation of microRNA-17-5p improves cardiac function after myocardial infarction via attenuation of apoptosis in endothelial cells. *Mol. Genet. Genom.* **2018**, *293*, 883–894. [CrossRef] [PubMed]

57. Kaucsár, T.; Révész, C.; Godó, M.; Krenács, T.; Albert, M.; Szalay, C.I.; Rosivall, L.; Benyó, Z.; Bátkai, S.; Thum, T.; et al. Activation of the miR-17 family and miR-21 during murine kidney ischemia-reperfusion injury. *Nucleic Acid Ther.* **2013**, *23*, 344–354. [CrossRef]
58. Fang, L.; Ellims, A.H.; Moore, X.L.; White, D.A.; Taylor, A.J.; Chin-Dusting, J.; Dart, A.M. Circulating microRNAs as biomarkers for diffuse myocardial fibrosis in patients with hypertrophic cardiomyopathy. *J. Transl. Med.* **2015**, *13*, 314. [CrossRef]
59. Wu, J.; Du, K.; Lu, X. Elevated expressions of serum miR-15a, miR-16, and miR-17-5p are associated with acute ischemic stroke. *Int. J. Clin. Exp. Med.* **2015**, *8*, 21071–21079.
60. Chen, J.; Xu, L.; Hu, Q.; Yang, S.; Zhang, B.; Jiang, H. MiR-17-5p as circulating biomarkers for the severity of coronary atherosclerosis in coronary artery disease. *Int. J. Cardiol.* **2015**, *197*, 123–124. [CrossRef]
61. Mendell, J.T. miRiad roles for the miR-17-92 cluster in development and disease. *Cell* **2008**, *133*, 217–222. [CrossRef] [PubMed]
62. Brock, M.; Samillan, V.J.; Trenkmann, M.; Schwarzwald, C.; Ulrich, S.; Gay, R.E.; Gassmann, M.; Ostergaard, L.; Gay, S.; Speich, R.; et al. AntagomiR directed against miR-20a restores functional BMPR2 signalling and prevents vascular remodelling in hypoxia-induced pulmonary hypertension. *Eur. Heart J.* **2014**, *35*, 3203–3211. [CrossRef] [PubMed]
63. Zhu, Y.; Tian, F.; Li, H.; Zhou, Y.; Lu, J.; Ge, Q. Profiling maternal plasma microRNA expression in early pregnancy to predict gestational diabetes mellitus. *Int. J. Gynaecol. Obstet.* **2015**, *130*, 49–53. [CrossRef] [PubMed]
64. Dickinson, B.A.; Semus, H.M.; Montgomery, R.L.; Stack, C.; Latimer, P.A.; Lewton, S.M.; Lynch, J.M.; Hullinger, T.G.; Seto, A.G.; et al. Plasma microRNAs serve as biomarkers of therapeutic efficacy and disease progression in hypertension-induced heart failure. *Eur. J. Heart Fail.* **2013**, *15*, 650–659. [CrossRef] [PubMed]
65. Rodosthenous, R.S.; Burris, H.H.; Sanders, A.P.; Just, A.C.; Dereix, A.E.; Svensson, K.; Solano, M.; Téllez-Rojo, M.M.; Wright, R.O.; Baccarelli, A.A. Second trimester extracellular microRNAs in maternal blood and fetal growth: An exploratory study. *Epigenetics* **2017**, *12*, 804–810. [CrossRef] [PubMed]
66. Sekar, D.; Venugopal, B.; Sekar, P.; Ramalingam, K. Role of microRNA 21 in diabetes and associated/related diseases. *Gene* **2016**, *582*, 14–18. [CrossRef]
67. Suárez, Y.; Fernández-Hernando, C.; Pober, J.S.; Sessa, W.C. Dicer dependent microRNAs regulate gene expression and functions in human endothelial cells. *Circ. Res.* **2007**, *100*, 1164–1173. [CrossRef]
68. Dong, S.; Ma, W.; Hao, B.; Hu, F.; Yan, L.; Yan, X.; Wang, Y.; Chen, Z.; Wang, Z. microRNA-21 promotes cardiac fibrosis and development of heart failure with preserved left ventricular ejection fraction by up-regulating Bcl-2. *Int. J. Clin. Exp. Pathol.* **2014**, *7*, 565–574.
69. Liu, Y.; Nie, H.; Zhang, K.; Ma, D.; Yang, G.; Zheng, Z.; Liu, K.; Yu, B.; Zhai, C.; Yang, S. A feedback regulatory loop between HIF-1α and miR-21 in response to hypoxia in cardiomyocytes. *FEBS Lett.* **2014**, *588*, 3137–3146. [CrossRef]
70. Zhang, J.; Xing, Q.; Zhou, X.; Li, J.; Li, Y.; Zhang, L.; Zhou, Q.; Tang, B. Circulating miRNA-21 is a promising biomarker for heart failure. *Mol. Med. Rep.* **2017**, *16*, 7766–7774. [CrossRef]
71. Long, B.; Gan, T.Y.; Zhang, R.C.; Zhang, Y.H. miR-23a Regulates Cardiomyocyte Apoptosis by Targeting Manganese Superoxide Dismutase. *Mol. Cells* **2017**, *40*, 542–549. [CrossRef] [PubMed]
72. Wang, S.; He, W.; Wang, C. MiR-23a Regulates the Vasculogenesis of Coronary Artery Disease by Targeting Epidermal Growth Factor Receptor. *Cardiovasc. Ther.* **2016**, *34*, 199–208. [CrossRef] [PubMed]
73. Cong, X.; Li, Y.; Lu, N.; Dai, Y.; Zhang, H.; Zhao, X.; Liu, Y. Resveratrol attenuates the inflammatory reaction induced by ischemia/reperfusion in the rat heart. *Mol. Med. Rep.* **2014**, *9*, 2528–2532. [CrossRef] [PubMed]
74. Gao, J.; Liu, Q.G. The role of miR-26 in tumors and normal tissues. *Oncol. Lett.* **2011**, *2*, 1019–1023. [CrossRef] [PubMed]
75. Zheng, L.; Lin, S.; Lv, C. MiR-26a-5p regulates cardiac fibroblasts collagen expression by targeting ULK1. *Sci. Rep.* **2018**, *8*, 2104. [CrossRef] [PubMed]
76. Ye, Y.; Hu, Z.; Lin, Y.; Zhang, C.; Perez-Polo, J.R. Downregulation of microRNA-29 by antisense inhibitors and a PPAR-gamma agonist protects against myocardial ischaemia-reperfusion injury. *Cardiovasc. Res.* **2010**, *87*, 535–544. [CrossRef] [PubMed]
77. Moraes, L.N.; Fernandez, G.J.; Vechetti-Júnior, I.J.; Freire, P.P.; Souza, R.W.A.; Villacis, R.A.R.; Rogatto, S.R.; Reis, P.P.; Dal-Pai-Silva, M.; Carvalho, R.F. Integration of miRNA and mRNA expression profiles reveals

microRNA-regulated networks during muscle wasting in cardiac cachexia. *Sci. Rep.* **2017**, *7*, 6998. [CrossRef] [PubMed]
78. Zhao, Y.; Yuan, Y.; Qiu, C. Underexpression of CACNA1C Caused by Overexpression of microRNA-29a Underlies the Pathogenesis of Atrial Fibrillation. *Med. Sci. Monit.* **2016**, *22*, 2175–2181. [CrossRef] [PubMed]
79. Widlansky, M.E.; Jensen, D.M.; Wang, J.; Liu, Y.; Geurts, A.M.; Kriegel, A.J.; Liu, P.; Ying, R.; Zhang, G.; Casati, M.; et al. miR-29 contributes to normal endothelial function and can restore it in cardiometabolic disorders. *EMBO Mol. Med.* **2018**, *10*, e8046. [CrossRef] [PubMed]
80. Moncini, S.; Salvi, A.; Zuccotti, P.; Viero, G.; Quattrone, A.; Barlati, S.; De Petro, G.; Venturin, M.; Riva, P. The role of miR-103 and miR-107 in regulation of CDK5R1 expression and in cellular migration. *PLoS ONE* **2011**, *6*, e20038. [CrossRef] [PubMed]
81. Huang, L.; Li, L.; Chen, X.; Zhang, H.; Shi, Z. MiR-103a targeting Piezo1 is involved in acute myocardial infarction through regulating endothelium function. *Cardiol. J.* **2016**, *23*, 556–562. [CrossRef] [PubMed]
82. Wang, J.X.; Zhang, X.J.; Li, Q.; Wang, K.; Wang, Y.; Jiao, J.Q.; Feng, C.; Teng, S.; Zhou, L.Y.; Gong, Y.; et al. MicroRNA-103/107 Regulate Programmed Necrosis and Myocardial Ischemia/Reperfusion Injury Through Targeting FADD. *Circ. Res.* **2015**, *117*, 352–363. [CrossRef] [PubMed]
83. Deng, B.; Du, J.; Hu, R.; Wang, A.P.; Wu, W.H.; Hu, C.P.; Li, Y.J.; Li, X.H. MicroRNA-103/107 is involved in hypoxia-induced proliferation of pulmonary arterial smooth muscle cells by targeting HIF-1β. *Life Sci.* **2016**, *147*, 117–124. [CrossRef] [PubMed]
84. Trajkovski, M.; Hausser, J.; Soutschek, J.; Bhat, B.; Akin, A.; Zavolan, M.; Heim, M.H.; Stoffel, M. MicroRNAs 103 and 107 regulate insulin sensitivity. *Nature* **2011**, *474*, 649–653. [CrossRef]
85. Shaham, L.; Binder, V.; Gefen, N.; Borkhardt, A.; Izraeli, S. MiR-125 in normal and malignant hematopoiesis. *Leukemia* **2012**, *26*, 2011–2018. [CrossRef]
86. Tiedt, S.; Prestel, M.; Malik, R.; Schieferdecker, N.; Duering, M.; Kautzky, V.; Stoycheva, I.; Böck, J.; Northoff, B.H.; Klein, M.; et al. RNA-Seq Identifies Circulating miR-125a-5p, miR-125b-5p, and miR-143-3p as Potential Biomarkers for Acute Ischemic Stroke. *Circ. Res.* **2017**, *121*, 970–980. [CrossRef]
87. Jia, K.; Shi, P.; Han, X.; Chen, T.; Tang, H.; Wang, J. Diagnostic value of miR-30d-5p and miR-125b-5p in acute myocardial infarction. *Mol. Med. Rep.* **2016**, *14*, 184–194. [CrossRef]
88. Wei, M.; Gan, L.; Liu, Z.; Kong, L.H.; Chang, J.R.; Chen, L.H.; Su, X.L. MiR125b-5p protects endothelial cells from apoptosis under oxidative stress. *Biomed. Pharmacother.* **2017**, *95*, 453–460. [CrossRef]
89. Bayoumi, A.S.; Park, K.M.; Wang, Y.; Teoh, J.P.; Aonuma, T.; Tang, Y.; Su, H.; Weintraub, N.L.; Kim, I.M. A carvedilol-responsive microRNA, miR-125b-5p protects the heart from acute myocardial infarction by repressing pro-apoptotic bak1 and klf13 in cardiomyocytes. *J. Mol. Cell. Cardiol.* **2018**, *114*, 72–82. [CrossRef]
90. Wu, X.J.; Zhao, Z.F.; Kang, X.J.; Wang, H.J.; Zhao, J.; Pu, X.M. MicroRNA-126-3p suppresses cell proliferation by targeting PIK3R2 in Kaposi's sarcoma cells. *Oncotarget* **2016**, *7*, 36614–36621.
91. Hsu, A.; Chen, S.J.; Chang, Y.S.; Chen, H.C.; Chu, P.H. Systemic approach to identify serum microRNAs as potential biomarkers for acute myocardial infarction. *Biomed. Res. Int.* **2014**, *2014*, 418628. [CrossRef]
92. Olivieri, F.; Spazzafumo, L.; Bonafè, M.; Recchioni, R.; Prattichizzo, F.; Marcheselli, F.; Micolucci, L.; Mensà, E.; Giuliani, A.; Santini, G.; et al. MiR-21-5p and miR-126a-3p levels in plasma and circulating angiogenic cells: Relationship with type 2 diabetes complications. *Oncotarget* **2015**, *6*, 35372–35382. [CrossRef]
93. Jansen, F.; Stumpf, T.; Proebsting, S.; Franklin, B.S.; Wenzel, D.; Pfeifer, P.; Flender, A.; Schmitz, T.; Yang, X.; Fleischmann, B.K.; et al. Intercellular transfer of miR-126-3p by endothelial microparticles reduces vascular smooth muscle cell proliferation and limits neointima formation by inhibiting LRP6. *J. Mol. Cell. Cardiol.* **2017**, *104*, 43–52. [CrossRef] [PubMed]
94. Liang, H.W.; Yang, X.; Wen, D.Y.; Gao, L.; Zhang, X.Y.; Ye, Z.H.; Luo, J.; Li, Z.Y.; He, Y.; Pang, Y.Y.; et al. Utility of miR-133a-3p as a diagnostic indicator for hepatocellular carcinoma: An investigation combined with GEO, TCGA, meta-analysis and bioinformatics. *Mol. Med. Rep.* **2018**, *17*, 1469–1484. [CrossRef] [PubMed]
95. Wang, J.; Xu, R.; Lin, F.; Zhang, S.; Zhang, G.; Hu, S.; Zheng, Z. MicroRNA: Novel regulators involved in the remodeling and reverse remodeling of the heart. *Cardiology* **2009**, *113*, 81–88. [CrossRef] [PubMed]
96. van Rooij, E.; Olson, E.N. MicroRNAs: Powerful new regulators of heart disease and provocative therapeutic targets. *J. Clin. Investig.* **2007**, *117*, 2369–2376. [CrossRef]
97. Kukreja, R.C.; Yin, C.; Salloum, F.N. MicroRNAs: New players in cardiac injury and protection. *Mol. Pharmacol.* **2011**, *80*, 558–564. [CrossRef] [PubMed]

98. Duisters, R.F.; Tijsen, A.J.; Schroen, B.; Leenders, J.J.; Lentink, V.; van der Made, I.; Herias, V.; van Leeuwen, R.E.; Schellings, M.W.; Barenbrug, P.; et al. miR-133 and miR-30 regulate connective tissue growth factor: Implications for a role of microRNAs in myocardial matrix remodeling. *Circ. Res.* **2009**, *104*, 170–178. [CrossRef] [PubMed]
99. Liu, W.; Ling, S.; Sun, W.; Liu, T.; Li, Y.; Zhong, G.; Zhao, D.; Zhang, P.; Song, J.; Jin, X.; et al. Circulating microRNAs correlated with the level of coronary artery calcification in symptomatic patients. *Sci. Rep.* **2015**, *5*, 16099. [CrossRef] [PubMed]
100. Taganov, K.D.; Boldin, M.P.; Chang, K.J.; Baltimore, D. NF-kappaB-dependent induction of microRNA miR-146, an inhibitor targeted to signaling proteins of innate immune responses. *Proc. Natl. Acad. Sci. USA* **2006**, *103*, 12481–12486. [CrossRef]
101. Paterson, M.R.; Kriegel, A.J. MiR-146a/b: A family with shared seeds and different roots. *Physiol. Genom.* **2017**, *49*, 243–252. [CrossRef] [PubMed]
102. Zhang, X.; Ye, Z.H.; Liang, H.W.; Ren, F.H.; Li, P.; Dang, Y.W.; Chen, G. Down-regulation of miR-146a-5p and its potential targets in hepatocellular carcinoma validated by a TCGA- and GEO-based study. *FEBS Open Bio* **2017**, *7*, 504–521. [CrossRef] [PubMed]
103. Li, S.H.; Chen, L.; Pang, X.M.; Su, S.Y.; Zhou, X.; Chen, C.Y.; Huang, L.G.; Li, J.P.; Liu, J.L. Decreased miR-146a expression in acute ischemic stroke directly targets the Fbxl10 mRNA and is involved in modulating apoptosis. *Neurochem. Int.* **2017**, *107*, 156–167. [CrossRef] [PubMed]
104. Wang, X.; Ha, T.; Liu, L.; Zou, J.; Zhang, X.; Kalbfleisch, J.; Gao, X.; Williams, D.; Li, C. Increased expression of microRNA-146a decreases myocardial ischaemia/reperfusion injury. *Cardiovasc. Res.* **2013**, *97*, 432–442. [CrossRef] [PubMed]
105. Quan, X.; Ji, Y.; Zhang, C.; Guo, X.; Zhang, Y.; Jia, S.; Ma, W.; Fan, Y.; Wang, C. Circulating MiR-146a May be a Potential Biomarker of Coronary Heart Disease in Patients with Subclinical Hypothyroidism. *Cell. Physiol. Biochem.* **2018**, *45*, 226–236. [CrossRef]
106. Sun, X.; Sit, A.; Feinberg, M.W. Role of miR-181 family in regulating vascular inflammation and immunity. *Trends Cardiovasc. Med.* **2014**, *24*, 105–112. [CrossRef]
107. Hulsmans, M.; Sinnaeve, P.; Van der Schueren, B.; Mathieu, C.; Janssens, S.; Holvoet, P. Decreased miR-181a expression in monocytes of obese patients is associated with the occurrence of metabolic syndrome and coronary artery disease. *J. Clin. Endocrinol. Metab.* **2012**, *97*, E1213–E1218. [CrossRef] [PubMed]
108. Lozano-Bartolomé, J.; Llauradó, G.; Portero-Otin, M.; Altuna-Coy, A.; Rojo-Martínez, G.; Vendrell, J.; Jorba, R.; Rodríguez-Gallego, E.; Chacón, M.R. Altered Expression of miR-181a-5p and miR-23a-3p Is Associated With Obesity and TNFα-Induced Insulin Resistance. *J. Clin. Endocrinol. Metab.* **2018**, *103*, 1447–1458. [CrossRef]
109. Du, X.; Yang, Y.; Xu, C.; Peng, Z.; Zhang, M.; Lei, L.; Gao, W.; Dong, Y.; Shi, Z.; Sun, X.; et al. Upregulation of miR-181a impairs hepatic glucose and lipid homeostasis. *Oncotarget* **2017**, *8*, 91362–91378. [CrossRef]
110. Nabih, E.S.; Andrawes, N.G. The Association Between Circulating Levels of miRNA-181a and Pancreatic Beta Cells Dysfunction via SMAD7 in Type 1 Diabetic Children and Adolescents. *J. Clin. Lab. Anal.* **2016**, *30*, 727–731. [CrossRef]
111. Wu, J.; Fan, C.L.; Ma, L.J.; Liu, T.; Wang, C.; Song, J.X.; Lv, Q.S.; Pan, H.; Zhang, C.N.; Wang, J.J. Distinctive expression signatures of serum microRNAs in ischaemic stroke and transient ischaemic attack patients. *Thromb. Haemost.* **2017**, *117*, 992–1001. [PubMed]
112. Zhu, J.; Yao, K.; Wang, Q.; Guo, J.; Shi, H.; Ma, L.; Liu, H.; Gao, W.; Zou, Y.; Ge, J. Circulating miR-181a as a Potential Novel Biomarker for Diagnosis of Acute Myocardial Infarction. *Cell. Physiol. Biochem.* **2016**, *40*, 1591–1602. [CrossRef] [PubMed]
113. He, J.F.; Luo, Y.M.; Wan, X.H.; Jiang, D. Biogenesis of MiRNA-195 and its role in biogenesis, the cell cycle, and apoptosis. *J. Biochem. Mol. Toxicol.* **2011**, *25*, 404–408. [CrossRef] [PubMed]
114. You, X.Y.; Huang, J.H.; Liu, B.; Liu, S.J.; Zhong, Y.; Liu, S.M. HMGA1 is a new target of miR-195 involving isoprenaline-induced cardiomyocyte hypertrophy. *Biochemistry* **2014**, *79*, 538–544. [CrossRef] [PubMed]
115. Zampetaki, A.; Attia, R.; Mayr, U.; Gomes, R.S.; Phinikaridou, A.; Yin, X.; Langley, S.R.; Willeit, P.; Lu, R.; Fanshawe, B.; et al. Role of miR-195 in aortic aneurysmal disease. *Circ. Res.* **2014**, *115*, 857–866. [CrossRef] [PubMed]
116. Du, J.; Zheng, R.; Xiao, F.; Zhang, S.; He, K.; Zhang, J.; Shao, Y. Downregulated MicroRNA-195 in the Bicuspid Aortic Valve Promotes Calcification of Valve Interstitial Cells via Targeting SMAD7. *Cell. Physiol. Biochem.* **2017**, *44*, 884–896. [CrossRef] [PubMed]

117. Li, Y.; Yang, C.; Zhang, L.; Yang, P. MicroRNA-210 induces endothelial cell apoptosis by directly targeting PDK1 in the setting of atherosclerosis. *Cell. Mol. Biol. Lett.* **2017**, *22*, 3. [CrossRef]
118. Zaccagnini, G.; Maimone, B.; Di Stefano, V.; Fasanaro, P.; Greco, S.; Perfetti, A.; Capogrossi, M.C.; Gaetano, C.; Martelli, F. Hypoxia-induced miR-210 modulates tissue response to acute peripheral ischemia. *Antioxid. Redox Signal.* **2014**, *21*, 1177–1188. [CrossRef]
119. Diao, H.; Liu, B.; Shi, Y.; Song, C.; Guo, Z.; Liu, N.; Song, X.; Lu, Y.; Lin, X.; Li, Z. MicroRNA-210 alleviates oxidative stress-associated cardiomyocyte apoptosis by regulating BNIP3. *Biosci. Biotechnol. Biochem.* **2017**, *81*, 1712–1720. [CrossRef]
120. Li, T.; Cao, H.; Zhuang, J.; Wan, J.; Guan, M.; Yu, B.; Li, X.; Zhang, W. Identification of miR-130a, miR-27b and miR-210 as serum biomarkers for atherosclerosis obliterans. *Clin. Chim. Acta* **2011**, *412*, 66–70. [CrossRef]
121. Zhao, D.S.; Chen, Y.; Jiang, H.; Lu, J.P.; Zhang, G.; Geng, J.; Zhang, Q.; Shen, J.H.; Zhou, X.; Zhu, W.; et al. Serum miR-210 and miR-30a expressions tend to revert to fetal levels in Chinese adult patients with chronic heart failure. *Cardiovasc. Pathol.* **2013**, *22*, 444–450. [CrossRef] [PubMed]
122. Lou, Y.L.; Guo, F.; Liu, F.; Gao, F.L.; Zhang, P.Q.; Niu, X.; Guo, S.C.; Yin, J.H.; Wang, Y.; Deng, Z.F. miR-210 activates notch signaling pathway in angiogenesis induced by cerebral ischemia. *Mol. Cell. Biochem.* **2012**, *370*, 45–51. [CrossRef]
123. Wang, L.; Xu, L.; Xu, M.; Liu, G.; Xing, J.; Sun, C.; Ding, H. Obesity-Associated MiR-342-3p Promotes Adipogenesis of Mesenchymal Stem Cells by Suppressing CtBP2 and Releasing C/EBPα from CtBP2 Binding. *Cell. Physiol. Biochem.* **2015**, *35*, 2285–2298. [CrossRef]
124. Collares, C.V.; Evangelista, A.F.; Xavier, D.J.; Rassi, D.M.; Arns, T.; Foss-Freitas, M.C.; Foss, M.C.; Puthier, D.; Sakamoto-Hojo, E.T.; Passos, G.A.; et al. Identifying common and specific microRNAs expressed in peripheral blood mononuclear cell of type 1, type 2, and gestational diabetes mellitus patients. *BMC Res. Notes* **2013**, *6*, 491. [CrossRef] [PubMed]
125. Eissa, S.; Matboli, M.; Bekhet, M.M. Clinical verification of a novel urinary microRNA panal: 133b, -342 and -30 as biomarkers for diabetic nephropathy identified by bioinformatics analysis. *Biomed. Pharmacother.* **2016**, *83*, 92–99. [CrossRef] [PubMed]
126. Cheng, S.; Cui, Y.; Fan, L.; Mu, X.; Hua, Y. T2DM inhibition of endothelial miR-342-3p facilitates angiogenic dysfunction via repression of FGF11 signaling. *Biochem. Biophys. Res. Commun.* **2018**, *503*, 71–78. [CrossRef] [PubMed]
127. Hezova, R.; Slaby, O.; Faltejskova, P.; Mikulkova, Z.; Buresova, I.; Raja, K.R.; Hodek, J.; Ovesna, J.; Michalek, J. microRNA-342, microRNA-191 and microRNA-510 are differentially expressed in T regulatory cells of type 1 diabetic patients. *Cell. Immunol.* **2010**, *260*, 70–74. [CrossRef]
128. Khalyfa, A.; Kheirandish-Gozal, L.; Bhattacharjee, R.; Khalyfa, A.A.; Gozal, D. Circulating microRNAs as Potential Biomarkers of Endothelial Dysfunction in Obese Children. *Chest* **2016**, *149*, 786–800. [CrossRef]
129. ACOG Practice Bulletin. Diagnosis and management of preeclampsia and eclampsia. *Obstet. Gynecol.* **2002**, *99*, 159–167.
130. Figueras, F.; Gratacos, E. Stage-based approach to the management of fetal growth restriction. *Prenat. Diagn.* **2014**, *34*, 655–659. [CrossRef]
131. Baschat, A.A. Neurodevelopment following fetal growth restriction and its relationship with antepartum parameters of placental dysfunction. *Ultrasound. Obstet. Gynecol.* **2011**, *37*, 501–514. [CrossRef] [PubMed]
132. Nardozza, L.M.; Caetano, A.C.; Zamarian, A.C.; Mazzola, J.B.; Silva, C.P.; Marçal, V.M.; Lobo, T.F.; Peixoto, A.B.; Araujo Júnior, E. Fetal growth restriction: Current knowledge. *Arch. Gynecol. Obstet.* **2017**, *295*, 1061–1077. [CrossRef] [PubMed]
133. Vyas, S.; Nicolaides, K.H.; Bower, S.; Campbell, S. Middle cerebral artery flow velocity waveforms in fetal hypoxaemia. *Br. J. Obstet. Gynaecol.* **1990**, *97*, 797–803. [CrossRef] [PubMed]
134. Cohn, H.E.; Sacks, E.J.; Heymann, M.A.; Rudolph, A.M. Cardiovascular responses to hypoxemia and acidemia in fetal lambs. *Am. J. Obstet. Gynecol.* **1974**, *120*, 817–824. [CrossRef]
135. National High Blood Pressure Education Program Working Group on High Blood Pressure in Children and Adolescents. The fourth report on the diagnosis, evaluation, and treatment of high blood pressure in children and adolescents. *Pediatrics* **2004**, *114*, 555–576. [CrossRef]
136. Livak, K.J.; Schmittgen, T.D. Analysis of relative gene expression data using real-time quantitative PCR and the 2(-Delta Delta C(T)) Method. *Methods* **2001**, *25*, 402–408. [CrossRef] [PubMed]

137. Vandesompele, J.; de Preter, K.; Pattyn, F.; Poppe, B.; Van Roy, N.; de Paepe, A.; Speleman, F. Accurate normalization of real-time quantitative RT-PCR data by geometric averaging of multiple internal control genes. *Genome Biol.* **2002**, *3*, research0034. [CrossRef]
138. Shapiro, S.S.; Wilk, M.B. An Analysis of Variance Test for Normality (Complete Samples). *Biometrika* **1965**, *52*, 591–611. [CrossRef]

© 2019 by the authors. Licensee MDPI, Basel, Switzerland. This article is an open access article distributed under the terms and conditions of the Creative Commons Attribution (CC BY) license (http://creativecommons.org/licenses/by/4.0/).

MDPI
St. Alban-Anlage 66
4052 Basel
Switzerland
Tel. +41 61 683 77 34
Fax +41 61 302 89 18
www.mdpi.com

International Journal of Molecular Sciences Editorial Office
E-mail: ijms@mdpi.com
www.mdpi.com/journal/ijms

www.ingramcontent.com/pod-product-compliance
Lightning Source LLC
LaVergne TN
LVHW070249100526
838202LV00015B/2197